Pharmacogenomics and Personalized Medicine

Nadine Cohen
Johnson and Johnson Pharmaceutical Research and Development, L.L.C.,
Raritan, NJ, USA

Editor

Humana Press

Editor
Nadine Cohen
Johnson and Johnson Pharmaceutical Research
and Development, L.L.C.,
Raritan, NJ, USA
ncohen2@prdus.jnj.com

Series Editor
Y. James Kang
University of Louisville School of Medicine
511 South Floyd Street
Louisville, KY, USA
yjkang01@louisville.edu

ISBN 978-1-61737-921-5 e-ISBN 978-1-59745-439-1
ISSN 1557-2153
DOI: 10.1007/ 978-1-59745-439-1

Cover illustration: (Background) Src kinase overexpression in breast cancer (Fig. 4, Chapter 14).

Printed on acid-free paper

9 8 7 6 5 4 3 2 1

springer.com

Preface

Some of the challenges the pharmaceutical industry faces in the current research and development processes are: (1) a lengthy process that takes, on average, approximately 11 years from target identification to the development of a new medicine; (2) an ever increasing costly process; (3) an inefficient process where too many drugs fail before they reach the market because of a lack of efficacy or unacceptable toxicity, as well as postmarketing withdrawal due to rare serious adverse events; (4) drug--drug interactions or toxicity is not uncommon; (5) the increasing difficulty in identifying novel drug targets; and (6) the mode of action for many compounds is often unknown. This is a depressing reality. Where are the improvements in both quality and efficiency often claimed in the drug development process? Why haven't the advances in science and technology made a greater impact? How can improvements in the process reduce the already high cost of drug development generally?

To address some of these issues, the pharmaceutical industry is actively exploring the relationships between human genetics and drug responsiveness, susceptibility to disease, and disease severity. While research approaches and emphases may vary from company to company, the overarching goal of the industry is largely consistent: to discover and develop new medicines based on an improved understanding of patient response to drugs (positive or negative) and of diseases etiology. Pharmacogenomic (PGx) methods are aimed at determining the contribution of genetic differences in ADME, drug target, and disease genes to drug response, thereby improving the safety and efficacy of drug therapy through use of genetically guided treatments, an approach called *personalized medicine. Personalized medicine* is both one of the newest disciplines of medicine currently being used and very much an ongoing work in progress. Many drug companies have incorporated genetic research, such as the collection of genetic samples, into their drug development programs. And while only a few examples of true success stories have emerged during the past few years of research, it is clear that the current landscape is driving us toward a more widespread acceptance of personalized medicine. Currently many questions arise regarding the appropriate implementation of this technology: how can the industry go about delivering true business value while recognizing that the ability to address patients' demand for safer and more efficient novel drugs might be met by engaging this technology more fully. There are concerns within the pharmaceutical industry about generating data that might be difficult to interpret in a regulated environment. There is also a growing appreciation for the challenges in translating this new information into clinical utility, including scientific, commercial, ethical, and policy challenges.

Pharmacogenomics and Personalized Medicine, which is part of the *Methods in Pharmacology and Toxicology* series, comprises chapters on selected aspects of pharmacogenomics and personalized medicine. Our overall intent is to assist both novice and experienced investigators in understanding the current scientific challenges in applying PGx to discovery and clinical development and in making appropriate decisions to engage in and interpret PGx research. Designed to share the experiences of leading experts in the field, the book is a useful guide for conducting PGx research--from discovery to the market, but we also aim to present a realistic perspective on the challenges, practicalities, and obstacles in applying pharmacogenomics. Generally, the book avoids statements such as "Pharmacogenomics is going to revolutionize the practice of medicine," which are neither realistic nor particularly useful to anyone.

The book presents an industry perspective on the implementation of PGx in research and development, in drug discovery, and in clinical trials, including recommendations for a systematic approach for assessing the feasibility and added value of PGx studies in clinical trials. It also provides guidance on the key logistical issues required to prepare the pharmacogenomics protocol and an informed consent form for sample collection and analysis, the strategies and resources for SNP marker selection, and genotyping in genetic association studies, and the study design and statistical methodologies for data analysis in PGx research. We have included an interesting view of the effect of genetic variation, as well as a description of recent PGx applications in drug metabolism, adverse drug reactions, and in a few selected therapeutic areas (epilepsy, Alzheimer's disease, psychiatry, oncology, HIV, cardiovascular diseases). Additional key topics,s such as the current regulatory environment and drug label implications, biomarker qualification and trial design, the co-development of drugs and diagnostics, and the translation of genomics biomarkers into clinical utility, are also covered. Furthermore, two chapters describe the current state of knowledge of PGx in rare and monogenic disorders and in children, which are currently less well covered in the published literature but deserve attention.

Pharmacogenomics and Personalized Medicine focuses on DNA data and associated analytical methodologies that are currently the more mature components of the evolving constellation of genomic sciences. However, complementary RNA-based studies are also being considered in some chapters. It is important to also acknowledge that remarkable progress is being made in complementary methodological areas such as *proteomics*, *metabolomics,* and *imaging*. Given the layered complexities of biological regulation, it is likely that reliable markers will be hybrids that will cross methodological disciplines. A program of persistent innovation is being required from the industry to balance near-term profit with the need to accommodate the increasingly competitive and changing landscape. Education and cooperation among experts from the scientific community, industry, and government are recognized as integral to greater success in personalized medicine. It is my hope that the knowledge we share here regarding DNA information may be leveraged to create a useful foundation for further progress in personalized medicine, using other approaches that will benefit the pharmaceutical industry overall, and most importantly the patients.

Experts from the pharmaceutical industry, scientific community, and government have been invited to contribute their experience to this book. I would like to express my gratitude to all contributors for their enthusiasm to this work. Without their time and energy, *Pharmacogenomics and Personalized Medicine* would not have been possible.

Nadine Cohen, PhD

Contents

Contributors

Martin Armstrong, PhD
Research and Development Genetics, AstraZeneca, Cheshire, UK

Hind Berrahmoune, PhD
Inserm University Henri Poincaré Nancy, France

Ramón Cacabelos, MD, PhD, DMSc
Biotechnology and Genomics, Camilo José Cela University, Madrid, Spain

Nadine Cohen, PhD
Department of Pharmacogenomics, Johnson and Johnson Pharmaceutical Research and Development, L.L.C., Raritan, NJ

Ann K. Daly, PhD
School of Clinical and Laboratory Sciences,
Newcastle University Medical School, Newcastle, UK

Chantal Depondt, PhD
Service de Neurologie, Université Libre de Bruxelles, Belgium

Reyna Favis, PhD
Department of Pharmacogenomics, Johnson and Johnson Pharmaceutical Research and Development, L.L.C., Raritan, NJ

Monique Franc, PhD
Department of Pharmacogenomics, Johnson and Johnson
Pharmaceutical Research and Development, L.L.C., Raritan, NJ

Theresa Frangiosa, MBA
Commercial Marketing, Johnson and Johnson Pharmaceutical Research and Development, L.L.C., Raritan, NJ

Felix W. Frueh, PhD
Office of Clinical Pharmacology, Center for Drug Evaluation and Research, Food and Drug Administration, Silver Spring, MD

Dong-Jing Fu, PhD
Department of Pharmacogenomics, Johnson and Johnson Pharmaceutical Research and Development, L.L.C., Raritan, NJ

Struan F. A. Grant, PhD
The Center for Applied Genomics and Division of Human Genetics, the Abramson Research Center of the Joseph Stokes Jr. Research Institute, Department of Pediatrics, The Children's Hospital of Philadelphia of the University of Pennsylvania School of Medicine, Philadelphia, PA

Hakon Hakonarson, MD, PhD
The Center for Applied Genomics and Division of Human Genetics, the Abramson Research Center of the Joseph Stokes Jr. Research Institute, Department of Pediatrics, The Children's Hospital of Philadelphia of the University of Pennsylvania School of Medicine, Philadelphia, PA

Shiew-Mei Huang, PhD
Office of Clinical Pharmacology, Center for Drug Evaluation and Research, Food and Drug Administration, Silver Spring, MD

Myong-Jin Kim, PharmD, PhD
Office of Clinical Pharmacology, Center for Drug Evaluation and Research, Food and Drug Administration, Silver Spring, MD

Todd Lencz, PhD
Department of Psychiatry Research, The Zucker Hillside Hospital, Glen Oaks, NY

Lawrence J. Lesko, PhD
Office of Clinical Pharmacology, Center for Drug Evaluation and Research, Food and Drug Administration, Silver Spring, MD

Qingqin S. Li, PhD
Department of Pharmacogenomics, Johnson and Johnson Pharmaceutical Research and Development, L.L.C., Raritan, NJ

Paul D. Maher, MD, MPH
Office of Orphan Products Development, Food and Drug Administration, LCDR, United States Public Health Service, Rockville, MD

Anil K. Malhotra, MD
Department of Psychiatry Research, The Zucker Hillside Hospital, Glen Oaks, NY

Jean-Brice Marteau, PhD
Inserm University Henri Poincaré Nancy, France

Nathalie Malo, PhD
Scripps Genomic Medicine, The Scripps Research Institute, La Jolla, CA

Duncan McHale, MD, PhD
Medical Director, Personalized Healthcare AstraZeneca, Stage3 F347, Alderley House, Alderley Park, Macclesfield, Cheshire, UK

George Mulligan, PhD
Millennium Pharmaceuticals, Cambridge, MA

Atiqur Rahman, PhD
Office of Clinical Pharmacology, Center for Drug Evaluation and Research, Food and Drug Administration, Silver Spring, MD

Deborah Sokol Ricci, PhD
Department of Pharmacogenomics, Johnson and Johnson Pharmaceutical Research and Development, L.L.C., Raritan, NJ

Jeffrey S. Ross, MD
Department of Pathology and Laboratory Medicine, Albany Medical College, Albany, NY

Nicholas J. Schork, PhD
Scripps Genomic Medicine, The Scripps Research Institute, La Jolla, CA

Gerard Siest, PharmD, PhD
Inserm University Henri Poincaré Nancy, France

Richard Simon, DSc
Biometric Research Branch, National Cancer Institute, Bethesda, MD

Nicole Soranzo, PhD
Wellcome Trust Sanger Institute, Cambridge, UK

Amalio Telenti, MD, PhD
Institute of Microbiology, University Hospital Center, University of Lausanne, Lausanne, Switzerland

Eric J. Topol, MD
Scripps Genomic Medicine, The Scripps Research Institute, La Jolla, CA

William L. Trepicchio, PhD
Millennium Pharmaceuticals, Cambridge, MA

Sophie Visvikis-Siest, PhD
Inserm University Henri Poincaré Nancy, France

Chapter 1
Challenges, Opportunities, and Evolving Landscapes in Pharmacogenomics and Personalized Medicine

An Industry Perspective

Nadine Cohen and Theresa Frangiosa

Contents

Abstract Pharmacogenomics (PGx) is the study of the genetic basis of variability among individuals in response to drugs. It is the newest discipline of medicine and is becoming a very active area of research, with the pharmaceutical industry gaining experience applying it, integrating it into the drug development process, and also learning to better manage the expectations of the medical community. Personalized medicine (PM), based on the genetic makeup of a patient, may result in not only an improved therapeutic response but also a clinically important reduction in adverse drug reactions. The experience to date is mixed, with a few successes but many frustrations. This chapter provides an industry perspective on the emergence of the field of PGx focusing on the more mature DNA technologies. Specifically, the chapter will: (1) give a brief description of the history of PGx, (2) provide definitions of key terms, (3) look at the elements in the current healthcare

Nadine Cohen
Johnson and Johnson Pharmaceutical Research and Development, L.L.C., 1000 Route 202, Raritan, NJ 08869
ncohen2@prdus.jnj.com

N. Cohen (ed.) *Pharmacogenomics and Personalized Medicine*,

and commercial environment that are driving us to personalized medicine, (4) consider the challenges (strategic/commercial, scientific, regulatory, implementation) that need to be addressed to make PGx and personalized medicine (PM) a reality, and finally, (4) provide a few practical recommendations from an industry perspective for improved success in this area.

Keywords pharmacogenomics, personalized medicine, DNA, commercial, pharmaceutical industry, challenges, landscape, recommendations

1 Introduction

Approximately 50 years ago, Watson and Crick elucidated the structure of DNA; and in 2003, the human genome sequence was published, capturing the imagination and raising the expectations, among both the medical community and the public, of "revolutionary" clinical applications in the near future. Key experts in genomics have publicly expressed that we will soon see drug therapies that are highly personalized and linked to DNA-based diagnostic tests. However, the experience to date is rather depressing, being a mix of a few successes but many frustrations. The average age of the population, particularly in the developed world, is rising, causing increased demands for drugs to treat late-onset illnesses, such as Alzheimer's disease, cancer, and cardiovascular diseases. There is an imperative need for the pharmaceutical industry to discover and market drugs that will allow patients to live longer and healthier lives. However, the pharmaceutical industry is facing a huge problem and some key challenges. The cost of drug development is rising, mostly due to attrition, and the number of drugs approved is falling. At present, fewer than one in ten candidate drugs that enter clinical trials are approved. Drugs fail the regulatory process due to issues with efficacy or clinical or preclinical safety. Furthermore, a substantial number of approved drugs have had to be withdrawn from the market due to unexpected and serious safety concerns. Such emerging safety issues are extremely difficult to address, as they are hardly ever observed during preapproval clinical trials. Regulatory authorities are also being scrutinized because of safety issues, and as a result approvals of new compounds are becoming tougher to obtain. Other challenges include generic competition for blockbuster medicines, insufficient drugs in development, patent challenges, and pressure to reduce prices. There is also an unrealistic demand on the pharmaceutical industry for double-digit profit growth, and this might be an explanation for the significant job cuts seen in some of the big pharmaceutical companies.

Thus the pharmaceutical industry is in desperate need of innovation, increased productivity, ways to better differentiate compounds from competitive compounds, and ways to bring better, safer, more efficient drugs to the market with lower costs of development. The patients themselves are also demanding better and safer drugs. The field of PGx, the study of the genetics of drug response, presents undeniable promise to change this depressing reality, to guide drug development and drug therapy, and to improve therapeutics by "personalizing therapy." Whether this promise of PGx will be fulfilled remains to be seen. However, there is also a growing appreciation of the challenges, both scientific and nonscientific, in translating this new knowledge into clinical applications. Increasingly and in a relatively short time, sponsors of new drugs have been integrating PGx into their drug development programs, despite a relative paucity of guidelines, regulations, and global harmonization. The outcome of this integration presents challenges to the traditional paradigms for drug development, regulatory evaluation of safety and efficacy, and clinical use of drugs. Ethical, legal, and pharmacoeconomic issues are also expected to weigh in heavily.

The intent of this chapter is to (1) give a brief description of the history of PGx, (2) provide definitions of key terms, (3) look at the elements in the current healthcare and commercial environment that are driving us to personalized medicine, (4) consider the challenges that need to be addressed, including the commercial, regulatory, scientific, and implementation issues involved with integrating PGx into the drug development process, and finally, (4) provide a few recommendations from an industry perspective on how to achieve improved success in this area.

2 History of Pharmacogenomics

Sir Archibald Garrod, in his 1902 studies, was probably the first to realize the inherited predisposition of certain individuals to alcaptonuria and phenylketonuria *(1)*. J.B.S. Haldane in 1949 made observations about unusual reactions to drugs on the basis of biochemical individuality *(2)*. These isolated observations preceded the arrival of pharmacogenetics and were followed by several other isolated findings summarized by Kalow, one of the pioneers of pharmacogenetics *(3)*. Pharmacology and genetics are two very old and independent sciences that combined into "pharmacogenetics" in the late 1950s when it was clearly established that genetic factors can be responsible for altered drug responses in some patients. One of the first findings involved patients with a genetic lack of butyrylcholinesterase, who died following a succinylcholine injection during anesthesia *(4)*. Another case in 1957 *(5)* described the genetic deficiency of N-acetyltransferase, an enzyme that destroyed the antituberculosis drug isoniazid. In 1959, the term "pharmacogenetics" was introduced by Vogel *(6)*, describing a new scientific discipline that dealt with inherited differences in the response to drugs. Further interest in pharmacogenetics in the clinic was created by subsequent findings, such as the discovery of genetic variation in the metabolism of debrisoquine *(7)* and of sparteine *(8)*. These findings were followed by observations about the absence of the cytochrome liver enzyme CYP2D6, and the involvement of this enzyme in the metabolism of more than 60 drugs *(9)*. By 2001, at least 42 drug metabolizing enzymes were known to be genetically variable *(10)*. Other determinants of drug response were also found to be genetically variable, including drug receptors (e.g., serotonin, dopamine) *(11)*, transporters (e.g., P-glycoprotein) *(12)*, and neuro-transmitter enzymes (e.g., COMT) *(13)*. Soon it became clear that drug effects tended to differ also between populations, not only between individuals *(14)*. Most of these initial pharmacogenetic studies were investigations of single-gene mutations between individuals and their consequences on pharmacological effects. However, advances in genomics technologies led to the understanding that most differences in drug responses between people or populations were not caused by the mutation of a single gene but by the altered function of numerous genes, combined with interacting environmental factors. Thus most variable drug responses appear to be "multifactorial." This realization led to the extension of pharmacogenetics into pharmacogenomics.

Pharmacogenomics investigations require an increased use of methods designed to study many genes or gene patterns, looking simultaneously at the structure and expression of whole sets of genes. At the same time, the biotech industry has very rapidly provided multiple technology platforms enabling the performance of low-, medium-, or large-scale genotyping or expression analysis using DNA or RNA chips, some of these tools being customized for this purpose. Next generation sequencing will gradually replace genotyping. These revolutionary achievements create the weighty obligation of responsibly translating genetic information derived from research studies into clinical applications in a manner that is both medically sound and in the best interests of patients.

3 Definitions of Key Terms and Basic PGx Principles

Pharmacogenetics is generally defined as the study of inherited factors (DNA variations) and their influence on interindividual variation in drug response. In contrast, pharmacogenomics encompasses the role of the whole genome in pharmacology and drug design. The terms are often used interchangeably. In this chapter, we will use the term pharmacogenomics (PGx) research—which refers to the use of appropriate DNA methodologies to develop reliable markers to predict drug response, adverse reactions, dose requirements, disease susceptibility, and disease stage—as we consider those technologies which are currently the more mature components of the evolving constellation of genomic sciences. PGx research is applicable to activities such as drug discovery, drug development, and clinical practice. Drug response includes drug disposition (pharmacokinetics, PK) and drug effect (pharmacodynamics, PD). Pharmacokinetic effects are due to interindividual differences in absorption, distribution, metabolism, or excretion of the drug. Inappropriate concentrations of the pharmaceutical agent, or inappropriate metabolites, or both, can result in lack of efficacy or in toxicity. Such PK effects have been seen mostly with the cytochrome P450 enzyme family as described in many reviews *(15, 16)*, but also with membrane transporters such as MDR-1 *(17)*, or the purine-analog-metabolizing enzyme, thiometyl-purine-transferase *(18)*. In contrast, pharmacodynamic effects may lead to interindividual differences in a drug's effect despite the presence of appropriate concentrations of the active drug compound at the intended site of action. In this case, DNA-based variation in the target molecule's genes or downstream mechanistic pathway genes can explain the variability among subjects in response to drugs.

PGx studies are based, in large part, on the "genotype-to-phenotype" principle—examining relationships between genetic information (genotype) and clinical information (phenotype). Genetic information may be generated using a candidate gene approach or a genome-wide screen approach. It may exist in the form of ***genotypes*** or ***haplotypes*** (for DNA); it may also include information on gene products (e.g., mRNA or protein expression). Phenotypic information includes PK or PD endpoints, efficacy or safety endpoints, or disease/disease states, among other endpoints generated in clinical trials. A relationship between a genotypic and a phenotypic endpoint may suggest a role for a given gene in the clinical outcome. In some cases, a gene may be a mere (although valuable) biomarker of response, without necessarily playing a direct role in that outcome. By relating variability in genotype to variability in phenotype, it is possible to identify the genes responsible for a given clinical outcome. PGx is not limited to genotype-to-phenotype information. In some cases (particularly in drug discovery), genetic information can be used directly in the absence of phenotypic information to guide target prioritization, among other uses.

In this chapter, the term "personalized medicine" refers in the first place to pharmacogenetics-based individualized pharmacotherapy—the ability to offer the appropriate treatment to the right person as needed. The term is sometimes misleading, and may be interpreted to mean that drugs are developed for individual patients. Another term often used is "stratified medicine"—proactively testing and selecting subsets of populations for treatment based on a likely positive or negative therapeutic response. Stratification is driving a trend away from the development of "blockbuster" drugs to that of "nichebusters," which could fundamentally alter the nature of competition in the biomedical industry. In principle, genotype-based, individually targeted prescribing ought to be more effective at improving response rates and decreasing the burdens of adverse drug reactions.

Other terms of relevance to PGx research have been defined in the FDA's recently published "guidance" for the submission of PGx data *(19)*. A **known valid biomarker** is defined as a genetic biomarker measured in an analytical test system with well-established performance characteristics *and* for which there is widespread agreement in the scientific community about the physiologic, pharmacologic, or clinical significance of the results. A **probable valid biomarker** is defined as a genetic biomarker measured in an analytical test system with well-established performance characteristics *and* for which there is a scientific framework or body of evidence that appears to elucidate the physiologic, pharmacologic, or clinical significance of the results. This accommodates biomarkers for which:

i. data are highly suggestive of significance, but may not be conclusive;
ii. independent replication may not have occurred; or
iii. data are generated within a single company and not available for public scrutiny.

4 Current Applications

Pharmacogenomics has the potential to (1) improve the discovery of drugs targeted to human disease, (2) improve proof of principle for efficacy trials and salvage drugs, (3) identify optimal dosing, (4) improve drug safety and understand adverse events in development and postapproval, and (5) improve the identification of patients who will benefit from genetically-defined therapy, thereby avoiding futile therapeutic attempts. These applications are shown in Fig. 1.1

Genetic research is generally being done in two main areas in the pharmaceutical industry: 1) the genetics of drug responsiveness (drug metabolizing enzymes, targets, and exploratory pharmacogenetics) and 2) the genetics of disease characteristics (genes associated with a disease, disease state, or disease prognosis).

1) Genetics of Drug Responsiveness (Pharmacogenetics)

The goal of the first area is to generate an understanding that will aid in making safe and more effective drugs for the specific individuals for whom they are prescribed. Variations in ADME genes (including transporters) and drug targets (and associated genes) may result in the absence of protein or the production of protein with altered or no activity. There are several described cases of genetic variation in ADME genes, mainly accounting for the variation in plasma drug concentration in patients following a fixed dose, as well as cases of genetic variation in the target genes affecting clinical outcomes. Among the polymorphic drug metabolizing enzymes most extensively investigated are the cytochrome P450s (CYPs). The clinical significance of these variations depends primarily on the contribution of the specific pathway to the overall metabolism of the drug and the therapeutic index of the drug, as well as the activity of its metabolites.

2) Genetics of Disease Characteristics (Disease Genetics)

The goal of the second area of study is to understand the contribution of genes to chronic diseases (and the biologic pathways of these diseases) in order to create therapies that are better tailored to the diseases under study. There is clearly potential overlap between disease genetics and pharmacogenetics, since subentities of a disease may well explain part of the differential response to a drug (e.g., the disease-causing gene is also the drug target). One of the familiar examples of disease genetics applied to medical practice is the APOE genotype and the clinical response to tacrine treatment in Alzheimer's disease *(20)*.

Many genetic research studies in these two areas are currently part of clinical trials within various pharmaceutical companies to address pharmacokinetics, efficacy, or safety issues. Often the information is used as an inclusion or exclusion criterion in

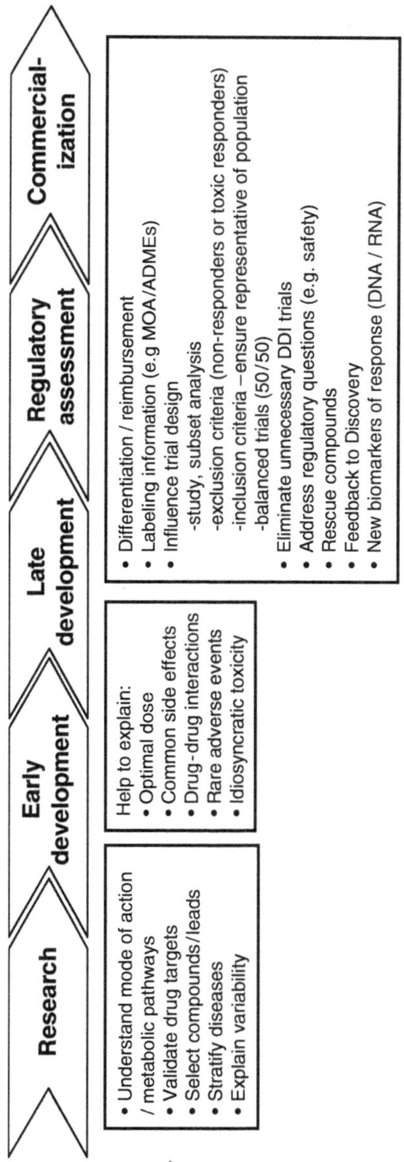

Fig. 1.1 Biomarkers in the pharmaceutical lifecycle: pharmacogenomics opportunities

prescreening studies or for decision making as described in Chapter 5. In most cases, genetic research studies are exploratory in nature, to proactively or retroactively test hypotheses or to generate new hypotheses. Pharmacogenetics is also incorporated early in the drug discovery pipeline to ensure that discovery efforts are directed at developing drugs against the most common target variants and against targets that display a manageable degree of genetic variation as described in Chapter 4.

Currently, a number of pharmaceutical and biotech companies are working towards the goal of producing medicines that will be correctly administered to the patients expected to respond to treatment. The most classic example of personalized medicine is the development of Herceptin (trastazumab). Herceptin is a targeted therapy that inhibits the proliferation of human tumor cells that overexpress HER2 *(21)*. This occurs in 24–30% of primary breast cancers. Labeling of Herceptin requires that patients be screened for HER2 overexpression by one of two available tests: The Hercep test which measures overexpression of the HER2 protein, or the PathVysion test which measures gene amplification by FISH. Only patients that have overexpression of HER2 should be treated with Herceptin, as it has been proven in previous clinical studies that they will respond to this drug. Erbitux (cetuximab) is an additional example of a drug with in its drug label, a requirement for testing patients with colorectal cancer for EGFR expression prior to treatment *(22)*. There are a number of other examples of personalized medicine which have been used either to identify patients that will respond to treatment (such as Gleevec and Tarceva) *(23)*, *(24)* or to identify patients that will develop severe toxicities (6-Mercaptopurin, irinotecan, and Straterra) *(25–27)*. In these latter examples, either pharmacogenomics information or a recommendation about pharmacogenomics testing is included on the drug label. It is noteworthy that the drug label of Irinotecan has been updated based upon data that were generated postmarketing and not by its drug developer. Recently warfarin's drug label has also been modified to point out that genetic variations in the CYP2C9 and VKORC1 enzymes are one of the factors that may influence the response of the patient to warfarin *(28)*. The pharmacogenomics section of the labeling includes a discussion of studies showing that the gene variants are associated with lower dose requirements. These approved labeling changes are further steps showing the FDA commitment to personalized medicine. The current regulatory landscape is further discussed later in this chapter and in Chapter 3.

5 The Current Healthcare Landscape Driving the Pharmaceutical Industry to Personalized Medicine

When thinking about the future of PGx, it is relevant to consider the current healthcare landscape and why it is driving us to personalized medicine (PM). We will elaborate on the following elements: the need for innovation and for increased productivity, the competitive pressure, and the interests of the regulators, legislators, and payers. We do not elaborate in this section on the huge progress in genomics technology and the demands of the patients for better and safer drugs, which also represent powerful drivers to (PM).

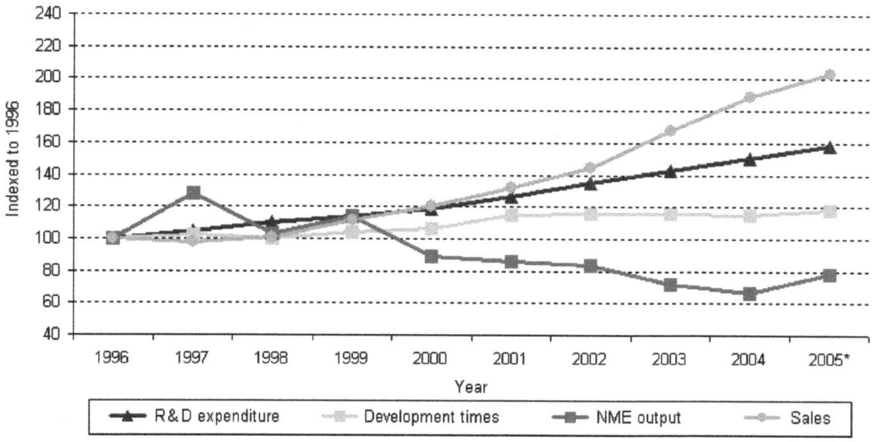

Fig. 1.2 Global R&D expenditure, development times, global pharmaceutical sales and new molecular entity output, 1996-2005. Source: The Centre for Medicines Research (CMR) International Ltd. (2006) *NME output lifts from 20 year low,* Thomson Scientific Knowledge Link Newsletter

5.1 The Need for Innovation

Several key concerns highlight the need for innovation to drive long-term success (ultimately via the identification of novel mechanisms). The CMR International Institute for Regulatory Science has presented data through 2002 showing that over the preceding ten years, both R&D investment and sales of pharmaceuticals have almost doubled, as shown in Fig. 1.2 *(29)*. However, during the same period the output of new molecular entities has fallen by 25%. Development times also display a disappointing trend—despite industry-wide efforts to speed up the drug development process, development times of drugs launched recently are on a par with those launched at the start of the 1990s. More recent surveys, such as the 2006 Tufts study, point to similar trends in recent years *(30)*. The FDA Critical Path Initiative further highlights the dramatic increase in biomedical research spending levels over a 10-year period from 1993 to 2003 and compares that to a significant decrease in major drug or product submissions to the FDA over the same time period *(31)*.

A combination of higher regulatory hurdles (efficacy and safety) and longer development times has resulted in significant challenges to achieving new goals in offering lower risk/higher benefit therapies. The recent postmarketing withdrawals of Vioxx and other compounds highlights the growing importance of a strong risk/benefit proposition *(32)*. Further, an examination of pipelines for key therapeutic areas reveals the need for newly identified novel mechanisms. Both efficacy and safety challenges have resulted in difficulties in identifying relevant innovative targets or testing in new areas.

One final point to raise in conjunction with the lessened novelty in pharmaceutical pipelines is the increasing levels of generic products on the market. As more and more compounds become generic, pharmaceutical company belts will tighten even further. A key question to ask is, "How great is the risk that companies cannot sustain the pace of innovation to keep up with research demands?" PGx is a logical approach that has the potential to drive innovation and to improve the productivity of the pharmaceutical industry.

5.2 Competitive Pressures

For some pharmaceutical companies, competitive initiatives may fuel the desire to develop a PGx program. While some organizations may not be driven to invest in spending programs in which there is significant uncertainty, they may become compelled to do so when it becomes clear that competitors are making relevant advances. A review of the competitive landscape highlights the fact that pharmaceutical companies are becoming interested in PGx activities in a big way. Virtually all companies have made deals and are beginning to establish an internal pharmacogenomic presence. Oncology is a field where many companies are investing in and applying PGx. An internal analysis from Johnson & Johnson reveals over 700 PGx deals, found through deals databases and newswires. Additionally, many companies already have internal structures that facilitate biomarker identification and diagnostic development. There were also 275 federally funded grants identified and several public/private partnerships initiated. Most companies have invested in biomarker identification and utilize PGx in clinical trials and drug discovery (target identification and/or validation). According to publicly available information, a number of the companies surveyed seem to focus their deals on particular aspects of PGx, including diagnostics, biomarkers, and SNP identification/validation.

There are several factors driving this growing interest in PGx approaches. The first consideration is the desire to meet patients' unmet medical needs. Another likely issue is competitive pressure and the importance of product differentiation in achieving market share and reimbursement in increasingly crowded markets in many therapeutic areas. In fact, payer pressures may be stronger drivers in some markets. It should be noted that as competitors engage in PGx analyses to support approval and formulary acceptance, they are "raising the bar" for all future market entrants. It may become an expectation of global regulatory authorities that all compounds will deliver similar analysis.

5.3 Legislators

Additionally, legislators have indicated an interest in providing universal health coverage that personalizes treatment. This topic promises to be an interesting area of debate in Congress. In fact, in 2006, Senator Barack Obama circulated for feedback some proposed legislation that addressed the provision of incentives to pharmaceutical companies for conducting PGx research resulting in pharmacoeconomic benefit *(33)*. This highlights the visibility and attractiveness of personalized medicine approaches to our nation's legislators. Such incentives, if coupled with a regulatory framework, would make it easier for the pharmaceutical industry to justify postmarketing PGx programs.

The Secretary's Advisory Committee on Genetics, Health, and Society (SACGHS) released a draft report to Health and Human Services (HHS) Secretary Leavitt titled *Realizing the Promise of Pharmacogenomics: Opportunities and Challenges.* This report focuses on opportunities and challenges in three areas of pharmacogenomics: research and development; "gatekeepers," or those involved in facilitating the progression of PGx; and the implementation of PGx to improve outcomes in clinical and public health practices. The report includes draft recommendations in each of these areas. Among its recommendations, SACGHS suggests that HHS improve efforts to translate new scientific knowledge into clinically useful PGx technologies and to assess their clinical validity and utility; encourage the FDA to finalize the codevelopment guidance on PGx drugs and diagnostics; and ensure that clinically validated PGx test results are included in electronic medical record systems to enhance appropriate test use and interpretation.

5.4 Payers

The view of payers about pharmacogenomic approaches does not appear to be clear or consistent yet. Different groups within payer organizations may be responsible for drug budgets versus diagnostic budgets versus hospitalization costs. It is likely that over time compelling arguments will be waged that will enable these disparities to be addressed. For example, improved communication and education directed to this customer base may be influential in highlighting the benefits of PGx approaches, especially if they influence the payer's bottom line. Diagnostics could be provided as a "loss leader," and risk-sharing opportunities may emerge.

5.5 Regulatory Agencies

The FDA has clearly communicated that it is encouraging PGx work and has undertaken several initiatives to facilitate the integration of PGx into drug development and clinical practice, as described by Kim et al. in Chapter 3 *(34)*. Open dialogue is possible between regulators, the pharmaceutical industry, and academic centers involved in PGx research, and this has led to several key initiatives. These have included the white paper entitled "Innovation or Stagnation: Challenge and Opportunity on the Critical Path to New Medical Products" *(31)* [U.S. FDA 2004a, http://www.fda.gov/oc/initiatives/criticalpath/whitepaper.html] and the "Guidance for Industry on Pharmacogenomics Data Submission" (November 2005) *(19)*. In 2005, the U.S. Food and Drug Administration (FDA) distributed for comment a draft concept paper on drug-diagnostic codevelopment, which describes a process for developing a diagnostic to determine the later use of a particular drug *(35)*. Other regulatory bodies around the world have also communicated the desire to see PGx data in product package submissions. The European Medicines Agency (EMEA) also started to become active in this area *(36)*, and the Pharmacogenetics Working Party issued guidelines for its briefing meetings and for biobanking. The EMEA and the FDA have also issued recently a joint procedure for the voluntary submission of PGx data *(37)*. In 2006, the ICH issued a draft consensus guideline regarding terminology in pharmacogenomics (E15), agreed upon by the regulatory authorities of the European Union, Japan, and the USA *(38)*.

Additionally, the recent nonapprovable for Arcoxia (etoricoxib), an NSAID in development by Merck & Co., *(39)* highlights the growing importance of better characterization of compounds before they receive marketing approval. Regulators have indicated that for a new NSAID to be considered for U.S. marketing approval, the drug must fill an unmet need for patients. The pharmaceutical industry is hoping that incentives such as fast-track approvals resulting in innovative drug development will be offered by regulatory agencies for compounds that are appropriately characterized through PGx approaches *(41)*.

5.6 Creation of Pharmacogenomics/Biomarkers Consortia and Task Forces

It is noteworthy that several pharmacogenomics networks and consortia involving various industry companies, the scientific community, and government agencies such as the FDA have been recently created. This is due to the realization that collaboration, where resources are being pooled on scientifically challenging projects, is required for increased success. For example, the PhRMA Biomarker Consortium *(40)*, the Predictive Safety Testing Consortium *(41)*, which was created under the auspices of the Critical Path Institute, and the Serious Adverse Event Consortium, involving industry *(42)*, the FDA, and academic groups, were formed to execute biomarker or PGx research that no single company could carry out on its own. The Industry Pharmacogenomics Working Group (I-PWG, http://www.i-pwg.org/cms/) is an association of 18 pharmaceutical companies engaged in both drug development and pharmacogenomics research *(43)*. This group has published several papers on noncompetitive topics such as terminology *(44)*, points to consider in informed consent forms for genetic research *(45)*, and points to consider in the return of genetic data to patients *(46)*. PWG recently initiated discussions regarding the preparation of educational material for prescribing physicians and of potential guidelines for pharmacogenetic study design and analyses. The Personalized Medicine Coalition (PMC) is another independent, nonprofit group that works to advance the understanding and adoption of personalized medicine for the ultimate benefit of patients *(47)*. Its diverse members include payers, patient advocacy groups, healthcare providers, governmental agencies, pharmaceutical companies, and biotech, diagnostic, and academic institutions—all working together to educate opinion leaders and the public about the issues that will shape how personalized medicine develops and how quickly all of us, particularly the patients, can benefit from it.

These recent activities and formations continue to illustrate the prominent role PGx will play in moving drug development and therapy from a population-based to an individualized paradigm.

6 The Challenges

PGx is one of the newest disciplines in medicine in the context of drug development, and is a true work in progress. The pharmaceutical industry, having gained experience in this field, and also having a greater appreciation of the hurdles in applying it, is starting to set more realistic expectations regarding the implications of this research. Some of the challenges regarding the appropriate implementation of this technology to deliver the greatest value to the pharmaceutical industry overall—and, more importantly, to benefit the patients—are discussed below.

6.1 Strategic and Commercial Considerations

There are concerns in the pharmaceutical industry about generating potentially uninterpretable PGx results in a regulated environment. This has led sometimes to a "let's not generate data that we do not fully understand" attitude in relation to PGx research on pharmaceutical compounds. This attitude is gradually going away in view of the recognition that many of the PGx data generated are exploratory and probabilistic in nature, extremely difficult to replicate and to translate into clinical practice, and that in the long term more information, particularly about drug safety, is better.

When thinking about the commercial attractiveness of PGx, critics often suggest that a more targeted approach to the identification of patients who might respond to therapy would "niche" those drugs, leading to a reluctance to embark on a given PGx study. In fact, utilizing a stratified approach (to identify the group of patients who might benefit from a particular therapy) may reduce new patient trials for some therapies. But this initial sales reduction may be offset by better compliance rates, ultimately higher product use, and pricing strategies that consider market size. One key variable is ensuring that PGx work is initiated sufficiently early to optimize a proactive approach to integration into development. Generally, the establishment of biomarker-driven endpoints within early phase clinical development may enable more efficient clinical trial design. Additionally, prospective introduction of PGx clinical endpoints can enhance the prospects for expedited drug approval, reduce development costs, and improve attractiveness to payers and prescribing physicians. Therefore, in the short term, a PGx approach may provide a competitive advantage for pharmaceutical compounds and support better treatment practices through drug-linked diagnostics. But commercial viability may not be a question of what is gained or lost by moving forward with the development of biomarkers; rather, it may center around what is at stake by not moving forward with these approaches. While pipelines for many therapeutic areas are shrinking, a landscape review highlights the increasing infrastructure development in PGx and the initiation of product-specific work across a variety of therapeutic areas, indicating the awakening of the pharmaceutical industry. So in the longer term, the utilization of biomarkers may improve prospects for significant new product development, in a time when there are fewer novel compounds in the pharmaceutical pipelines. Finally, as external groups apply more pressure on pharmaceutical companies to develop valuable new offerings, it may become a requirement to provide information that helps the regulatory agencies to ascertain which patient populations might benefit from the availability of a new drug. PGx is one means for providing such information to regulators and payers.

6.2 Regulatory Considerations

As indicated above, the FDA has been the first agency to put a regulatory framework around the submission of pharmacogenomics data and the codevelopment of drugs and linked diagnostics. In spite of these efforts, the codevelopment of drugs and diagnostics is extremely difficult because of regulatory and time constraints, and also because of the complexity of the science. However, this concept emphasizes the need to start developing hypotheses as early as possible, with a decision point at the end of phase II on whether a diagnostic will be developed—which is rarely the case. The drug developers are still lacking guidance on (1) when and how to collect DNA/RNA samples in clinical trials; (2) the type of data that is necessary to bring the PGx information to the drug label, and whether or not this will lead to a test requirement or recommendation for dose adjustment or patient selection prior to treatment (3) how PGx data should be analyzed; and (4) on laboratory repuirements for PGx testing (e.g. CLIA versus GLP). Additional guidelines from FDA currently in progress might shed lights on some of those issues. A table of valid genomic biomarkers has been created by the FDA, providing a reference for these biomarkers on labels of FDA-approved drug products *(48)*. There are only a few examples of drugs where PGx data including a requirement for a test are part of the drug label as prescribed (e.g., Herceptin, Erbitux). Other examples of drugs with PGx data include either descriptive information or recommendations but no requirements for a test (e.g., Strattera, 6-mercaptopurine, irinotecan, warfarin).

Overall, in spite of recent changes in the labels of a few drugs, there is still a lack of dosing instructions associated with label information. Many questions about the standards required to validate genotype-phenotype associations in order to determine optimal dosing in clinical practice or for regulatory policies regarding label updates are undergoing intense debate among the key stakeholders, as described by Lesko *(49)*. It is expected that within the next few years, we will see an increase of investment in PGx research by the pharmaceutical industry coupled with more evidence of clinical relevance for PGx data, and this will lead to more examples of drugs with prescribing labels.

6.3 Complexity of Science and Technology Considerations

This section describes some of the huge progress made in genomics technology and the availability of tests and presents a discussion of some of the current scientific hurdles. Genetic testing does not represent a barrier anymore to personalized medicine (PM), with a multitude of reagents (DNA chips) and pharmacogenomics services available as home brew tests from diagnostic laboratories. Home brew tests are being actively marketed to physicians or even directly to patients via the Internet; and while they are not generally regulated by the FDA, they are however being scrutinized. Furthermore, pharmacogenomics tests have recently been approved by the FDA that would allow physicians and patients to make more personalized treatment decisions. They include, for example, the Roche Molecular Systems's Amplichip, which detects polymorphisms in CYP2C19 and CYP2D6. These enzymes are responsible for metabolizing over 25% of currently marketed drugs. The results from this test could be used to determine the correct dose in patients. Genzyme's invader UGT1A1 molecular assay has also recently been approved. This technology is able to detect polymorphisms in UGT1A1, and subsequently dosing decisions can be made for patients taking irinotecan or other drugs thought to be metabolized by UGT1A1. Another test, the Visible Genetics TRUEGENE HIV-1 genotyping kit, uses sequencing technology to identify variation in HIV sequences, which could allow physicians to determine which drug would treat the HIV infection effectively. The Cell Search Technology from Veridex, one of Johnson and Johnson's diagnostic companies, has been approved by the FDA in cases of metastatic breast cancer to predict progression-free survival and overall survival in patients. In February 2007, the FDA approved the first microarray-based test, called the MammaPrint test, to determine the likelihood of breast cancer returning within 5–10 years after a woman's initial cancer. Currently there is no point-of-care pharmacogenomic testing, but some research is being done in this area. Dr. Yusuke Nakamura, for example, has reported the development of a prototype commercial instrument that would allow physicians to check the status of metabolism genes and how patients would respond to an individual drug *(50)*.

There is no shortage of science and data; as a matter of fact, we are almost overwhelmed by the massive amount of data we can now generate easily using, for example, the DNA chips from Affymetrix or Illumina. Pharmaceutical companies are investing more and more on data management and information technology infrastructure in which clinical data, genotyping data, and data from other types of biomarker technologies (such as RNA, protein, metabolomics, and imaging) can be mined. We are just starting to learn how to analyze these massive amounts of data with the help of statisticians, bioinformatics specialists, and epidemiology experts. We all recognize the need to have better tools to diagnose complex disorders and disease progressions, in order to stratify them into subcategories of a broader phenotype. As more and more data are generated, the gap between bench and bedside continues to grow, with possibly the missing link being effective translational medicine.

As indicated by Lesko *(49)*, "better science is the way to personalized medicine and there are numerous opportunities to utilize the core principles of clinical pharmacology to address the concerns, difficulty of interpretation surrounding the associations between genes, SNP, and clinical phenotypes, and to provide a biological, mechanistic framework for future decision making in PGx." If the technology does not seem anymore to be a barrier, the science of pharmacogenomics remains highly challenging. Identifying and replicating valid associations is difficult because of statistical considerations, sample size, and their inherent biological complexity. Clinical trials are generally not tailored to PGx studies. Sample size in early development trials are typically low; this stage of research is often used for hypothesis generation, and occasionally for hypothesis testing, if candidate markers emerging from either literature or preclinical studies have been identified. Meta-analysis combining data from several trials enables the generation of data on larger numbers of samples. Studies using large numbers of genes or genome-wide screens are likely to be seriously underpowered, resulting in the risk of false negatives or false positives. Replication of data is essential; however, too many genetic associations have no evidence of replication in independent populations. In Phase III trials, sample sizes are generally large enough to allow the generation of hypotheses or to test hypotheses generated in earlier PGx research. In the case of safety biomarkers, the statistical challenges are even greater because of the rarity of adverse drug reactions, and hence the fact that only a small number of samples will be available to carry PGx research. Initiatives such as the Serious Adverse Event (SAE) consortium, in which samples and resources will be pooled, are necessary and hopefully will greatly facilitate the understanding of the genetic basis of SAEs.

For some compounds, the mechanism of response is known and related to the mode of action (MOA) of the compound (Herceptin, Iressa, Tarceva). However, we continue to use drugs with not enough understanding of their mode of action or of the molecular mechanisms which cause the disease, or how to determine which patient is at risk for an adverse event, or which patient will respond to a drug. It is likely that despite the hype and high expectations that PGx will provide personalized care and will apply to all drugs, it will only apply to a fraction of the drugs being developed. Instead, we foresee that more precise diagnosis of diseases into molecular subtypes will occur, based on a better understanding of pathology at the molecular level. This will lead to a PGx scenario of stratified medicine, in which the right drug will be found for the disease subtype, rather than the scenario of finding the right drug for the right patient.

6.4 Implementation

6.4.1 Lack of Education

In spite of the fact that FDA-approved tests have become available in recent years, the use of PGx testing in clinical medical practice has remained limited, largely due to the lack of evidence for its clinical utility compared to the usual care. Providing the scientific evidence presents a significant challenge. However, in the case of Herceptin and the HER2 protein test, the uptake into clinical practice for the treatment of HER2 overexpressing metastatic breast cancer was rapid, most probably because the FDA recommended the testing prior to prescribing the drug, and because the results of the test led to an actionable decision on selecting the most appropriate treatment. In contrast, when the label of a previously approved drug such as the immunosuppressant 6-MP has been updated, as with genetic information on TPMT, it is possible that the uptake of TPMT testing to guide dosing has been minimal because the knowledge gap for physicians was less, since they were used to dosing patients and monitoring their absolute neutrophile count. In this latter case, testing was recommended but not required. It is very possible that uptake into clinical practice will also be given stimulus if the regulatory agencies recommend testing prior to prescribing the drug, and if pharmaceutical companies or patient groups would advocate for the use of the test.

Despite the significant progress, a critical factor in bringing PGx from the bench to the bedside is educating the prescribing physicians and other healthcare professionals about the benefits of using genomics information to individualize drug therapy. The rapid pace of the science, combined with the relative paucity of professional training in pharmacogenetics, leaves many providers without satisfactory answers for their patients. It is likely that organizations such as the National Coalition for Health Professional Education in Genetics (NCHPEG) *(51)*, I-PWG, and the Personalized Medicine Coalition will play a key role in promoting health professional education and access to information about advances in pharmacogenomics. Guidelines directing the clinical use of PGx test results and explaining drug labels should be developed for PGx tests shown to improve patient care. Since another challenge is reimbursement for the tests, more information on cost effectiveness and cost consequences should be provided to facilitate reimbursement by insurance companies and implementation of the tests into clinical practice. With information technology making it possible for physicians to access complete patient medical records, new medical practice models in which physicians would spend more time with each patient will need to be established in order to provide the necessary infrastructure for personalized medicine (PM). It is likely that patients and their advocacy groups will also play a key role as they become more educated about PM and PGx.

6.4.2 Ethical Aspects of Pharmacogenomics

Ethical issues in relation to PGx have been discussed extensively in several reviews and reports *(52, 53)*. DNA samples need to be collected in order for PGx research to be carried out. Obtaining, storing, and analyzing DNA samples has always been perceived to be special and more problematic than in the case of other types of samples, and they do receive particular attention from ethics committees and regulatory agencies. Privacy and confidentiality issues remain as a challenge to gaining the trust of all consumers. The voices of patients and their advocacy groups has yet to be heard. There currently are overarching expectations for a higher level of stringency in maintaining confidentiality and preventing unintended access to or release of genomic samples and data. The pharmaceutical industry in general has developed stringent and appropriate procedures to routinely collect samples for pharmacogenomic applications in clinical trials. In the last few years, the industry Pharmacogenomics Working Group (I-PWG) has made much progress in standardizing the nomenclature and informed consent forms used in clinical trials *(44, 45)*, In general, this has led to a more consistent approach to the approval of ICF and protocols for PGx clinical trials by ethics committees and regulatory bodies in different countries. On an international level, some countries have developed laws and regulations about DNA sampling which create some confusion and make sample collection more cumbersome, while it is easier in other countries. Current efforts are ongoing towards the harmonization and standardization of regulations and practices applicable to pharmacogenomic collections globally. However, it is anticipated that harmonization will not happen in the near future and that much work will be required to bring about consensus among the nations. Chapter 2 presents an overview of those considerations for sample collections intended for PGx analyses. Another topic of debate within the PGx community has been whether and how individual genetic research results should be returned to the study participants. A paper from the PWG *(46)* has summarized the key points to be considered when making those decisions.

7 Recommendations—The Way Forward

Statements such as "Personalized medicine is going to revolutionize medicine," which we see too often in publications, websites, or newspapers, are unrealistic and more damaging than useful. It is important to make a remark on personalized medicine. The practice of medicine is personalized by definition, as it aims to meet individual needs by seeking to provide optimum treatment for individual patients. Therefore, personalized medicine in a way is not particularly a new concept. It is likely to become increasingly important in drug discovery and development, as knowledge of the importance of genetic factors helps to identify optimal populations for a particular medicine.

In practical terms, several large pharmaceutical companies are making efforts to integrate pharmacogenomics into their development programs by expanding their internal capabilities, and also by outsourcing some of the work using service providers such as CRO (Quintiles, Covance), or biotech companies providing various genotyping services. Such capabilities include the development of laboratory infrastructure in the spirit of Good Laboratory Practice (GLP) or Clinical Laboratory Improvement Amendments (CLIA) processes for clinical trials DNA samples handling, collection, genotyping. Increasingly, investment in data management, bioinformatics, pharmacoepidemiology and biostatistics capabilities to analyze and interpret pharmacogenomics data are being made. In addition, a few pharmaceutical companies, such as Johnson & Johnson, Abbott, and Roche already have both internal pharmaceutical and diagnostic capabilities.

Below are some recommendations based upon the authors' experiences in applying pharmacogenomics in a pharmaceutical industry setting, with the hope they will help others in similar circumstances.

For drug developers, the long term vision is to integrate pharmacogenomics into clinical and nonclinical studies in order to provide value to pharmaceutical R&D by supplementing the information from these studies. The goal is to provide safer and more efficient medicines, combined with diagnostics, in order to meet the needs of patients. An integrated, scientific-based approach is recommended, beginning at the non-clinical stage: learn (identification of genes involved in PK and PD) and continuing throughout clinical development: continue to learn in earlier phase and confirm/validate in late phase (PG_X testing of clinical samples in various ethnic populations) and post-marketing studies: apply information to drug label; product differentiation for fast followers. Data generated in late-phase development and in the postmarketing phases can then be fed back into the discovery process to improve preclinical screening and the development of backup compounds. A decision whether to continue clinical development with or without diagnostics should ideally be made at the end of Phase II. It is strongly recommended that DNA samples from clinical trials be routinely collected and archived to permit PGx analysis either during trials or even postmarketing (as issues emerge). This strategy best exploits the power of PGx to contribute to successful compound submissions and be part of label claims. The various steps involved in pharmacogenomics research in the R&D programs of drug developers include development of a strategy, preparation of informed consent forms and protocols, design of the study, collection and genotyping of DNA samples, and preparation of the statistical analysis plan and report. Several aspects of this activity are described in subsequent chapters of this book.

The key elements to consider when establishing a PGx infrastructure in a pharmaceutical industry setting are the following:

1. Develop stringent procedures to enable routine collection of samples in clinical trials and either the de-identification or anonymization of the samples for long-term storage to ensure the privacy and confidentiality of the subjects. Develop informed consent forms and PGx protocol templates which meet high ethical and regulatory standards.

2. Develop laboratory capabilities, including a biobank, with stringent and standardized procedures and an adequate data management system to store information about DNA samples, genotyping, and clinical data. This also applies to other types of samples such as RNA, tissues and biopsies.
3. Develop bioinformatics and biostatistics capabilities to create tools to mine and analyze the genetic data and to generate reports.
4. Develop a PGx strategy as part of a clinical development plan involving a multifunctional team—PGx and discovery scientists, clinical pharmacologists, physicians, statistics/bioinformatics specialists, commercial/marketing experts, and regulatory affairs and diagnostic consultants. Such a team would assess the feasibility and added value of PGx studies in the clinical program using a multiattribute decision analysis approach prior to embarking on a program, as described for example in Chapter 13.
5. PGx Implementation
   a. Collecting samples in all trials is highly recommended for the following reasons:
      i. It enables post hoc analysis of unexpected findings, e.g., PK outliers, responder subpopulation, safety.
      ii. Large sample collection enables one to conduct drug response and disease genetics studies, to develop new disease diagnostics, and to stratify diseases into molecular subgroups. It enables both exploration and validation of data and creates a potential for DNA diagnostics. Samples can also be used to validate prospective drug targets.
      iii. Sampling enables continued research into improving medicines as new PGx findings are discovered and published by both academia and industry.
      iv. Retrospective sampling/re-consent is difficult, costly, and often not feasible.
   b. Where possible, use genomics information to guide trial design.
   c. Include PGx as early as possible in the overall development program and examine the feasibility of linkage of the drug to a companion diagnostic as early as possible.
   d. Where a candidate gene approach is inadequate, evaluate the feasibility of a genome wide screen approach.
   e. Do not limit application of PGx to biomarker identification. Exploit PGx to identify or support mode of action in vivo, and to optimize discovery processes and clinical trials.
   f. Consider both DNA and RNA markers, as well as other types of (e.g. imaging, proteomics) when appropriate.
6. PGx in clinical trials should be a balancing act of experiments where hypotheses are being generated and tested. The ideal biomarker strategy needs to have the right balance between the use of known biomarkers and exploratory biomarker research. The advantage of using known biomarkers is that they have a degree of validation that allows them to be used in decision making.

Hypotheses should be tested and known valid biomarkers should be genotyped if candidate markers emerging from either the literature or preclinical studies have been identified. An exploratory biomarker could still inform one's strategy by indicating more about pathophysiology, and by showing that the drug works in a subpopulation, rather than just doesn't work. However, discovering a biomarker during clinical development reduces the chance of using it for clinical decision-making purposes until later in the development cycle or post-marketing, because the biomarker is not validated. Exploratory analysis under research mode, including small-, medium-, and large-scale candidate gene studies or genome-wide screens, should be considered for hypothesis generation if the number of samples is sufficient. The replication of new associations is essential.

7. The use of pharmacogenomics in drug discovery can improve the decision-making process and provide substantial cost savings by reducing timelines and promoting the judicious allocation of resources. Pharmacogenomics insights can help select targets that have manageable genetic variations, identify genes associated with diseases, and validate drug targets. Pharmacogenomics can facilitate interactions between drug discovery and clinical development, supporting synergy and advancing both ends of the drug pipeline. In drug discovery, genetic variability analysis should be performed as soon as a prospective target is identified. Potential benefits of early analysis include avoiding targets with unmanageable variability, and selecting the variant(s) that are most prevalent in human populations, thus improving the likelihood of success in clinical trials.
8. Early development PGx work is most important. PGx initiatives will not have an impact on currently marketed products with more imminent patent expiry. This knowledge highlights the point that advanced and continued planning can be utilized to optimize the commercial impact of PGx activities. As noted above, there are many potential commercial implications from PGx approaches. One obvious opportunity to limit risk is to begin implementation of this work as early as possible in a product's life cycle. To do so would facilitate rapid, more efficient development, with potentially quicker discontinuation of some development programs, and salvaging of other compounds. While not proven, the hope is that PGx will enhance productivity through new approaches and research models. Additionally, it is envisioned that the use of PGx biomarkers will improve predictability in preclinical/clinical assessments. At the earliest phases in compound development, the key benefit of PGx activities is to feed back on attractive drug targets. Once a compound is adequately characterized, early integration of PGx biomarkers into development can ideally lead to faster development, approval, adoption, and penetration, and will in turn lead to commercial advantages that will outweigh the disadvantages of smaller eligible patient populations. Additionally, earlier opportunity assessment can facilitate a company's potential to adequately differentiate a compound and strengthen its value proposition for pricing and reimbursement authorities. This activity would pave the way for potential drug-linked diagnostic offerings.

8 The Vision for Pharmacogenomics

As depicted in the following chart (Fig. 1.3), today we live in a world where PGx, molecular diagnostics, and even companion diagnostics are becoming a reality. Pipelines in several key therapeutic areas are sparse. Further, a few drugs already have PGx data in their package inserts, and some of them, such as Herceptin, represent both medical and commercial success. There appears to be an initiation of significant industry development and interest within regulatory groups. Consortia are being created between industry, governmental groups, and academia. These partnering initiatives are an effort to address some significant challenges by the pooling of limited resources. It will be necessary to build basic competency for long-term gains.

In the mid term (5 to 10 years), a significant increase in PGx activities may be seen as an innovative way to provide competitive advantage through product differentiation. With increased learning and identification of genes and drug targets, there should be increased acknowledgement that PGx is a key path toward drug innovation. It can be envisioned that drug development programs will be routinely implemented with the inclusion of biomarker-driven endpoints. More and more collaborations are expected to arise, to overcome the need for major resource pooling in order to complete key PGx analyses. It may become more apparent that other forms of resourcing will be critical in expediting organizational learning around PGx, in order to realize gains sooner. Government and payers can be expected to require more PGx information.

In the longer term (10+ years), biomarker-driven disease stratification and modification strategies will become more prevalent. When it becomes possible, it is conceivable that drug-linked diagnostics may become a regulatory requirement. Ideally, learnings gained from preliminary analysis will be channeled back into discovery efforts to fuel new innovation.

9 In Conclusion

Challenges to pharmaceutical development, commercialization, and reimbursement are increasing. PGx represents an innovative area for product differentiation, competitive advantage, and R&D productivity enhancement; and the pharmaceutical industry is learning how to best apply it in its R&D programs. Recent activities and initiatives, such as the formation of a variety of biomarker-focused consortia, several new regulatory guidance documents, the introduction of legislative bills, and high-profile safety concerns continue to illustrate the prominent role PGx will play in moving drug development and therapy from a population-based to an individualized paradigm. Genetic markers will likely play a major role, in spite of the challenges of identifying valid associations and of inherent biological complexity. Our capacity to experience future progress is limited only by our skepticism about

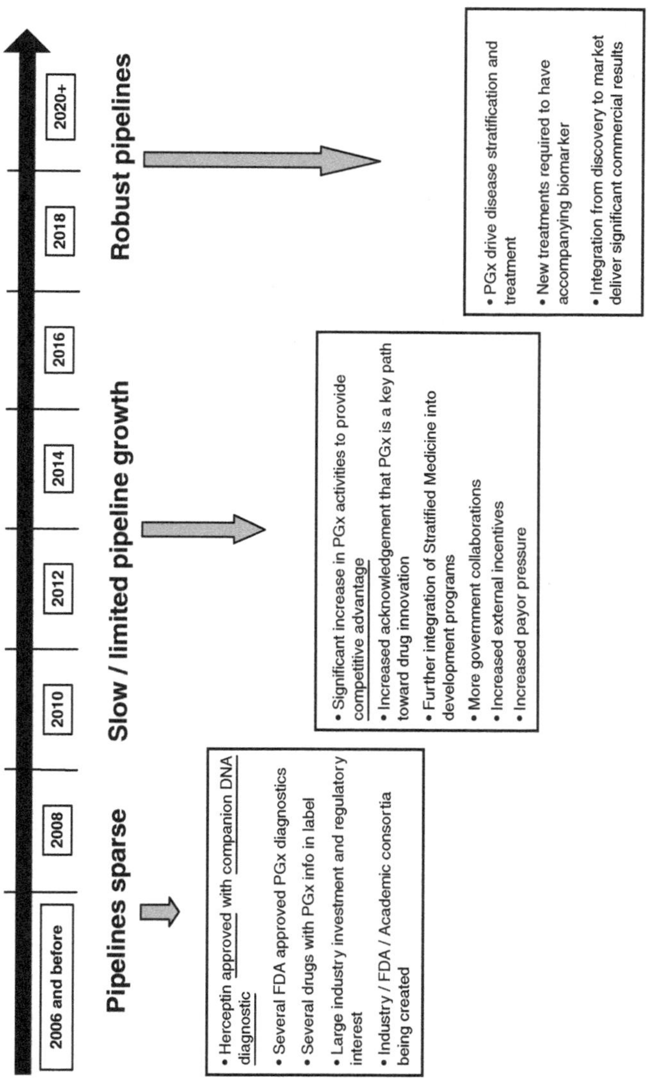

Fig. 1.3 Pharmacogenomics vision

partnering with other agencies, groups, and even competitors, in the coming decades. The fear of the loss of blockbusters, concerns about potential regulatory risks to drug development programs, and skepticism about the true value that PGx will bring to the pharmaceutical industry are likely to fade away as organizations continue to gain experience with this field, and as the regulatory framework for this research continues to grow. In the meantime, PGx research deserves further support and investments from all concerned, but without unrealistic expectations.

References

1. Garrod AE (1902) The incidence of alkaptonuria. A study in chemical individuality. Lancet, pp 1616–1620.
2. Haldane, JBS (1949) Disease and evolution. Ric Sci 19:68–75.
3. Kalow W (2006) Pharmacogenetics and pharmacogenomics: origin, status, and the hope for personalized medicine. Pharmacogenomics J 6:162–165.
4. Kalow W (1956) Familial incidence of low pseudocholinesterase level. Lancet pp 576
5. Bonicke R, Lisboa BP (1957) Über die Erbbedingtheit der intraindividuellen Konstanz der Isoniazidausscheidung beim Menchen. Naturwissenschaften 44:314–320.
6. Vogel F (1959) Moderne Probleme der Humangenetic. Ergeb Inn Med Kinderheikd 12:52–125.
7. Mahgoup A, Dring L, Idle JR, Lancaster R, Smith RL (1977) Polymorphic hydroxylation of debrosiquine in man. Lancet 2:584–586.
8. Eichelbaum M, Spanbrucker N, Steinke B, Dengler HJ (1997) Defective N-oxydation of spartein in man: a new pharmacogenetic defect. Eur J Clin Pharmacol 16:183–187.
9. Maraz D, Legrand M, Sabbagh N et al. (1997) Polymorphism of the cytochrome P450 CYP2D6 in a European population: characterization of 48 mutations and 53 alleles, their frequencies and evaluation. Pharmacogenetics 7:197–202.
10. Kalow W (2001) Interethnic differences in drug response. In: Kalow W, Meyer UA, Tyndale RF (eds) Pharmacogenomics. Marcel Dekker Inc., New York, pp 109–134.
11. Weber WW (2001) Pharmacogenetics-receptors. In: Kalow W, Meyer UA, Tyndale RF (eds) Pharmacogenomics. Marcel Dekker Inc., New York, pp 51–80.
12. Ho RH, Kim RB (2005) Transporters and drug therapy: implications for drug disposition and disease. Clin Pharmacol Ther 78:260–277.
13. Bondy B (2005) Pharmacogenetics in depression and antidepressants. Dialogues Clin Neurosci 7:223–230.
14. Kalow W (1982) Ethnic differences in drug metabolism. Clin Pharmacokinet 7:373–400.
15. Dickins M, Ducker G (2001) Drug disposition: to phenotype or genotype. Int J Pharm Med 15:70–73.
16. Evans WE, Relling MV (1999) Pharmacogenomics: translating functional genomics into rational therapies. Science 206:487–491.
17. Fellay J et al. (2002) Response to antiretroviral treatment in HIV-1 infected individuals with allele variants of the multidrug resistance transporter 1: a pharmacogenetics study. Lancet 359:30–36.
18. Dubinsky M et al. (2000) Pharmacogenomics and metabolite measurement for 6-mercaptopurine therapy in inflammatory bowel disease. Gastroenterology 118:705–713.
19. U.S. FDA. Guidance for industry: pharmacogenomic data submissions. http://www.fda.gov/cder/guidance/6400fnl.pdf. Accessed July 25, 2007.
20. Farlow MR, Lahiri DK, Poirier J, Davignon J, Hui S (1996) Apolipoprotein E genotype and gender influence response to tacrine therapy. Ann N Y Acad Sci. 802:101–110.
21. Herceptin product label. http://www.fda.gov/cder/biologics/products/trasgen092598.htm. Accessed July 25, 2007.

22. Erbitux product label. http://www.fda.gov/Cder/drug/infopage/erbitux/default.htm Accessed February 12, 2004.
23. Gleevec revised product label. http://www.fda.gov/CDER/drug/infopage/gleevec/default.htm. Accessed October 30, 2006.
24. Tarceva product label. http://www.fda.gov/cder/foi/label/2004/021743lbl.pdf. Accessed July 25, 2007.
25. Camptosar product label. http://www.fda.gov/cder/foi/label/2006/020571s030lbl.pdf. Accessed July 25, 2007.
26. Strattera product label. http://www.fda.gov/cder/foi/label/2007/021411s004s012s013s015s021lbl.pdf. Accessed July 25, 2007.
27. Purinethol product label. http://www.fda.gov/cder/foi/label/2004/09053s024lbl.pdf. Accessed July 25, 2007.
28. Coumadin product label. http://www.fda.gov/cder/foi/label/2006/009218s102lbl.pdf. Accessed July 25, 2007.
29. Centre for Medicines Research (CMR) International Ltd. (2006) NME output lifts from 20 year low. Thomson Scientific KnowledgeLink Newsletter.
30. Tufts Center for the Study of Drug Development, Outlook 2006.
31. U.S. FDA. Innovation or stagnation: challenge and opportunity on the critical path to new medical products. http://www.fda.gov/oc/initiatives/criticalpath/whitepaper.html. Accessed on July 25, 2007.
32. Vioxx withdrawal. Merck press release. http://www.vioxx.com/vioxx/documents/english/vioxx_press_release.pdf.
33. Bill S.3822. Genomics and personalized medicine act of 2006. Introduced in U.S. Senate by Barak Obama.
34. Kim MJ et al. (2008) Pharmacogenomics: the regulatory environment and labeling implication. In: Cohen N (ed) Pharmacogenomics and personalized medicine. Humana Press (Springer) Chapter 3.
35. Gutman S, Hackett J (2006) Search for shortcuts on the critical path to market: US FDA perspectives from the diagnostic side. Pharmacogenomics 7(8):1223–1227.
36. EMEA Pharmacogenomics Working Party. http://www.emea.europa.eu/pdfs/human/pharmacogenetics/10159204en.pdf.
37. Guiding principles: processing joint FDA-EMEA voluntary genomic data submissions (VGDSs) within the framework of the confidentiality arrangement. http://www.emea.europa.eu/pdfs/general/direct/pr/FDAEMEA.pdf.
38. ICH terminology in pharmacogenomics (E15). http://www.fda.gov/cder/guidance/7619dft.pdf.
39. Arcoxia non–approvable. http://www.merck.com/newsroom/press_releases/research_and_development/2007_0427.html.
40. PhRMA Biomarker Consortium. http://www.innovation.org/index.cfm/NewsCenter/Briefings/The_Biomarkers_Consortium.
41. Predictive Safety Testing Consortium. http://www.fda.gov/bbs/topics/news/2006/NEW01337.html.
42. Serious Adverse Event Consortium (www.saeconsortium.org).
43. Industry-Pharmacogenomics Working Group. http://www.i-pwg.org/cms/.
44. Spear B, Heath-Chiozzi M, Barnes D, Cheeseman K, Shaw P, Campbell D (2001) Terminology for sample collection in clinical genetic studies. Pharmacogenomics J 1:101–3.
45. Anderson C, Gomez- Mancilla B, Spear B et al. (2002) Elements of informed consent for pharmacogenetic research: perspective of the Pharmacogenetics Working Group. Pharmacogenomics J 2(5):284–92.
46. Renegar G, Webster C, Stuerzebecher S et al. (2006) Returning genetic research results to individuals: points to consider. Bioethics 20(1):24–36.
47. Personalized Medicine Coalition. http://www.personalizedmedicinecoalition.org/communi cations/overview.php.
48. U.S. FDA. Genomics at FDA: table of valid genomic biomarkers in the context of approved drug labels. http://www.fda.gov/cder/genomics/genomic_biomarkers_table.htm. Accessed July 25, 2007.

49. Lesko LJ. (2007) Personalized medicine: elusive dream or imminent reality? Clin Pharmacol Ther 81:807–816.
50. Point of Care Diagnostic Dr Nakamura accessed at http://www.twt.com/company/press-releases/2006/March_2_2006.htm.
51. National Coalition for Health Professional Education in Genetics (NCHPEG). http://www.nchpeg.org/.
52. Council for International Organizations of Medical Sciences (CIOMS) (2002) International Ethical Guidelines for Biomedical Research Involving Human Subjects accessed at http://www.cioms.ch/frame_guidelines_nov_2002.htm.
53. Nuffield council report on bioethics of pharmacogenetics. http://www.nuffieldbioethics.org/filelibrary/paf1/pharmacogenetics_report.pdf.

Chapter 2
Implementation of Pharmacogenomic Sample Collection in Clinical Trials

Deborah Sokol Ricci and Monique Franc

Contents

Abstract This chapter is intended to provide an overview of the operational considerations and potential obstacles that can be anticipated during the implementation of pharmacogenomic research in clinical trials. Particular attention is given to the elements of the protocol and of the informed consent and the considerations for collection of different sample types on a global level. The goal is to provide the reader with an appreciation for the study design elements on an operational level rather than on a scientific or statistical study design level. Educational efforts by various working groups to harmonize global standards are also outlined and will provide the reader with an overview of the ongoing efforts to promote global genomic research in the present day.

Keywords biomarker, genomics, pharmacogenomics, global sample handling, genetics, global regulations, local regulations, sample coding, exploratory research

---

Deborah Sokol Ricci
Johnson and Johnson Pharmaceutical Research and Development, L.L.C., 1000 Route 202, Raritan, NJ 08869
dricci@prdus.jnj.com

Glossary

AAPS Pharmacogenetics and Pharmacogenomics Focus Group	A focus group working towards information exchange for developments in pharmacogenomics and pharmacogenetics.
Adverse event	In pharmacology, any unexpected or dangerous reaction to a drug.
Anonymization	Samples are double coded and labeled with a unique second number. The link between the clinical study subject number and the unique second number is deleted.
Assay validation	Optimization of an assay protocol with respect to sensitivity, dynamic range, signal intensity, and stability.
Comparative genome hybridization (CGH)	Comparative genomic hybridization (CGH) measures DNA copy number differences between a reference genome and a sample genome.
Complementary DNA (cDNA) library	A collection of cDNAs, each of which has been inserted in a DNA vector (e.g., a circular DNA plasmid) and replicated in a bacterium such as *E. coli*.
CPT tubes	Cell preparation tubes with sodium heparin, utilized for the separation of mononuclear cells from whole blood.
De-identification	Samples are double coded and labeled with a unique second number. The link between the clinical study subject number and the unique second number is maintained, but unknown to investigators and patients.
Deoxyribonucleic acid (DNA)	A molecule that encodes genetic information.
EDTA	A crystalline acid, $C_{10}H_{16}N_2O_8$, that acts as a strong chelating agent.
European Federation of Pharmaceutical Industries and Associations (EFPIA)	A focus group with a pharmacogenomics task force; this group has overlap with the Pharmacogenetics Working Group.
Exploratory analyses	General exploratory or research information collected from studies such as broad gene expression screening, whereby the markers studied have not reached the status of a probable valid biomarker.
Formalin fixation	Tissue fixation in a solution containing formalin.
Formalin fixed paraffin embedded (FFPE)	A method of preserving tumor tissue for pathological and other analyses.
Laser capture microdissection (LCM)	A method to collect a specific subset of cells from a slice of tumor tissue captured on a slide.
Loss of heterozogosity (LOH)	The loss of one parent's contribution to part of the cell's genome.
Paraffin embedding	A method of preserving fixed tissue (see formalin fixation).
PAXgene™	The PAXgene™ Blood RNA System consolidates and integrates the key steps of whole blood collection, nucleic acid stabilization, and RNA purification. By minimizing the unpredictability associated with RNA processing, the system provides enhanced accuracy of intracellular RNA analysis.
Pharmacogenetics for Every Nation Initiative (PGENI)	An initiative to enhance the understanding of pharmacogenetics in the developing world.
Pharmacogenetics Research Network	Enables a network of multidisciplinary research groups to conduct studies addressing research questions in pharmacogenetics and pharmacogenomics with a goal to populate a knowledge base with data.

(continued)

Glossary (continued)

Pharmacogenetics Working Group	A voluntary and informal association of pharmaceutical companies engaged in research in the science of phamacogenetics.
Pharmacogenomics	The study of how variations in the human genome affect the response to medications.
Polymerase chain reaction (PCR)	A method to enzymatically replicate DNA.
Definitive analysis	Preplanned and prespecified research analyses.
Protein	Proteins are fundamental components of all living cells and include many substances, such as enzymes, hormones, and antibodies, that are necessary for the proper functioning of an organism.
Real time quantitative PCR (qRT-PCR)	A method to quantify low abundance messenger RNA (mRNA), enabling a researcher to quantify relative gene expression at a particular time, or in a particular cell or tissue type.
Regulations	A legal restriction promulgated by government administrative agencies through rulemaking supported by a threat of sanction or a fine.
Ribonucleic acid (RNA)	RNA serves as the template for the translation of genes into proteins.
RNALater	A reagent used to immediately stabilize RNA from tissues.
Sample coding	A method to label samples whereby personal identifiers are not present.
SELDI-TOF	Surface Enhanced Laser Desorption/Ionisation Time of Flight mass spectrometry. A methodology utilized for proteomic analyses.
The Council for International Organizations in Medical Sciences Pharmacogenetics Working Group.	A working group formed to consider issues related to pharmacogenetics with respect to drug development and regulatory, ethical, educational, and economic issues.

1 Introduction

The value of pharmacogenomics in clinical trials has become increasingly recognized, not only by the pharmaceutical industry, but also by regulatory agencies (as evidenced by a growing regulatory framework for pharmacogenomic research) *(1–3)* and by the general public (as evidenced by the increasing media attention on "personalized medicine") *(4)*. In a relatively short time, there has been significant evolution in the acceptance of this science as both a supplement and in some cases an alternative to the classical paradigm of the drug development process; and this despite a relative paucity of guidelines, regulations, and global harmonization. Nevertheless, with the appropriate procedures, it is now possible to routinely collect samples for pharmacogenomic applications in clinical trials, although apprehensions and hurdles still linger in some locales. On an international level, it is predicted that genomic sample collection will become more mainstream in some jurisdictions and more cumbersome in others as knowledge, experience, and familiarity increase and as laws and regulations are implemented and revised. Current efforts are ongoing to educate various bodies toward harmonization and standardization of regulations and practices applicable to pharmacogenomic collections globally. However, it is anticipated that harmonization will not happen in the near future and that a lot of work will be required to bring consensus across the nations.

It has become evident that there is no one-size-fits-all solution for implementing pharmacogenomic sample collections when operating in a global environment. Not only do requirements vary from country to country, but they frequently vary on state, provincial, and local levels. This requires a great degree of flexibility, since adjustments are often necessary at individual sites. However, the considerations described herein should allow the researcher to efficiently implement the collection of pharmacogenomic samples in clinical trials on an international level while maximizing the use and value of the collected samples and maintaining stringent standards for subject privacy.

The term "genomic" used throughout refers to both DNA and RNA. It can be debated whether RNA deserves the same level of stringency for sample and data handling as does DNA, or for that matter, whether either of these molecular endpoints should be handled any differently than any other biochemical or clinical endpoints (i.e., "genetic exceptionalism"). However, the reality today is that these endpoints *are* viewed as "special" and *do* receive unique attention by regulatory agencies. There currently are overarching expectations for a higher level of stringency for maintaining confidentiality and preventing unintended access to or release of genomic samples and data. Since both DNA and RNA are captured together in the recent flood of pharmacogenomic guidelines released by regulatory agencies (U.S. Food and Drug Administration [FDA], European Medicines Agency [EMEA], and Japan Ministry of Health, Labor, and Welfare [MHLW]), both molecular endpoints are treated in tandem in this chapter; although it is acknowledged that privacy and confidentiality expectations may not always be as strict for RNA-based research as they are for DNA-based research. Because proteomic analyses often accompany genomic-based research, methods to increase sample integrity are mentioned. However, since regulations around these analyses are not as stringently controlled, they are not addressed herein. A glossary of useful terms is provided on page 28.

2 Protocol

As is true with all clinical trial procedures, pharmacogenomic research on human subjects must be described in a protocol, whether harmonized within the clinical protocol itself or as a stand-alone document. In developing protocols for pharmacogenomic studies, there are a number of practical study design elements that are dictated by the goals of the trial and of the pharmacogenomic study, notably: i) whether participation will be optional or mandatory, ii) whether genomic endpoints are already known or will only be defined over the course of the trial according to emerging clinical issues, and iii) whether samples will be analyzed within the context of the trial only or will also be retained for future research. Each of these parameters is associated with varying degrees of operational, ethical, and regulatory implications described below.

2.1 Optional Versus Mandatory Subject Participation

Most commonly, pharmacogenomics is integrated as an "add-on" component to the clinical trial, although increasingly, pharmacogenomic parameters are being factored into trial design. The pharmacogenomic component usually does not have a direct impact on patient medical care. It is, however, accompanied by sensitivities around privacy and the potential for discrimination. For these reasons, a decision must be made whether the provision of samples for genomic research is required of subjects enrolling in a clinical trial or whether it is sufficient to offer this to subjects as an optional component. When referring to subject participation, the term "optional" should be distinguished from "voluntary," since in a legitimate clinical trial, by definition, every procedure is "voluntary"—meaning that a person cannot be forced to undergo any procedure against his/her will (or that of his/her legally acceptable representative, as applicable). This is true for both optional and mandatory components of the trial. However, for optional procedures, refusal to consent would not compromise eligibility for the trial, whereas for mandatory procedures, refusal to consent would result in ineligibility for the trial.

Optional Participation

Optional subject participation in pharmacogenomic research is currently the most common and straightforward pharmacogenomic study design option. It generally is appropriate when there are no definitive genomic analyses to be performed, or when pharmacogenomic results are not critical to the outcome or design of a study, or when the proposed analyses are purely exploratory. Operationally, optional participation has no impact on the rate of enrollment or on the duration of the screening period. The rate of participation will largely be dependent on i) whether subjects are healthy volunteers or diseased patients, ii) the specific disease under investigation, iii) the delivery of the informed consent process, iv) the geographical location, and v) the specific patient population (e.g., pediatric). Although there are exceptions, agreement to participate in genomic research is often higher in healthy volunteers than in diseased patients, presumably since subjects have a somewhat different focus and motivation for their involvement in the trial. With the appropriate informed consent process, a participation rate for optional pharmacogenomic research of 80% or greater should be readily achievable in studies involving healthy volunteers. Participation rates tend to be lower in diseased patients, although not necessarily for all disease indications. The attitude of the investigator administering the informed consent also can have an appreciable influence on participation rates, owing to the impressionability of subjects in the face of perceived authority figures. The opinion of one or a few other participants can similarly have a significant impact on participation rates, particularly in the case of group consent procedures owing to the groupthink phenomenon of human behavior. Acceptance may be dictated by cultural background, personal experience, and level of education of the subjects. Education of investigators, study coordinators, regional monitors, and local trial managers is of the utmost importance in maximizing participation rates while simultaneously avoiding the coercion of subjects. The degree of pushback from ethics committees on optional participation is minor except in occasional cases, such as when the term "optional" is deemed to imply "unimportant" and therefore "unnecessary;" but this can usually be readily resolved through education on the value of genomic sample collections in clinical trials. The obvious and most important limitation of optional participation is that it is possible that not all subjects enrolled in the trial will agree to provide genomic samples, and thus any unusual clinical outcome occurring in non-consenting individuals (e.g., adverse events) could not be investigated using a pharmacogenomic approach (unless the subjects were approached again retrospectively for their consent). However, in the absence of specific analyses that are critical to the success of the trial, the limitation of having samples from less than 100% of the subjects is generally outweighed by the operational and ethical impediments that can be expected by imposing mandatory participation.

Mandatory Participation

Mandatory participation may be necessary in some cases, notably when genomic results are i) used to determine eligibility for the trial (i.e., inclusion/exclusion criterion; e.g., exclusion of CYP2D6 poor metabolizers), ii) are critical to the successful analysis of the clinical data (e.g., EGFR stratification), or iii) are requested by regulatory authorities (e.g., valid biomarkers known to be relevant to the compound under investigation). Mandatory participation may pose a number of operational challenges. Site selection will be affected, since some countries do not permit collection or export of genomic samples. Therefore, mandatory participation would preclude the execution of clinical trials in certain countries, and consequently in corresponding ethnic groups. Even within countries that authorize genomic sample collection, local regulations may preclude it, and therefore necessary assurances that genomic sample collection is permissible should be sought before sites are selected. Ethics committees will generally approve the mandatory requirement if the rationale is explicit and justified; they generally will not approve it in the absence of definitive analyses (see below). Subject enrollment rates may be compromised to varying degrees, since some prospective subjects may be uncomfortable with the idea of genomic research being conducted on their samples. Importantly, these subjects would be denied access to the trial and to the potential benefits of treatment with a novel drug; however this may not be an issue if alternative therapies are available. Subjects should be clearly informed that refusal to consent or subsequent withdrawal of consent to conduct research on their genomic sample would result in ineligibility for continued participation in the trial, although ethical decisions may override this requirement. Where genetic data are intended to be used to determine eligibility, the impact on the duration of the screening period should be anticipated. This will be dictated primarily by the prevalence (frequency) of the genomic result of interest, the turnover time for generating the data, and the overall sample size. The advantages of mandatory participation are that samples are available for each and every subject (assuming no samples are lost due to mishandling), and that studies can be designed and optimized based on genomic information.

2.2 *Definitive Versus Tentative Analyses*

Definitive analyses refer to preplanned and prespecified genomic endpoints that are committed to being analyzed in a clinical trial. Tentative analyses refer to analyses that may be performed only as necessary, if it is hypothesized that this might help to resolve unanticipated issues with the clinical data. The terminology "definitive analyses" is used here preferentially over "prospective analyses" or "hypothesis testing," which can have statistical or trial design connotations.

In principle, a clinical protocol should provide a thorough description of all endpoints to be measured in a clinical trial. For definitive analyses, this may consist of specific genes, genetic loci, or transcripts, whether few or many. However, by its inherent nature, pharmacogenomics is frequently utilized to help address unexpected clinical results (e.g., pharmacokinetic outliers, variable efficacy, adverse events). Therefore, room must be made to accommodate this valuable application by allowing for tentative analyses in the absence of a specific preexisting hypothesis. There are several points for consideration when collecting samples, even if only for tentative analyses. The operational aspects include: establishment of contracts, coordination with central or local laboratories, logistics for shipment, education of investigators and site staff, sample and consent tracking, additional informed consent procedures, and time for collection of the additional specimen(s). The cost associated with the collection, handling, and potential long-term storage of the sample must also be taken into consideration, but is generally nominal compared to retrospective sample collections. For example, the cost of a DNA collection (from whole blood), including disposables (e.g., collection tubes/kits), phlebotomy, sample shipping and handling, DNA extraction, and sample and data management, can currently be estimated at approximately US$50–100 per sample, excluding costs associated with long-term sample management. Costs are higher for DNA obtained from various tissues (e.g., tumors), because of the more involved process of sample acquisition and preparation. Similar procedures for RNA extraction are also more costly. It may be challenging to justify this cost, particularly in very large Phase III or Phase IV trials, in the absence of a definitive analysis to be performed. However, this must be weighed against the risk and cost associated with not having the samples in the event of an emerging issue, as well as the lost opportunity to conduct large-scale pharmacogenomic research on banked samples (e.g., genomic studies of disease, rare adverse events, drug class effects). Retrospective collection of DNA from subjects may be an option, but is exceedingly more costly (as high as tenfold) and more logistically challenging than is prospective DNA collection, and is associated with potentially significant delays in attempts to address emerging issues. Ethics committee resistance may sometimes be encountered if the collection for tentative analysis is not viewed as being critical or necessary for the success of the trial, since there is reluctance to collect human biological samples if they may sit endlessly in a freezer, never to be analyzed. Increasingly, however, ethics committees are conscious of the "insurance value" of precautionary genomic sample collection and will normally approve collection for the purpose of tackling unanticipated issues, if this rationale is clearly stated. The justification is further reinforced if samples are also intended for storage for future research. Since open-ended proposals for research on genomic samples is generally viewed unfavorably by ethics committees, the listing of candidate genes/loci/transcripts that may potentially be analyzed will ordinarily satisfy committee needs for a definition of the scope and boundaries of the possible use of the samples. This list will ordinarily include genomic endpoints relevant to pharmacokinetics, potential adverse events, mode of action, and the disease under investigation (as appropriate). To accommodate situations in which ethics committees do not approve genomic sample collections, it is advisable to state explicitly in the protocol that the clinical protocol can be approved independently of the pharmacogenomic component. The qualifier "where local regulations permit" throughout is useful for this purpose and avoids the need for protocol amendments.

2.3 Sample Banking for Future Research

Since the value of genomic samples generally increases as sample sizes increase, it is recommended that the protocol be conceived to allow for long-term sample storage for the purpose of future research in order to maximize the potential value of the samples, particularly in clinical trial settings where clinical data collection is standardized and of high quality. As scientific discoveries are made and as science evolves, valuable research can be done in the future on samples collected today. Some study participants may not be comfortable with long-term storage of their samples, particularly if future uses are unknown. Therefore, processes that introduce two levels of participation, i.e., one for research specifically related to the trial (including both definitive and tentative analyses) and another for storage of samples for future research of broader scope, offer a higher degree of flexibility and help to maximize subject participation rates. Although most ethics committees are agreeable to the banking of samples for future research, many will require the delineation of boundaries and limitations for the scope of the research that may be conducted on the samples. For instance, research may be limited to that which is relevant to the drug or drug class and/or the disease or therapeutic area under investigation. Many ethics committees will permit the indefinite storage of samples; some insist on sample destruction after a predefined storage period; and others will not approve of this application at all. Processes should therefore allow for tracking timelines for sample destruction.

Ethics committees and subjects will generally be amenable to long-term sample storage for future research, provided that there are sufficient assurances that stringent processes and standards for patient privacy/confidentiality are in place. Patient privacy can be achieved by measures that minimize the possibility of linking genetic data back to a subject's identity. This can be accomplished by a number of methods, including i) de-identification of samples such that a coded sample is relabeled with a unique second code, while maintaining a link between the two codes (i.e., double-coded); or ii) anonymization of the samples such that the link between the two codes of a double-coded sample is permanently deleted. Anonymization offers the maximum achievable level of security, while still allowing for genotype-to-phenotype correlative analyses to be undertaken. The deletion of the coding key linking the sample(s) to the subject's study identifier provides an additional level of security over de-identified data, as it renders obsolete the coding key used for the re-identification of subjects via their original subject identifier. The purpose of anonymization is to express the deliberate intent to not re-identify subjects. This is in contrast to de-identification which maintains the intent to link back to the subject identifier, if necessary. Consequently, actions such as returning results, sample withdrawal, clinical monitoring, or patient follow-up cannot be undertaken on anonymized samples. A common misconception is that anonymization severs the link between the sample and the corresponding clinical data for a given subject; when, in fact, what is lost is the ability to link the new subject identifier to the original subject identifier. Anonymization does not interfere in any way with relating genotype data to phenotype data, since genomic samples and data are coupled to the clinical data prior to anonymization. Consequently, it is critical that all relevant clinical data be fed into the anonymization procedure since, by definition, anonymization is a permanent, irreversible process that does not allow retrospective addition of data. It is not unusual to find that the level of participation in sample storage for future research is generally slightly lower than for research that is directly relevant to the trial, although this would depend on the assurances offered for protection of patient confidentiality. Interestingly, some subjects will choose to participate only in the storage for future research component because of the fact that the risk of linking genetic data back to their identity is lessened through the anonymization/de-identification process (as applicable).

It is recognized that anonymization can be susceptible to reconstruction of the link between anonymized genetic data and a study subject identifier by means of comparing an anonymized dataset with a separate dataset that contains the subject identifier. The reason for this is that the clinical data set can serve as a "clinical barcode" or "clinical fingerprint" that uniquely identifies a subject. For this reason, the term "*not possible*" is not accurate as it relates to the ability or possibility to link anonymized samples/data back to a subject *(5)*. Anonymization should therefore always be accompanied by specific policies or standard operating procedures (SOPs) prohibiting reconstruction of any kind of link between genetic data and the original study subject identifier. In addition, access to datasets ideally should be restricted, and no one individual should have access to all information necessary to re-establish a patient's identity. It should be noted that anonymization may have regulatory consequences, because currently, data generated from anonymized samples may not always be used for regulatory decision-making. It should also be noted that whereas some countries require anonymization of samples prior to storage, others do not permit anonymization. Therefore, a means of tracking country of origin is essential.

3 Informed Consent

With few exceptions, obtaining legally effective, voluntary informed consent is a fundamental prerequisite for conducting research on human beings. Surprisingly, despite a long history of medical research, there is no single universally accepted list of basic elements of informed consent, although the International Conference on Harmonization (ICH) has significantly improved harmonization of informed consent requirements on a global level. The policies and regulations which allow informed consent to be legally effective vary on national, state, and local levels, which poses a challenge to clinical research that is conducted on an international level as is commonly encountered in clinical trials *(6)*. Institutional review boards (IRBs) and independent ethics committees (IECs) serve as gatekeepers to ensure compliance with requirements and regulations.

It is important to appreciate that informed consent is a process, not just a form for the subject to sign. A key requirement for informed consent is that the information be presented in a manner that is understood by the prospective subject (or legally acceptable representative), and that it enable the individual to voluntarily decide whether or not to participate. Regrettably, informed consent forms are more often geared toward legal protection of the investigator and study sponsor than toward providing information to the subject in a manner that is truly understandable, educational, and meaningful. In the absence of a test to ascertain the true degree of understanding by the subject, every effort must be made to simplify the informed consent process and to strike a balance between providing sufficient information for a subject to make a reasoned decision about whether to participate while simultaneously protecting the legal interests of those conducting the study. The specific elements of consent and the verbiage selected are equally important.

3.1 Readability and Understanding

There is currently no universal standard for assessing how much information is understood or retained by a prospective study participant *(7, 8)*. Readability algorithms such as Flesch Reading Ease *(9, 10)* and Flesch-Kincaid Grade Level, which are based on scientific linguistics that calculate average sentence length and number of syllables per word to generate an index of difficulty, may prove valuable in the design of the informed consent form. However, readability should not be confused with understandability and there is some debate about whether readability statistics do indeed result in improved understandability and retention *(11–13)*. Oversimplification of sentences and words can reach a point of diminishing return and actually make understanding more difficult, in part by unnecessarily lengthening the overall text *(14, 15)*. However, a combination of techniques, including the use of short sentences, monosyllabic words, simple phrases, active voice, paragraphs no longer than four to five sentences, sentence structure in subject-predicate position, use of ample white space between paragraphs, left justification with right ragged margins, minimum 10-point font size, avoidance of nouns created from verbs, avoidance of multiple negatives, and limitations on the total amount of information provided, can work synergistically in creating an informed consent document that is understandable by the average subject. By whatever means achieved, a readability level approximately equivalent to that of a 12-year-old child, or comparable to that of a typical newspaper, would be suitable for the average layperson (16). The goal is to communicate the information in a thorough, clear, and concise way, while avoiding information overload.

Owing to the sensitivities surrounding genomic research (whether perceived or real), and the corresponding unique considerations applicable to genomic samples and data that are generally not necessary for other samples types (e.g., implications for family members due to the heritability of DNA), it is not uncommon for separate informed consent forms, one for the clinical trial and one for genomic research, to be used. This allows for the general details of the trial to be more effectively communicated without distraction by the specific details and sensitivity issues that are associated with the genomic samples. A subject might otherwise be overwhelmed trying to decipher which conditions apply to which samples in which parts of the trial. The dual consent format can improve readability and understanding by allowing the subject to consider the issues presented in each consent form separately. Since participation in genomic research is more commonly offered as optional, and since local regulations may preclude genomic sample collection at some investigational sites, the dual consent model allows a subject or site to readily opt out of genomic research. This model also helps to make it clear that the pharmacogenomic component is a separate substudy and that agreement or refusal to participate is unrelated to eligibility for the trial (as applicable). For clinical trials involving mandatory participation in genomic research, it would be reasonable to merge the genomic ICF with the clinical ICF; however, for ease of readability, the details pertaining specifically to the genomic component would best be contained within one section rather than interwoven with the main clinical ICF.

3.2 Elements of Informed Consent

In the United States, the Code of Federal Regulations (CFR) 21 CFR 50.25 (2007) lists eight basic elements of informed consent, and six additional elements to be included where applicable (17). In contrast, the Council for International Organizations of Medical Sciences (CIOMS) Guideline 5 recommends 26 basic elements, many but not all of which are an extension of the eight basic elements of informed consent from the CFR (see Table 1) (18). To date, there are no internationally recognized regulations that dictate the basic elements of informed consent for

Table 2.1 CIOMS essential information for prospective research subjects (Guideline 5 of the International Ethical Guidelines for Biomedical Research Involving Human Subjects (18))

Before requesting an individual's consent to participate in research, the investigator must provide the following information, in language or another form of communication that the individual can understand:

1. that the individual is invited to participate in research, the reasons for considering the individual suitable for the research, and that participation is voluntary;
2. that the individual is free to refuse to participate and will be free to withdraw from the research at any time without penalty or loss of benefits to which he or she would otherwise be entitled;
3. the purpose of the research, the procedures to be carried out by the investigator and the subject, and an explanation of how the research differs from routine medical care;
4. for controlled trials, an explanation of features of the research design (e.g., randomization, double-blinding), and that the subject will not be told of the assigned treatment until the study has been completed and the blind has been broken;
5. the expected duration of the individual's participation (including number and duration of visits to the research centre and the total time involved) and the possibility of early termination of the trial or of the individual's participation in it;
6. whether money or other forms of material goods will be provided in return for the individual's participation and, if so, the kind and amount;
7. that, after the completion of the study, subjects will be informed of the findings of the research in general, and individual subjects will be informed of any finding that relates to their particular health status;
8. that subjects have the right of access to their data on demand, even if these data lack immediate clinical utility (unless the ethical review committee has approved temporary or permanent nondisclosure of data, in which case the subject should be informed of, and given, the reasons for such nondisclosure);
9. any foreseeable risks, pain or discomfort, or inconvenience to the individual (or others) associated with participation in the research, including risks to the health or well-being of a subject's spouse or partner;
10. the direct benefits, if any, expected to result to subjects from participating in the research;
11. the expected benefits of the research to the community or to society at large, or contributions to scientific knowledge;
12. whether, when, and how any products or interventions proven by the research to be safe and effective will be made available to subjects after they have completed their participation in the research, and whether they will be expected to pay for them;
13. any currently available alternative interventions or courses of treatment;
14. the provisions that will be made to ensure respect for the privacy of subjects and for the confidentiality of records in which subjects are identified;
15. the limits, legal or other, to the investigators' ability to safeguard confidentiality, and the possible consequences of breaches of confidentiality;
16. policy with regard to the use of results of genetic tests and familial genetic information, and the precautions in place to prevent disclosure of the results of a subject's genetic tests to immediate family relatives or to others (e.g., insurance companies or employers) without the consent of the subject;
17. the sponsors of the research, the institutional affiliation of the investigators, and the nature and sources of funding for the research;
18. the possible research uses, direct or secondary, of the subject's medical records and of biological specimens taken in the course of clinical care (see also Guidelines 4 and 18 Commentaries);
19. whether it is planned that biological specimens collected in the research will be destroyed at its conclusion, and, if not, details about their storage (where, how, for how long, and final disposition) and possible future use, and that subjects have the right to decide about such future use, to refuse storage, and to have the material destroyed (see Guideline 4 Commentary);

(continued)

Table 2.1 (continued)

20. whether commercial products may be developed from biological specimens, and whether the participant will receive monetary or other benefits from the development of such products;
21. whether the investigator is serving only as an investigator or as both investigator and the subject's physician;
22. the extent of the investigator's responsibility to provide medical services to the participant;
23. that treatment will be provided free of charge for specified types of research-related injury or for complications associated with the research, the nature and duration of such care, the name of the organization or individual that will provide the treatment, and whether there is any uncertainty regarding funding of such treatment;
24. in what way, and by what organization, the subject or the subject's family or dependants will be compensated for disability or death resulting from such injury (or, when indicated, that there are no plans to provide such compensation);
25. whether or not, in the country in which the prospective subject is invited to participate in research, the right to compensation is legally guaranteed;
26. that an ethical review committee has approved or cleared the research protocol.

genomic research. The industry's Pharmacogenetics Working Group has prepared an elegant and comprehensive compilation of elements of informed consent for consideration in pharmacogenomic research studies (19), the essence of which is captured below, in addition to that of the authors' experience. The specific consent elements selected for a particular pharmacogenomic study and the details thereof will generally be a reflection of the policies or standard operating procedures of the sponsor, the specific trial design, the alignment with local laws and regulations, and the concessions made for readability and understanding.

It is beyond the scope of this chapter to evaluate the validity of concerns held by study participants, government bodies, ethical review boards, or investigators regarding risks or potential risks associated with the generation, use, and disclosure of genomic data. The major concerns undoubtedly stem from the heritable nature of DNA, the potential misuse and misinterpretation of genomic data, the shortage of policies and laws regarding the use and misuse of genetic information, and the fear of potential stigmatization and discrimination (20). Additionally, the banking of samples for future use of potentially unknown scope also raises some legitimate concerns for obtaining truly valid informed consent *(21, 22)*. In response to these concerns, activities related to genomic research are generally conducted under a higher level of stringency with regard to privacy protection and confidentiality.

The eight elements of informed consent of the U.S. Code of Federal Regulations (CFR) are presented below and are used as a framework for additional considerations for informed consent for pharmacogenomic research. The 26 basic elements of consent from CIOMS are presented in Table 2.1. A balance must be sought between the number of elements to include in order to adequately inform the subject and to comply with local regulations, while maintaining an acceptable level of readability and avoiding information overload.

CFR Element 1: A statement that the study involves research, an explanation of the purposes of the research and the expected duration of the subject's participation, a description of the procedures to be followed, and identification of any procedures which are experimental.

Specific considerations for pharmacogenomic studies:

A definition of "DNA" and "genes" and the heritable nature thereof should be presented in simple terms. For RNA-based studies, the nonheritable nature of RNA should be stated, although the direct derivation of RNA from DNA should be acknowledged.

A statement explaining the reason that DNA/RNA is being collected and how this will bring value to the clinical trial or to science in general, both in the short term and in the long term, should be included. In the case of definitive analyses, some key highlights on the relevance of specific endpoints that will be analyzed should be provided. If the samples are only being collected for tentative analyses, subjects should not leave with the impression that their samples will definitely be analyzed. Some subjects may feel that the additional sample collection is not justified and may opt not to participate on these grounds. It should be clear that the results from the research will not be used in the subject's medical care (where applicable). In the case of prescreening for trial eligibility, subjects should be informed that results of the genetic tests will be used to determine eligibility for the trial.

Although not part of the classical definition of pharmacogenomics, disease-genetics studies may overlap with pharmacogenomic studies since genetic factors that determine disease etiology or subtype may influence response to drugs. It should therefore be clearly stated if research related to disease genes/loci will be conducted.

The procedure for collecting the genomic sample (e.g., blood draw, buccal swab, tumor or tissue biopsy), including the volume or size of the sample and the timing of sampling should be described. For RNA studies, it is often necessary to collect samples at multiple time points; therefore the number of samples, time points, and volume at each time point should be defined.

The scope of the intended use of the samples should be stated in order to define the boundaries of what can be done with the samples. This can range from the analysis of one or a few candidate genes/loci/transcripts that are related to the drug(s) or indication(s) under investigation to broader research that is not directly relevant to the trial. It is insufficient to state that "genetic research will be done on the samples." Some ethics committees may require that these specific endpoints be listed in the informed consent, whereas others take the position that gene names are not meaningful to the nonexpert. One compromise is to make available the list of genes only upon a subject's request. If large-scale or genome/transcriptome-wide investigations might be conducted, this should be stated. In such cases, it is generally sufficient to state that "thousands of genes/RNAs will be analyzed in relation to…." It can be useful in the case of commercially available analytical platforms to include the name of the platform and/or web link to allow easy access to the list of specific genes/transcripts that will be analyzed.

If the samples will be retained for research in the future, this must be clearly stated, including both known uses and potentially unknown uses (if applicable). There have been many ethical discussions about the validity of consent for future unknown research on human tissue and samples from DNA biobanks *(21, 22)*. Since there are still many unknowns associated with the information contained within the genetic code, subjects should be made aware that there is uncertainty about the information the samples could potentially yield in the future. Ideally and where possible, subjects should be given the opportunity to agree separately to the storage of samples for future research. The duration of sample retention, whether finite or indefinite, should be specified, as well as any possibility of the perpetuation of samples (e.g., whole-genome amplification, creation of immortalized cell lines, etc.).

A statement describing the degree to which the tests can or cannot be used to make a diagnosis or treat a person for a certain disease should be included. For research-grade tests that cannot be used to make any diagnosis, the term "DNA research" is recommended over "genetic testing" since the latter comes with a diagnostic connotation (e.g., "genetic testing" for cystic fibrosis).

If additional clinical information is to be collected exclusively for the purpose of the pharmacogenomic research component (e.g., ethnicity information, family history, etc.), this should be stated, and the additional information should only be collected from subjects who choose to participate in DNA research.

CFR Element 2: A description of any reasonably foreseeable risks or discomforts to the subject.

Specific considerations for pharmacogenomic studies:

Physical risks: The physical risks associated with genomic sample collection are generally minor, since sampling customarily involves a blood draw or buccal swab, but should still be stated. If a more invasive sampling technique is required (e.g., tumor or tissue biopsy) the physical risks must be disclosed. Often, pharmacogenomic samples can be collected in tandem with other sample collections in the trial. However, any added risks associated with the collection of additional sample volumes/amounts intended specifically for pharmacogenomic purposes (if any) should be stated.

Emotional, psychological, financial, and social risks: The greatest perceived risk of genomic research is that of the potential for misuse of genetic information consequent to intentional or unintentional disclosure to third parties or to the subjects themselves (or their relatives). For instance, genetic results revealing a higher risk for a certain disease for the subject or subject's family can potentially be worrisome to some participants and, in theory, could have implications for insurability, employability, or eligibility for adoption, among other things. These potential risks should be stated, but should also be represented realistically and not be an overexaggeration that causes unnecessary alarm, which could have an unfounded negative impact on the conduct of the intended pharmacogenomic studies. Where genomic analyses are not of diagnostic grade, the potential for discrimination from misuse of the data is greatly reduced. Exploratory pharmacogenomic research generally does not fall under the category of "genetic testing" as understood by insurance companies (with some exceptions). In such a case, subjects should be informed that they would not need to inform insurance companies that they had previously undergone genetic testing, a parameter that is used in underwriting in some jurisdictions.

Ethics committee opinions vary considerably regarding the amount of detail to include under the risks section of the informed consent. However, as per the ICH *(23)* and the U.S. CFR *(17)*, stated risks should be "reasonably foreseeable" and not an exhaustive list of what in theory could happen, particularly when there is no concrete history or evidence of such risks. Nevertheless, risks exceeding those of everyday life must be included in the consent process *(17)*, although a statement that "the chance of this happening is very small," may be appropriate.

CFR Element 3: A description of any benefits to the subject or to others which may reasonably be expected from the research.

Specific considerations for pharmacogenomic studies:

Pharmacogenomic studies generally offer limited direct benefit to the sample donor since investigations i) are not customarily conducted as part of clinical care, ii) are generally exploratory in nature, and iii) are not intended for the purpose of making diagnoses (with some exceptions). It should therefore be explained in the consent process that the information from the pharmacogenomic study may benefit others in the future by leading to the discovery of safer and more effective drugs or better understanding of the disease. The sense of helping the population at large should be highlighted. It cannot be ignored that clinical designs, such as dose selection based on genotype, could potentially benefit the patient by optimizing the dose for that patient, or by excluding subjects who might otherwise suffer predictable adverse events (e.g., excluding CYP2C9 poor metabolizers in a warfarin drug-drug interaction study). It is also conceivable that subjects who request their data may also follow up on these results in an accredited diagnostic setting and eventually learn information that could benefit them in the future (e.g., knowing one's *CYP2C9* and *VKORC1* genotype in the event of future warfarin therapy). The use of diagnostic-caliber assays may also be of direct benefit to subjects. However, more commonly, analyses are conducted in research mode and the potential to benefit the subject is nominal. Rather, the likely benefit is to the scientific community or to the drug development process.

CFR Element 4: A disclosure of appropriate alternative procedures or courses of treatment, if any, that might be advantageous to the subject.

Specific considerations for pharmacogenomic studies:

Generally, for pharmacogenomic studies, the only alternative is not to participate. Where participation is mandatory, the alternative may be to participate in another trial for which there is no mandatory pharmacogenomic component.

CFR Element 5: A statement describing the extent, if any, to which confidentiality of records identifying the subject will be maintained and that notes the possibility that the FDA may inspect the records.

Specific considerations for pharmacogenomic studies:

Information on sample coding and storage procedures should be described but should not be a lengthy discourse on processes (e.g., how a sample and corresponding data are anonymized). A description of the impact of these procedures on patient privacy is more useful and should be the emphasis. For example, in the case of anonymization, it would be sufficient to explain to participants that their sample will be labeled with a new number that is not linked to their original study number, which makes it very difficult (but not impossible) to link their genomic sample and data back to them.

Examples of safeguards to prevent unauthorized access to or loss of the samples should be provided, e.g., building card-key access, locked freezers, etc. It is not advisable to simply state that samples and data will be maintained securely and that confidentiality will be maintained.

Since the value of genomic samples increases with the number of samples, it has become common for samples to be shared or pooled among research groups. Policies for the sale, loan, donation, or transfer of samples to third parties, including research partners, biobanks, service providers, and commercial entities, should be stated. The type of research that may be conducted by these parties should also be mentioned as well as the possibility that samples will be sent to countries where privacy regulations may not be as stringent (if applicable, see below).

The degree to which access to data will be safeguarded, including a list of parties who will or will not have access to the data and measures to control this access (e.g., secure databases, passwords, locked archives, policies, etc.) should be briefly stated.

A statement on publication and presentation of data, including the possibility of uploading genetic and clinical data into public databases, should be included.

The extent to which pharmacogenomic data and documentation will be segregated from medical records should be addressed.

CFR Element 6: For research involving more than minimal risk, an explanation as to whether any compensation and an explanation as to whether any medical treatments are available if injury occurs and, if so, what they consist of, or where further information may be obtained.

Specific considerations for pharmacogenomic studies:

Pharmacogenomic studies usually do not involve more than minimal physical risk, unless a tissue or biopsy sample is being collected exclusively for this purpose, in which case details of compensation or medical treatments in the event of injury should be stated. Otherwise, in keeping with improved readability and to avoid unnecessary repetition, it would be sufficient to explain in the pharmacogenomic informed consent that any medical injury sustained from the collection of the pharmacogenomic sample will be handled in the same way as described for the main clinical trial. Since pharmacogenomic research potentially could involve other non-physical risks, an explanation of what compensation would consist of in such a case, if any, should be provided.

CFR Element 7: An explanation of whom to contact for answers to pertinent questions about the research and research subjects' rights, and whom to contact in the event of a research-related injury to the subject.

In general, there are no specific considerations for pharmacogenomic studies.

CFR Element 8: A statement that participation is voluntary, that refusal to participate will involve no penalty or loss of benefits to which the subject is otherwise entitled, and that the subject may discontinue participation at any time without penalty or loss of benefits to which the subject is otherwise entitled.

Specific considerations for pharmacogenomic studies:

In addition to stating that participation is voluntary, it is also important to specify whether participation is optional or mandatory.

A description of the process for withdrawal of consent and implications for eligibility for the trial should be provided. Where participation is mandatory, it must be clear that withdrawal of consent from pharmacogenomic research would result in ineligibility for continued participation in the trial (if applicable).

The time frame during which a subject can withdraw from the pharmacogenomic component of the study should be defined, with mention of any conditions that would not allow sample destruction upon withdrawal from the trial (e.g., anonymization or pooling of samples or data). The available options for the fate of the samples upon withdrawal should be offered (e.g., samples will be maintained according to original consent, or samples will be destroyed).

An additional element of informed consent for pharmacogenomic studies that is commonly required by IECs and IRBs is a description of procedures for the return of research data to subjects and the implications thereof. The Pharmacogenetics Working Group has published detailed recommendations on the return of pharmacogenetic research data to research subjects *(24)*. In brief, some important considerations are i) the subjects' right to know and their right not to know; ii) the extent to which the data are interpretable and the ability to make a diagnosis; iii) the conditions under which the data will be generated (research versus diagnostic) and the consequent need to have tests repeated by an accredited diagnostic laboratory, noting that diagnostic-caliber tests may not be available for the endpoints analyzed; iv) the implications of knowing one's results (risks and benefits); v) the potential impact on family members should they learn of these results; and vi) access to genetic counseling. It is beyond the scope of this chapter to address each of these points. However, on a practical level, the overall approach that is currently most broadly accepted by ethics committees is to provide genomic research results to subjects only upon their explicit request, and this only after the limitations of the interpretability of the results have been clearly explained during the informed consent process. If results are to be returned to subjects, the conditions under which this would occur, who might see these data, the risk of the data turning up in subjects' medical files, and the degree of interpretability of the data and the potential impact on family members should be stated, including a statement about whether genetic counseling would be provided. In compliance with local regulations in some countries, ethics committees will not allow the return of genomic results to subjects unless the data were generated under conditions that allow clinically relevant interpretations to be drawn. In such cases, subjects should be informed upfront that they will not be entitled to receive their data, including the reason for this restriction.

The informed consent requirements in the U.S. CFR regulations are not intended to preempt any applicable federal, state, or local laws which require additional information to be disclosed for informed consent to be legally effective *(17)*. Additional elements may include any of the 26 elements of informed consent from CIOMS or any other requirement that satisfies local laws and regulations *(25)*. Ethics committees are entitled to impose additional requirements to ensure compliance with institutional policy and local law.

The implementation of pharmacogenomic research in clinical trials does not end with the protocol and informed consent; additional documentation and infrastructure are required to successfully implement these studies in the context of clinical trials. Additional documentation minimally includes forms for withdrawal of consent, forms for coordinating data return to subjects, and templates for the accurate and consistent reporting of data. Also necessary are case report forms to capture consent status as well as information on local requirements (e.g., limitations on duration of storage) or any additional phenotypic data collected exclusively for the pharmacogenomic component. Obviously, SOPs supporting sample and data processing and handling, anonymization, and data return, and other relevant aspects, are recommended.

4 Considerations for Sample Collections

Because pharmacogenomic studies are being increasingly used to create and validate diagnostic and prognostic signatures and to support toxicological and functional studies that underlie the regulatory filings for new drug submissions, it is increasingly important to create standardized and robust methods for sample procurement and processing in addition to the parameters listed above. Correct sample identification requires error-free handling during all stages of sample collection and storage. Informatics systems should be specifically designed to register and track samples in addition to housing genomic and other data in a robust manner. All procedures related to sample acquisition intended for genomic research should be accompanied by guidelines or formal SOPs to ensure the quality and integrity of the samples and related data collected for these purposes. The following sections will outline processes that should ensure quality standards for sample procurement that will enable accurate and predictable data generation. Standardized procedures for sample collections during the conduct of clinical studies will significantly improve the reliability of the results obtained, while standardized isolation procedures for DNA, RNA, and protein will improve the overall quality of the results. The following sections describe multiple aspects to consider when collecting samples from multicenter clinical trials with the intent of conducting robust genomic and proteomic analyses worldwide.

4.1 Blood Samples

Blood samples are an excellent source of large amounts of DNA that can be used for genetic testing, either via candidate gene or genome-wide screens. In general, whole blood is collected under standard conditions into vacutainer tubes containing EDTA and kept at room temperature or 4°C for overnight shipments for processing and/or storage. Alternatively, immediate processing and storage can be done at temperatures ranging from -20°C to -70°C, although this method is not convenient for multicenter clinical trials. DNA yields are optimal when whole blood samples are immediately processed to isolate DNA. Whole blood samples stored at ambient temperatures for six days can be expected to produce up to 50% less DNA compared to fresh sample processing *(26)*. A 30–40% decrease in DNA yield was observed in samples stored for three to seven days at 4°C, compared to fresh extractions *(26–29)*. Gustineich et al. *(27)* reported that DNA yield decreased by 30–40% if the blood was frozen at -20°C while Cushwa et al. *(29)* observed a 41% decrease in DNA yield in samples stored at -20°C. DNA yields of samples stored at -70°C were shown to be comparable to yields from samples immediately isolated *(26)*, *(30)*, *(31)*; however, Ross and coworkers observed a 25% decrease in DNA yield after similar storage of samples at -70°C *(32)*. In general, 150–250 μg of DNA can be isolated from 10 mL of whole blood *(33)*, although some laboratories have noted higher yields (e.g., 100–200 μg/5mL whole blood) *(34)*.

RNA can also be isolated from blood samples. For blood collection and preservation, PAXgene™ (PreAnalytiX GmbH, Switzerland) and CPT™ tubes (Becton Dickinson, NJ) have been widely used for whole blood and peripheral blood mononuclear cell (PBMC) collections *(35)* intended for RNA isolation. Extensive mRNA changes are eliminated or markedly reduced when whole blood is stored in preservatives contained in the PAXgene™ tubes *(36)*. The PAXgene™ system offers a number of potential advantages that makes it highly attractive for multicenter clinical studies, the primary one being ease of use *(36)*. However, some investigators have shown *(37)* that there is increased noise and reduced responsiveness in the gene expression profiles derived from whole blood compared with a leukocyte isolation protocol. These authors concluded that erythrocytes or reticulocytes and other nonleukocyte sources contribute an appreciable number of mRNA species in the whole blood collection system; but that simply removing the overabundant hemoglobin mRNA species does not result in a response pattern identical to that seen from leukocyte isolations.

The goal of any RNA isolation procedure is to recover an RNA population that mirrors the biology of the sample at the time of collection. Problems associated with the extraction of biologically representative RNA arise primarily from the susceptibility of RNA to degradation by ubiquitous and catalytically potent RNases. Therefore, RNA preservatives should be added, since many RNA transcripts change gene expression levels when stored (e.g., in EDTA) within hours (36, 38–40). It is important to note that the purity of the RNA as measured by A260/A280 is very consistent, even after extended storage of whole blood at ambient temperatures; and often the intactness of ribosomal RNA bands is also well maintained, although the underlying representation of many genes may have changed dramatically *(41)*. As noted previously, it may be important to reduce the globin mRNA population *(42)* contributed from the reticulocytes portion of whole blood samples, especially since the globin mRNA can contribute significantly to background noise in microarray experiments.

4.2 Tumor Biopsies

Paraffin embedded tumor samples are also utilized for pharmacogenomic studies. Formalin fixation and paraffin embedding is the standard tissue processing method used in many histopathology laboratories. This method allows for permanent preservation of tissues, easy storage, and optimal histological quality. However, formalin fixation may compromise the analysis of biomolecules, including DNA, mRNA, and proteins. Fresh frozen or immediately preserved tumor samples are preferred; however, samples prepared in this manner are not widely available.

A problem with the analysis of tumor samples is contamination of the samples by stromal cells (e.g., fibroblasts, myofibroblasts, and endothelial cells) and the surrounding normal cells. Even the most sophisticated genetic testing methods will be of limited value if the input material (nucleic acids) is not derived from sufficiently pure populations of the cells of interest. To address this problem, Emmert-Buck and colleagues introduced the laser capture microdissection (LCM) system *(43)* in 1996. LCM can be used to specifically obtain tumor tissue from surrounding normal tissue, whereby each laser pulse selectively transfers one small focal region of tissue or cell cluster to film contained on a slide *(43)*. This methodology does not adversely affect the ability to perform polymerase chain reaction (PCR) or other enzyme activity assays *(43)*. The success of LCM is illustrated by the large number of studies utilizing this technique for a broad range of downstream applications, such as loss of heterozygosity analysis (LOH), comparative genome hybridization (CGH) array analysis, methylation specific PCR, real-time (RT) quantitative (q)-PCR, expression microarrays, cDNA library construction, etc. In oncology, the genetic analysis of premalignant lesions has potential clinical implications, since these mutations represent an intermediate step of tumor progression from normal cells to cancer and may provide information with respect to malignant transformation. Analysis of these samples may also allow identification of multiple mutations (signatures or classifiers) that are associated with response to drug treatment.

RNA analyses can also be performed on samples obtained from LCM sections; however, the RNA yield is generally low and control of RNA quality is necessary to avoid misinterpretation of the gene expression results. Additionally, the elevated temperatures required for paraffin embedding are known to reduce the quality and yields of RNA. The use of different fixatives also has a significant effect on RNA integrity. Ethanol fixation and paraffin embedding of tissue specimens is not optimal for high-throughput mRNA expression analysis *(44)*; however, RT-PCR for specific genes can be performed on these samples. Kim et al. *(45)* showed that methacarn, a combination of methanol, chloroform, and acetic acid, was the optimal fixative for RNA studies; while Vincek et al. *(46)* showed that RNA can be adequately preserved in a new universal molecular fixative (UMFIX, Sakura Finetek USA, Inc., Torrance, CA). Other factors that can alter the integrity of RNA are the age of the paraffin block and the length of time that the samples have been stored. RNA extracted from archived FFPE blocks that are older than 10 years is typically about 100 nucleotides in length. However, newer microarray designs for genome-wide profiling of FFPE samples from vendors such as Affymetrix allow the interrogation of smaller target sequences compared to standard gene chip arrays *(42)*.

Fresh tumor tissue can also be preserved by flash freezing in liquid nitrogen or by the use of RNALater™ (PreAnalytix GmbH, Switzerland). RNALater is more convenient for multicenter clinical trials, since tissue can be stored in RNALater at room temperature for up to three days without introducing any systematic changes in gene expression as measured in microarray experiments *(47)*. Protection of RNA in tumor samples has been previously accomplished by immediate lysis using high concentrations of detergents and/or chaotropic agents and organic solvents such as TRI reagent® (Applied Biosystems, CA). These methods are complex to use at the point of care and suffer from low sample throughput. Flash freezing of samples in liquid nitrogen and transport on dry ice are impractical in most clinical settings as well.

4.3 Serum/Plasma (Proteomic Analyses)

Proteomic analyses often complement genomic analyses and include interrogation of the entire proteome or portions of the proteome. The impact of preanalytical variables, ranging from patient posture to sample timing and tube type, on the quality of laboratory results for many protein measurements is well recognized *(48)*. In addition, other preanalytical aspects, such as centrifugation (speed, time, and temperature), storage time and temperature, and exposure to freeze-thaw cycles, are important. The direct effect of tube additives such as silicones, surfactants, and plasticizers on some analyses may be factors as well *(49)*.

These issues were focused on in the HUPO Plasma Proteome Project *(50)*. Within this project, comparison of serum and plasma specimens was done with respect to the human proteome. Serum samples were clotted by glass/silica-based activation and plasma specimens were derived using the three most common anticoagulants, namely, potassium-EDTA, lithium-heparin, and sodium citrate. The effects of storage were tested under various time and temperature conditions, and it was found that no major differences were observed between storage at −20°C, −80°C, and liquid nitrogen over two months time as detected by surface-enhanced laser desorption/ionization time-of-flight mass spectrometry (SELDI-TOF); however, there were differences at both room temperature and refrigerated storage. Since serum generation relies on a biochemical process, it is reasonable to expect that various parameters, such as temperature after sample collection, time for sample processing/clot formation, or medication of patients, can alter the peptide content of serum. These issues are difficult to standardize in routine clinical practice.

Therefore, the use of serum samples for peptidomic mono/oligo-biomarker discovery should be avoided in most cases. Serum peptide patterns have been used for prediction of early stage cancers, and a debate about this approach is ongoing *(51–54)*. At this time it is not clear whether the proteomic patterns reflect directly disease related peptides, or peptides that are generated due to secondary effects during *ex vivo* coagulation. The choice of sample type is dependent on downstream analyses. Each of the individual sample types, serum, EDTA-plasma, heparin-plasma, and citrate plasma, exhibit shortcomings. EDTA forms soluble complexes with metal ions and should not be utilized if the endpoint measurement involves assays requiring divalent cations such as Mg2+ or Ca2+. Heparin can interfere in affinity processes such as SELDI-TOF analysis since it competes for binding of molecules to charged surfaces. Citrate can bind calcium and may falsely lower immunoassay measurements of multiple analytes *(55–57)*. Protease inhibitors may protect plasma proteins as early as phlebotomy procedures, and protease inhibitor use seems likely to provide a more reproducible sample. However, some inhibitors have the potential to alter proteins, and thus consideration of the desired analytical outcome is important.

5 Global Regulatory Considerations for Sample Collections

5.1 Country-Related Regulatory Considerations

Consideration of all the parameters discussed in the previous section should lead to standard collection procedures for sample procurement that will allow more robust downstream analyses. Emphasis on the quality measures taken for sample procurement may also assist with obtaining approval from relevant regulatory bodies for the intended genomic or proteomic research. As addressed in previous sections, many issues may be encountered in the pharmacogenomic protocol approval process. Other questions that may potentially arise relate to the processes surrounding sample acquisition and the degree of validation of the assay that will be used to analyze the samples. Efforts are currently ongoing to harmonize regulations for genomic sample collections; however, it may be well into the future before harmonization does occur. Because country-specific, local, and regional regulations continually change, it is recommended that one acquire and review specific country-related regulations prior to implementing a pharmacogenomic study at a particular site. Some countries regulate sample importation or exportation to stimulate commerce or to control data generation from ethnically derived sample sets. Some countries require importation or exportation application procedures that can be lengthy, and delays in sample procurement should be anticipated in these cases. Additionally, limits can be placed on the type of research, location of sample storage, coding of samples, and the rights to sample data. The following barriers can be expected to be encountered, either because of local regulations superseding country-level regulations or because of differences in the interpretation of specified regulations:

- Limitations on exploratory research: Argentina, Canada
- Prohibition of mandatory research: Korea, Spain
- Requirements for decriptions of research: Chile (requires gene listing)
- Requirements for a separate protocol describing research: Brazil, Thailand

- Separate approval bodies that require extensive time for review and approval: Australia, France, Israel, Netherlands
- Prohibition of anonymization: Brazil, Italy
- Limitations to location for sample banking: Iceland, Sweden
- Limitations to length of storage time: Italy, Netherlands
- Prohibition of sample storage: Malaysia, Taiwan, Thailand
- Requests for length of sample storage: Australia, Belgium
- Limitations or applications necessary for export: China, India, Spain
- Limitations to length of time samples can be outside country: Sweden
- Allowances for subject to request results of research: Brazil

5.2 Ongoing Efforts for Education and Policy Change Related to Sample Acquisition

To address some of these specific issues concerning global sample acquisitions, various groups have emerged to provide information in public forums that may assist in leading to harmonization of regulations across countries. These groups include (but are not limited to) the Pharmacogenetics Working Group, the European Federation of Pharmaceutical Industries and Associations, the Pharmacogenetics Research Network, the Council for International Organizations in Medical Sciences Working Group on Pharmacogenetics, the AAPS Pharmacogenetics and Pharmacogenomics Focus Group, and the Pharmacogenetics for Every Nation Initiative. The activities of these groups are described below.

The Pharmacogenetics Working group (PWG, http://www.pharmacogenetics working group.org) is a voluntary and informal association of pharmaceutical companies engaged in research in the science of pharmacogenetics. This group initially formed in response to regulatory requests for noncompetitive information from the industry. It provides information intended to promote a better public understanding of pharmacogenetic research and its development *(19, 24, 58, 59)*. The PWG works with the U.S. FDA, the EMEA, and regulators and various policy groups to provide information on noncompetitive issues related to pharmacogenetic research. The European Federation of Pharmaceutical Industries and Associations (EFPIA) has a pharmacogenomics task force. There is overlap in the membership between the EFPIA task force and the PWG. This task force does not currently have a separate website.

The Pharmacogenetics Research Network (http://www.nigms.nih.gov/pharma cogenetics, http://www.pharmgkb.org/), associated with NIH-NIGMS (National Institutes of Health-National Institute of General Medical Science), enables a network of multidisciplinary research groups to conduct studies addressing research questions in pharmacogenetics and pharmacogenomics in order to ultimately populate a knowledge base (PharmGKB) with data. The long-term goal of this group is to translate this knowledge and identify safe and effective drug therapies for individual patients. Among its other goals is to interact with and influence the wider community of scientists in academia, industry, and government regulatory agencies in order to advance the field of pharmacogenetics.

Another group of interest is the Council for International Organizations in Medical Sciences, Working Group on Pharmacogenetics (CIOMS, http://www.cioms.ch). Of note, CIOMS has issued the "International Ethical Guidelines for Biomedical Research Involving Human Subjects" (developed in conjunction with WHO), which was published in 1993. The Working Group on Pharmacogenetics, which includes senior scientists from ten drug regulatory authorities and ten pharmaceutical companies, plus experts from WHO and academia, formed to consider drug development and the regulatory, ethical, educational, and economic issues related to pharmacogenetics. The findings and recommendations of the CIOMS-WGP have been presented at many international conferences in Europe, Japan, and the U.S.

The goal of the AAPS Pharmacogenetics and Pharmacogenomics Focus Group (http://www.aapspharmaceutica.com/inside/focus_groups/PGX/index.asp) is to provide a forum for information exchange on developments in pharmacogenetics and pharmacogenomics. They do this by generating yearly themes in these areas in the *AAPS Journal*, and by organizing symposia, workshops, roundtables, and guest speaker programs. The goals are to develop a knowledge base in pharmacogenetics and pharmacogenomics research, and to facilitate communication between academia, biotechnology, genomics firms, pharmaceutical companies, and regulatory agencies.

Finally, the Pharmacogenetics for Every Nation Initiative (PGENI, http://pgeni.unc.edu) has formed with four goals: i) to enhance the understanding of pharmacogenetics in the developing world, ii) to help build local infrastructure for future pharmacogenetic research studies, iii) to provide guidelines for medical prioritization for individual countries using pharmacogenetic information, and iv) to promote the integration of genetic information into public health decision making processes.

These and many other organizations are working towards the goal of providing comprehensive knowledge in the fields of pharmacogenetics and pharmacogenomics. It is anticipated that the activities of these groups may influence regulations applicable to genomic research, leading to harmonization of those regulations for samples intended for genomic analysis, as described above. It is hoped that such harmonization will occur in the near future, especially considering that a vast amount of genomic information is being captured and interpreted with the intent of personalizing medicine, in order to reduce unnecessary adverse events and to increase drug efficacy in individual patients.

In conclusion, many regulatory and operational considerations should take precedence over study start-up activities, when the intent is to acquire as many samples of high quality as possible for pharmacogenomic analysis. As discussed above, specific issues that may be encountered in the pharmacogenomic protocol approval process include inquiries related to:

- the intended use of samples collected for pharmacogenomic analyses,
- the length of time samples will be stored,
- sample coding procedures,

- management of the data collected,
- the maintenance of subject privacy and confidentiality,
- the physical sample storage location and the conditions under which samples are stored,
- allowance for and limitations on withdrawal of consent and sample destruction,
- limits on access to the sample data,
- reporting of results to individual subjects (and potentially genetic counseling),
- publication policies and the dissemination of results.

Since country-specific, local, and regional regulations continually change, it is recommended that one acquire and review specific regulations prior to placing a pharmacogenomic study. In addition, emphasis should be placed on standardizing global sample acquisition and handling procedures to ensure acquisition of samples of the highest quality and integrity for all intended downstream genomic applications.

References

1. EMEA, http://www.emea.europa.eu/
2. FDA, http://www.fda.gov/cder/
3. MHLW, http://www.mhlw.go.jp/english/index.html
4. PMC, http://www.personalizedmedicinecoalition.org/communications/overview.php
5. Eriksson S, Helgesson G (2005) Potential harms, anonymization, and the right to withdraw consent to biobank research. Eur J Hum Genet 13(9):1071–6.
6. Rivera R, Borasky D, Rice R, Carayon F, Wong E (2007) Informed consent: an international researcher's perspective. Am J Public Health 97(1):25–30.
7. Miller CK, O'Donnell DC, Searight HR, Barbarash RA (1996) The Deaconess Informed Consent Comprehension Test: an assessment tool for clinical research subjects. Pharmacotherapy 16(5):872–8.
8. Daugherty C, Ratain MJ, Grochowski E, et al (1995) Perceptions of cancer patients and their physicians involved in phase I trials. J Clin Oncol 13(5):1062–72.
9. Flesch R (1978) A new readability yardstick. J Appl Psychol 32:221–33.
10. Flesch R (1979) How to write plain English. Harper, New York.
11. Baker MT, Taub HA (1983) Readability of informed consent forms for research in a Veterans Administration medical center. JAMA 250(19):2646–8.
12. Duffy T, Kabance P (1982) Testing a readability writing approach to text revision. J Educ Psychol 74:733–48.
13. Eaton ML, Holloway RL (1980) Patient comprehension of written drug information. Am J Hosp Pharm 37(2):240–3.
14. Irwin J (1991) Teaching reading comprehension process, 2nd ed. Prentice Hall, New Jersey.
15. Vacca R, Vacca J (1989) Content area reading, 3rd ed. Scott Foresman, Illinois.
16. Kirsch I, Jungeblut A, Jenkins L, Kolstad A (1993) Adult literacy in America., U.S. Department of Education, Washington.
17. Regulations USCoF (2007) United States Code of Federal Regulations. In: 21 CFR 50.25.
18. Sciences CfIOoM (2002) International ethical guidelines for biomedical research involving human subjects. Geneva, ISBN 92-9036-075-5.
19. Anderson C, Gomez-Mancilla B, Spear B et al (2002) Elements of informed consent for pharmacogenetic research: perspective of the Pharmacogenetics Working Group.Pharmacogenomics J 2(5):284–92.
20. Wertz DC (2002) Genetic discrimination—an overblown fear? Nat Rev Genet 3(7):496.

21. Shickle D (2006) The consent problem within DNA biobanks. Stud Hist Philos Biol Biomed Sci 37(3):503–19.
22. Hoeyer K, Olofsson BO, Mjorndal T, Lynoe N (2004) Informed consent and biobanks: a population-based study of attitudes towards tissue donation for genetic research. Scand J Public Health 32(3):224–9.
23. ICH Harmonized Tripartite Guideline E6(R1): Good Clinical Practice: Consolidated Guideline, 1996.
24. Renegar G, Webster C, Stuerzebecher S et al (2006) Returning genetic research results to individuals: points to consider. Bioethics 20(1):24–36.
25. Bhutta ZA (2004) Beyond informed consent. B World Health Organ 82(10):771–7.
26. Madisen L, Hoar D, Holroyd C, Crisp M, Hodes M (1987) DNA banking: the effects of storage of blood and isolated DNA on the integrity of DNA. Am J Med Genet 27:379–90.
27. Gustincich S, Manfioletti G, Del Sal G, Schneider C, Carninci P (1991) A fast method for high-quality genomic DNA extraction from whole human blood. Biotechniques 11:298–300.
28. McCullough J, Carter S, Quie P (1974) Effects of anticoagulants and storage on granulocyte function in bank blood. Blood 43:207–17.
29. Cushwa W, Medrano J (1993) Effects of blood storage time and temperature on DNA yield and quality. Biotechniques 14:204–7.
30. Polakova H, Kadasi L, Zelinkova M (1989) The yield and quality of DNA extracted from blood samples stored under various conditions. Bratisl Lek Listy 90:844–7.
31. Bomjen G, Raina A, Sulaiman I, Hasnain S, Dogra T (1996) Effect of storage of blood samples on DNA yield, quality and fingerprinting: a forensic approach. Ind J Exp Biol 34:384–6.
32. Ross K, Haites N, Kelly K (1990) Repeated freezing and thawing of peripheral blood and DNA in suspension: effects on DNA yield and integrity. J Med Genet 27:569–70.
33. Ellsworth D, Manolio T (1999) The emerging importance of genetics in epidemiologic research. I. Basic concepts in human genetics and laboratory technology. AEP 9(1):1–16.
34. McIndoe R, Linhardt M, Hood L (1995) Single tube genomic DNA isolation from whole blood without pre-isolating white blood cells. BioTechniques 19(1):30–2.
35. Fan H, Hedge P (2005) The transcriptome in blood: challenges and solutions for robust expression profiling. Curr Mol Med 5:3–10.
36. Rainen L, Oelmueller U, Jurgensen S et al (2002) Stabilization of mRNA expression in whole blood samples. Clin Chem 48:1883–90.
37. Feezor R, Baker H, Mindrinos M et al (2004) Whole blood and leukocyte RNA isolation for gene expression analyses. Physiol Genomics 19:247–54.
38. Haskill S, Johnson C, Eierman D, Becker S, Warren K (1988) Adherence induces selective mRNA expression of monocyte mediators and proto-oncogenes. J Immunol 140:1690–4.
39. Pahl A, Brune K (2002) Gene expression changes in blood after phlebotomy: implications for gene expression profiling. Blood 100:1094–5.
40. Tanner M, Berk L, Felten D, Blidy A, Bit S, Ruff D (2002) Substantial changes in gene expression level due to the storage temperature and storage duration of human whole blood. Clin Lab Haematol 24:337–41.
41. Davidson T, Johnson C, Andruss B (2006) Analyzing micro-RNA expression using microarrays. Method Enzymol 411:1–14.
42. Madabushi L, Latham G, Andruss G (2006) RNA extraction for arrays. Method Enzymol 411:1–14.
43. Emmert-Buck M, Bonner R, Smith P et al (1996) Laser capture microdissection. Science 274:998–1001.
44. Perlmutter M, Best C, Gillespie J et al (2004) Comparison of snap freezing versus ethanol fixation for gene expression profiling of tissue specimens. J Mol Diagn 6(4):371–7.
45. Kim J, Hwang M, Shin H et al (2003) Differential expression analysis using paraffin-embeded tissues after laser microdissection. J Cell Biochem 90:998–1006.
46. Vincek V, Nassiri M, Nadji M, Morales A (2003) A tissue fixative that protects macromolecules (DNA, RNA, and protein) and histomorphology in clinical samples. Lab Invest 90:1427–35.

47. Mutter G, Zahrieh D, Liu C et al (2004) Comparison of frozen and RNALater solid tissue storage methods for use in RNA expression microarrays. BMC Genom 5:88.
48. Guder W, Narayanan S, Wisserh H, Zawta B (2003) Samples: from the patient to the laboratory: the impact of preanalytical variables on the quality of laboratory results, 3rd ed. Wiley, New York. p 106.
49. Drake S, Bowen R, Remaley A, Hortin G (2004) Potential interferences from blood collection tubes in mass spectrometric analysis of serum polypetides. Clin Chem 50:2398–401.
50. Rai A, Gelfand C, Haywood B et al (2005) HUPO plasma proteome project specimen collection and handling: towards the standardization of parameters for plasma proteome samples. Proteomics 5:3262–77.
51. Villanueva J, Philip J, Entenberg D et al (2004) Serum peptide profiling by magnetic particle-assisted, automated sample processing and MALDI-TOF mass spectrometry. Anal Chem 76:1560–70.
52. Petricoin E, Ardekani F, Hitt A, Levine B (2002) Use of proteomic patterns in serum to identify ovarian cancer. Lancet 359:572–7.
53. Check E (2004) Proteomics and cancer: running before we can walk. Nature 429:496–7.
54. Diamandis E (2004) Mass spectrometry as a diagnostic and a cancer biomarker discovery tool. Proteomics 3:367–78.
55. Rai A, Stemmer J, Zhang Z et al (2005) Analysis of human proteome organization plasma proteome project (HUPO PPP) reference specimens using surace enhanced laser desorption/ionization-time of flight (SELDI-TOF) mass spectrometry: multi-institution correlation of spectra and identification of biomarkers. Proteomics 5:3467–74.
56. Haab B, Geierstanger B, Michailidis B et al (2005) Immunoassay and antibody microarray analysis of the HUPO plasma proteome project reference specimens: systematic variation between sample types and calibration of mass spectrometry data. Proteomics 5:3278–91.
57. Tubes and Additives for venous blood specimen collection: approved standard-fifth edition, NCCLS. In. Wayne, PA; 2003:33.
58. Spear B, Heath-Chiozzi M, Barnes D, Cheeseman K, Shaw P, Campbell D (2001) Terminology for sample collection in clinical genetic studies. Pharmacogenomics J 1:101–3.
59. Lesko L, Salerno R, Spear B et al (2003) Pharmacogenetics and pharmacogenomics in drug development and regulatory decision making: report of the first FDA-PWG-PhRMA-Drug Safe Workshop. J Clin Pharmacol 43(4):342–58.

Chapter 3
Pharmacogenomics

The Regulatory Environment and Labeling Implications

Myong-Jin Kim, Shiew-Mei Huang, Atiqur Rahman, Felix W. Frueh, and Lawrence J. Lesko

Contents

Abstract The use of pharmacogenomic information has opened new opportunities in drug discovery and development. The FDA has undertaken several initiatives to promote and exchange ideas in the field of pharmacogenomics as a key opportunity for the critical path. In this chapter, a regulatory science perspective of pharmacogenomics is discussed addressing the critical aspects of pharmacogenomics in drug development, drug therapy, regulatory decision making, and labeling implications.

The mission of the U.S. Food and Drug Administration (FDA) is to protect and advance the public health, and encourage scientific innovations to develop safe and effective drugs *(1)*. However, the FDA's efforts to achieve this critical mission can be challenging because of rapidly emerging science and technology. To bridge the potential gap between scientific innovations and translating them into clinical use, the FDA has undertaken several initiatives to promote and exchange ideas and information in the field of pharmacogenomics. The FDA's "personalized medicine" initiatives make use of pharmacogenomics—the science that predicts a response to drugs based on a patient's genetic makeup.

Individualized therapy based on pharmacogenomics could be important in drug development. Pharmacogenomics has the potential to identify sources of interindividual variability in drug responses that affect the efficacy and safety of drugs. In addition,

---

Myong-Jin Kim
WO 21, Room 4610, 10903 New Hampshire Avenue, Silver Spring, Maryland 20993
myongjin.kim@fda.hhs.gov

N. Cohen (ed.) *Pharmacogenomics and Personalized Medicine*,

pharmacogenomics/pharmacogenetics can provide a key opportunity to improve the safety outcomes of existing therapies. For example, drugs with a narrow therapeutic range, such as warfarin and irinotecan, can benefit from this emerging science. By integrating the use of pharmacogenomics into routine clinical practice, pharmacogenomics can help to individualize therapy with the intent of maximizing effectiveness and minimizing risk (i.e., improve the benefit/risk ratio) *(2)*.

In this chapter, a regulatory science perspective on pharmacogenomics will be discussed to address the critical aspects of pharmacogenomics in drug development, drug therapy, and regulatory decision making.

Keywords FDA, Personalized Medicine, Critical Path, Pharmacogenomics, Pharmacogenetics

1 The Integration of Pharmacogenomics into the Continuum of Drug Development

The "productivity problem" *(3)*, as mentioned in the FDA's critical path whitepaper entitled "Innovation or Stagnation" *(4)*, is evident by the number of new drug and biologic applications submitted to the FDA. During the last several years, this number has declined significantly (Fig. 3.1) *(4)*. In 2006, only 23 new drugs were approved by

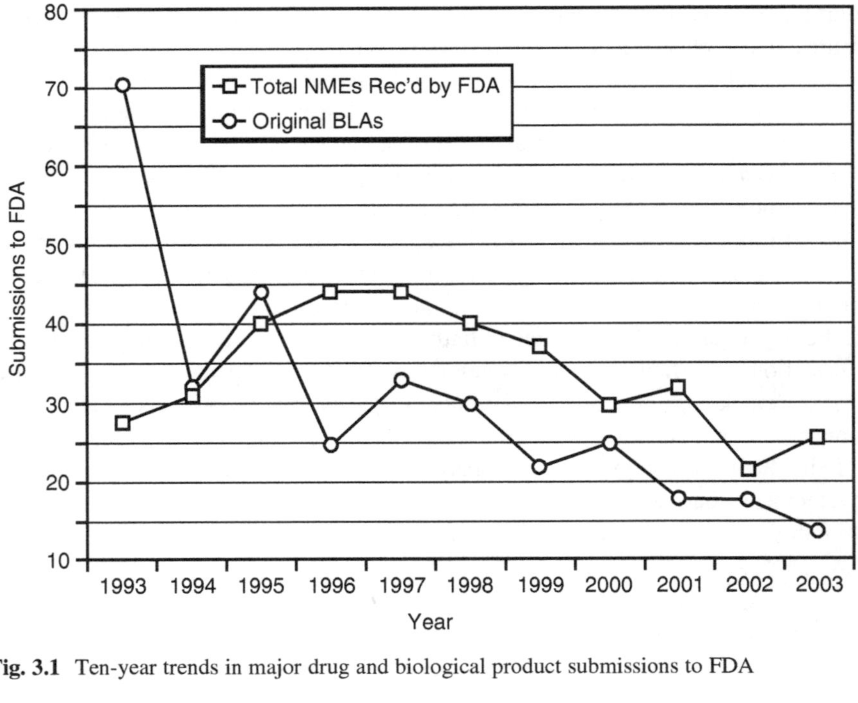

Fig. 3.1 Ten-year trends in major drug and biological product submissions to FDA

the FDA *(5)*. However, the costs of these product developments have increased over the last decade *(4)*, *(6)*. This is indicative of the applied sciences lagging behind the tremendous advances in the basic sciences. So the question is, can greater use of pharmacogenomics and pharmacogenetics help to reduce the "productivity problem"? There are alternative strategies that have the potential to lead to improved productivity by using molecular biomarkers to enrich clinical trials with known responders, to exclude those at risk for serious adverse events, and to individualize dosing to genetic profiles of individuals *(5)*. Pharmacogenomic biomarkers can be used to identify potential responders of a drug product. By stratifying patients by biomarker status in a dose-finding study, a target dose for a specific population can be obtained for phase 2, and subsequently phase 3, efficacy trials, thereby increasing the probability of success and regulatory approval of the drug. Therefore, genetic and genomic factors together with environmental factors can be useful in determining interindividual variability in drug responses and can help in optimizing drug development.

2 The FDA's Initiatives to Facilitate Use of Pharmacogenomics in Drug Development and Clinical Practice

The integration of pharmacogenomics into routine clinical practice remains a major challenge. The FDA has undertaken several initiatives to facilitate such integration. In 2002, the agency published a paper that described a regulatory perspective on the opportunities and challenges of integrating pharmacogenomics into drug development and regulatory decision-making *(7)*. In May 2002, the agency held a workshop, cosponsored by pharmaceutical industry groups, to identify key issues associated with the application of pharmacogenetics and pharmacogenomics to drug development. Subsequently, the FDA published a draft "Guidance for Industry: Pharmacogenomic Data Submissions" in November 2003 and received public comment on it. Additionally, the FDA has coordinated its efforts with the pharmaceutical and biotechnology industry groups to convene a series of public pharmacogenomic workshops (8–10). The objective of these workshops was to discuss the status of pharmacogenomic technology, the use of pharmacogenomics in drug development, and the specific strategies that are most needed for using pharmacogenomics as a tool to facilitate more efficient and effective research along the critical path of drug development.

2.1 FDA Critical Path Initiatives

In March 2004, the FDA released a white paper entitled "Innovation or Stagnation: Challenge and Opportunity on the Critical Path to New Medical Products" *(4)*. The concept of this white paper was to bring attention and focus to the need for targeted scientific efforts to modernize the tools, techniques, and methods used to evaluate the safety, efficacy, and quality of drug products. The critical path is defined as the path from candidate selection to product launch, and it defines the potential bottlenecks in bringing a product to market. The focus of the critical path initiative is to identify ways to update the product development infrastructure for drugs, biologics, and devices, and the evaluative tools currently used to assess the safety and efficacy of new medical products. It describes the urgent need to build bridges among constituencies, including the FDA, other government agencies such as the National Institutes of Health, and the academic or private sectors, to modernize the development process for medical products—the critical path—to make product development more predictable and less costly. As a scientific opportunity to improve the critical path, the use of pharmacogenomics can provide insights into the stage of a disease, disease progression, drug response, and drug dose requirements, and thereby lead to the development of tests to predict clinical outcomes more reliably *(6)*.

3 The Use of Pharmacogenomics and Pharmacogenetics in Drug Development

3.1 New Drug Development

The FDA, as a regulatory agency, has a responsibility to provide a consistent policy and framework for pharmacogenomic data collection, submission, and assessment. In order to address this much needed guidance for stakeholders, the agency published "Guidance for Industry: Pharmacogenomic Data Submissions" in March 2005 *(2)*. The main purpose of this guidance is to promote the use of pharmacogenomics in drug development and to encourage open and public sharing of data and information on pharmacogenomic test results. In general, the guidance addressed the following: (a) when to submit pharmacogenomic data to the Agency; (b) what format and content to provide for submissions; and (c) how and when the genomic data would be used in regulatory decision making.

More specifically, this guidance laid out the cases when the regulations required pharmacogenomic data to be submitted and when the submission of such data would be on a voluntary basis. Depending on the cases, a complete report of pharmacogenomic studies, an abbreviated report, or a synopsis would be submitted. In addition, the guidance addressed when the pharmacogenomic data would be considered sufficiently reliable to serve as the basis for regulatory decision making, when it would be considered only supportive to a decision, and when the data would not be used in regulatory decision making.

The guidance defined categories of biomarkers as exploratory, probably valid, and known valid biomarkers. Although most pharmacogenomic measurements are not considered valid biomarkers, many of those related to drug metabolism have well established mechanistic and clinical significance and are currently being integrated into drug development and clinical practice (Table 3.1) *(11)*. These valid biomarkers are defined as being measured in an analytical test system with well established performance characteristics. They have an established scientific

Table 3.1 DNA-based biomarkers of enzyme activities considered as valid biomarkers

Enzyme	Model drugs	Outcome measures	Study results
CYP2C9	Warfarin	Maintenance dose, Time to reach stable dosing	Patients with *2 and *3 maintained with lower doses and took longer time to reach stable dosing
CYP2C19	Proton pump inhibitors	Plasma levels	Higher in PM (20 mg)
		Gastric pH	
		Gastroesophageal reflux disease cure rate	Higher dose (40 mg) showed no difference
CYP2D6	Codeine	Morphine formation Analgesic effects	Higher in EM
	Atomoxetine	Pharmacokinetic measure	PM higher AUC (10-fold)
UGT1A1	Irinotecan	Grade 3/4 neutropenia	UGT1A1 7/7 and 6/7 more frequent than 6/6
		Pharmacokinetic parameters (AUC ratio of SN38G/SN38)	UGT1A1 *28 and *6 with reduce ratios
TPMT	6-MP	Dose-limiting hematopoietic toxicity	More in TPMT deficiency or heterozygosity

UGT 1A1: uridine diphosphate glucuronosyl transferase 1A1; TPMT: thiopurine methyl transferase; SN-38: an active metabolite of ironotecan: SN-38G: a glucuronide metabolite of SN-38.

framework or body of evidence that elucidates the physiologic, pharmacologic, toxicologic, or clinical significance of the test results. A probably valid biomarker is a biomarker that is measured in an analytical test system with well established performance characteristics and for which there is a scientific framework or body of evidence that appears to elucidate the physiologic, toxicologic, pharmacologic, or clinical significance of the test results. Table 3.2 shows the list of DNA-based biomarkers of enzyme or transporter activity currently considered as exploratory biomarkers.

The guidance gives three decision algorithms or decision trees based on the categories of biomarkers and the stage of drug development. These decision trees can be used to determine when genomic data can be submitted voluntarily, and when submissions of the data are required by FDA regulations. One of the decision trees from the guidance that illustrates the process for submitting pharmacogenomic data to an Investigational New Drug Application (IND) is shown as an example (Fig. 3.2) *(2)*.

In addition, the guidance describes the format for submitting such data. The following is a hypothetical scenario in which a full report of pharmacogenomic data is required for a New Drug Application (NDA) submission *(11)*.

A sponsor conducted a phase 3 clinical trial of a New Molecular Entity (NME) in patients with the target indication. The NME is metabolized primarily by CYP2D6 to an active metabolite equipotent to the parent molecule. The sponsor genotyped a randomly selected subset of the patients for their CYP2D6 alleles to explore the association between genotype, drug dosing, and clinical outcome. The results showed minor differences in clinical outcomes among the genotypes. The information was included in the proposed labeling in the NDA submission.

Table 3.2 DNA-based biomarkers of enzyme or transporter activity currently considered as exploratory biomarkers

Enzyme/ transporter	Model drugs	Outcome measures	Study results
CYP3A4	Testosterone	In vitro metabolism rate	*17 lower activity while *18 higher activity
CYP3A5	Tacrolimus Cyclosporine	Pharmacokinetic parameters	*3 (non-expressor) associated with higher trough plasma concentrations
CYP2B6	Efavirenz	Pharmacokinetic parameters	*6 homozygous associated with higher plasma concentrations
CYP2C8	Repaglinide	Pharmacokinetic parameters	*3 associated with lower plasma concentrations
CYP2A6	Nicotine	Pharmacokinetic parameters	*7, *10 associated with higher nicotine and lower cotinine plasma concentrations
ABCB1 (MDR1)	Digoxin	Pharmacokinetic parameters	TT homozygous C3435T associated with higher plasma concentrations
	Fexofenadine	Pharmacokinetic parameters	TT homozygous C3435 associated with lower plasma concentrations
	Nelfinavir Efavirenz	Pharmacokinetic parameters & Immune recovery	TT homozygous C3435 associated with lower plasma concentrations, and greater rise in CD4 responses
	Antiepileptic drugs	Clinical responses	CC homozygous C3435 associated with drug-resistant epilepsy
ABCA1	Atorvastatin, Simvastatin, Pravastatin	LDL-cholesterol lowering	Higher adjusted mean change in certain HAP markers
OATP-C	Pravastatin	Pharmacokinetic parameters	*15 associated with lower clearance

ABCB1: ATP-binding cassette family (ABC) B1, multi-drug resistance. (MDR1) a human gene that encodes P-glycoprotein; MRP: multi-drug resistance protein. OATP-C: organic anion transporting peptide-C.

4 Examples of How Genetic Information Can Be Used in the Product Labels

As one way to protect public health, the FDA provides safety and efficacy information of drugs in the product package inserts. Several examples of drug labels with pharmacogenetic information are discussed below.

4.1 Labeling Implications

Labeling of approved drug products must be in the format prescribed by the Code of Federal Regulations (21 CFR 201.56). In a final rule of physician labeling, new

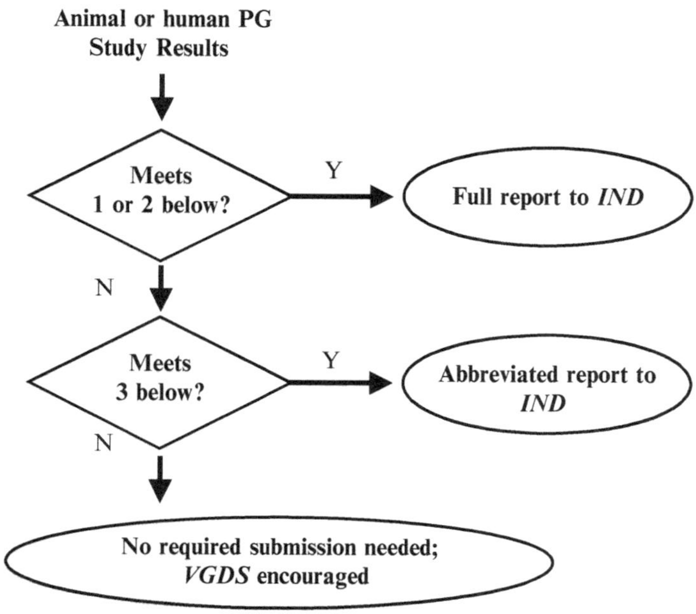

Fig. 3.2 An example of a decision tree for submitting pharmacogenomic data during the IND stage

Pharmacogenomic data must be submitted to the IND under § 312.23 if ANY of the following apply:

1. The test results are used for making decisions pertaining to a specific clinical trial, or in an animal trial used to support safety (e.g., the results will affect dose selection, entry criteria into a clinical trial safety monitoring, or subject stratification).
2. A sponsor is using the test results to support scientific arguments pertaining to, for example, the pharmacologic mechanism of action, the selection of drug dosing, or the safety and effectiveness of a drug.
3. The test results constitute a known, valid biomarker for physiologic, pathophysiologic, pharmacologic, toxicologic, or clinical states or outcomes in humans, or is a known valid biomarker for a safety outcome in animal studies or a probable valid biomarker in human safety studies. If the information on the biomarker (example, human CYP2D6 status) is not being used for purposes 1 or 2 above, the information can be submitted to the IND as an abbreviated report.
   Submission to an IND is NOT required, but voluntary submission is encouraged (i.e., information does not meet the criteria of § 312.23) if
4. Information is from exploratory studies or is research data, such as from general gene expression analyses in cells/animals/humans, or single nucleotide polymorphism (SNP) analysis of trial participants.
5. Information consists of results from test systems where the validity of the biomarker is not established.

content and format requirements are described for the labeling of human prescription drug and biological products *(12)*. Pharmacogenomic data and related information can be described in the following sections as appropriate: Indications and Usage, Dosage and Administration, Contraindications, Warnings and Precautions, Adverse Reactions, Clinical Pharmacology, Drug Interactions, and Use in Specific Populations.

If evidence is available to support the safety and effectiveness of the drug only in selected subgroups of the larger population with a disease, the labeling shall describe the evidence and identify specific tests needed for selection and monitoring of patients who need the drug (21 CFR 201.57).

When patients of a certain genotype show different clinical responses to drugs or biologic products, relevant genomic information may be included in the different sections of labeling. If a genetic test is required prior to prescribing a drug or biologics for a patient or to select a particular dose, pharmacogenomic information may be included in the "Indications and Usage" section (e.g., Herceptin). Other relevant information should be placed in the different sections of the label as appropriate (e.g., HER2 testing under "Precautions," HER2 detection under "Clinical Studies"). When dose reduction is recommended for the specific genotype groups, genetic information can be placed in the "Dosage and Administration" and "Warnings" sections (e.g., Purinethol) with relevant information in other sections such as "Clinical Pharmacology," "Laboratory Test," and "Adverse Reactions." For drugs with no serious adverse events associated with genetics, the genetic information in the package insert can still add useful information so that a patient may avoid or be aware of non-serious adverse events through genetic testing. Such information may be placed in the "Clinical Pharmacology," "Drug Interactions," "Laboratory Test," "Special Populations," or "Adverse Events" sections of the label (e.g., Strattera) *(11)*.

The knowledge of pharmacogenomics can be applied in drug development, but many approved drugs can also benefit from it by understanding how genetics may affect the benefit/risk ratio of the drug. Examples of approved drugs that could benefit from applying pharmacogenetic information into clinical practice are 6-mercaptopurine (6-MP), azathioprine, irinotecan, and warfarin. These drugs have a narrow therapeutic range, wide interindividual variability in dosing requirements, and serious adverse events *(6)*. In recent years, the product labels of 6-MP, azathioprine, irinotecan, and warfarin have been revised to include genetic information. The relabeling efforts to include pharmacogenetics in the product labels are important, since one of the Agency's missions is to protect public health in subgroups of the population who may benefit from the drug as mandated by the regulation.

In recent years, there have been an increased number of product labels with pharmacogenomic information *(13)*. Some of the examples are described below to show how pharmacogenetics can help to optimize the benefit/risk ratio and improve safety profiles.

4.1.1 Azathioprine and 6-Mercaptopurine (6-MP)

Azathioprine (Imuran®) is indicated as an adjunct for the prevention of rejection in renal homotransplantations, and for the management of active rheumatoid arthritis to reduce signs and symptoms *(14)*. 6-MP (Purinethol®) is indicated for maintenance therapy of acute lymphatic (lymphocytic, lymphoblastic) leukemia as part of a combination regimen *(15)*. Azathioprine is metabolized to 6-MP, a substrate of thiopurine methyltransferase (TPMT). TPMP is a polymorphic enzyme and it is responsible for converting 6-MP into **inactive metabolite, methyl-6-MP (6-MeMP). About 10% of Caucasians and African-Americans have intermediate TPMT activity whereas 0.3% of them have low or absent activity. Patients with intermediate or low/absent TPMT activity are at increased risk of myelotoxicity if a conventional dose of azathioprine or 6-MP is administered.** It is important to continue monitoring white blood cell counts in patients receiving azathioprine and 6-MP. TPMT testing, when combined with other tests and observations, can lead to higher-quality decisions about drug selection and drug dosing that will further decrease the risk of severe and preventable bone-marrow toxicity and yet provide the desired benefit from the therapy.

In July 2003, the FDA Pediatric Subcommittee of the Oncology Drug Advisory Committee (ODAC) discussed the pharmacogenetics of 6-MP and whether relabeling with genetic information was warranted *(16)*. Based on the evidence presented, the subcommittee recommended that the label of 6-MP should be updated with TPMP genetic information. According to the ODAC recommendation, Purinethol and subsequently, Imuran product labels were revised to include TPMT genetic information in July 2004 and July 2005, respectively. For the Imuran product label, pharmacogenetic information about TPMP was included in the "Clinical Pharmacology," "Warnings," "Adverse Events," and "Dosage and Administration" sections of the label *(14)*.

Clinical Pharmacology

6-MP undergoes two major inactivation routes. One is thiol methylation, which is catalyzed by the enzyme thiopurine S-methyltransferase (TPMT), to form the inactive metabolite methyl-6-MP (6-MeMP). TPMT activity is controlled by a genetic polymorphism. For Caucasians and African Americans, approximately 10% of the population inherit one non-functional TPMT allele (heterozygous) conferring intermediate TPMT activity, and 0.3% inherit two TPMT non-functional alleles (homozygous) for low or absent TPMT activity. Non-functional alleles are less common in Asians. TPMT activity correlates inversely with 6-TGN levels in erythrocytes and presumably other hematopoietic tissues, since these cells have negligible xanthine oxidase (involved in the other inactivation pathway) activities, leaving TPMT methylation as the only inactivation pathway. Patients with intermediate TPMT activity may be at increased risk of myelotoxicity if receiving conventional doses of IMURAN. Patients with low or absent TPMT activity are at an increased risk of developing severe, life-threatening myelotoxicity if receiving conventional doses of IMURAN. TPMT genotyping or phenotyping (red blood cell TPMT activity) can help identify patients who are at an increased risk for developing IMURAN toxicity.

Warnings

Patients with intermediate thiopurine S-methyl transferase (TPMT) activity may be at an increased risk of myelotoxicity if receiving conventional doses of IMURAN. Patients with low or absent TPMT activity are at an increased risk of developing severe, life-threatening myelotoxicity if receiving conventional doses of IMURAN. TPMT genotyping or phenotyping can help identify patients who are at an increased risk for developing IMURAN toxicity.

Laboratory Tests, TPMT Testing
It is recommended that consideration be given to either genotype or phenotype patients for TPMT. Phenotyping and genotyping methods are commercially available. The most common non-functional alleles associated with reduced levels of TPMT activity are *TPMT*2, TPMT*3A and TPMT*3C.* Patients with two non-functional alleles (homozygous) have low or absent TPMT activity and those with one non-functional allele (heterozygous) have intermediate activity. Accurate phenotyping (red blood cell TPMT activity) results are not possible in patients who have received recent blood transfusions. TPMT testing may also be considered in patients with abnormal CBC results that do not respond to dose reduction.

Adverse Reactions, Hematologic
TPMT genotyping or phenotyping can help identify patients with low or absent TPMT activity (homozygous for nonfunctional alleles) who are at increased risk for severe, life-threatening myelosuppression from IMURAN. Death associated with pancytopenia has been reported in patients with absent TPMT activity receiving azathioprine.

Dosage and Administration
TPMT genotyping or phenotyping can be used to identify patients with absent or reduced TPMT activity. Patients with low or absent TPMT activity are at an increased risk of developing severe, life-threatening myelotoxicity from IMURAN if conventional doses are given. Physicians may consider alternative therapies for patients who have low or absent TPMT activity (homozygous for non-functional alleles). IMURAN should be administered with caution to patients having one non-functional allele (heterozygous) who are at risk for reduced TPMT activity that may lead to toxicity if conventional doses are given. Dosage reduction is recommended in patients with reduced TPMT activity.

4.1.2 Irinotecan

Irinotecan (Camptosar) is an antineoplastic agent of the topoisomerase I inhibitor class. It is indicated as a component of first-line therapy in combination with 5-fluorouracil and leucovorin for patients with metastatic carcinoma of the colon or rectum. It is also indicated for patients with metastatic carcinoma of the colon or rectum whose disease has recurred or progressed following initial fluorouracil-based therapy *(17)*. Irinotecan is hydrolyzed by carboxylesterase enzymes to its active metabolite, SN-38. Enzyme UDP-glucuronosyl transferase 1A1 (UGT1A1) is primarily responsible for inactivation of SN-38, and formation of a glucuronide metabolite. UGT1A1*28, a variant gene, is associated with decreased enzyme activity, and patients with this variation in the UGT1A1 gene are at increased risk of neutropenia from Irinotecan treatment. In November 2004, an FDA Advisory

Committee for Pharmaceutical Science—Clinical Pharmacology Subcommittee (CPSC) meeting was held to discuss the pharmacogenetics of irinotecan *(18)*. Based on the FDA CPSC recommendation, the label of irinotecan was updated in 2005 to include genetic information in the "Clinical Pharmacology," "Warnings," and "Dosage and Administration" sections of the label. Patients who are homozygous for UGT1A1*28 alleles are recommended to start the therapy with a reduced dose *(17)*.

Clinical Pharmacology, Metabolism and Excretion
*The metabolic conversion of irinotecan to the active metabolite SN-38 is mediated by carboxylesterase enzymes and primarily occurs in the liver. SN-38 is subsequently conjugated predominantly by the enzyme UDP-glucuronosyl transferase 1A1 (UGT1A1) to form a glucuronide metabolite. UGT1A1 activity is reduced in individuals with genetic polymorphisms that lead to reduced enzyme activity such as the UGT1A1*28 polymorphism. Approximately 10% of the North American population is homozygous for the UGT1A1*28 allele. In a prospective study, in which irinotecan was administered as a single-agent on a once-every-3-week schedule, patients who were homozygous for UGT1A1*28 had a higher exposure to SN-38 than patients with the wild-type UGT1A1 allele.*

Warnings
Patients with Reduced UGT1A1 Activity
Individuals who are homozygous for the UGT1A1*28 allele are at increased risk for neutropenia following initiation of CAMPTOSAR treatment. A reduced initial dose should be considered for patients known to be homozygous for the UGT1A1*28 allele. Heterozygous patients (carriers of one variant allele and one wild-type allele which results in intermediate UGT1A1 activity) may be at increased risk for neutropenia; however, clinical results have been variable and such patients have been shown to tolerate normal starting doses.

Dosage and Administration
Dosage in Patients with Reduced UGT1A1 Activity
When administered in combination with other agents, or as a single agent, a reduction in the starting dose by at least one level of CAMPTOSAR should be considered for patients known to be homozygous for the UGT1A1*28 allele. However, the precise dose reduction in this patient population is not known and subsequent dose modifications should be considered based on individual patient tolerance to treatment (See Tables 10–13).

4.1.3 Atomoxetine

One of the recent examples of labeling a new drug product with pharmacogenetic information is atomoxetine (Strattera). Atomoxetine, a selective norepinephrine reuptake inhibitor, was approved in November 2002 for the treatment of attention-deficit/hyperactivity disorder (ADHD) *(19)*. It is primarily metabolized by cytochrome P450

2D6 (CYP2D6), a polymorphic enzyme, to 4-hydroxyatomoxetine with a clearance of 0.35 L/hr/kg in CYP2D6 extensive metabolizers (EM) and 0.03 L/hr/kg in CYP2D6 poor metabolizers (PM). About 7% of Caucasians and 2% of African-Americans are PMs of CYP2D6. Patients with reduced CYP2D6 activity (PMs) have higher plasma concentrations of atomoxetine compared with EMs. The area-under-the-curve (AUC) and peak concentrations of atomoxetine are about ten- and fivefold higher in PMs compared with EMs, respectively. The sponsor analyzed the efficacy and safety data in patients identified retrospectively as EMs and compared these data with those identified as PMs. The frequencies of adverse events, such as decreased appetite, insomnia, and sedation, were higher in PMs compared with those of EMs. There were no major differences in serious adverse events between PMs and EMs.

The label of atomoxetine mentions the role of CYP2D6 in the "Clinical Pharmacology," "Precautions," "Laboratory Tests," and "Adverse Reactions" sections of the label. It is stated that "poor metabolizers (PMs) of CYP2D6 have a tenfold higher AUC and a fivefold higher peak concentration to a given dose of Strattera compared with extensive metabolizers (EMs)." Although a pharmacogenetic test for CYP2D6 was not specifically recommended before prescribing the drug, the labeling did provide descriptive information that could be used along with other observations (for example, an adverse event) to guide clinician decisions about an individual's need for dosing adjustment. This example demonstrates that pharmacogenetic information in a package insert including knowledge related to genotype (e.g., CYP2D6*1/*4), phenotype (e.g., PMs), and clinical outcomes (e.g., adverse events) can increase the quality of a clinician's decision about individualizing drug treatment *(6)*, *(19)*.

4.1.4 Warfarin

Warfarin, a widely used anticoagulant with a narrow therapeutic index, was approved in 1954 for the prevention and/or treatment of venous thrombosis, pulmonary embolism, and thromboembolic complications associated with atrial fibrillation and other chronic conditions *(20)*. It is a difficult drug to use, since the optimal dose varies and depends on many clinical and environmental factors including age, gender, diet, and concomitant medications. The major adverse event associated with warfarin therapy is bleeding *(21)*. The risk of bleeding rises with increasing intensity of anticoagulation. There is evidence that genetic testing of cytochrome P450 2C9 (CYP2C9) and vitamin K epoxide reductase complex 1 (VKORC1) will reduce the uncertainty associated with the variability to warfarin response during the induction phase of therapy. Therefore, warfarin dosing could be guided by the knowledge of CYP2C9 and VKORC1 genotypes.

The *S*-enantiomer of warfarin is mainly metabolized to 7-hydroxywarfarin by CYP2C9. Patients with at least one variant allele of CYP2C9*2 or *3 have lower clearance of S-warfarin compared to patients with the wild-type allele (CYP2C9*1). This low clearance results in the need for a lower daily warfarin dose requirement in patients with one or more variant alleles compared to patients with the wild-type allele. Warfarin interferes with clotting factor synthesis by inhibition of VKORC1, thereby reducing the regeneration of vitamin K1 epoxide. Single nucleotide polymorphisms in the VKORC1 gene are associated with reduction in warfarin dose. Together with other empirical risk factors such as age, sex, and body weight, CYP2C9 and VKORC1 can explain as much as 56% of the variability in dose response. Continued monitoring of prothrombin time is important, even with these improvements in dosing. Based on the FDA CPSC recommendation in November 2005 *(22)*, the warfarin label was revised to include pharmacogenetic information on CYP2C9 and VKORC1.

4.1.5 Other Examples

Other examples of product labels with pharmacogenetic information are trastuzumab (Herceptin), erlotinib (Tarceva), cetuximab (Erbitux), rituximab (Rituxan), imatinib (Gleevec), and lapatinib (Tykerb). Trastuzumab, a recombinant DNA-derived humanized monoclonal antibody, is indicated for the treatment of human epidermal growth factor receptor 2 protein (HER2) positive metastatic breast cancer. It is the first drug to be approved on the basis of pharmacogenomic testing. The drug is to be prescribed only if HER2/neu is overexpressed in the tumor *(23)*. Another recent example is the label for erlotinib (Tarceva), which is indicated for the treatment of non-small-cell lung cancer. It is an epidermal growth factor receptor (EGFR) inhibitor. The label states that an apparent larger survival effect in patients with EGFR-positive tumors was observed based on exploratory univariate analyses *(24)*.

These examples demonstrate that pharmacogenetics can contribute to drug safety by guiding healthcare providers with appropriate dosing. However, translating pharmacogenetic information from research to clinical practice is still a challenge for many approved drugs. This is addressed later in the chapter.

5 The Need for Education in Pharmacogenomics

The effort of education about pharmacogenomics should be matched with successful internal efforts within regulatory agencies at training reviewers on the appropriate use and applications of pharmacogenomics *(25)*. This should facilitate the integration of pharmacogenomics into regulatory process, as the FDA scientists and reviewers are more prepared to take on this task. As a part of ongoing training, the FDA held several lecture series and reviewer training courses to educate FDA scientists on the latest developments and research in pharmacogenomics. In addition to offering an introduction on the basic principles of genomics, the courses were designed to promote and create regulatory consensus based on appropriate scientific and regulatory interpretation of genomic data *(25)*. The FDA offers weekly scientific seminars or rounds on various topics, including pharmacogenomics. On a regular basis, the FDA invites speakers from diagnostic and pharmaceutical industries, academia, and institutions such as the National Institutes of Health, to provide different aspects of pharmacogenomics from their own perspectives. It is a valuable experience for the FDA reviewers to participate in these educational programs. Such training opportunities can help the reviewers to implement the use of pharmacogenomics into their review process in a positive manner.

6 What Are the Challenges?

There are several challenges that pharmaceutical industries, regulatory agencies, and healthcare providers face in translating pharmacogenomic information from research into clinical practice. The types of genomic data (e.g., which alleles, what genotypes) that need to be evaluated is one of the critical issues in drug development and regulatory review *(26)*. Additionally, consideration of racial/ethnic differences in the distribution of various alleles with null or reduced metabolic activity to evaluate dose-response relations is important *(11)*. Other potential challenges for translating pharmacogenomic information into the clinical setting are the lack of readily available access to genetic tests, and education for general practitioners. Recently published studies have shown that the extent of drug interactions can be affected by the genotype status of certain metabolic enzymes (Table 3.3) *(11, 27)*. Differences in the extent of drug-drug interactions based on the genotype or phenotype status have been observed, and this type of information has started to appear on the product label. For example, the product label of atomoxetine has the following recommendation: "Dosage adjustment of STRATTERA in EMs may be necessary when coadministered with CYP2D6 inhibitors, e.g., paroxetine, fluoxetine, and quinidine." However, there are no similar precautions for PMs of CYP2D6. The label indicates that "in vitro studies suggest that co-administration of cytochrome P450 inhibitors

Table 3.3 The effects of genotypes on the extent of drug interactions

Substrate (enzyme)	Inhibitor or inducer	Outcome (changes in plasma AUC or concentrations of substrates)
Atomoxetine (CYP2D6)	Fluoxetine, Paroxetine	AUC increase 6–8 fold in EM; no change in PM expected
Metoprolol (CYP2D6)	Diphenhydramine	Higher inhibition in EM vs. PM
Tamoxifen (CYP2D6)	Paroxetine	Greater reduction in plasma levels of endoxifen (active metabolite of tamoxifen formed via CYP2D6) in homozygous EM as compared to patients with at least one variant allele
Diazepam (CYP2C19)	Omeprazole	No inhibition in PM
Omeprazole (CYP2C19)	Fluvoxamine	AUC increased 3–6 fold in EM; no changes in PM
Omeprazole (CYP2C19)	Gingko Bloba	Higher induction in EM

to PMs will not increase the plasma concentrations of atomoxetine," and no dosage adjustments in PM were recommended *(11, 19)*. In order for general practitioners to use such genetic information to consider the different extents of drug interactions, easy access to genetic tests as well as readily available interpretation of the results should be provided at the time of prescribing. Some of the more specific challenges are listed below *(6)*.

- What is the best way to educate healthcare providers about the advantages and limitations of using a genetic test for a drug that they have been using for many years, but still with many adverse events (e.g., warfarin)?
- How should the dosing of a drug (e.g., 6-MP) be adjusted, based on genotype, when there is an absence of prospective clinical trials to demonstrate the efficacy of the reduced dose?
- What alleles should be studied in drug development, and how should this information be translated into a product's package insert?
- How should pharmacogenetic information be reported on the label? This raises two subissues: whether to report only phenotype data (for example, PMs and EMs), or specific alleles of CYP2D6 as well (for example, *3, *4, and *5). And who will interpret the significance of these data with respect to dosing, safety, and efficacy?

Conclusions

The FDA is responsible for protecting the public health by assuring the safety and efficacy of drugs, biological products, medical devices, and food. In addition, the FDA is responsible for advancing the public health by promoting innovations that make medicines and foods more effective, safer, and more affordable; and by helping the public get the accurate, science-based information they need to use medicines and foods to improve their health *(1)*. To fulfill its mission as a public health Agency, the FDA has become a proactive and thoughtful advocate of pharmacogenomics. The FDA is supportive of promoting the use of pharmacogenomics in drug development, and of translating its use into clinical practice. The key initiatives and strategies adopted by the FDA—the critical path white paper, and its advocacy of pharmacogenomics and pharmacogenetics, should be helpful for sponsors considering the submission of genomic data to the agency.

The FDA is aware that despite significant scientific progress, a critical factor in bringing pharmacogenomics "from the bench to the bedside" is educating healthcare professionals about the logistics and benefits of using genetic and genomic information to individualize drug therapy *(11)*. Other challenges are test availability, reimbursement, biomarker validation, and the adoption of pharmacogenomic and pharmacogenetic tests into clinical practice. The FDA will continue to foster genomic-based research and drug development, and the translation of the resulting scientific data to clinical practice.

"Personalized medicine" is the future, with the only remaining question being how soon it will come about *(3)*. "Personalized medicine" will finally become reality when medicine no longer needs to be called personalized medicine to indicate that prescriptions are routinely written for patients based on the unique genetic patterns of polymorphisms in their genes—it will simply be called "medicine" *(5)*.

References

1. U.S. FDA's Mission Statement. http://www.fda.gov/opacom/morechoices/mission.html. Accessed on July 25, 2007.
2. U.S. FDA. Guidance for industry: pharmacogenomic data submissions. http://www.fda.gov/cder/guidance/6400fnl.pdf. Accessed on July 25, 2007.
3. Woodcock J (2007) The prospects for "personalized medicine" in drug development and drug therapy. Clin Pharmacol Ther 81:164–169.
4. FDA. Innovation or stagnation: challenge and opportunity on the critical path to new medical products. http://www.fda.gov/oc/initiatives/criticalpath/whitepaper.html. Accessed on July 25, 2007.
5. Lesko LJ (2007) Personalized medicine: elusive dream or imminent reality? Clin Pharmacol Ther 81:807–816.
6. Lesko LJ, Woodcock J (2004) Translation of pharmacogenomics and pharmacogenetics: a regulatory perspective. Nat Rev Drug Discov 3:763–769.
7. Lesko LJ, Woodcock J (2002) Pharmacogenomic-guided drug development: regulatory perspective. Pharmacogenomics J 2:20–24.
8. Lesko LJ, Salerno RA, Spear BB, Anderson DC, Anderson T, Brazell C, Collins J, Dorner A, Essayan D, Gomez-Mancilla B, Hackett J, Huang SM, Ide S, Killinger J, Leighton J, Mansfield E, Meyer R, Ryan SG, Schmith V, Shaw P, Sistare F, Watson M, Worobec A (2003) Pharmacogenetics and pharmacogenomics in drug development and regulatory decision making: report of the first FDA-PWG-PhRMA-DruSafe workshop. J Clin Pharmacol 43: 342–358.
9. Ruaño G, Collins JM, Dorner AJ, Wang SJ, Guerciolini R, Huang SM (2004) Pharmacogenomic data submissions to FDA: clinical pharmacology case studies. Pharmacogenomics 5:513–517.
10. Salerno RA, Lesko LJ (2006) Three years of promise, proposals, and progress on optimizing the benefit/risk of medicines: a commentary on the 3rd FDA-DIA-PWG-PhRMA-BIO pharmacogenomics workshop. Pharmacogenomics J 6:78–81.
11. Huang SM, Goodsaid F, Rahman A, Frueh F, Lesko LJ (2006) Application of pharmacogenomics in clinical pharmacology. Toxicol Mech Methods 16:89–99.
12. U.S. FDA. Physician labeling, new content and format requirements: FR notice 2006. http://www.fda.gov/cder/regulatory/physLabel/default.htm. Accessed on July 25, 2007.
13. U.S. FDA. Genomics at FDA, table of valid genomic biomarkers in the context of approved drug labels. http://www.fda.gov/cder/genomics/genomic_biomarkers_table.htm. Accessed on July 25, 2007.
14. Imuran product label. http://www.fda.gov/cder/foi/label/2005/016324s030,017391s013lbl.pdf. Accessed on July 25, 2007.
15. Purinethol product label. http://www.fda.gov/cder/foi/label/2004/09053s024lbl.pdf. Accessed on July 25, 2007.
16. U.S. FDA. Pediatric Subcommittee of the Oncology Drug Advisory Committee, 6-MP. http://www.fda.gov/OHRMS/DOCKETS/AC/03/transcripts/3971T1.pdf. Accessed on July 25, 2007.
17. Camptosar product label. http://www.fda.gov/cder/foi/label/2006/020571s030lbl.pdf. Accessed on July 25, 2007.

18. U.S. FDA. Clinical Pharmacology Subcomitte of the Advisory Committe for Pharmaceutical Science. Camptosar. 2004. http://www.fda.gov/ohrms/dockets/ac/04/briefing/2004-4079b1.htm. Accessed on July 25, 2007.
19. Strattera product label. http://www.fda.gov/cder/foi/label/2007/021411s004s012s013s015s021lbl.pdf. Accessed on July 25, 2007.
20. Coumadin product label. http://www.fda.gov/cder/foi/label/2006/009218s102lbl.pdf. Accessed on July 25, 2007.
21. Wysowski DK, Nourjah P, Swartz L (2007) Bleeding complications with warfarin use: a prevalent adverse effect resulting in regulatory action. Arch Intern Med 167:1414–1419.
22. U.S. FDA. Clinical Pharmacology Subcommittee of the Advisory Committee for Pharmaceutical Science. Warfarin. 2005 http://www.fda.gov/ohrms/dockets/ac/cder05.html#PharmScience. Accessed on July 25, 2007.
23. Herceptin product label. http://www.fda.gov/cder/biologics/products/trasgen092598.htm. Accessed on July 25, 2007.
24. Tarceva product label. http://www.fda.gov/cder/foi/label/2004/021743lbl.pdf. Accessed on July 25, 2007.
25. Frueh FW, Goodsaid F, Rudman A, Huang SM, Lesko LJ (2005) The need for education in pharmacogenomics: a regulatory perspective. Pharmacogenomics J 5:218–220 .
26. Andersson T, Flockhart DA, Goldstein DB, Huang SM, Kroetz DL, Milos PM, Ratalin MJ, Thummel K (2005) Drug-metabolizing enzymes: evidence for clinical utility of pharmacogenomic test. Clin Pharmacol Ther 78:559–581.
27. Huang SM, Lesko LJ (2005) Application of pharmacogenomics in clinical pharmacology. In: Knablein J and Muller RH, ed. Molecular Medicine, Correlation between genes, diseases and biopharmaceuticals, in "Modern Biopharmaceuticals-Design, Development and Optimization, vol. 1. VCH: Wiley, 49–70.

Chapter 4
Applications of Pharmacogenomics in Drug Discovery

Dr. Duncan McHale

Contents

Abstract The last decade has seen the increasing use of genetics and genomics tools in the pharmaceutical industry, and much of this use has been in the drug discovery process. These tools are now becoming part of the standard discovery armamentarium and are being used across a range of areas from novel target identification to early predictors of intersubject variability. As with many innovations in the drug discovery process, the true value of pharmacogenomics will take many years to determine, as the new range of molecularly targeted and assessed compounds go through development. The expectation is that the use of the techniques described in this chapter will reverse the current trend of high drug failure rates and hence ensure that the next wave of innovative medicines reaches the waiting patient population.

Keywords drug discovery, CCR5, druggable genome, indication discovery, drug targets, drug metabolising enzymes, toxicogenomics, chemical, compound

1 Introduction

The last decade has seen the application of genomics throughout the drug discovery process. This chapter will cover the use of genomics tools from the very start of the process, with the choice of target, to the choice of chemical lead, and onto preclinical

---

Dr. Duncan McHale
AstraZeneca, Stage3 F347, Alderley House, Alderley Park, Macclesfield, Cheshire, UK
Duncan.McHale@astrazeneca.com

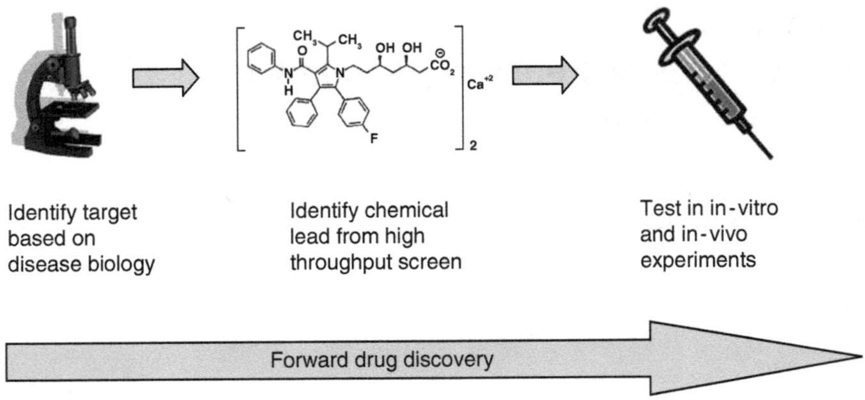

Fig. 4.1 Forward drug discovery process

testing and informing clinical development, finishing with the identification of new diseases for compounds successfully transitioned into the clinic.

Most drug programs follow a straightforward approach starting with the disease of interest, identifying a target based on knowledge of the biology, and screening a compound library for a chemical which will interact with the target, producing the desired effect (Fig. 4.1). This lead is then refined using combinatorial chemistry until a compound can be found with the right combination of properties in terms of affinity for the target, selectivity over closely related proteins, and the physicochemical properties to ensure bioavailability. The chemical is then tested in a range of in vitro and in vivo models to establish its efficacy in disease models and safety in toxicology studies. These tests are then followed by phase 1 studies to establish toleration and pharmacokinetics in humans. At least 2/3 of compounds die before efficacy can be established in the diseases of interest in humans, confirming the target selection was correct. The attrition of unprecedented mechanisms can be as high as 49 in 50 compounds tested, so the majority of compounds will not become drugs.

The single most important decision in all drug discovery programs is the choice of target. The publication of the genome sequence dramatically increased the number of potential targets from approximately 500 that had been worked on for the previous century to over 3000 druggable targets *(1)*. Druggability is defined as being a member of a gene family in which there was at least one established chemical entity. However, it is estimated that only half of these may have disease relevance, and within only a subset of these will pharmacological intervention be safe and well tolerated. The choice of targets is therefore of paramount importance, and genetics and genomics are becoming well established tools in this process. Multiple examples of the success of this approach, e.g., Herceptin, Glivec, Maraviroc, are emerging.

In addition to being the key determinant of the likelihood of success of a drug program, improved understanding of the role of the drug target in the disease aetiology will allow an assessment of likely variability in the drug program. It is possible to use this information to inform the early development plan in order to establish the magnitude of this effect.

Variability in drug response is universally seen with all therapies, regardless of the choice of disease *(2)*. Once the target has been established, then the choice of chemical is the next major determinant of the likely variability in response to the drug. Historically, work to understand this variability has waited until the drug has been tested in humans. Over the last decade technologies have been developed which allow the testing of compounds preclinically in order to predict the likely variability observed in the clinic, allowing plans to minimise its impact, either through the choice of compound or the choice of clinical trial participants in exploratory development.

The development of approximately 20% of all nominated compounds is terminated in preclinical toxicology *(3)*. A further 10% are terminated preclinically due to ADME issues. A further 15% of all compounds entering the clinic fail for safety and toxicity reasons. Pharmacogenomics is being used increasingly to try and predict these toxicity issues early, reducing costs both in terms of animals used and financial costs. Additionally, pharmacogenomics is also being used to understand the mechanisms of adverse reactions in order to determine species specificity and develop risk management plans.

The combination of the increased number of putative drug targets afforded by the genome project and the advances in combinatorial chemistry has resulted in a large rise in potential drug programs. Testing of all these opportunities using a traditional approach is not feasible, due to the large financial costs of running multiple large phase 2b programs before clear efficacy has been established. There is therefore an increasing demand for establishing efficacy early in smaller phase 2a and even 1b studies. One way of increasing the potential for early detection of efficacy is to enrich the early studies with subjects "most likely" to respond to therapy. This enrichment approach requires an improved understanding of the disease biology and the pharmacokinetic variability of the new compound. This knowledge allows enrichment of small efficacy studies by identifying those subjects based on genetic or genomic profiles that will give the most robust efficacy signal. Failure to demonstrate efficacy in this "enriched" group would suggest that efficacy in a wider population is highly unlikely.

Finally, the concept of using genomic approaches to identify new indications for either approved drugs or compounds in development will be briefly discussed.

2 Drug Discovery

The drug discovery process has had a steady evolution over the last 50 years from a pharmacologically driven process to a chemically driven process and now towards a biologically driven process. As a pharmacologically driven process, chemicals were tested across a range of tissues looking for hints of the pharmacological properties required, e.g., smooth muscle relaxation. This approach required no knowledge of the underlying action of the target, and many of these compounds interacted with more than one protein. As biological and chemical techniques developed, so these drugs were improved by improving selectivity for the active drug targets and pharmacokinetic profiles. This reverse drug discovery approach, whereby compounds are selected for their effect on the physiological system of interest, and the drug target it is interacting with is only discovered later, is rarely used now.

Today the majority of drug design is in the forward direction, with the identification of the drug target based on the biological understanding of the disease in question, which is then followed by a series of chemical screens and the development of potential lead material (Fig. 4.1). This forward approach has the distinct advantage that the specific drug target is known, and assays can be designed to establish selectivity from all close family members prior to going into preclinical and clinical testing. This should reduce the number of surprises that are observed in early testing due to off-target pharmacology, and increase our confidence in observing efficacy and safety in later studies.

2.1 Choosing the Target

The choice of drug target is the first and most important decision of any drug discovery and development program. Prior to the publication of the human genome sequence in 2001, the pharmaceutical industry as a whole had worked on approximately 500 different drug targets, and produced licensed drugs based on approximately 120 of these. The publication of the DNA sequence of the human genome revealed that the total number of targets amenable to small chemicals is between 3000 and 5000, although only half of these may have any disease relevance. As the DNA sequence is now freely available, the choice of targets depends upon our biological understanding of the physiology and pathophysiology of the disease process.

Human genetics and genomics approaches are now being broadly used to aid in the choice of targets. The chief advantage of using human tissues is that the data generated is from the diseases that the eventual therapies are hoping to treat. The disadvantages are that many tissues are difficult to access in humans, making mRNA expression studies logistically impossible; and for genetic studies, the available genetic variation is dependent on polymorphisms present in the population.

Genetic studies provide evidence of a causal relationship between the drug target and the disease of interest. Both family-based and population-based approaches have been used, and although there are limited examples of approved drugs where human genetics prospectively predicted therapeutic efficacy, an association between the drug target and the disease has been demonstrated retrospectively in several of today's top selling drug classes, e.g., angiotensin converting enzyme inhibitors and hypertension, Beta agonists and asthma, and serotonin reuptake inhibitors and depression. In addition, several new mechanisms of action currently in late stage development have been triggered by human genetic data, e.g., CCR5 antagonists for HIV therapy and Jak3 Kinase inhibitors for transplant rejection. It is hypothesised that compounds with positive human genetic evidence will have a much greater chance of demonstrating efficacy than compounds identified through animal studies, but this remains to be tested.

In most complex traits and diseases, genetic variation represents minor changes in function in the encoded protein, resulting in changes within normal physiological parameters. It is therefore difficult to estimate the magnitude of effect a potential therapeutic agent will have, since pharmacological blockade or agonism is generally significantly greater than the physiological differences resulting from genetic variation. However, in some instances where clear evidence of the functional effects of a genetic variation are known, a qualitative assessment of the likely therapeutic effect of a pharmacological agent can be estimated. This is most often the case where the variant results in a major impact on the function of the protein, e.g., NaV 1.7 and pain. Major mutations in the SCN9A gene which encodes the voltage gated sodium channel (Na 1.7) have been shown to cause congenital insensitivity to pain and paroxysmal extreme pain *(4)*. Additional work has confirmed that insensitivity to pain is caused by mutations which result in no functional protein, and paroxysmal extreme pain by mutations which result in a hyperexcitable channel. Hence full blockade of the Nav 1.7 channel with a specific antagonist should result in complete analgesia.

The evidence of a statistical association between a genetic variant in the putative drug target and the proposed disease is rarely sufficient on its own to start a drug discovery program. Data demonstrating function, either directly through protein studies or mRNA expression levels, or indirectly through transgenic studies, are usually required. Messenger RNA expression studies are a powerful way of demonstrating the role of a target (or pathway) in a disease process. This is most powerful when human tissue can be used, but in many cases this is not possible and animal model experiments are performed. An increase or decrease in the expression of a particular drug target in the appropriate human tissue, or from a well validated animal model, can significantly strengthen the rationale for that drug target. However, the presence of altered expression provides no evidence of causality, and may just represent downstream changes which, if targeted, would offer no therapeutic value. Hence the combination of genetic and transcriptional data represents the most powerful approach, since it provides evidence of function and causality.

Using genetics and genomics to drive the choice of drug targets in particular indications is not new. The chemokine Receptor 5 (CCR5) antagonist, maraviroc, was based on human genetic data showing that reducing the function of CCR5 via naturally occurring genetic variation (del 32 polymorphism) protects individuals carrying two copies of this polymorphism from HIV infection *(5)*. In addition, we can obtain insights into the safety of reducing the function of CCR5 by studying these subjects who naturally have no functional CCR5 receptor. Maraviroc blocks the entry of HIV through the CCR5 receptor by pharmacologically inhibiting the function of this receptor, thus mimicking the loss-of-function polymorphism known to protect subjects from HIV infection. Phase 3 trials have recently confirmed its efficacy and safety in large populations of subjects infected with HIV.

2.2 *Picking the Right Sequence*

Once a target has been chosen and a suitable biological assay developed, then high throughput screening (HTS) can commence. High throughput screening involves putting millions of chemicals into an assay to see if any interact with the target. This is an expensive process, and it is vital that the most common genetic variant of the target is used, as this is generally only performed once and is often performed in a cloned expression system. Genetic variation is present in all drug targets, although the functional relevance of most of these variants is unknown. Genetic variation can alter either the amino acid sequence of a protein and hence its function, or the levels of expression of the drug target, through either increased or decreasing mRNA production or stability (Fig. 4.2). For HTS purposes, alterations in amino acid sequence are more problematic than changes in expression level, as amino acid substitutions can result in different binding affinities.

Although all drug targets have some genetic variation, 23% of targets have no amino acid changing polymorphisms, whilst 41% have between one and two, and 36% more than two (Fig. 4.3). All putative drug targets should be screened for polymorphic amino acid variation in all populations of interest. The most relevant

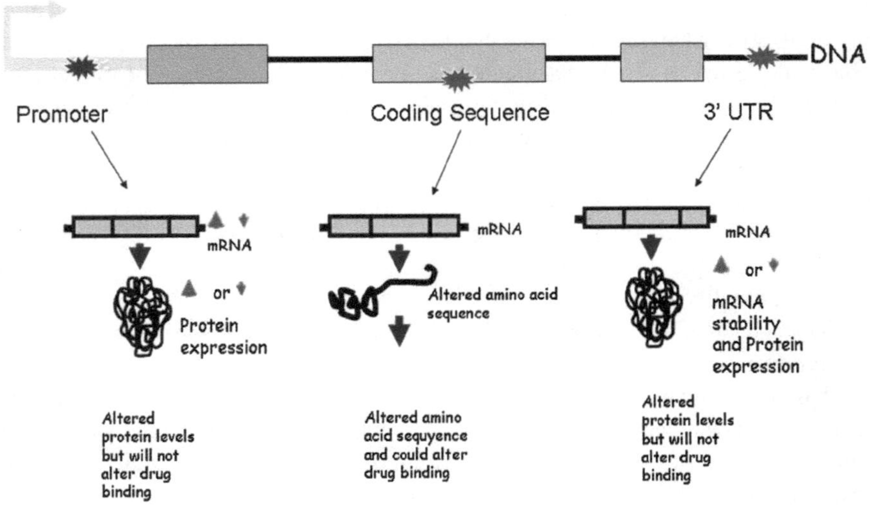

Fig. 4.2 Types of genetic variation and their effects

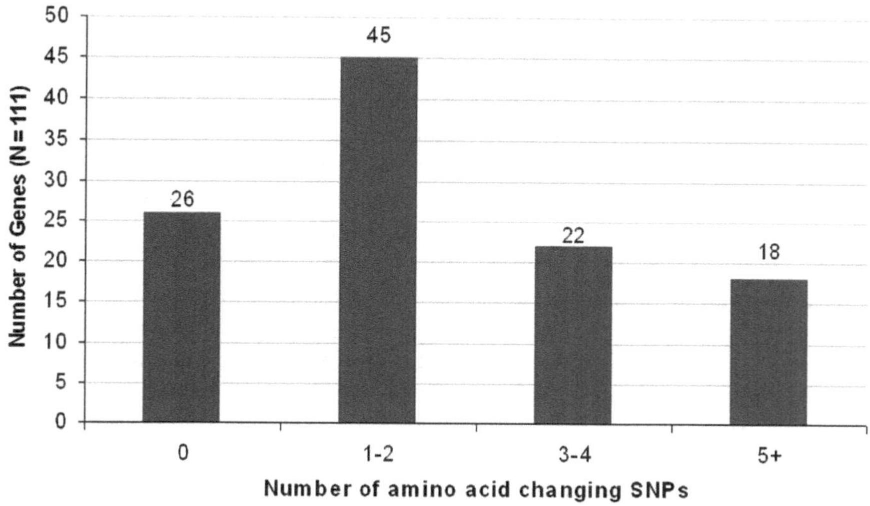

Fig. 4.3 Frequency of amino acid changing polymorphisms in drug target

(usually common) variant should then be chosen for HTS, with additional common variants screened in lead development. The screening of additional common variants against the final chemical chosen is important, since it may provide valuable information to the clinical team, as there may be certain variants against which the binding affinity is so low as to make effective treatment extremely unlikely. It is still unclear as to how often this is likely to be the case, but if assayed prior to clinical development, then the appropriate clinical experiments can be designed to test efficacy across the range of common variants.

2.3 *Choosing the Right Chemical*

The ideal chemical is one which is highly selective for the drug target, has physicochemical properties suited to the particular mode of delivery, has limited pharmacokinetic variability, and binds with similar affinity to all the common protein variants. The first two properties are directly attributable to the chemical structure, whilst the third and fourth result from the interaction between the individual and the chemical. Genetic variation can directly impact this interaction, resulting in variability in drug response. Whilst the true impact of this can only be measured in the clinic, it is possible to do experiments preclinically to identify compounds at increased risk of significant interactions. Since the frequency of the genetic variants responsible for altering the host chemical interaction varies across ethnic groups, the resultant differences in safety and/or efficacy have in the past often been attributed to interethnic variation.

2.4 Understanding the Impact of Common Variation

The most simple pharmacogenomic experiment that can be performed in an effort to understand and/or predict variable drug response is to sequence the drug target. This sequencing needs to be across all ethnic groups likely to receive the drug, and needs to be in a minimum of 25 individuals per ethnic group. This equates to 50 chromosomes per group, which will be sufficient to detect >90% of all SNPs with a frequency of >5%. Genetic variation is routinely seen in all drug targets sequenced with differing distributions across ethnic groups. As would be expected, greater variation is seen in African populations and lesser in Asian. The vast majority of these polymorphisms do not alter the encoded amino acid sequence and probably have no functional effect. Approximately 75% of drug targets sequenced by Pfizer have at least one amino acid changing genetic variant, with >35% having more than three variants. The sequence polymorphism highlights the potential for variability in chemical target interactions, but the true magnitude of this effect can only be tested using in vitro or in vivo models (including clinical trials). When possible, in vitro models should be performed to assess the binding affinities for the common variants. Where this is not possible due to resource or reagent constraints, further refinement may be gained by mapping the position of the variant onto the 3D structure of the drug target and, where known, comparing it to the position of the drug binding site. This can be a powerful tool, but it must be remembered that the 3D structure mapping may not be accurate, as it is often estimated from other protein family members—e.g., the crystal structure of rhodopsin is currently generally used as the base structure for all other GPCR mapping. This approach can be used as a filter with only high risk variants examined in in vitro assays.

3 Toxicogenomics

3.1 Potential Target Organs for Toxicity

Drug toxicity is a major cause of attrition, with approximately 20% of compounds with unprecedented mechanisms failing in preclinical toxicology testing (Fig. 4.4). A further 15% of compounds fail in clinical testing due to unacceptable safety or tolerability findings, despite showing no significant toxicological effects on those with a clear safety margin in animal testing (Fig. 4.4). An ability to predict these events would enable early assessment of the likelihood of developing specific toxicities and rational decision making based on the likely benefits when weighed against the predicted toxicological effects. Pharmacogenomics can aid in this decision making in several ways.

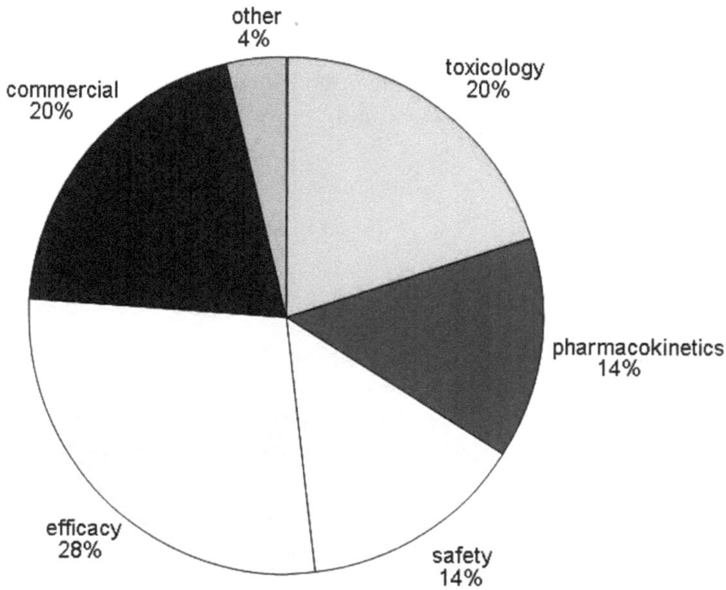

Fig. 4.4 Causes of attrition in drug development

3.2 Early Detection of Toxicity

Toxicogenomics is the use of mRNA profiling to identify specific toxicities, usually in preclinical experiments. The expectation is that by using multiple RNA measurements, greater sensitivity will be gained over more traditional approaches, e.g., histopathology. Recent work has highlighted potential RNA profiles which correlate and predict hepatotoxic, renotoxic, and vasculitic compounds. As more compounds are profiled, then the sensitivity and specificity of these approaches will increase, reducing drug failures due to clinical toxicity.

Toxicogenomics can also be used to identify species specific toxicity, which can be a major problem when toxicological findings are observed in only one of the two species tested in regulatory toxicology studies. An ability to demonstrate that the toxicological effect was confined to the species, offers the opportunity to go on and develop a chemical which would otherwise have been halted.

Pharmacogenomics is also used to identify and then target specific organs for additional study based on expression profiling. Drug toxicity can be divided into mechanistic and structure-based toxicities. The potential for mechanism-based toxicities can be identified through expression profiling with careful histological examination in all organs expressing the target. Structure-based toxicity is due to interactions of the target with other proteins, and is also termed off-target pharmacology, or structure activity related. mRNA profiling can be used in some instances to determine the mechanism of toxicity by identifying the biological pathways that are altered following drug exposure and identifying the likely actual protein(s) binding to the chemical, hence uncovering the mechanism of toxicities. This will become an increasingly powerful tool as our understanding of biological pathways improves.

3.3 Theoretical Safety Concerns

As well as adding confidence in the rationale for drug efficacy, disease genetics can also be used to aid confidence in safety or highlight potential safety concerns. The chemokine receptor 5 (CCR5) antagonist maraviroc was discovered and then developed following the identification of CCR5 as a key coreceptor required for HIV infection. Approximately 1% of Caucasians are homozygous for a major mutation in the CCR5 gene (CCR5 del 32) and produce no CCR5 protein *(5)*. These subjects are very resistant to HIV infection but are otherwise healthy. This data provides both confidence in the rationale of this target for HIV therapies and confidence in the safety of the approach. However, genetic associations have been reported demonstrating an increased risk of infection with West Nile virus in subjects heterozygous and homozygous for the mutation *(6)*. This data suggests that increased rates of infection with West Nile virus could be seen in cohorts of subjects treated with CCR5 antagonists, but this theoretical risk is still to be proven.

The identification of individuals who have congenital insensitivity to pain because they have no functioning Nav 1.7 has provided a strong rationale for the development of NaV 1.7 antagonists as an analgesic agent. The lack of any other clinically significant abnormality provides strong support for this also being a safe mechanism to target, with a low likelihood of mechanistic side effects. However, the expression pattern of Nav 1.7 includes the autonomic nerves creating a theoretical risk of autonomic dysfunction following treatment with a Nav 1.7 antagonist, and this will need to be addressed in the clinical program.

4 Drug Metabolism and Drug Transporters

The human body has evolved a whole range of mechanisms to protect itself from exogenous and toxic compounds. Active transport mechanisms such as the MDR transporter are present on key membrane barriers, e.g., the gut wall and blood brain barriers, and are able to rapidly excrete many diverse chemical structures. Similarly, enzymes have evolved to metabolise a broad range of chemicals which the body comes into contact with daily. These enzymes are broadly split into those catalysing phase 1 reactions, which are typically oxidation, reduction, or hydrolysis reactions;

and phase 2 reactions, which are conjugating reactions (usually with glucuronic acid, sulfonates, glutathione, or amino acids).

4.1 Phase 1 Reactions

Phase 1 reactions are a very common route of drug metabolism and predominantly involve the cytochrome P450 family of enzymes. Drugs may be metabolised by none, one, or more of these enzymes. Genetic variation is commonly observed in the genes encoding these enzymes, and this variation shows marked ethnic diversity. It is not surprising that there is such diversity in these genes, as they are a key defence against exogenous toxins, which vary by location. Selection for variants which increase or reduce the activity of particular enzymes presumably conferred a significant selection advantage in that environment (Fig. 4.5). A good example of this is cytochrome p450 2D6, which is absent in approximately 10% of Caucasians and overexpressed in 20% of Ethiopians. It is unclear what environmental toxins drove this selection, but it results in marked differences in compound metabolism where Cyp 2D6 is the predominant metabolic route. The metabolic route of new compounds is initially established in in vitro assays. The key role of specific cytochrome p450 pathways can be clearly established before administering the drug to humans, but the impact of genetic variation in the metabolic pathway cannot be reliably confirmed using these assays. Therefore, whilst preclinical experiments can highlight which polymorphisms could be important in understanding pharmacokinetic variability, it is not possible to reliably quantify this in vitro.

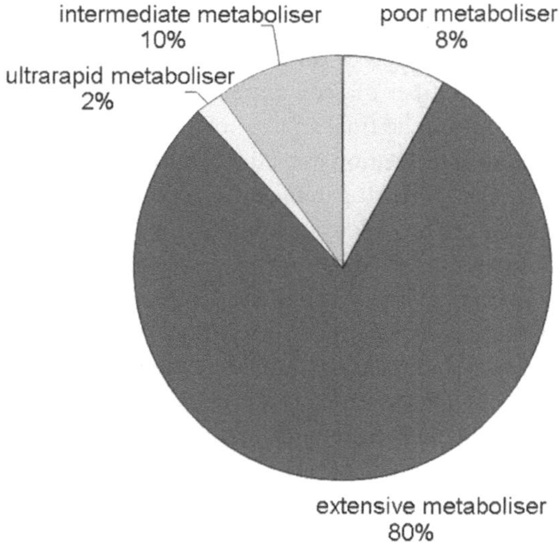

Fig. 4.5 Frequency of Cyp 2D6 phenotypes in caucasians

4.2 Phase 2 Reactions

The vast majority of drugs require some metabolic transformation in order to convert them from lipophilic molecules (desirable for absorption) to more water-soluble molecules (desirable for excretion). The phase 2 reactions are a key component of this process with glucuronidation, acetylation, and sulfonation being the most common routes. These reactions are catalysed by a range of enzymes, many of which are polymorphic. Major polymorphic variation is described in both acetylation and glucuronidation, leading to altered plasma exposures and in some cases adverse events. As with the phase 1 reactions, whilst it is now possible to identify the presence of these metabolic routes, the effect of polymorphic metabolism in these pathways can only be clearly established in man.

4.3 Summary

Preclinical assessment of the metabolic pathways due either to phase 1 reactions or to phase 2 reactions generally predicts the common pathways reliably. However, the impact of genetic variation in these pathways on the interindividual variability in pharmacokinetics can only be accurately measured in the clinical development program.

5 Making the Most Out of Your Chemicals

5.1 Druggable Genome

The intersection of the proportion of the human genome that is tractable to chemical intervention and the number of drug targets that are relevant to human disease may be as few as 600–1500. The final subset not considered in this analysis is those where pharmacological intervention would be tolerated—the pharmacologically tolerant genome. This is a difficult parameter to estimate, as our willingness to tolerate adverse effects of drugs varies considerably depending on the disease being treated and the seriousness of the adverse event. Even if we are optimistic, our ability to tolerate pharmacological intervention of these targets may reduce the total number of tractable targets by a further third (Fig. 4.6).

The high attrition rates and relatively limited number of drug targets highlight the need to ensure that all potential diseases which could be treated by a new mechanism of action are identified, once the safety of the prototype compound has been established. Identifying new indications for proven drugs has been used with great success in the past, meeting significant areas of medical need, and adding billions of dollars to the commercial value of products. On average, 40% of sales from blockbuster drugs are derived from alternative indications. Good examples include gabapentin, originally developed as an antiepileptic medication which subsequently showed

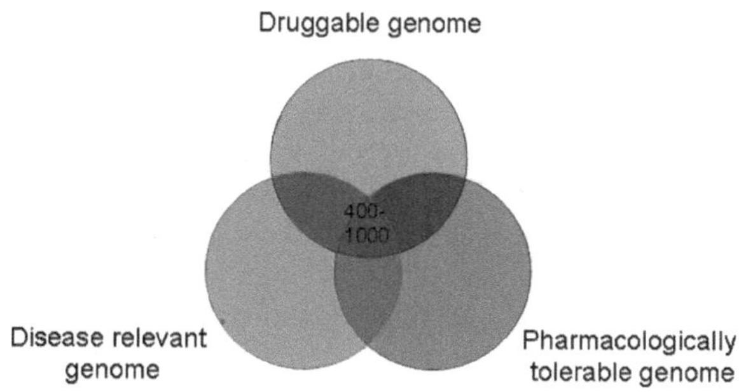

Fig. 4.6 Number of likely drug targets for small chemical intervention

efficacy in neuropathic pain; and sildenafil, developed for erectile dysfunction and subsequently demonstrated to offer a major advance in the treatment of primary pulmonary hypertension. Some of these alternative indications are initially identified in small studies run by independent academics following drug approval, and others are from case reports detailing unexpected benefits of therapies. The challenge is how to systematically identify and evaluate these opportunities earlier in the drug development and approval process. A key advantage of this cross-disease application is the ability to discover novel associations linking a particular drug being studied in one disease area to that of an unrelated disease, and where the only major attrition risk left is lack of efficacy. Attrition due to lack of efficacy represents approximately 1/3 of the total risk in developing drugs to unprecedented targets. Historical data would suggest therefore that these targets have approximately a 1 in 15 probability of success compared with a only a 1 in 50 probability of a novel chemical with a new mechanism of action. Only empirical data will enable us to measure whether this approach will impact attrition in development. Nonetheless, there is precedence for this approach resulting in significant clinical benefit. If sufficient efficacy is observed in only one of these indications, it will still represent a huge return on investment.

5.2 Genetic Approaches

Genetics can be used to find new indications for drugs in development (or post approval) by studying the effect of genetic variation in the drug target and correlating this with disease risk across a wide range of diseases.

The general approach is to study the genetic variation of the proposed target using DNA samples from well characterised sets of patients in all diseases of interest. It is now well accepted that for there to be confidence in the data resulting from these types of studies, they need to be well powered (often with sample sizes exceeding 1000 subjects), clinically well characterized, and the results replicated independently. As described earlier, most targets screened (>75%) have polymorphisms which result in amino acid changes. As well as these nonsynonymous changes, all drug targets are genetically polymorphic at the DNA level, and although these changes do not alter the protein sequence, many reside in regions of conserved sequence and could potentially influence RNA regulation. It is therefore possible to use this genetic variation as a surrogate for protein function (activity or levels) and compare that to disease risk across a whole range of diseases. This can be done by taking an individual target approach, or more broadly by evaluating genetic variation in large numbers of targets (and pathways), defined either by chemical doability representing the druggable genome, or a subset of the chemical genome defined by the availability of lead matter. This candidate gene approach can then be used to look for genetic associations across all diseases of interest for the company in question. Specific high density genotyping chips can be designed and built, to allow multiple experiments to be performed.

The density of the SNP coverage of these indication discovery chips is often greater than that used in whole genome scan experiments, and allows a greater coverage of rarer variants. This is important for a set of genes, where even a small effect could highlight a major benefit if pharmacological blockade was used rather than the naturally occurring variation assayed using human genetics. As the density of the whole genome scan chips increases, and the techniques are developed to impute rare variants from this data, then the value of custom designed chips will reduce. For the initial experiments, a minimum of 500 cases and 500 matched controls is used per case control experiment, and 1000 subjects for quantitative traits. Even with these numbers, many real associations will not stand up to rigorous statistical corrections for multiple testing, and false discovery rates will be high. Hence it is vital that replication approaches are considered early and put in place to add confidence to the initial experiment. The "replication" may not necessarily be a second genetic association study, since some diseases have animal models which can be used on a smaller number of compounds, and many genes now have published transgenic phenotype data available, providing insight into the biological consequences of up or down regulation. The genetic association literature also offers a source of replication data, which will become more useful as the quality of these studies improves. Use of the literature data must be done with care, as there is huge variation in the quality of the published experimental data, and a considered meta-analysis of all available studies will be required *(7)*.

5.3 Genomic Approaches

Transcription approaches can also be used to identify additional indications, and this is likely to be a very powerful tool when human tissue can be obtained from the diseased organ, e.g., oncology and inflammation. The challenge will be to identify those changes which are driving the pathology and hence will be important to target, versus secondary changes.

6 Summary

Pharmacogenomics is defined as the investigation of variations of DNA and RNA characteristics as related to drug response. The impact of interindividual variation of DNA and RNA characteristics on drug response can only be truly established in clinical studies, but preclinical work can be done to predict these effects. Genomics can improve decision making, from the earliest decision of which target to process, through choice of chemical lead, and finally to choice of patient population. This can be divided into understanding the molecular pathology of the disease, understanding the interactions between the compound and the genetic variants of the drug target and its metabolic pathway, and predictions of the likely variability in clinical trials and optimal early populations. Early considerations and experiments allow the predictions of these effects, leading to informed clinical development plans and reduced attrition. The goal of getting the right drug to the right patient at the right dose starts early in discovery and is most efficiently performed when it is integrated early into the discovery and development plans.

7 References

1. Hopkins AL, Groom CR (2002) The druggable genome. Nat Rev Drug Discov. 1(9):727–30.
2. Silber BM (2000) Pharmacogenomics, biomarkers and the promise of personalised medicine. In: Sadée W (ed) Pharmacogenetics-Pharmacogenomics. American Association of Pharmaceutical Scientists.
3. Kola I, Landis J (2004) Can the pharmaceutical industry reduce attrition rates? Nat Rev Drug Discov 3:711–5.
4. Cox JJ, Reimann F, Nicholas AK, Thornton G, Roberts E, Springell K, Karbani G, Jafri H, Mannan J, Raashid Y, Al-Gazali L, Hamamy H, Valente EM, Gorman S, Williams R, MchHale DP, Wood JN, Gribble FM, Woods CG (2006) An SCN9A channelopathy causes congenital inability to experience pain. Nature 444(7121):894–8.
5. Samson M, Libert F, Doranz BJ et al (1996) Resistance to HIV-1 infection in Caucasian individuals bearing mutant alleles of the CCR-5 chemokine receptor gene. Nature 382(6593):722–5.
6. Glass WG, McDermott DH, Lim JK, Lekhong S, Yu SF, Frank WA, Pape J, Cheshier RC, Murphy PM (2006) CCR5 deficiency increases risk of symptomatic West Nile virus infection. J Exp Med 203(1):35–40.
7. Wheeler J, McHale M, Jackson V, Penny M (2007) Assessing theoretical risk and benefit suggested by genetic association studies of CCR5: experience in a drug development programme for maraviroc. Antivir Ther 12(2):233–45.

Chapter 5
Applications of Pharmacogenomics in Clinical Trials

Monique Franc

Contents

Abstract Despite some initial resistance, pharmacogenomics is now finding widespread use and application throughout all phases of clinical drug development in many pharmaceutical companies. Applications, feasibility, and deliverables of pharmacogenomic studies are largely dictated by sample sizes, availability of clinical (phenotypic) endpoints, and existence of working hypotheses, and therefore vary with the phase of clinical development. Variability in a given clinical endpoint is the main driver and prerequisite for pharmacogenomic investigations. Applications can therefore readily be classified into three broad categories of clinical endpoint: pharmacokinetics, efficacy, and safety, although there may be overlap among categories depending on underlying mechanisms. Applications range from mechanistic, regulatory, trial design (inclusion/exclusion), product differentiation, companion diagnostics, and portfolio decision-making. The promise of pharmacogenomics has been advertised for some time. We are gradually beginning to see the fruits of our labors in the context of the pharmaceutical industry, as apprehensions surrounding this technology fade in favor of recognition that a better understanding of our compounds is beneficial in the long run. In an industry that is hungry for innovation, alternative approaches, even if associated with some unknowns and some risks, are imperative. More developments are expected as experience with the application of pharmacogenomics grows (including both successes and failures) and as the industry continues

Monique Franc
Johnson and Johnson Pharmaceutical Research and Development, L.L.C., 1000 Route 202, Raritan, NJ 08869
mfranc@prdus.jnj.com

N. Cohen (ed.) *Pharmacogenomics and Personalized Medicine*,

to work both competitively and collaboratively to realistically apply this technology toward therapeutic innovation and evolution of the basic science.

Keywords Pharmacogenomics, applications, clinical trials, pharmaceutical industry

1 General Introduction

Despite the relatively short history of pharmacogenomics in pharmaceutical drug development, this science has become increasingly accepted as a means of better understanding data generated in the context of classical drug development and as a tool for innovation in this highly competitive arena. Variability in drug response, be it relevant to pharmacokinetics, efficacy, or safety, may be influenced, in part, by genetic variability in genes encoding proteins involved in drug metabolism, drug mode of action (i.e., intended targets), off-target mechanisms (i.e., unintended targets), or in disease susceptibility/etiology. In simple terms, pharmacogenomics is the investigation of the relationship between genetic variability in these pathways and variability in clinical parameters following drug exposure. This chapter is intended to provide a broad overview of opportunities for pharmacogenomic studies in clinical trials involving human subjects. It is not intended to be a review of the successful applications of pharmacogenomics reported in the literature, nor is it intended to fuel the hype of the promise of pharmacogenomics to revolutionize the pharmaceutical industry. Rather, it is an overview of the current application of this methodology based on the author's experience with the evolution of pharmacogenomics in an industry setting.

2 Phases of Drug Development and Potential Pharmacogenomic Opportunities

The goals and applications of pharmacogenomic studies in clinical trials will tend to parallel those of the stage of clinical development. A paradigm that applies to early development studies may not be appropriate in later stages, and vice versa. Applications and deliverables will depend largely on sample size, availability of clinical endpoints, and the existence of working hypotheses. It goes without saying that the availability of genomic samples and appropriate corresponding informed consent is a prerequisite for the conduct of pharmacogenomic research in clinical trials. The four phases of drug development (I, II, III, IV) each have their own focus and consequently offer different opportunities for pharmacogenomic contributions, described below.

- Phase I clinical trials are primarily intended to assess pharmacokinetic (PK) properties and preliminary safety of investigational new drugs. These trials are customarily conducted in healthy volunteers and include single ascending dose, multiple ascending dose, bioavailability/bioequivalency, drug-drug interaction (DDI), food effect, metabolite profiling (using radio-labeled drugs), QT-prolongation, and special populations (hepatic and renal impairment, geriatric, and ethnicity bridging). The focus of pharmacogenomics in Phase I is therefore on drug metabolism/disposition and on safety. Owing to small sample sizes that are characteristic of Phase I studies, pharmacogenomic analyses often are hypothesis-generating in nature and may include i) explaining unexpected variability in pharmacokinetic data, ii) supporting metabolic pathway information from preclinical studies, iii) eliminating concern for classical polymorphic enzymes on drug exposure, or iv) helping to explain adverse events. Pharmacogenomics may also be applied prospectively as an inclusion/exclusion criterion. In the interest of maximizing efficiency, Phase I trials will occasionally incorporate surrogate efficacy endpoints that are measurable even in healthy volunteers (e.g., cholesterol levels for lipid-lowering drugs, sleep-wake cognition for sleep disorder drugs; blood pressure for cardiovascular drugs). Therefore, it is possible to encounter pharmacodynamic-related pharmacogenomic studies in Phase I. Pharmacogenomic information can lead to development decisions such as dose selection and prediction of drug-drug interactions or to the generation of hypotheses for further expansion in later phases of development. The greatest limitation to pharmacogenomics in Phase I is sample size, which can be overcome in some cases through meta analysis of data across trials.

- Phase II clinical trials are therapeutic exploratory trials designed to establish efficacy and assess short-term safety/tolerability and pharmacokinetics (dose finding). These trials may be conducted in the intended diseased population or in human models of the disease (e.g., CCK4 treatment of healthy subjects for the investigation of anxiolytic drugs). Phase II trials may also be conducted to explore secondary indications while the primary indication is undergoing Phase III development. The inclusion of pharmacogenomic analyses in Phase II may be used to develop hypotheses to i) help explain unexpected variability in the pharmacokinetic or pharmacodynamic data, ii) provide preliminary support for mode of action *in vivo*, iii) identify responder subgroups for better decision-making in Phase III trials, and iv) help to explain safety outcomes. The use of pharmacogenomics at this stage may influence attrition (positively or negatively), particularly for compounds with variable efficacy.
- Phase III clinical trials (also referred to as late development trials) are therapeutic confirmatory studies designed to assess efficacy and safety in large numbers of patients in order to generate the required data for drug registration. The focus of pharmacogenomic studies will therefore be on efficacy and safety, although pharmacokinetic endpoints may also be investigated if sparse PK sampling is conducted. Inclusion of pharmacogenomics in this phase of development is especially useful to identify new genetic markers or to confirm hypotheses emerging from earlier phases. With the significantly larger sample sizes, the power to detect genetic associations is greatly improved, although it may still be necessary to pool data across trials in a meta-analysis. Outcomes may include i) label information, ii) focused approval for targeted populations, iii) differentiation from competitors, and iv) identification of novel pathways for the development of next-generation

compounds. Depending on the application, trials that are prospectively designed to test a pharmacogenomic hypothesis with sufficient power may be required by regulatory agencies.

- Phase IV clinical trials may be undertaken for additional product differentiation, pharmacoeconomics, or to assess long-term safety. Pharmacogenomic studies in Phase IV may therefore potentially be applied to extend patent life for unique subpopulations within the general treatment population, or to address pharmacoeconomic concerns held by payers and government bodies in the case of marginal drug efficacy. Regrettably, the current lack of incentives or regulatory framework to facilitate these applications has made it more challenging to justify pharmacogenomic research post-marketing. However, preliminary signs that incentives are imminent have already emerged, e.g., proposed bill to improve and expand the use of molecular genetic tests and therapies; (Senator Barack Obama, 109th congress, 2nd session, 2006).

Since each phase of drug development can involve the evaluation of pharmacokinetics, efficacy, or safety measurements, the detailed applications of pharmacogenomics described herein are partitioned according to these three phenotypic categories. However, it should be recognized that there may be overlap among categories. For example, variability in pharmacokinetics may be a key determinant of efficacy or of safety. Similarly, a safety event may be the byproduct of agonism/antagonism of the intended drug target (i.e., extension of the efficacy). For simplicity, applications related to efficacy below will refer primarily to target-related pathways (i.e., mode of action) and safety will refer primarily to unintended pharmacodynamic pathways. Pharmacokinetics will be described separately, regardless of the consequent impact on efficacy or safety, or lack thereof.

3 Applications to Pharmacokinetics

Pharmacogenomic studies related to pharmacokinetics involve the analysis of genes encoding proteins that are known or hypothesized to be involved in absorption, distribution, metabolism, and elimination (ADME) of a given drug. It is not uncommon to encounter the declaration that, "*This drug is not metabolized by a polymorphic enzyme, therefore no pharmacogenomic investigations are necessary*". Unfortunately this blanket statement can lead to lost opportunities. The key operative terms are *not metabolized by* and *polymorphic enzyme*. Regarding the former, it should be appreciated that, more often than not, drug metabolism will involve multiple enzymes, each contributing a fraction to the overall metabolism. Both major and minor routes of metabolism may be involved. Although major routes of metabolism may be the key determinants of exposure to the parent compound, minor routes of metabolism may also be important. A classical example is the metabolism of the prodrug codeine to the active moiety morphine. It is via a minor route of metabolism (O-demethylation via CYP2D6, that accounts for less than 10% of codeine metabolism) that morphine is formed *(1)*. When analyzed in relation to CYP2D6 metabolizer status, the impact of genetic polymorphisms on codeine exposure is not detectable (since this is a minor route of metabolism), whereas when analyzed in relation to the minor metabolite exposure (morphine), the pharmacogenomic relationship becomes very apparent and has clinical implicatons for efficacy and for risk of developing dependence *(2–8)*. Furthermore, it is well known that minor routes of metabolism can have important safety implications (e.g., due to formation of minor reactive metabolites). Investigations should therefore not be limited to parent-compound exposure. Where metabolites that are hypothesized to have clinical implications are measured, the impact of genetic polymorphism on metabolite formation should be considered. Regarding the latter term, *polymorphic enzyme*, this term is often used to refer exclusively to the classical polymorphic enzymes CYP2D6, CYP2C9, and CYP2C19. It is important to recognize that there are other drug metabolising enzymes that carry polymorphisms that are of clinical consequence (e.g., NAT2 and sulfamethazine, GSTM1 and GSTT1 and tacrine, SULT1A1 and tamoxifen, UGT1A1 and irinotecan, ADH1B/ALDH2 and ethanol, to name a few). Genotyping of the genes encoding these enzymes should therefore be considered for drugs that are known or hypothesized to be metabolized via these pathways.

3.1 Help Explain Outliers or Variability in Pharmacokinetic Data

Some of the original applications of pharmacogenomics were to explain variability in drug metabolism that could not be explained by other factors. Since variability in pharmacokinetics can have implications for efficacy and safety, it is desirable to minimize and understand the factors that contribute to PK variability. Variability may refer to a small number of outliers or to a wide spread in the distribution of the pharmacokinetic data. Pharmacogenomics can also find a use in ruling out a role for genetics in PK variability. For example, genetic causes may need to be ruled out in support of other suspected explanations for unexpected variability (e.g., suspected noncompliance). Understanding the mechanisms of variability in drug exposure can help to customize drug dosing to enhance the safety and efficacy profiles of new therapeutic agents.

3.2 Support Metabolic Pathway Information from In Vitro Studies

Drug-drug interactions are a significant factor contributing to the early termination of drug candidates or to the withdrawal of therapeutic agents after their introduction to the market. Over the past two decades, a number of preclinical and *in vitro* methodologies such as cDNA expression systems and microsomal models have allowed early identification of the specific CYP450 isoforms that likely play a role in the disposition of drugs. Preclinical drug metabolism studies provide a valuable qualitative indication of the potential fate of drugs in humans. However, the quantitative scaling of *in vitro* data to the clinically relevant context is limited. In addition, the scope of preclinical drug metabolism studies usually focuses on CYP450 isoforms or select drug transporters such as P-glycoprotein. Some drug metabolizing enzymes (notably the glucuronidating enzymes) are not as amenable to *in vitro* assays. The knowledge of isozyme-specific metabolism patterns of a drug may also contribute to predictions involving selection of concomitant medications that may precipitate mechanism-based drug-drug interactions. In accordance with these theoretical and conceptual predictions, regulatory authorities and the pharmaceutical industry are keenly aware of the need for adequate and early characterization of drug metabolism in humans.

It is against this background that clinical pharmacogenomic studies of drug-metabolizing enzymes offer an additional and complementary perspective on the nature of metabolic routes and their quantitative significance for disposition in the clinical setting. One of the key features of pharmacogenomic analyses in clinical trials is that the information generated is relevant to the human context. Genotyping for polymorphic drug metabolizing enzymes and subsequent correlation with interindividual variability in pharmacokinetic endpoints can discern whether, and to what extent, a given drug-metabolizing enzyme or drug transporter contributes to drug disposition in humans. There are a number of potential paradigms for the application of pharmacogenomics and the selection of candidate genes to support metabolic pathway information from preclinical studies (described below). There is no one correct approach. Selection will often reflect the corporate climate and investment in pharmacogenomics.

- **Strong candidate gene(s):** This strategy is guided by preclinical drug metabolism data. It proposes a threshold value (e.g., 30%) for the fraction metabolized by a given polymorphic isozyme to warrant genotyping of a candidate gene.
- **All candidate genes:** This strategy proposes genotyping of any ADME gene shown *in vitro* or speculated (based on metabolite profiling) to be involved in metabolism/disposition of the drug. There are no quantitative thresholds in this approach.
- **Standard panel of classically polymorphic ADMEs or ADMEs that metabolize most pharmaceuticals:** This approach involves the routine screening of a short panel of genes encoding enzymes/transporters that metabolize/transport most drugs and are known to harbor functional polymorphisms (e.g., *CYP2C9, CYP2C19, CYP2D6, CYP2A6, CYP2B6, CYP3A5, UGTs,* and *ABCB1*). This approach allows for the identification of clinically relevant pathways that may not otherwise have been explored based on preclinical information. It may also help with the forecasting of variability in drug exposure in the different ethnic populations since the distribution of ADME polymorphisms across ethnicities is known.

- **Broad screen of a large panel of ADME genes:** Some companies have opted to routinely genotype subjects for a large number of ADME genes using available ADME gene chip technologies. The question of overgeneration of potentially uninterpretable data is a legitimate one. However, the broad screen approach does offer a unique opportunity to yield novel hypotheses that are independent of preexisting information.

3.3 Subject Enrollment (Inclusion/Exclusion)

- **Exclusion Criterion:** The overall goals of subject exclusion by genotype include i) the efficient testing of clinical trial hypotheses, ii) smaller trial sizes, and iii) unnecessary exposure of subjects who would otherwise not contribute to the objectives of the trial. Subject selection by genotype during prescreening may be desirable when it is known that certain genotype subtypes would not contribute to the objective of the trial. For example, in ADME-DDI trials that make use of a probe drug (e.g., dextromethorphan/CYP2D6, tolbutamide/CYP2C9, omeprazole/CYP2C19) to evaluate the metabolism by or induction/inhibition of a given isozyme by an investigational drug, subjects having no enzyme activity (i.e., poor metabolizers) would not yield useful data toward the hypothesis being tested in the trial. Excluding poor metabolizers from such a trial would not mean that this metabolizer phenotype would need to be excluded from all future studies since the reason for exclusion is unique to the objective of the study. In contrast, the exclusion of subjects may not be appropriate in comedication-DDI studies that are intended to investigate the potential interaction between two drugs that are expected to be taken in tandem in the eventual intended population since it is important to generate pharmacokinetic and safety data in subjects carrying all genotypes that would be encountered in the general population receiving these two drugs. However, if a specific genetic subgroup of subjects is systematically excluded from a clinical program, a corresponding diagnostic test may be a prerequisite for prescribing the drug.
- **Inclusion Criterion:** Subject selection by genotype during prescreening can be used to ensure adequate enrollment of subjects of a particular genotype for statistical reasons, or to create a balanced population to ensure that all metabolizer subtypes are captured in the clinical trial. One form of balanced population includes proportions of subjects from each genetic subgroup that are genetically representative of the targeted population. For example, approximately 7% of Caucasians are poor metabolizers (PMs) of CYP2D6. One can envision a scenario in which, by chance, no poor metabolizers get enrolled in a clinical trial. It may therefore be desirable to ensure that the appropriate ratio of metabolizer subtypes (7% PMs to 93% non-PMs) be enrolled in order to estimate the drug pharmacology in a representative

population. Alternatively, one can envision a situation in which, by chance, a disproportionate number of poor metabolizers are enrolled in a trial, thus significantly compromising the interpretation of the data and the outcome of the trial. Another form of a balanced population may involve equal numbers of all known metabolizer categories in order to thoroughly evaluate clinical outcomes in these genetic subgroups. The benefit of using the genotype as an inclusion criterion is ensuring that clinical evaluations are conducted in appropriate genetic subpopulations, thus avoiding the need for additional trials.

3.4 Summary of Deliverables for Pharmacokinetics

- Explain observed outliers or pharmacokinetic variability for improved interpretation of the data.
- Adjust dose based on genetic variability in drug metabolism.
- Address regulatory concerns about pharmacokinetic variability, dosing, and safety.
- Forecast the pharmacokinetic variability in different ethnic populations.
- Identify key isozymes involved in the metabolism of a drug in humans.
- Maximize trial efficiency by excluding subjects who would otherwise not contribute to the goals of the trial (e.g., in ADME-DDI studies).
- Ensure that drug pharmacokinetics were indeed examined in poor and extensive (and other) metabolizers alike.

4 Applications to Efficacy

Pharmacogenomic studies related to efficacy are based on the reality that drugs are generally not effective in 100% of patients. The percentage of responders to non-responders deemed acceptable is largely dependent on the severity of the indication and the availability of alternative therapies. Drug responsiveness may have an underlying genetic component and can originate at several levels i) pharmacokinetics (discussed above), ii) pharmacodynamics (i.e., intended drug target or pathway-related), or iii) disease etiology/subtype. There are numerous reports in the literature of genetic associations between polymorphisms in drug targets and pharmacologic responses, some replicated, others not, and yet others with contradictory results. Examples include i) ß-adrenoceptor *ADRB2* and bronchodilation by albuterol in the treatment of asthma *(9–13)*, ii) angiotensin-converting enzyme *ACE* with sensitivity to ACE inhibitors in the treatment of hypertension *(14)*, iii) sodium channel subunit *SCN1A* and maximum doses for carbamazepine and phenytoin in the treatment of epilepsy *(15, 16)*, and iv) vitamin K epoxide reductase *VKORC1* and anticoagulation by acenocoumarol *(17, 18)*, to name a few. The genotyping of drug targets, where these are known for an investigational drug, can provide several opportunities in a drug development setting. Disease etiology/subtype has also been shown to influence efficacy and can similarly be explored to stratify subjects according to response *(19, 20)*. Regardless of the origin or nature of the marker, an efficacy-related marker may demonstrate either that efficacy is i) not appreciably influenced by genetic variability in candidate pathways, ii) lesser in a given genetic subgroup, but not sufficiently compromised to influence treatment decisions, iii) insufficient in a given subgroup to warrant treatment with a particular drug, or iv) better in a given subgroup than average (i.e., super-responders). It should be recognized that most pharmacogenomic biomarkers are probabilistic in nature and generally are not absolute predictors of response. Therefore, the terms "responders" and "nonresponders" should be defined with this consideration in mind. The principles of sensitivity, specificity, positive and negative predictive value, and prevalence that are relevant to other biochemical biomarkers are also applicable to pharmacogenomic biomarkers.

4.1 Informed Strategic Decisions (Go/No-Go Decisions)

Investigating and understanding the genetic factors that contribute to variability in efficacy does not inevitably imply that a diagnostic test will be required for a drug to be prescribed. It is noteworthy that, to date, there are only two examples of biomarker tests that are prerequisites for prescription, namely, the test for HER2 overexpression for treatment of breast cancer with Herceptin® (trastuzumab), and the test for EGFR expression for treatment of colorectal cancer with Erbitux® (cetuximab); all other current valid biomarkers are either merely "recommended" or "for information only" according to U.S. Food and Drug Administration (FDA) classification *(21)*. Furthermore, replication and validation of genetic associations are necessary to generate results that are sufficiently robust to yield a diagnostic test. Consequently, the lingering apprehensions around embarking on pharmacogenomic research to identify biomarkers related to efficacy are generally unjustified.

Putative genetic associations with efficacy are already being used in the pharmaceutical context to contribute to strategic go/no-go decisions about whether to terminate or to rescue a compound that demonstrates variable, borderline, or insufficient efficacy. On the one hand, a decision may be made to terminate development if it is determined that a diagnostic biomarker would likely be a prerequisite for prescription and therefore not commercially viable in a particular therapeutic area. On the other hand, a decision may be made to attempt to rescue a drug or a secondary indication that otherwise would not survive the go/no-go decision to transition into late development. Such decisions involve a number of considerations, including the severity of the indication the availability of existing therapies, the competitor landscape, and diagnostic development capabilities, among others. The ability to rescue a compound in early development generally requires some assumption- and judgment-making, and a certain degree of risk-taking, since sample sizes in Phase II are generally too small to draw firm conclusions about the validity of genetic associations. However, understanding the factors that contribute to variability in efficacy in early development helps to avoid surprises later in development after significant investments have been made. Evidence that efficacy is not appreciably influenced by genetic variability in candidate pathways (i.e., lack of apparent genetic association) may also afford an added level of confidence in the product profile and contribute to prioritization of compounds or indications. It is anticipated that the "*it's better not to know*" attitude, as it relates to the generation of research data in the pharmaceutical context, will continue to fade and shift toward the recognition that data and information, particularly when generated early, do more good than harm in the long run.

4.2 Focused Approval for Targeted Populations—Opportunity for Drug-Diagnostic Co-Development

The choice between blockbuster and personalised medicine is more complex than often expected and is addressed in detail in Chapter 13. The stratification of patients by genotype can provide a higher resolution to detect efficacy that may otherwise have gone undetected due to a dilution effect by nonresponders in an unstratified cohort. This allows efficacy to be demonstrated in patient subgroups for drugs that might not have been considered effective in the general population. Drugs developed in genetically stratified trials, once on the market, would, by definition, only be indicated for the genetically identified subset of patients.

In 2005, the U.S. Food and Drug Administration (FDA) released a draft concept paper on drug-diagnostic co-development *(22)*, which describes a process for developing a diagnostic to determine later use of a particular drug. The development of the diagnostic is described as proceeding smoothly in parallel with the development of the drug, beginning as early as drug discovery (Fig. 5.1). It is recognized that this is perhaps an overly idealized situation, since rare will be the case that a sufficiently

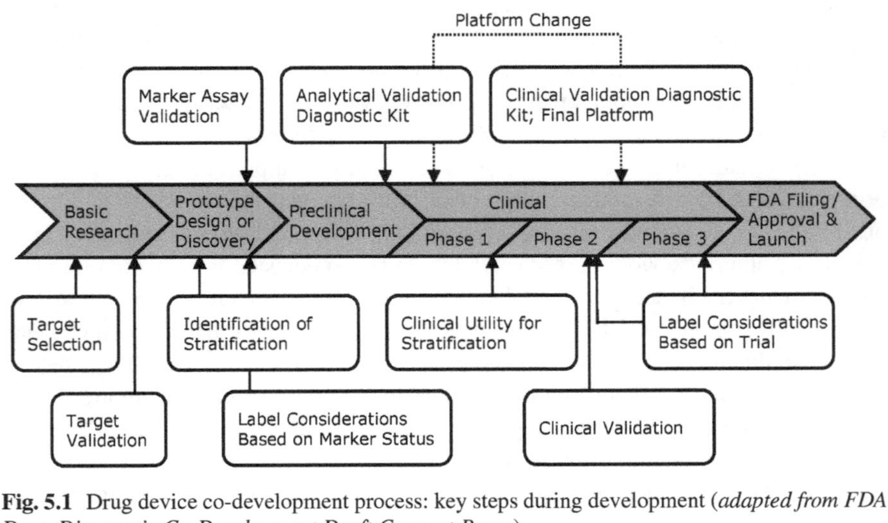

Fig. 5.1 Drug device co-development process: key steps during development (*adapted from FDA Drug-Diagnostic Co-Development Draft Concept Paper*)

robust hypothesis will be available so early in development. Nevertheless, the concept paper highlights the importance of developing hypotheses as early as possible, despite the general lack of statistical power, if the window of opportunity to co-launch a drug and diagnostic is not to be missed. Therefore, it is recommended that the screening of drug targets be considered as soon as pharmacodynamic endpoints are available, which can occur as early as Phase I for studies that include surrogate efficacy endpoints, although Phase II trials would be the more common entry point for efficacy-related investigations. The goal should be to focus early on the appropriate patient population(s), while maximizing flexibility around labelling alternatives before Phase III work is initiated. The information available at the time of entry into Phase III is often a main driver for the label; labels are often drafted before Phase III studies are implemented or finalized. Some may advocate the routine pharmacogenomic screening of drug targets where these are known for an investigational drug, even if polymorphisms in these genes have not been previously characterized for functional consequences. In such cases, tagging SNP approaches may be utilized to assess the overall genetic variability in a drug target (see Chapter 8). Although exploratory, these analyses offer a key opportunity for innovation—something desperately needed in the pharmaceutical industry today. In the current environment, we cannot limit ourselves to the paradigm of retrospective investigations, i.e., waiting to see "how the data look" before considering an efficacy biomarker strategy. Proactive pharmacogenomic investigations of pathways related to efficacy should be encouraged.

4.3 Improved Understanding of Drug Mode of Action

Pharmacogenomic analysis of drug targets can also be applied to validate drug targets *in vivo*, i.e., to support the known or hypothesized mode of action or identification of an as yet unknown mode of action *(23, 24)*. Although it is not a prerequisite that the mode of action be known for a drug to be marketed, information on mode of action can be used to predict possible drug interactions and side effects, or to differentiate a product from its competitors by providing evidence for a novel mode of action. Obviously, drugs that have a single simple mode of action are more amenable to this pharmacogenomic dissection. The underlying assumption and requirement for such mechanistic applications is that genetic polymorphisms in the target(s) lead to variability in efficacy. A genetic association with drug response for a candidate drug target therefore provides supporting evidence for that mechanism in the human context. For drugs with unknown targets, exploratory candidate gene or genome-wide studies should be considered to identify candidate pathways.

4.4 Super-Responders

Strategies have been developed around the identification of super-responders (i.e., extreme responders). One obvious marketing goal is the clinician's preferential selection of a novel drug over competitor's drug, which is particularly important in highly competitive areas where many therapeutic options are available (e.g., depression, epilepsy). If a diagnostic marker can show that particular subjects are likely to respond extremely well to a novel drug, this drug may be preferentially selected over its well-established competitors as a first line treatment in these subjects. This is particularly relevant in indications that may have grave consequences if left ineffectively treated. A biomarker for super-responders would not mean that a diagnostic test would be required for prescription of the drug, but rather that it would be used to optimize treatment decisions at the discretion of the physician on a case-by-case basis. The identification of genes associated with super-response may also find use in drug discovery for the development of next-generation compounds.

4.5 *Optimizing Clinical Trial Design*

A final motivation for pharmacogenomics in the area of efficacy is the cost associated with each additional patient enrolled in a clinical trial. In an effort to improve the probability of success and reduce development costs (particularly in Phase III), pharmacogenomics is already being used in a variety of ways to attempt to optimize trial design. Four general study designs are briefly mentioned below.

Classical Design: The fundamental difference between the classical trial design and the other designs is the timing at which pharmacogenomic testing is performed with respect to randomization. The classical design does not require genotyping for randomization; genotyping is performed during or after the trial. Data are therefore only generated for particular genetic subgroups if groups happen to be enrolled in the trial. The trial may or may not be powered to detect significant genetic associations.

The advantages of this conventional design are that it i) is operationally straightforward, with no additional time or burden to screen subjects; ii) is a more traditional design and therefore tends to be more familiar to both sponsors and regulators; and iii) requires minimal trial design modifications. The main drawback is that statistical association analyses hinge on the genetic subgroups being enrolled (or not enrolled) in the trial by chance; therefore the power to detect associations is often insufficient.

Inclusion/Exclusion Design: This design excludes subjects who are predicted, based on an existing hypothesis, to be non-responders (i.e., test negative subjects). In an initial pharmacogenomic screening, all test negative subjects are excluded from the efficacy trial. There must be a clear, well-defined knowledge that test negative subjects are not likely to respond to the drug and/or may be at greater risk for toxicity. The advantages are i) the increased probability of demonstrating efficacy in the enrolled population; ii) smaller trial sizes; and iii) the prevention of unnecessary exposure and untoward events in subjects who would not respond to the drug anyway. Drawbacks are that i) no data are generated in excluded patients; ii) a pharmacogenomic test must be available for market approval of the drug;

iii) a smaller overall phase III program could reduce the probability of detecting rare SAEs; iv) for a pharmacogenomic test having mediocre sensitivity, some true responders would not have the opportunity of being prescribed an effective treatment; and v) the additional operational burden of performing a pharmacogenomic testing prior to randomization.

Balanced Design: This trial design ensures balance between treatment groups with respect to genotype rather than relying on conventional randomization; the latter which can occasionally result in overrepresentation of one genetic group in a given treatment arm and can introduce bias and decrease power. As described for pharmacokinetics, balance can refer to a "50–50" scenario, in which equal proportions of the genetic subgroups are enrolled in the trial; or it can refer to a "representative population" scenario, in which enrollment aims to achieve proportions of genetic subgroups that are representative of the intended population. In contrast to the inclusion/exclusion design, the balanced design generates data for the test negative patients. The balanced design allows the exact patient numbers to be enrolled to meet the powered statistical analysis plan. Advantages include i) not having to perform additional trials, by ensuring that the trial is conducted in the appropriate population; ii) improving the ability to demonstrate efficacy; iii) being statistically powered; iv) reducing bias; and v) allowing a possibly smaller sample size. Drawbacks include i) the possible requirement for a pharmacogenomic test for market approval (depending on the outcomes); ii) a smaller overall phase III program, which can reduce the probability of detecting rare SAEs; and iii) the additional operational burden of performing pharmacogenomic testing prior to randomization.

Adaptive Design: The adaptive design is a flexible design that allows for the modification of various aspects of the trial during the trial, in order to achieve the planned goals without undermining the validity of the trial. Modifications are based on interim results, and may include sample size re-estimation, patient allocation, or early termination *(25, 26)*. This design allows for the preservation of power when the initial estimations of treatment effect and variability were inaccurate. For example, when a trial is designed based on an estimate of variance for a given variable, an increase or decrease in the true variability could significantly affect the power. By monitoring variability during the trial, the sample size can be adjusted to achieve the desired power. Adaptive trial design has been the subject of numerous discussions by regulatory authorities who have expressed openness to novel trial designs *(26)*. Several methods and study designs are available *(25)*, the elaboration of which is beyond the scope of this chapter. As it relates to pharmacogenomics, the basic principle involves the selection of genomically classified patient subsets mid-trial in order to increase probability of trial success. Genomic biomarkers that can identify subsets of patients who are more likely to respond may allow studies to be enriched for these patients. The main advantages include i) ethical and cost benefits, since fewer patients are exposed to the less effective therapy; and ii) improved chances of clinical trial success and drug registration. Disadvantages include i) the introduction of bias when interim unblinded results are used for patient selection; ii) the complexity of the design, analysis, and implementation; iii) the lack of familiarity with how to appropriately implement; and iv) the lack of a regulatory framework to accommodate these designs.

4.6 *Summary of Deliverables for Efficacy*

- Opportunity for innovation.
- Opportunity for drug-diagnostic development.
- Informed strategic decisions (go/no-go decisions), including compound termination and rescue.
- Increased understanding of drug mode of action, which might enable therapeutic and commercial differentiation from competitors.
- Preferential selection of novel drugs over established competitors.
- Feedback of information to drug discovery for next-generation compounds.
- Optimization of design of large and expensive Phase III trials to maximize likelihood of success.

5 Applications to Safety

Drugs that show sufficient efficacy may be rejected, withdrawn, or limited in their use because of rare but serious adverse drug reactions (ADRs). Examples are the antiepileptic felbamate, the atypical antipsychotic clozapine, and several drugs withdrawn because of prolongation of the QT-interval (e.g., cisapride). These rare events are believed to be multifactorial including environmental, immunologic, and genetic factors, and are therefore difficult to predict and characterize mechanistically. Many drugs also exhibit common side effects, some of which may not pose health risks to subjects, whereas others may be potential indicators of more severe toxicities (e.g., alanine aminotransferase (ALT) elevations that may signal potential hepatotoxicity).

Although many drug reactions are difficult to prevent, recent developments suggest that some reactions may be avoidable through individualization of drug therapies based on genetic information (e.g., dose adjustment of warfarin). If pharmacogenomic predictors of adverse events could prevent drug exposure of genetically vulnerable patients and preserve even a single drug, the costs of any large-scale research efforts could be fully recovered. Clinical care would be improved by limiting the treatment to patients that are least likely to experience adverse events or by adjusting dose regimens.

Identification of biomarkers that can explain or predict serious adverse events is considered to be the "holy grail" for the pharmaceutical industry. Some current areas of priority include drug-induced liver injury (DILI); circulatory system irregularities (e.g., QT prolongation, anemias, and neutropenias); immune system reactions (e.g., acute hypersensitivity and skin rash); retinopathy; and renal failure. The main challenges in the area of adverse events are i) the often very low frequency of serious adverse events and consequent grossly insufficient sample size; ii) the idiosyncratic nature of many adverse events that may involve multiple mechanisms working together to culminate in a susceptibility to treatment-related adverse events; iii) the paucity of working hypotheses for off-target related adverse events; and iv) the sometimes compound-specific nature of adverse events. ADRs may occur at any phase, but may not be observed until phases III-IV.

The most feasible adverse events to tackle from a pharmacogenomic perspective are those related to pharmacokinetics (due either to variability in exposure or formation of minor metabolites) or those related to pharmacodynamics (i.e., target-related), since working hypotheses are more readily conceived. For example, an obvious scenario is one in which a genetic polymorphism in the gene encoding a drug target had been previously reported in the literature as associated with an adverse event that was observed in the drug development (e.g., cardiovascular adverse events observed for a drug that targets the α-adrenoceptor). Many of the concepts related to PK and PD have already been described in the previous sections. More challenging are adverse events related to off-target events or complex mechanisms.

5.1 *Identify Predictive Biomarkers of Toxicity*

A number of predictive biomarkers for adverse events have already been identified and are in clinical use. Classical examples include i) the increased risk of azathiopurine-induced myelotoxicity in subjects with thiopurine methyltransferase (TPMT) deficiency or lower activity due to genetic polymorphism. TPMT testing is recommended and consideration should be given to either genotyping or phenotyping patients for TPMT; ii) the increased risk for irinotecan-induced neutropenia in subjects who are homozygous for the *UGT1A1*28* polymorphism *(27)*. This association was discovered by an independent group post-marketing, and required revision of the label, highlighting the importance of exploring candidate pathways during drug development; and iii) the increased risk for carbamazepine-induced severe skin rash (Stevens-Johnsons Syndrome [SJS] and toxic epidermal necrolysis [TEN]) in subjects carrying the HLA-B*1502 allele. Significant advances in the area of safety are anticipated in the near term as technologies catering to toxicologically relevant pathways become available, notably, SNP chips containing broad panels of ADME genes or SNP chips capturing the major histocompatability complex (HLA) locus, both of which may find particular use in the area of drug-induced liver injury for which PK-based and immunology-based hypotheses exist. Evidence of the potential for liver injury based on classical liver function tests (LFTs) including serum alanine aminotransferase (ALT), alkaline phosphatase (ALP), and total bilirubin (TB), has an important impact on compound attrition rate, despite these markers not being reliable predictors of *bona fide* hepatotoxicity. Nevertheless, these red flags can weigh heavily on the decision whether to proceed or not with compound development. Elevations in liver enzymes can occur at both low and at high frequencies, the latter offering an opportunity for pharmacogenomics even in early development. Identifying the culprit pathway(s) associated with the susceptibility to liver enzyme elevations may serve as an important factor in the decision to move forward with the development of a compound. Such investigations are already underway. The byproduct of these investigations will be a growing body of knowledge of the mechanisms underlying aberrant liver function tests.

5.2 Confirm Suspected Preexisting Diagnosis and Address Regulatory Questions

A pharmacogenomic approach can also be applied to support claims that a particular adverse event is not treatment-related. In this situation, a known disease-related biomarker may be analyzed to verify whether a subject harbored a pre-existing condition that went undiagnosed at the time of enrollment in the trial.

5.3 Demonstrate Improved Safety Profile over Competitors

It is generally felt that a pharmacogenomics test that could achieve a reduction in the incidence of adverse events to meet that of a competitor drug is of limited value. Although the drug might be approved, it is unlikely that it would be used as first line therapy because of the need to perform pharmacogenomic testing. However, a pharmacogenomic test that could reduce the probability of an adverse event (AE) significantly below that of a competitor drug with equivalent efficacy would be an important element in the approval and marketing of the drug.

5.4 Rare Adverse Events and Collaborative Models

Although there is a need for pharmacogenomic tests to predict rare safety events, the feasibility of clinically validating the predictive power of such a marker is questionable. The incidence of rare adverse events (AEs) is defined as an observed frequency of $<0.1\%$, therefore the number of rare AEs in a typical clinical development program of 5000–10,000 patients will be approximately 5–10 cases. For rare adverse events, different post-marketing surveillance scenarios have been described with regard to validating test findings. Assessing the seriousness and frequency of the AEs would drive the need for a pharmacogenomic test. It is more likely that pharmacogenomics will find its greatest use in helping to explain more common AEs observed in clinical trials, as well as to improve our mechanistic understanding of these AEs.

The industry is now realizing the need to join efforts in a collaborative mode to pool resources including samples, technology, scientific input, and funding and to share risks if any significant headway is to be made in the area of rare but serious adverse events. One example is the recent creation of the Serious Adverse Events Consortium (SAEC), which is a non-profit partnership of industry, academia, and government in a global effort to identify genetic markers related to harmful drug reactions. The short-term priorities of the SAEC are drug-induced liver injury and serious skin rash, to be followed by other serious adverse events such as QT prolongation. This is a major step forward in understanding the basic science underlying drug-induced toxicity and, if successful, will benefit the pharmaceutical industry overall, but more importantly, will benefit patients.

5.5 Summary of Deliverables for Safety

- Identification of predictive safety biomarkers.
- Addressing regulatory questions.
- Opportunity to rescue a compound that would otherwise fail to be commercialized due to safety concerns. Such a strategy would usually lead to the marketing of a compound with a companion diagnostic test.
- Increased understanding of drug safety. This may, in some cases, enable therapeutic differentiation from competitive compounds by adding information to the drug label.
- Dose adjustment in susceptible patients.

Concluding Remarks

A combination of scientific reasoning, trial and error, and some risk-taking has led to rapid growth in our understanding of how pharmacogenomics can best be applied to clinical development programs. This experience has helped to reset realistic expecations and squelch the hype associated with the application of this approach to the industry. There is no one-size-fits-all solution to pharmacogenomic strategy development. The greatest value can be obtained by synergizing pharmacogenomic research with clinical development plans. When pharmacogenomics is no longer viewed as a novel and innovative approach to drug development but rather is considered a core component of conventional drug development, a new era in pharmaceutical development will have been reached.

References

1. Dayer P, Desmeules J, Leemann T, Striberni R (1988) Bioactivation of the narcotic drug codeine in human liver is mediated by the polymorphic monooxygenase catalyzing debrisoquine 4-hydroxylation (cytochrome P-450 dbl/bufI). Biochem Bioph Res Co 152(1):411–6.
2. Johansson I, Yue QY, Dahl ML et al (1991) Genetic analysis of the interethnic difference between Chinese and Caucasians in the polymorphic metabolism of debrisoquine and codeine. Eur J Clin Pharmacol 40(6):553–6.
3. Mikus G, Bochner F, Eichelbaum M, Horak P, Somogyi AA, Spector S (1994) Endogenous codeine and morphine in poor and extensive metabolisers of the CYP2D6 (debrisoquine/sparteine) polymorphism. J Pharmacol Exp Ther 268(2):546–51.
4. Mortimer O, Persson K, Ladona MG et al (1990) Polymorphic formation of morphine from codeine in poor and extensive metabolizers of dextromethorphan: relationship to the presence of immunoidentified cytochrome P-450IID1. Clin Pharmacol Ther 47(1):27–35.
5. Persson K, Sjostrom S, Sigurdardottir I, Molnar V, Hammarlund- Udenaes M, Rane A (1995) Patient-controlled analgesia (PCA) with codeine for postoperative pain relief in ten extensive metabolisers and one poor metaboliser of dextromethorphan. Brit J Clin Pharmacol 39(2):182–6.
6. Sindrup SH, Poulsen L, Brosen K, Arendt- Nielsen L, Gram LF (1993) Are poor metabolisers of sparteine/debrisoquine less pain tolerant than extensive metabolisers? Pain 53(3):335–9.
7. Tyndale RF, Droll KP, Sellers EM (1997) Genetically deficient CYP2D6 metabolism provides protection against oral opiate dependence. Pharmacogenetics 7(5):375–9.
8. Yue QY, Alm C, Svensson JO, Sawe J (1997) Quantification of the O- and N-demethylated and the glucuronidated metabolites of codeine relative to the debrisoquine metabolic ratio in urine in ultrarapid, rapid, and poor debrisoquine hydroxylators. Ther Drug Monit 19(5):539–42.
9. Cho SH, Oh SY, Bahn JW et al (2005) Association between bronchodilating response to short-acting beta-agonist and non-synonymous single-nucleotide polymorphisms of beta-adrenoceptor gene. Clin Exp Allergy 35(9):1162–7.
10. Choudhry S, Ung N, Avila PC et al (2005) Pharmacogenetic differences in response to albuterol between Puerto Ricans and Mexicans with asthma. Am J Resp Crit Care Med 171(6):563–70.
11. Israel E, Chinchilli VM, Ford JG et al (2004) Use of regularly scheduled albuterol treatment in asthma: genotype-stratified, randomised, placebo-controlled cross-over trial.[see comment]. Lancet 364(9444):1505–12.
12. Israel E, Drazen JM, Liggett SB et al (2001) Effect of polymorphism of the beta(2)-adrenergic receptor on response to regular use of albuterol in asthma. Int Arch Allergy Imm 124(1–3):183–6.
13. Lima JJ, Thomason DB, Mohamed MH, Eberle LV, Self TH, Johnson JA (1999) Impact of genetic polymorphisms of the beta2-adrenergic receptor on albuterol bronchodilator pharmacodynamics. Clin Pharmacol Ther 65(5):519–25.
14. Arnett DK, Claas SA, Glasser SP (2006) Pharmacogenetics of antihypertensive treatment. Vasc Pharmacol 44(2):107–18.
15. Tate S, Singh R, Hung C et al (2006) A common polymorphism in the SCN1A gene associates with phenytoin serum levels at maintenance dose. Pharmacogenet Genom 16(10):721–6.
16. Tate SK, Depondt C, Sisodiya SM et al (2005) Genetic predictors of the maximum doses patients receive during clinical use of the anti-epileptic drugs carbamazepine and phenytoin. P Natl Acad Sci USA 102(15):5507–12.
17. Bodin L, Verstuyft C, Tregouet DA et al (2005) Cytochrome P450 2C9 (CYP2C9) and vitamin K epoxide reductase (VKORC1) genotypes as determinants of acenocoumarol sensitivity. Blood 106(1):135–40.
18. Schalekamp T, Brasse BP, Roijers JF et al (2007) VKORC1 and CYP2C9 genotypes and phenprocoumon anticoagulation status: interaction between both genotypes affects dose requirement. Clin Pharmacol Ther 81(2):185–93.

19. Bartsch H, Dally H, Popanda O, Risch A, Schmezer P (2007) Genetic risk profiles for cancer susceptibility and therapy response. Recent Res Cancer 174:19–36.
20. Cacabelos R (2002) Pharmacogenomics in Alzheimer's disease. Mini-Rev Med Chem 2(1):59–84.
21. Table of Valid Genomic Biomarkers within the Context of Approved Drug Labels: http://www.fda.gov/cder/genomics/genomic_biomarkers_table.htm
22. Drug-Diagnostic Co-Development Concept Paper - Draft: http://www.fda.gov/cder/genomics/pharmacoconceptfn.pdf.
23. Kalow W (2005) A pharmacogeneticist's look at drug effects and the drug development process: an overview. Expert Opin Pharmaco 6(8):1299–303.
24. McMahon FJ, Buervenich S, Charney D et al (2006) Variation in the gene encoding the serotonin 2A receptor is associated with outcome of antidepressant treatment. Am J Hum Genet 78(5):804–14.
25. Chang M (2005) Adaptive design for clinical trials. In: International symposium on applied stochastic models and data analysis. France.
26. Gottleib S (2006) Adaptive trial design. http://wwwfdagov/oc/speeches/2006/trialdesign0710 html.
27. Irinotecan HCl Drug Label: http://www.fda.gov/medwatch/SAFETY/2005/Jun_PI/Camptosar_PI.pdf.

Chapter 6
Pharmacogenomics Applications in Drug Metabolism

From Genotyping to Drug Label-Challenges?

Ann K. Daly

Contents

Abstract There is increasing recognition that pharmacogenetic polymorphisms affecting drug metabolism are valid biomarkers affecting drug safety and efficacy. This is shown by the inclusion of information about genetic polymorphisms affecting drug metabolism on drug labels with, in some cases, a recommendation that testing for the polymorphism should be performed before prescription. However, in most cases, this information is for information only. It is likely that this is in part because testing for the relevant polymorphisms is unlikely to be available to patients being prescribed the drug, but also because clear advice about issues such as dose adjustment is not available, mainly since appropriate clinical trials have not yet been performed. Metabolic polymorphisms mentioned by the U.S. Food and Drug Administration (FDA) as valid biomarkers include those in thiopurine methyltransferase, the UDP-glucuronosyltransferase UGT1A1, the cytochromes P450 CYP2D6, CYP2C19, and CYP2C9, the N-acetyltransferase NAT2, and dihydropyrimidine dehydrogenase. Each of the above polymorphisms is considered here in detail, with particular reference to current knowledge and to their relevance to the drugs considered to be related to the individual polymorphisms.

Keywords Pharmacogenomics, Cytochrome P450, N-acetyltransferase, UDP-glucuronosyltransferase, Dihydropyrimidine dehydrogenase, Thiopurine methyltransferase, Vitamin K epoxide reductase

---

Ann K. Daly
School of Clinical and Laboratory Sciences Newcastle University Medical School
Framlington Place, Newcastle upon Tyne NE2 4HH, UK
A.K.Daly@ncl.ac.uk

N. Cohen (ed.) *Pharmacogenomics and Personalized Medicine*,

1 Introduction

Pioneering studies in the early 1960s resulted in the identification of the acetylation polymorphism (1). Since this initial recognition that drug metabolism is often subject to interindividual variation, it has been feasible to perform pharmacogenetic tests prior to drug prescription. Important further advances have included *(1)* the finding that common genetic polymorphisms result in interindividual variation in the levels of a number of different cytochromes P450, and *(2)* from the early 1990s, the development of PCR-based tests to enable genotyping for common genetic polymorphisms. Despite this knowledge, pharmacogenetic tests, especially those relevant to drug metabolism, are still seldom used in normal clinical practice. However, there is increasing recognition of the importance of pharmacogenetics/genomics in optimising drug safety and efficacy. In particular, about 10% of drug labels approved by the U.S. FDA now include pharmacogenomic information. The FDA also provides detailed recommendations, updated quarterly, about the use of pharmacogenomic tests prior to drug prescription *(2)*. Tests are classified as either required or recommended, or the information is provided for reference only. The drugs for which a test is required are all novel anticancer therapies, which target tumour phenotypes rather than agents subject to polymorphic metabolism. However, a test is recommended in relation to several drugs which undergo polymorphic metabolism; and, for a growing list of drugs, information on polymorphic metabolism is included for reference only (see Table 6.1).

This article focusses specifically on those metabolic polymorphisms now recognised by regulators as valid biomarkers for drug efficacy and safety by their inclusion

Table 6.1 Examples of genes relevant to drug metabolism and summary of current regulatory position with FDA

Gene	Drug	FDA-licensed test available	FDA recommendation for testing
TPMT	6-mercaptopurine	Yes	Recommended
	Azathioprine	Yes	Recommended
UGT1A1	Irinotecan	Yes	Recommended
CYP2D6	Atomoxetine	Yes	Information only
	Many other drugs (e.g., tricyclic antidepressants, antipsychotics, codeine, tamoxifen)	Yes	Information only
CYP2C19	Voriconazole	Yes	Information only
	Other drugs (e.g., proton pump inhibitors)	Yes	Information only
CYP2C9/ VKORC1	Warfarin	No	Information only
CYP2C9	Celecoxib	No	Information only
DPD	Capecitabine	No	Information only
NAT2	Isoniazid	No	Information only

From (2)

on this FDA list. Their recognition as biomarkers may enable more rapid progress to be made on making appropriate genotyping tests available prior to drug prescription.

2 Metabolism Genes Recommended as Genomic Biomarkers

2.1 Thiopurine methyltransferase

Thiopurine *S*-methyltransferase (TPMT) metabolizes the cytotoxic drug 6-mercaptopurine, widely used in the treatment of childhood acute lymphoblastic leukaemia, together with azathioprine, a 6-mercaptopurine precursor used as an immunosuppressant. Approximately 0.3% of Europeans have undetectable activity, and 11% have intermediate levels *(3)*. It is currently the metabolic polymorphism for which most progress has been made in performing testing prior to prescription, possibly because of the serious hematological toxicity seen in those with the deficiency. In individuals lacking TPMT, high concentrations of thioguanine nucleotides will be formed, resulting in toxicities such as myelosuppression, which can be life-threatening *(4)*. The molecular basis of the deficiency is now well understood, and the two main alleles associated with the absence of enzyme activity have been identified *(5)*. The most common defective allele, *TPMT*3*, results in two amino acid substitutions which either together or separately result in a complete absence of activity and account for approximately 75% of defective alleles. The clinical importance of this polymorphism has been demonstrated in a number of studies. For example, in one large study, individuals who were either homozygous or heterozygous for variant alleles were demonstrated to be at a significantly increased risk of toxicity when treated with 6-mercaptopurine *(6)*. TPMT deficiency has also been linked to an increased risk of second malignancies among patients with acute lymphoblastic leukemia *(7)*. In the U.S., drug labels for both 6-mercaptopurine and azathioprine now include information on the TPMT polymorphism and recommend determining patient phenotype or genotype prior to drug treatment *(2)*. Azathioprine is used in the treatment of several immune-related diseases including atopic eczema, Crohn's disease, and autoimmune liver disease *(8, 9)*; and, because these diseases are relatively common compared with childhood leukemia, it is used more widely than 6-mercaptopurine. TPMT status can be determined either by genotyping or by phenotyping, which involves the measurement of enzyme levels in erythrocytes, prior to azathioprine treatment with the appropriate dose adjustment then performed. Although generally 6-mercaptopurine is very useful in combination therapy of childhood leukaemia, providing the dosage is adjusted to take account of TPMT genotype, the response to azathioprine is more variable. It appears that while dose adjustment on the basis of genotype should prevent serious hematological toxicity, the response to azathioprine is rather variable, suggesting that other factors, possibly additional genetic polymorphisms, also contribute *(8)*. Reports in the literature suggest that TPMT testing prior to initiation of treatment with either

6-mercaptopurine or azathioprine is now common in many centres *(10, 11)*, but this does not appear to be universal. Nevertheless, TPMT is the best current example of a pharmacogenetic test involving a host genotype rather than a tumor genotype that is already in use clinically.

2.2 UGT1A1

The UDP-glucuronosyltransferases are the major enzyme superfamily carrying out phase II drug metabolism *(12)*. The active metabolite (SN-38) of the topoisomerase I inhibitor irinotecan is mainly metabolized by glucuronidation *(13)*. The enzyme responsible for this metabolism is UGT1A1, which is also the main enzyme responsible for the glucuronidation of bilirubin. Gilbert's syndrome, which is characterized by a raised serum bilirubin, is due to genetic defects in UGT1A1 *(14)*. The most common polymorphism is a 2 bp insertion in the promoter region (*UGT1A1*28* allele) but certain single nucleotide polymorphisms (SNPs) which result in amino acid substitutions can also give rise to the Gilbert's phenotype *(14)*. Individuals homozygous or heterozygous for polymorphisms associated with Gilbert's syndrome appear to be at increased risk of toxicity with irinotecan *(13)*. It has now been recommended in the FDA-approved drug label for the U.S. that genotyping should be performed prior to administration of this drug because of the increased risk of neutropenia in patients with Gilbert's syndrome *(2)*. The FDA has also licensed a genotyping test for *UGT1A1*28 (15)*. However, there are still some issues that need to be addressed regarding the value of UGT1A1 genotyping in patients receiving irinotecan. A review of all published studies linking the UGT1A1 genotype and either irinotecan pharmacokinetics or irinotecan-associated toxicity has recently been published *(13)*. In particular, the majority of pharmacokinetic studies found that possession of either *UGT1A1*28* or another "Gilbert's" allele was associated with a lower SN38-glucuronide over SN38 ratio, as expected because of lower rates of glucuronide formation. However, the various studies disagreed on whether *UGT1A1*28* was a risk factor for either severe diarrhoea or neutropenia; although there was some indication that *UGT1A1*28* might be associated with an increased risk of neutropenia, but with a decreased risk of diarrhoea. A possible reason for this lack of agreement could be that each study involved less than 100 patients in total, resulting in few patients with variant alleles being present. In addition, some of the studies involved more than one tumor type and drug regimens which included additional agents to irinotecan such as 5-fluorouracil. In addition to UGT1A1, other members of the UGT1A family can also glucuronidate SN38. Associations between toxicity and other UGT1A genotypes including UGT1A6, UGT1A7, and UGT1A9 have also been reported *(16, 17)*. Strong linkage disequilibrium within the UGT1A locus complicates interpretation of these studies, but it is possible that genotyping for additional SNPs may provide a better prediction of susceptibility to toxicity. Irinotecan is a second-line therapy for metastatic colorectal cancer in Europe as well as the U.S., but there is still a need for additional larger studies on the association between UGT1A genotype and toxicity. The frequency of *UGT1A1*28* is lower in non-European populations, but a number of other polymorphisms which give rise to the same phenotype are more common in those of non-Europe ethnic origin *(18)*. The current licensed genotyping assay does not detect these other alleles.

3 Genes Listed as Genomic Biomarkers for Information Only

3.1 CYP2C9

3.1.1 CYP2C9, VKORC1 and Oral Anticoagulants

Warfarin and other coumarin anticoagulants are very widely prescribed and are already subject to individualized prescribing, although not with a genetic test. The dose is currently set by initiating treatment using a standard protocol and then adjusting the dose on the basis of the patient's coagulation rate (INR). It has been known for some years that the genotype for the main warfarin metabolizing enzyme CYP2C9 contributes to the dose required. Two common CYP2C9 variant alleles, *CYP2C9*2* and *CYP2C9*3*, both encode enzymes with decreased catalytic activity towards warfarin compared with the wild-type *CYP2C9*1* allele (for a review see *[19]*). Individuals with one or two of these variants require a lower dose of warfarin on average, but it is also clear that other factors contribute to the dose requirement *(20)*. VKORC1, the gene encoding the warfarin target enzyme vitamin K epoxide reductase, has been identified quite recently. It has now been clearly demonstrated that the genotype for this gene is a slightly more important predictor than CYP2C9, especially in individuals of certain ethnic groups where the variant CYP2C9 alleles are rare *(21–24)*; and although it is not a drug metabolism gene, it needs to be considered alongside CYP2C9 in any discussion of oral anticoagulant pharmacogenetics. The main contributors to the effect of VKORC1 on dose requirement are genetic polymorphisms in the upstream sequence and in intron 1, which are in complete linkage disequilibrium and appear to affect levels of gene expression *(21)*.

Some limited clinical trials have been reported involving CYP2C9 genotyping prior to warfarin prescription to allow tailored dosing *(25)*. Current data indicate that a tailored dosing protocol will require consideration of both nongenetic and genetic factors. Several dosing algorithms based on patient VKORC1 and CYP2C9 genotype, together with age and either height, weight, or body surface area, have been proposed and should now be tested in clinical trials. VKORC1 and CYP2C9 genotyping requires only three single nucleotide polymorphisms to be analyzed *(22)*. This should facilitate the development of simple, rapid, and cheap genotyping assays for use at the point of care, so that a rapid decision on the warfarin dose can be made. For such an assay to be used widely, it will be necessary to demonstrate cost-effectiveness.

3.1.2 CYP2C9 and Other Drugs

CYP2C9 is also the main metabolizing enzyme for a number of nonsteroidal anti-inflammatory drugs. In the case of one of these, celecoxib, the FDA-approved U.S. label includes the information that known or suspected CYP2C9 "poor metabolizers" (essentially those homozygous for *CYP2C9*3*) should be administered the drug with caution *(2)*. There is clinical data confirming that individuals with this rare genotype show very high levels of celecoxib, but the effect of other CYP2C9 genotypes is still not clear *(26)*. The general question of the impact of the CYP2C9 genotype on cyclooxygenase inhibitors has been considered recently, with the conclusion that the clearance of only certain drugs would vary with the CYP2C9 genotype, and that with several of these (including celecoxib) the contribution of CYP3A4 should also be considered *(27)*.

3.2 CYP2D6

A polymorphism affecting the metabolism of the antihypertensive agent debrisoquine was described in 1977 *(28)*. Subsequent studies showed that the enzyme responsible for debrisoquine 4-hydroxylation was the cytochrome P450 CYP2D6, and that a number of other drugs, particularly tricyclic antidepressants and antipsychotic agents, were also subject to polymorphic metabolism, with individuals having an impaired ability to hydroxylate debrisoquine also showing impaired metabolism of these drugs. The genetic basis of impaired metabolism was also identified, and it is now possible to identify at least 95% of those lacking CYP2D6 activity by genotyping (for a review see [*(29)*]). A microarray-based system for assigning CYP2D6 genotype, the Amplichip *(30)*, has been approved by the FDA as a diagnostic test; although, because of its rather specialized nature, it may be better suited to use in a research environment than as a routine diagnostic test prior to prescription. Absence of CYP2D6 is inherited as a codominant effect, and those heterozygous for variant alleles also show impaired metabolism of some substrates. In addition to the absence of CYP2D6 in significant numbers of patients, the existence of unusually fast metabolism in some individuals, usually but not exclusively due to at least one additional copy of CYP2D6 being present in germ-line DNA, has been described *(31)*.

Despite the fact that the CYP2D6 polymorphism was initially identified almost 30 years ago and it has been possible to identify most of those with the genetic deficiency for the last 15 years, CYP2D6 genotyping has so far failed to enter routine clinical practice. There are a number of possible reasons for this, ranging from the general difficulty of introducing pharmacogenotyping into clinical practice to the facts that either a number of key CYP2D6 substrates have been withdrawn from the market because of the problems experienced by poor metabolizers (e.g., phenformin, perhexiline), or certain types of CYP2D6 substrates are less commonly used than when the polymorphism was first described. For example, most tricyclic antidepressants are metabolized mainly by CYP2D6; but selective serotonin reuptake inhibitors, in whose metabolism CYP2D6 has a role but is less important, are more widely used currently in the treatment of depression. Guidelines for dose adjustment for antidepressant drugs on the basis of the CYP2D6 genotype have been formulated but have not yet been tested in clinical trials *(32)*. The FDA-approved labels for atomoxetine and fluoxetine now include mention of CYP2D6; and the label for atomoxetine specificially mentions the possibility of higher plasma concentrations in poor metabolizers, although this is mentioned for information only and a test is neither required nor recommended *(2)*.

Codeine is an important CYP2D6 substrate. It is activated to morphine exclusively by CYP2D6 and it is generally accepted that this reaction is essential to achieve analgesia. Two recent case reports have appeared concerning excessive activation of codeine in ultrarapid metabolizers with one additional copy of CYP2D6. In the first, a patient who was prescribed a cough medicine containing codeine suffered life-threatening opioid intoxication *(33)*. This individual was found on genotyping to have at least three copies of CYP2D6 and was therefore clearly an ultrarapid metabolizer. The second report concerned the death of a breast-fed baby 13 days after birth *(34)*. His mother was prescribed codeine for pain post-delivery. Postmortem examination of stored breast milk samples showed a morphine level at least four times higher than expected, and the mother was found to have a CYP2D6 gene duplication with the infant an extensive metabolizer. A recent study on codeine administration to healthy volunteers of known CYP2D6 genotype showed that ultrarapid metabolizers were significantly more likely than extensive metabolizers to suffer sedation *(35)*. It appears that CYP2D6 genotyping in patients requiring treatment with codeine and related compounds, including tramadol, could be beneficial in avoiding both dangerous intoxication and lack of response.

Tamoxifen is an extremely successful and widely used treatment for hormone-receptor positive breast cancer. Its metabolism is complex, but it has been recently recognised that CYP2D6 produces a 4-hydroxy-N-desmethyltamoxifen metabolite (endoxifen) *(36, 37)*. Endoxifen is found at high plasma levels in many patients and appears to bind strongly to estrogen receptors, suggesting it is important in the biological response to tamoxifen *(38)*. Evidence is now emerging that patients positive for one or two CYP2D6 poor metabolizer alleles show an increased incidence of breast cancer relapse *(39, 40)*. As mentioned by the FDA *(2)*, tamoxifen is also a substrate for CYP3A and CYP2C9, and it may be necessary to also consider the effect of additional polymorphisms on tamoxifen metabolism before comprehensive recommendations can be formulated. In view of the availability of other effective treatments, such as aromatase inhibitors, CYP2D6 genotyping may be of value in determining the most appropriate treatment for hormone-receptor positive breast cancer.

3.3 CYP2C19

CYP2C19 is another cytochrome P450 with a relatively common polymorphism associated with complete absence of enzyme activity. Compared with CYP2D6, its role in drug metabolism is more minor, but it is possible to genotype for the common variants using the same Amplichip technology as for CYP2D6 *(30)*. The most widely prescribed CYP2C19 substrates include omeprazole and other proton pump inhibitors. Possession of one or more variant CYP2C19 alleles is associated with a better therapeutic response to proton pump inhibitors than in the case of wild-type individuals *(41)*. A recent study found that the antiplatelet agent clopidogrel was not effective in individuals with at least one variant CYP2C19 allele, probably because of a major role for CYP2C19 in the activation of this prodrug *(42)*. In addition, some benzodiazepines, including diazapam and clobazam, are CYP2C19 substrates, and individuals defective in CYP2C19 may be at risk of toxicities such as oversedation *(43)*. Voriconazole, a second generation triazole anti-fungal agent, is a CYP2C19 substrate with contributions to its metabolism by other P450s, particularly CYP3A4. The U.S. drug label mentions that individuals heterozygous for CYP2C19 have on average a twofold higher exposure level than homozygous wild-type individuals; but, as in the case of CYP2D6 and atomoxetine, this is for information only *(2)*.

3.4 NAT2

There are two *N*-acetyltransferase isoforms, termed *N*-acetyltransferase 1 and 2 (NAT1 and NAT2), which acetylate amino, hydroxyl, and sulfhydryl groups. The *NAT2* gene is subject to extensive polymorphism, with many individuals who are usually termed slow acetylators unable to acetylate a range of drugs, including isoniazid, sulphamethoxazole, and caffeine *(44)*. A number of different polymorphisms in NAT2 give rise to amino acid substitutions, and these have been demonstrated to result in absence of catalytic activity in vitro *(45)*. Screening for three variant alleles (*NAT2*5*, *NAT2*6*, and *NAT2*7*) results in the detection of the vast majority of Caucasian slow acetylators, although additional alleles are also common in some other ethnic groups *(46)*. The precise percentage of slow acetylators also varies with ethnic origin, ranging from 90% in North Africans to less than 10% in many Asian populations, with a frequency of 50% in Caucasians.

Few NAT2 substrates are widely used in modern medicine, although isoniazid remains an important drug in the treatment of tuberculosis, and sulphamethoxazole is used in the treatment of secondary infections in AIDS patients. With respect to isoniazid, the FDA states that “slow acetylation may lead to higher blood levels of the drug, and thus, an increase in toxic reactions” *(2)*. It is well established that slow acetylators are more likely to suffer side effects when prescribed isoniazid, although there is also evidence that these individuals’ overall response to therapy may be better because of their exposure to higher drug levels for longer *(47)*. Therefore, while offering genotyping for NAT2 is likely to be feasible, determining guidelines for dosage recommendations for slow and fast acetylators may not be completely straightforward, although some proposals for this have been put forward *(47)*.

3.5 Dihydropyrimidine Dehydrogenase

Dihydropyrimidine dehydrogenase (DPD) has a biochemical role in the catabolism of uracil and thymine and is not primarily a drug metabolizing enzyme. However, this enzyme is also responsible for the phase I metabolism of the anticancer drug 5-fluorouracil and related compounds such as capecitabine; and interindividual variation in the metabolism of this drug has been correlated with levels of dihydropyrimidine dehydrogenase in peripheral blood mononuclear cells *(48)*. Complete deficiency of dihydropyrimidine dehydrogenase has been linked to various physiological abnormalities. It is estimated that up to 3% of the population may be heterozygous for the deficiency and, although they do not suffer physiological abnormalities, it appears that these individuals are at increased risk of serious toxic effects if given 5-fluorouracil treatment. The FDA suggests that "rarely, unexpected, severe toxicity (e.g., stomatitis, diarrhea, neutropenia, and neurotoxicity) associated with 5-fluorouracil has been attributed to a deficiency of dihydropyrimidine dehydrogenase (DPD) activity. A link between decreased levels of DPD and increased, potentially fatal toxic effects of 5-fluorouracil therefore cannot be excluded" *(2)*. A number of polymorphisms that give rise to DPD deficiency have been identified, but these do not appear to explain all cases of low DPD activity, indicating the complex nature of the genetics of this enzyme *(49, 50)*. Measurement of DPD levels in peripheral blood mononuclear cells may therefore be a more useful predictor of 5-fluorouracil toxicity than genotyping.

4 Concluding Remarks

It is almost 20 years since the molecular basis of the CYP2D6 polymorphism was established; but, despite a wide range of studies demonstrating its relevance to the prescription of a number of drugs, genotyping for this polymorphism in the clinic is still uncommon. The original studies on CYP2D6 have served as a useful paradigm for similar studies on other metabolic genes; and our understanding of variability in these genes, especially the cytochromes P450, is considerably greater than for most other genes, including those encoding drug targets and those that may contribute to disease susceptibility. There is increasing recognition among drug regulators internationally that genotyping for certain pharmacogenomic polymorphisms may enable the safer use of a number of commonly used drugs. The FDA recommendations on pharmacogenomics biomarkers serve as a useful framework, especially if they are updated regularly. There are examples of additional genes that could be included: for example, CYP3A5 is relevant to immunosuppressive drugs, particularly tacrolimus; and CYP2B6 is an important contributor to antiretroviral drug metabolism. It is now important that effective mechanisms for the delivery of this recommended genotyping should be developed.

References

1. Evans DA, White TA (1964) Human acetylation polymorphism. J Lab Clin Med 63:394–403.
2. www.fda.gov/cder/genomics/genomic_biomarkers_table.htm.
3. Weinshilboum R, Sladek SL (1980) Mercaptopurine pharmacogenetics: monogenic inheritance of erythrocyte thiopurine methyltransferase activity. Am J Hum Genet 32:651–62.
4. Lennard L, Gibson BES, Nicole T, Lilleyman JS (1993) Congenital thiopurine methyltransferase deficiency and 6-mercaptopurine toxicity during treatment for acute lymphoblastic-leukemia. Arch Dis Child 69(5):577–9.
5. Szumlanski C, Otterness D, Her C et al (1996) Thiopurine methyltransferase pharmacogenetics: human gene cloning and characterization of a common polymorphism. DNA Cell Biol 15:17–30.
6. Relling MV, Hancock ML, Rivera GK et al (1999) Mercaptopurine therapy intolerance and heterozygosity at the thiopurine S-methyltransferase gene locus. J Natl Cancer Inst 91(23):2001–8.
7. Relling MV, Rubnitz JE, Rivera GK et al (1999) High incidence of secondary brain tumours after radiotherapy and antimetabolites. Lancet 354(9172):34–9.
8. Meggitt SJ, Gray JC, Reynolds NJ (2006) Azathioprine dosed by thiopurine methyltransferase activity for moderate-to-severe atopic eczema: a double-blind, randomised controlled trial. Lancet 367(9513):839–46.
9. Heneghan MA, Allan ML, Bornstein JD, Muir AJ, Tendler DA (2006) Utility of thiopurine methyltransferase genotyping and phenotyping, and measurement of azathioprine metabolites in the management of patients with autoimmune hepatitis. J Hepatol 45(4):584–91.
10. Gardiner SJ, Begg EJ (2005) Pharmacogenetic testing for drug metabolizing enzymes: is it happening in practice? Pharmacogenet Genom 15(5):365–9.
11. Woelderink A, Ibarreta D, Hopkins MM, Rodriguez-Cerezo E (2006) The current clinical practice of pharmacogenetic testing in Europe: TPMT and HER2 as case studies. Pharmacogenomics J 6(1):3–7.
12. Wells PG, Mackenzie PI, Chowdhury JR et al (2004) Glucuronidation and the UDP-glucuronosyltransferases in health and disease. Drug Metab Dispos 32(3):281–90.
13. Nagar S, Blanchard RL (2006) Pharmacogenetics of uridine diphosphoglucuronosyltransferase (UGT) 1A family members and its role in patient response to irinotecan. Drug Metab Rev 38(3):393–409.
14. Burchell B, Soars M, Monaghan G, Cassidy A, Smith D, Ethell B (2000) Drug-mediated toxicity caused by genetic deficiency of UDP-glucuronosyltransferases. Toxicol Lett 112–113:333–40.
15. http://www.twt.com.
16. Carlini LE, Meropol NJ, Bever J et al (2005) UGT1A7 and UGT1A9 polymorphisms predict response and toxicity in colorectal cancer patients treated with capecitabine/irinotecan. Clin Cancer Res 11(3):1226–36.
17. Girard H, Villeneuve L, Court MH et al (2006) The novel UGT1A9 intronic I399 polymorphism appears as a predictor of 7-ethyl-10-hydroxycamptothecin glucuronidation levels in the liver. Drug Metab Dispos 34(7):1220–8.
18. Hall D, Ybazeta G, Destro-Bisol G, Petzl-Erler ML, Di Rienzo A (1999) Variability at the uridine diphosphate glucuronosyltransferase 1A1 promoter in human populations and primates. Pharmacogenetics 9(5):591–9.
19. Daly AK, King BP (2006) Contribution of CYP2C9 to variability in vitamin K antagonist metabolism. Expert Opin Drug Metab Toxicol 2(1):3–15.
20. Daly AK, King BP (2003) Pharmacogenetics of oral anticoagulants. Pharmacogenetics 13(5):247–52.
21. Rieder MJ, Reiner AP, Gage BF et al (2005) Effect of VKORC1 haplotypes on transcriptional regulation and warfarin dose. N Engl J Med 352(22):2285–93.

22. Sconce EA, Khan TI, Wynne HA et al (2005) The impact of CYP2C9 and VKORC1 genetic polymorphism and patient characteristics upon warfarin dose requirements: proposal for a new dosing regimen. Blood 106(7):2329–33.
23. Veenstra DL, You JH, Rieder MJ et al (2005) Association of Vitamin K epoxide reductase complex 1 (VKORC1) variants with warfarin dose in a Hong Kong Chinese patient population. Pharmacogenet Genom 15(10):687–91.
24. Yuan HY, Chen JJ, Lee MT et al (2005) A novel functional VKORC1 promoter polymorphism is associated with inter-individual and inter-ethnic differences in warfarin sensitivity. Hum Mol Genet 14(13):1745–51.
25. Hillman MA, Wilke RA, Yale SH et al (2005) A prospective, randomized pilot trial of model-based warfarin dose initiation using CYP2C9 genotype and clinical data. Clin Med Res 3(3):137–45.
26. Lundblad MS, Ohlsson S, Johansson P, Lafolie P, Eliasson E (2006) Accumulation of celecoxib with a 7-fold higher drug exposure in individuals homozygous for CYP2C9*3. Clin Pharmacol Ther 79(3):287–8.
27. Rodrigues AD (2005) Impact of CYP2C9 genotype on pharmacokinetics: are all cyclooxygenase inhibitors the same? Drug Metab Dispos 33(11):1567–75.
28. Mahgoub A, Idle JR, Dring LG, Lancaster R, Smith RL (1977) Polymorphic hydroxylation of debrisoquine in man. Lancet 2(8038):584–6.
29. Daly AK (2003) Pharmacogenetics of the major polymorphic metabolizing enzymes. Fundam Clin Pharmacol 17(1):27–41.
30. http://www.roche-diagnostics.com/products_services/amplichip_cyp450.html.
31. Ingelman-Sundberg M (1999) Duplication, multiduplication, and amplification of genes encoding drug-metabolizing enzymes: evolutionary, toxicological, and clinical pharmacological aspects. Drug Metab Rev 31(2):449–59.
32. Kirchheiner J, Brosen K, Dahl ML et al (2001) CYP2D6 and CYP2C19 genotype-based dose recommendations for antidepressants: a first step towards subpopulation-specific dosages. Acta Psychiatr Scand 104(3):173–92.
33. Gasche Y, Daali Y, Fathi M et al (2004) Codeine intoxication associated with ultrarapid CYP2D6 metabolism. N Engl J Med 351(27):2827–31.
34. Koren G, Cairns J, Chitayat D, Gaedigk A, Leeder SJ (2006) Pharmacogenetics of morphine poisoning in a breastfed neonate of a codeine-prescribed mother. Lancet 368(9536):704.
35. Kirchheiner J, Schmidt H, Tzvetkov M et al (2006) Pharmacokinetics of codeine and its metabolite morphine in ultra-rapid metabolizers due to CYP2D6 duplication. Pharmacogenomics J, published online.
36. Desta Z, Ward BA, Soukhova NV, Flockhart DA (2004) Comprehensive evaluation of tamoxifen sequential biotransformation by the human cytochrome P450 system in vitro: prominent roles for CYP3A and CYP2D6. J Pharmacol Exp Ther 310(3):1062–75.
37. Jin Y, Desta Z, Stearns V et al (2005) CYP2D6 genotype, antidepressant use, and tamoxifen metabolism during adjuvant breast cancer treatment. J Natl Cancer Inst 97(1):30–9.
38. Lim YC, Li L, Desta Z et al (2006) Endoxifen, a secondary metabolite of tamoxifen, and 4-OH-tamoxifen induce similar changes in global gene expression patterns in MCF-7 breast cancer cells. J Pharmacol Exp Ther 318(2):503–12.
39. Goetz MP, Rae JM, Suman VJ et al (2005) Pharmacogenetics of tamoxifen biotransformation is associated with clinical outcomes of efficacy and hot flashes. J Clin Oncol 23(36):9312–8.
40. Goetz MP, Knox SK, Suman VJ et al (2007) The impact of cytochrome P450 2D6 metabolism in women receiving adjuvant tamoxifen. Breast Cancer Res Treat 101(1):113–21.
41. Klotz U, Schwab M, Treiber G (2004) CYP2C19 polymorphism and proton pump inhibitors. Basic Clin Pharmacol Toxicol 95(1):2–8.
42. Hulot JS, Bura A, Villard E et al (2006) Cytochrome P450 2C19 loss-of-function polymorphism is a major determinant of clopidogrel responsiveness in healthy subjects. Blood 108(7):2244–7.

43. Desta Z, Zhao X, Shin JG, Flockhart DA (2002) Clinical significance of the cytochrome P450 2C19 genetic polymorphism. Clin Pharmacokinet 41(12):913–58.
44. Evans DAP (1989) *N*-acetyltransferase. Pharmacol Ther 42:157–234.
45. http://www.louisville.edu/medschool/pharmacology/NAT.html.
46. Meyer UA, Zanger UM (1997) Molecular mechanisms of genetic polymorphisms of drug metabolism. Annu Rev Pharmacol Toxicol 37:269–96.
47. Kinzig-Schippers M, Tomalik-Scharte D, Jetter A et al (2005) Should we use N-acetyltransferase type 2 genotyping to personalize isoniazid doses? Antimicrob Agents Chemother 49(5):1733–8.
48. Gonzalez FJ, Fernandez-Salguero P (1995) Diagnostic analysis, clinical importance and molecular basis of dihydropyrimidine dehydrogenase deficiency. Trends Pharmacol Sci 16(10):325–7.
49. Collie-Duguid ES, Etienne MC, Milano G, McLeod HL (2000) Known variant DPYD alleles do not explain DPD deficiency in cancer patients. Pharmacogenetics 10(3):217–23.
50. van Kuilenburg AB, Haasjes J, Richel DJ et al (2000) Clinical implications of dihydropyrimidine dehydrogenase (DPD) deficiency in patients with severe 5-fluorouracil-associated toxicity: identification of new mutations in the DPD gene. Clin Cancer Res 6(12):4705–12.

Chapter 7
The Genetics of Adverse Drug Reactions

Promises and Problems

Martin Armstrong

Contents

Abstract There is increasing pressure from patients, health care providers, regulatory authorities, and pharmaceutical companies and their shareholders to bring safer drugs to the market. Despite highly regulated preclinical screening and clinical monitoring, drugs do still make it onto the market that have potentially serious safety issues. The reasons why only a small minority of exposed patients experience these adverse drug reactions (ADRs) are uncertain, but there is increasing interest in the study of genetics as one of the potential susceptibility factors. The following chapter reviews the major advances in this area, discusses how genetics can be used in understanding and mitigating ADR risk, highlights the major challenges associated with performing research in this area, and looks at some of the potential solutions.

Keywords Adverse drug reaction, drug safety, genetics, susceptibility, utility, challenges, solutions

1 Introduction

1.1 The Scale of the Problem

It has been reported that more than 6% of all hospital admissions in the UK are due to adverse drug reactions (ADRs). For over 2% of these admissions the ADR will prove fatal. This equates to approximately 5700 deaths/year in the UK directly

Martin Armstrong
Research and Development Genetics, AstraZeneca, Cheshire, UK

N. Cohen (ed.) *Pharmacogenomics and Personalized Medicine*,

attributable to ADRs (representing an overall fatality rate in the UK population of 0.15%). This could potentially rise to more than 10,000 deaths/year if ADRs occurring *whilst* patients are in hospital are included in these statistics. With a median bed-stay of 8 days, ADRs will cost the UK National Health Service more than £460 million/year *(1)*.

Drug safety concerns are one of the predominant reasons for drug withdrawal from the market. Of 583 new substances authorised in the UK between 1972 and 1994, 59 were withdrawn from market, 22 (37%) of which were for safety reasons (second only to commercial considerations at 59%) *(2)*.

Failures in late phase drug development and withdrawal of drugs from the market due to safety (and any other) concerns have significant financial implications for pharmaceutical companies and their shareholders. The withdrawal of the non-steroidal anti-inflammatory drug Vioxx in September 2004 by Merck, due to unexpected cardiovascular side effects, cut more than 25% from Merck's share price and erased $25 billion from its market value *(3, 4)*. Furthermore, in the present climate, the potential cost of litigation to a company must also be taken into account. Bayer, who withdrew their cholesterol-lowering statin, Baycol, from the market after 30 deaths from rhabdomyolysis, have subsequently paid more than $1 billion to settle nearly 3000 lawsuits and there presently remain around 6000 lawsuits pending *(5)*.

In addition to these direct costs, safety issues also impact the pharmaceutical industry in more subtle ways. Publicity over ADRs such as those suffered by volunteers in a phase I trial of TGN1412, a novel immunomodulatory monocolonal antibody under development for the treatment of B cell chronic lymphocytic leukaemia at Northwick Park in the UK in March 2006, and the withdrawal of Vioxx, has ensured that drug safety remains an issue in the public spotlight *(6)*. Such events contribute to a loss of reputation and confidence in the pharmaceutical industry within the general population.

Clearly, therefore, there are major drivers from the public, health care providers, regulatory authorities, pharmaceutical companies, and shareholders to ensure that safer drugs are brought to the market.

Despite the highly regulated preclinical safety requirements and clinical monitoring performed during drug development, this has proved a challenging goal. This is largely because during the clinical trial process a drug is tested on only a relatively small number of carefully selected patients, in a controlled manner, and over a limited time period. Once licensed, a greater number of less well controlled patients will be exposed to the drug for longer time periods, potentially in combination with other medications. Furthermore, the potential exists for off-label use in other indications, for inappropriate dosing (at both a prescription and individual level), and for inadequate patient monitoring. It is within this spectrum of circumstances that the relatively rare ADRs occur that are responsible for the major drug safety issues and withdrawals *(7)*. A well-known example of this trend was the drug cisapride, which was licensed in the US in 1993 for nocturnal heartburn, and within two years of launch five million prescriptions/year were being filed. Unfortunately, there were 50 reports of cardiac arrhythmia and four deaths attributed to the use of the drug. Despite the low incidence of ADRs associated with the drug, and the benefit received by millions of people, cisapride was finally removed from the market in 1999 *(8)*.

1.2 Idiosyncratic ADRs: The Root of the Problem

ADRs are classified according to their mechanisms of causation, as detailed in Table 7.1. Those ADRs primarily driving the major safety issues and drug withdrawals highlighted above generally fall into the Type B or "bizarre" classification.

These reactions are rare and usually serious or potentially life threatening events. They are also host-dependent events, as opposed to drug-dependent, and are, therefore, often referred to as "idiosyncratic." Such reactions do not show any simple relationship to dose and at present cannot be reliably predicted during either the preclinical or clinical phases of drug development.

In most cases the factors determining susceptibility to type B ADRs are uncertain. The fact that they are host-dependent suggests that individual genetic variation, and its interaction with the drug and the environment, may play a role in determining an individual's susceptibility to an ADR. This reasoning has led to an increasing interest in genetics as one of the potential susceptibility factors.

Table 7.1 Mechanistic classification of adverse drug reactions (Adapted from Park *et al. (56)* and Edwards and Aronson *(57)*)

Type of Reaction *mnemonic*	Features *Occurrence*	Example
Type A *Augmented*	Reactions predictable from the known pharmacology often representing exaggeration of the pharmacological effect of the drug. *Common*	Hypotension with anti-hypertensives
Type B *Bizarre*	Unpredictable from knowledge of the basic pharmacology of the drug. Show no simple dose-response relationship. *Uncommon*	Halothane hepatitis
Type C *Chronic*	Reactions whose biological characteristics can be either predicted or rationalised in terms of chemical structure of the drug. *Uncommon*	Acetaminophen hepatotoxicity
Type D *Delayed*	Become apparent some time after beginning use of the drug. Include carcinogenicity and teratogenicity. *Uncommon*	Fetal hydantoin syndrome with phenytoin
Type E *End of treatment*	Occur soon after drug withdrawal. *Uncommon*	Withdrawal seizures on stopping phenytoin
Type F *Failure*	Unexpected failure of therapy. Often dose-related and caused by drug interactions. *Common*	Inadequate oral contraceptive dosage, particularly when used with specific enzyme inducers

Type A reactions are predictable from the known pharmacology of the drug, showing a dose-response relationship *(9)*. Genetic factors leading to inappropriate exposure to the parent drug and/or its metabolites can also be an important determinant of ADRs, and have, perhaps, been the most studied in relation to the pharmacogenetics of ADRs.

The following chapter will review the evolving use of genetics to study ADRs and discuss the potential benefits, challenges, and issues associated with this research.

2 Promises: Potential Benefits of Studying the Genetics of ADRs

With drug safety issues taking on a growing importance for all parties involved in drug development, licensing, and use, any measures that can be taken to reduce risk will represent a significant advance for all concerned. With the increasing use of genetics to study the underlying causes and mechanisms of ADRs, it is anticipated that these efforts will increase the safety of drug development and prescription in a number of ways.

2.1 The Gold Standard: Predictive Biomarkers

The discovery of a predictive safety biomarker, identifying those at risk of specific ADRs prior to therapy, and allowing the prescription of alternative therapies or dosing regimens, is, perhaps, the greatest opportunity for pharmacogenetics, and is often regarded as the holy grail for this field. Whilst limited, there are a growing number of examples where this is now feasible from both a biomarker and technological perspective.

Irinotecan is a topoisomerase 1 inhibitor licensed as an anticancer therapy with potent activity against a number of human cancer types. Aside from its impressive efficacy, irinotecan does have potentially fatal dose limiting side effects, including neutropenia, diarrhoea, and a vascular syndrome *(10)*. The genetic biomarker for these ADRs is based on the metabolism of irinotecan, which is a prodrug that is converted to the active moiety, SN-38, by carboxylesterase 2, resulting in a 1000-fold increase in cytotoxic activity *(11)*. SN-38 is inactivated by glucuronidation via the enzyme uradine diphosphate-glucuronosyltransferase 1A1 (UGT1A1). The *UGT1A1* gene is subject to a polymorphism related to the number of TA dinucleotide repeats in the promoter region, with the minor allele (known as *UGT1A1*28*) having a series of 7 repeats as opposed to the 6 repeats present in the wild-type allele. *UGT1A1*28* homozygotes (7/7), which make up approximately 10% of a Caucasian population, have been shown to have reduced enzyme expression and a 1.8–3.9-fold lower glucuronidation of SN-38 when compared with homozygotes for the wild-type (6/6) gene, both *in vitro* and *in vivo (12, 13)*. A number of studies have shown an association between *UGT1A1*28* and an increased risk of developing neutropenia and diarrhoea with irinotecan treatment, with perhaps the definitive prospective study being provided by Innocenti *et al.*, who showed that patients with the 7/7 genotype had a 9.3-fold greater risk of leucopenia than patients carrying either the 6/6 or 6/7 genotype *(14)*.

An advisory committee to the US Food and Drug Administration (FDA) retrospectively reviewed the status of the research relating to the *UGT1A1* genotype and susceptibility to ADRs. On the basis of the advice from this committee, the irinotecan label was revised by the sponsor in consultation with, and approved by, the FDA *(15)*. Irinotecan's new labelling now recommends that clinicians consider reducing the dose in *UGT1A1*28* homozygous patients, and the FDA have cleared for marketing a genotyping test for *UGT1A1* status. The FDA, however, clearly state that the assay is an "aid" to treatment decisions. They go on to say that it is not a substitute for physician judgement and experience, and that other important factors that may affect dosing, such as age, concurrent medications, and liver and kidney function, should also be considered. In short, it is a recommended test and not mandatory.

Abacavir: Another recent example of a genetic biomarker able to predict patients at risk from a Type B ADR is HLA-B57 status as a marker for the potentially fatal hypersensitivity reactions observed in 4–8% of patients taking the HIV-1 reverse inhibitor, abacavir.

Several lines of evidence supported a genetic component to this ADR and pointed towards the involvement of the MHC region *(16)*. Typing of the MHC region in a primarily Caucasian Western Australian population identified an association between carriers of the *HLA-B*5701, HLA-DR7* and *HLA-DQ3* alleles and susceptibility to the ADR. When considering these alleles together, the positive predictive value ([PPV] probability that the patient has the ADR, when restricted to those patients who test positive) for hypersensitivity, was 100%; and the negative predictive value ([NPV], the probability that the patient will not have the ADR, when restricted to all patients who test negative) was 97%. Further studies confirmed the association between the *HLA-B*5701* allele and hypersensitivity in a mixed race North American population, albeit with a lower sensitivity, 46%, probably reflecting the fact that values for predictive markers will vary across different populations *(17)*. Data from subsequent studies have proven to be more variable and a meta-analysis has proposed PPVs and NPVs of 82% and 85%, respectively *(18, 19)*. Hence, although there are still relatively high predictive values associated with the biomarker, and despite the fact that routine preprescription pharmacogenetic testing was deemed to be cost effective, the test is used routinely only in Australia and has not been included on the drug label *(18)*.

This data has shown that it is, to a certain extent, feasible to predict individual susceptibility to ADRs based on a genetic biomarker test. However, the extent to which this will be accepted into clinical practice is uncertain. This, and the factors that determine uptake, will be discussed later.

2.2 *Part of the Jigsaw: Data Integration*

Figure 7.1 illustrates the potential interacting factors that will drive susceptibility to ADRs, indicating that development of predictive models will likely require the integration of data from a number of sources, including genetics. High quality phenotypic/clinical data will be essential if efforts in this area are to be successful. In this respect, as much effort needs to be invested into the clinical characterisation of ADR cases, determination of their causation, and collection of all available epidemiological/demographic information to be used as covariates within the analysis, as there is invested into the collection of the samples themselves. It is essential that this information be integrated with the genetic analysis.

2.2.1 ADR Follow up: Clinical and Demographic Data

Most pharmacogenetic studies are driven by association studies between relatively large sample sets and the derivation of a meaningful statistical p value. With only relatively small cohorts available to study the genetics of ADRs, there are still benefits to be gained from performing genetic studies. Studying limited numbers of cases, or even single cases, has utility in generating hypotheses to be tested in other sample sets, and can also provide additional data to explain individual ADR cases.

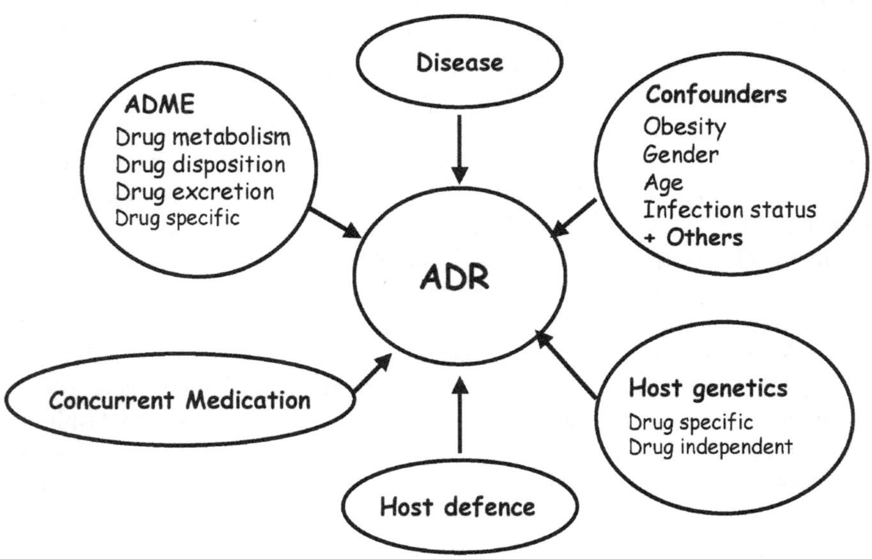

Fig. 7.1 Interacting factors determining susceptibility to ADRs.
Determining and predicting causation of ADRs will require integration of data from a number of sources, including genetics

One potential use of individual genetic analysis is to provide additional data for drug safety follow-up of specific ADR cases. Once an ADR is reported, causality is usually assessed by the company responsible for that drug. This involves the collection and review of data on the individual, such as concurrent medication, dosages, disease, infection status, and any other relevant confounding factors, in an attempt to understand and assign causation. Acquisition and analysis of a DNA sample at this stage could provide additional data for drug safety follow-up and could ultimately aid in explaining causation, delineating drug effects from individual susceptibility factors.

An example of the utility of this approach was a case study, published in 1999, of a single subject presenting with the ventricular arrhythmia *torsade de pointes* (TdP), with causation being assigned to the concomitant use of cisapride, the arrhythmogenic trigger drug, and the antibiotic clarithromycin. Under these circumstances it was proposed that clarithromycin would compete with cisapride for metabolic elimination via the drug metabolising enzyme CYP3A4, potentially raising plasma levels of the trigger drug *(20)*. Subsequent DNA collection and analysis of the genes responsible for the congenital form of the long QT syndrome (LQT) identified a SNP in the gene coding for the cardiac ion channel hERG that had previously been reported to be associated with acquired (drug-induced) LQT (21; see section 3.1.2. for a more complete discussion of genetics related to QT prolongation). It is now possible to piece together information relating to this individual ADR case, i.e., a potentially high circulating plasma level of cisapride, due to the concomitant use of clarithromycin, acting on a pharmacologically sensitive hERG channel to elicit an arrhythmia. Integration of genetic data in this way adds another piece of the jigsaw to help form the complete picture of interacting factors responsible for driving ADRs.

2.2.2 Molecular Data

With newer "omics" technologies, such as genomics, proteomics, and metabonomics becoming more robust and feasible for large-scale research, the integration of molecular and genetic data should facilitate mechanistic understanding and biomarker development. Despite such approaches being relatively new, some successes in this area are beginning to emerge.

Tacrine is a reversible acetlycholinesterase inhibitor for the treatment of Alzheimer's dementia (AD) that was withdrawn from the UK market due to a high incidence of raised alanine aminotransferase (ALT), a liver enzyme that is released into the bloodstream and which is used as a biomarker of liver damage. The factors determining individual susceptibility to the raised ALT levels associated with tacrine use are largely unknown. Carr *et al.* performed expression profiling on hepatic tissue derived from rats that had shown increased levels of ALT on treatment with tacrine *(22)*. From the expression profiles derived from the samples, there was evidence of an IL6-regulated acute phase response, with the response genes alpha-2-macroglobulin, fibronectin, and haptoglobin showing significant up-regulation.

IL6 was then taken forward as a candidate gene and studied in DNA samples obtained from AD patients with and without raised ALT levels as a result of tacrine treatment. Single SNP and haplotype analysis was performed and positive associations were identified between an IL6 haplotype and transaminitis (>2x upper limit of normal of ALT), maximum ALT, and AUC for ALT.

Although "omics" technologies are potentially powerful tools, derivation of samples for analysis are limited by the same constraints as those that apply to collection of DNA samples for ADR analysis, i.e., retrospective location of patients and accessibility of samples, with the added limitation of the analytes being transient over time (unless a marker was related to the underlying state of the individual and not transiently related to the ADR; for example disease-related). Their utility will, therefore, probably be limited to the use of samples derived from animal models, *in vitro* cell systems or clinical trial material.

With increasing information on biological pathways becoming available, the integration of genetic association data with pathway analysis may help point to perturbed pathways as a mechanism of ADRs and, therefore, to identification of novel (non-genetic) biomarkers that are relatively easy to develop into predictive biomarkers. With point of care genotyping still needing some development to become integrated into clinical decision-making, this could provide an additional use of genetics for the development of predictive biomarkers.

2.3 Front loading: Refining and Designing Pre-clinical Assays

Pre-clinical development is one of the most important stages of drug development, during which any potential safety issues of a candidate drug can be predicted and avoided. The aim of this testing is to determine any potential liabilities in candidate drugs before they are taken forward into clinical development. Using this information, a decision is taken as to whether or not to continue with the drug project; if so, to estimate a safe starting dose of the drug for clinical trials in humans; and to determine what monitoring (if any) should be incorporated into the trial designs to ensure patient safety. Such pre-clinical testing is obviously not able at present to detect all liabilities, since ADRs do still occur in the clinical trial and post-marketing settings. Hence any advances that give us the ability to sharpen these pre-clinical tools and to better predict and understand the nature of such liabilities prior to proceeding into human testing would undoubtedly result in safer drugs. Genetic testing is one of the approaches that may provide information on the molecular mechanisms and pathways related to toxicity, and it is feasible that this information could be used to define novel pre-clinical drug screening strategies (i.e., front-loading), and also refine existing front-loading efforts.

An example of this approach is the determination of any likelihood for a compound to cause prolongation of the cardiac QT interval, as a biomarker for the ventricular arrhythmic potential of a drug. This determination is now a regulatory requirement and is assessed by measuring the ability of the compound to block the activity of the cardiac channel, hERG, heterologously expressed in a cell line. The main question arising from this approach is, "Does it matter which hERG variant we screen against?" i.e., do genetically determined hERG variants have altered pharmacology that will predispose an individual to hERG block and subsequent QT prolongation, and should this be determined pre-clinically?

In AstraZeneca we have selected relevant genetic variants and created and expressed the variant channels in an *in vitro* expression system. Utilising high throughput electrophysiology platforms, we have assessed any alterations in the pharmacology of the variant channels against a diverse compound set, selected for its range of hERG liabilities, as well as assessing the biophysics of each variant channel. This strategy allows us to decide whether to include genetic variants in our preclinical screening to take account of differential channel liabilities related to genetic variation. (Similar strategies can also be considered when performing bridging studies into alternate ethnic groups to cover ethnic variation in consensus target sequences as a potential cause of safety liabilities.)

The US FDA has recently published guidelines for thorough QT evaluation of compounds in development and recommends that "genotyping patients who experience marked prolongation of the QT/QTc or TdP whilst on drug therapy should be considered" *(23)*. Whilst it is encouraging that the FDA recognises the potential of genetic variants to influence susceptibility to QT prolongation and arrhythmias, the long-term aim should be to avoid ADRs by designing out liabilities during pre-clinical screening.

Whilst the above example highlights where genetics can help in *refining* existing strategies, this approach could be extended to other genes shown to be involved in the mechanisms of ADRs in the future and could aid in *defining* new screening strategies via an insight into novel mechansisms. For example, the genetic basis of the group of hereditary cholestatic diseases, progressive familial intrahepatic cholestasis (PFIC), has been characterised as being due to variations within the hepatic canalicular transporter genes *ABCB11* (BSEP), *ATP8B1* (FIC1), and *ABCB4* (MDR3). A role for these canalicular transporters in drug-induced cholestasis is now beginning to emerge, with a number of drugs suspected to cause cholestasis via inhibition of BSEP *(24)*. Due to the similarity in clinical phenotypes elicited through perturbation of the transporters, screening for a candidate drug's ability to interact with and inhibit the activity of these transporters could be warranted to reduce the cholestatic potential of new drugs.

2.4 The Lazarus Effect: Is Drug Resurrection Possible?

The concept that a pharmacogenetics approach could be used to rescue or "resurrect" drugs that have previously failed due to efficacy or safety considerations, by re-positioning the drug with a genetic test to identify those subgroups of appropriate responders, has often been presented as one potential way in which genetics could add value to the drug development process. Although, in theory, this concept seems to offer an attractive opportunity for safety genetics, in practice there are no known examples in which a drug that has failed the drug development process, or that has been removed from market, has been resurrected with a companion genetic test, either by its own developers or by another company.

A possible explanation for this disconnect between theory and practice is provided in an analysis by Shah, who outlined the key criteria that would be needed for the genotype-based rescue of a drug *(25)*. These include high efficacy versus currently available alternatives, an understanding of the mechanism of toxicity (including whether it is the parent drug or metabolite that is primarily responsible for toxicity), evidence to support the involvement of genetic factors, and evidence that there were no obvious non-genetic risk factors in the majority of cases. Based on these criteria, Shah reviewed 38 drugs withdrawn from market due to safety issues between 1990 and 2006 and concluded that only one, the antianginal drug perhexiline, would be amenable to resurrection. Perhexiline was first introduced in the early 1970s but was withdrawn worldwide in 1988 due to peripheral neuropathy, papilloedema, and hepatotoxicity. In man, perhexiline is cleared by a single enzyme, CYP2D6, and there is a clear relationship between plasma concentrations and toxicity. The molecular basis for impaired CYP2D6 activity is well understood, and commercially available genotyping assays are available. Therapeutic and nontoxic plasma concentrations can be achieved by prescribing genotype specific doses that have already been firmly established. These factors, plus the fact that perhexiline is a highly effective antianginal drug, make resurrection based on a genetic test possible.

In Shah's review, the main reason for the inability to rescue drugs was that the mechanism of toxicity was not known, and therefore there were no obvious genetic loci related to the outcome. Whilst this may currently be true, it is likely that this balance will change over time due to the increasing efforts in this area, opening up the possibility of resurrection for a number of other drugs. Furthermore, it has also been suggested that opportunities in this area would be limited due to the restricted patent life of the drugs involved; and although this could theoretically be circumvented by a new patent related to the combined use of the drug/diagnostic, this has never been tested *(26)*.

Even if the above issues are addressed, this will not address the more pragmatic concerns in applying this concept in reality. Even assuming that sufficient DNA samples were available from subjects who experienced the ADR, along with sufficient numbers of appropriately matched and treated controls to allow pharmacogenetic research and identify genes associated with safety issues, it is difficult to imagine a situation in which drug development would be an economically viable prospect for a company once a drug had failed. Indeed, it is normal practice within pharmaceutical companies to develop follow-up or back-up drugs with improved safety and efficacy profiles that would already have entered the drug development pipeline. In addition, it has been suggested that there are presently so many opportunities in drug discovery that there is little need to return to old drugs, with pharmaceutical companies preferring to "bury" their failed drug projects *(27)*.

In conclusion, although drug resurrection could be considered in certain circumstances where there is still an unmet medical need not covered by alternative therapies, in the foreseeable future it is unlikely that there will be any drugs resurrected based on a pharmacogenetics test. The present challenge and focus of genetics should be on delivering improved risk:benefit ratios by prospectively applying pharmacogenetics to existing drugs or those in development, and in managing ADRs in the post-marketing setting.

3 Problems: The Challenges Associated with Studying the Genetics of ADRs

From the previous discussions it is obvious that there are a number of important considerations driving the increasing research into the genetics of ADRs and a huge potential benefit to be gained from being able to understand and predict these genetic (and other) factors. Aside from the normal challenges and considerations that apply to all pharmacogenetics studies, there are a number of challenges specific to studying the genetics of ADRs that need to be considered when reviewing this area.

3.1 Homogeneity and Phenotype Selection

Genetic association studies are ideally carried out on large, well-characterised, phenotypically homogeneous patient sets. ADRs, however, present specific challenges, since most cases occur in the post-marketing setting where factors such as assigning causation, off-label and appropriate use (dosage), concurrent medications, and other confounding host factors can serve to yield very heterogeneous sample sets. Furthermore, the fact that only small numbers of ADR samples resulting from a single drug may be available means that there are major decisions to be made in the design and execution of pharmacogenetic studies in this area.

3.1.1 Drug-Specific ADRs

In an attempt to reduce the heterogeneity within genetic ADR studies, the simplest approach in research is to establish collections of cases based around a single ADR with a single drug. Where such drugs are still licensed and in use, and where the ADR in question is relatively common, then this may represent a feasible approach.

Such a scenario exists with the treatment of arterial and venous thromboembolism with warfarin. Due to the lack of alternative therapies, warfarin is still widely used despite the difficulties in managing its use, a result of its narrow therapeutic window and high inter-individual variability in response. Bleeding events are the main ADR associated with warfarin use, affecting approximately 8% of patients *(28)*.

In a study of 2460 patients the average length of hospital stay associated with warfarin-induced bleeding episodes was 6 days, at an average cost of $15,988 *(29)*. The lack of alternative therapies, high incidence, and implications of the ADRs, as well as the associated costs, have encouraged genetic and non-genetic studies into determining the basis of the bleeding events. Genetic factors significantly associated with determining dosing levels and susceptibility to ADRs are polymorphisms within the *CYP2C9* gene (the enzyme responsible for the metabolism of warfarin), the vitamin K reductase complex subunit 1 (*VKORC1*) gene (the drug target for warfarin involved in the biotransformation of vitamin K), and the protein C (*PROC*) gene (involved in the vitamin K clotting process). A multiple regression model combining the above three genes with non-genetic predictors (age, bodyweight, drug interactions, and indication) jointly account for 62% of the variance in warfarin dose *(30)*. This could therefore provide a vital tool in determining the dose required for warfarin therapy.

Both the US FDA and the UK Department of Health have ongoing programmes to assess the effect of genotype on warfarin prescription. In the US, this is now part of the Critical Path Initiative, and a prospective trial is also being funded by the Department of Health within the UK. The FDA Clinical Pharmacology Subcommittee has recommended testing for variations in the *CYP2C9* and *VKORC1* genes in patients requiring warfarin therapy and the drug label has recently been altered to reflect this recommendation *(31)*.

When ADRs are not so common, or when a drug is rarely prescribed, sample sets restricted to a single phenotype elicited by a single drug may be very small. In this situation, detection of genetic associations relies on a strong genetic effect and a highly penetrant variant. Nevertheless, when these criteria apply there have been associations published (Table 7.2). Such small sample sets are, however, particularly prone to both false positive and false negative associations. False positive associations would ideally be dealt with by testing for replication in a second independent cohort; however, obtaining a single sample set for analysis is extremely challenging, making replication sample sets a very rare commodity in this field. False negative results may be even more difficult to quantify, since it is often difficult to publish negative results. A possible example of this is the report by Aithal *et al.* of a lack of the expected association between 24 diclofenac-induced hepatotoxicity cases and the CYP2C9 genotype, the major metabolic route for diclofenac *(32)*. In general, these small studies are best considered to provide hypotheses to be tested in the context of other efforts to establish collections (see sections 3.3.1 and 5).

Table 7.2 Drug-specific ADRs
Selected examples where ADR cohorts related to use of specific drugs have been established and used to study genetic susceptibility

Drug (ref)	ADR (cohort size)	Associated Gene	P value
Perhexiline *(66)*	Hepatotoxicity (4 cases, 70 controls)	CYP2D6	5×10^{-3}
Irinotecan *(67)*	Diarrhoea (26 cases, 92 controls)	UGT1A1	1×10^{-3}
Abacavir *(68)*	Hypersensitivity (14 cases, 167 controls)	HLA-B*57	1×10^{-4}
Carbamazepine *(69)*	Hypersensitivity (23 cases, 63 controls)	TNF	1×10^{-2}

3.1.2 ADR Phenotypes

The issue of restricted numbers available from studying a single drug can, in some cases, be circumvented by pursuing a specific phenotype elicited by a number of drugs. Whilst studying all samples as a single group will increase the availability and ease of case collection, this approach is based on the premise that any genetic factors driving the ADR are not drug–specific, and that there will be common underlying susceptibility factors detectable across all drug classes.

Such a hypothesis has driven genetic studies into the relatively rare phenomenon of acquired (drug-induced) QT prolongation (aLQT) that predisposes to the potentially fatal ventricular arrhythmia TdP. Approximately 60% of families with the congenital form of long QT syndrome (cLQT) have mutations in 1 of 6 different genes coding for cardiac ion channels and the associated proteins required for their correct functioning: hERG and MiRP1 (*KCNH2* and *KCNE2*), KvLQT1 and minK (*KCNQ1* and *KCNE1*), and SCN5a (*SCN5a*), as well as the membrane adaptor protein ankyrin-B (*ANKB*) *(33, 34, 35)*. Due to the low penetrance of the mutant alleles involved in cLQT it has been proposed that some individuals carry "forme fruste" (i.e., clinically inapparent) mutations within the cLQT genes *(36)*. Under normal circumstances, these individuals are clinically asymptomatic with normal QT intervals, but their cardiac ion channels may have altered pharmacology, making them more susceptible to block with certain drugs. In addition, it is known that hERG is a promiscuous channel, capable of being blocked by a large number of drugs from a range of classes. To date there are no examples of drugs that have caused TdP that do not block the hERG channel *(37, 38)*. Hence genetic pre-disposition may also play a role in susceptibility to aLQT. Individual case reports have appeared supporting the hypothesis that variation within the cLQT genes predisposes to aLQT *(20, 21)*.

The role of common susceptibility factors across different drugs has been addressed more recently in larger aLQT cohorts derived from cases triggered by a variety of drugs. Paulussen *et al.* analysed the *KCNH1, KCNE2, KCNQ1, KCNE1*, and *SCN5a* genes in 32 aLQT cases triggered by 9 different drugs versus 32 normal healthy controls *(21)*. Missense forme fruste mutations were identified uniquely in 4 of the 32 cases (12%). Other groups have also used similar heterogenous sample sets to study aLQT, and the results are similar, indicating that 5–12% of aLQT cases carry mutations in one of their cLQT genes that may be identifiable via screening (Table 7.3 *[39, 40, 41, 42]*).

As well as highlighting the utility of heterogeneous sample sets (from a causative drug perspective) in exploring certain ADRs with a common underlying mechanism, the data also suggest that there are other factors contributing to the determination of QT prolongation in the remaining cases. These factors are likely to be an interplay of both genetic factors (e.g., additional genes responsible for determining the cardiac action potential, and drug-specific genes determining individual drug disposition) and non-genetic factors (e.g., disease state/history, concurrent medication, gender, metabolic state); and this highlights the need to integrate data from all possible sources in order to determine causation on an individual level.

Table 7.3 Number of aLQTS patients in whom a disease-associated mutation was detected by screening of cLQT genes
Taken from Paulussen *et al.* (*[29]*, reproduced with kind permission of Springer Science+Business Media, LLC)

	Abbott *et al.* (37)	Sesti *et al.* (38) Yang *et al.* (39)	Chevalie *et al.* (40)	Paulussen *et al.* (20)
Genes screened				
ANKB (Ankyrin-B)	ns	ns	ns	ns
KCNE1 (Mink)	ns	0	0	2
KCNE2 (MiRP1)	1	4	0	1
KCNH2 (HERG)	ns	1	1	1
KCNQ1 (KvLQT1)	ns	1	0	0
SCN5A (SCN5A)	ns	3	ns	0
Number of aLQTS patients screened	20	92	16	32
Number of cases explained	1	9	1	4
Percentage of the investigated aLQTS patient population	5	9	6	12

ns = not studied

3.2 Analysis Strategies, and Sample Size

Whilst statistical considerations and discussions of the candidate gene (CGA) and whole genome analysis (WGA) approaches are covered elsewhere in this book, the choice of analysis strategy may have significant implications for collection strategies and sample sizes. Until recently, most studies investigating the genetics of ADRs have utilised CGA; i.e., the selection of genes based on prior knowledge of factors such as mechanism of action, pathways, on/off target effects, drug disposition, etc. Whilst this has the advantage of generally having a greater statistical power for a smaller sample size, success relies upon the ability to select the appropriate genes based on present knowledge. Availability of HapMap data and recent technological advances now mean that whole genome analysis (WGA) is becoming a more feasible and cost effective option, with the advantage that it is not restricted to any prior hypotheses or to known genes.

Although the vast majority of published pharmacogenetic studies have used CGA, a small number of publications are now starting to compare this approach with WGA. An example of this is the association between *UGT1A1* and hyperbilirubinaemia observed with the antirestenosis drug tranilast, which was originally identified by a CGA *(43)*. This data was amenable to subsequent modelling analysis to estimate the number of cases and controls, and the SNP coverage across the genome that would have been required to detect the same association using a WGA. The authors estimated that a genome map of only 100,000 SNPs would have been required to detect the association with the extended LD block containing the *UGT1A1* gene and, with a control cohort of 1085, only 10 cases would have been needed to identify the association with *UGT1A1* at $P < 0.05$ *(44)*. Whilst these numbers do reflect the large genetic effect involved in determining hyperbilirubinaemia and the powerful effect of the *UGT1A1* genotype on the phenotype; they are somewhat surprising, given that the WGA studies published to date advocate the use of larger sample sizes, even to detect relative risks that are larger than that of the *UGT1A1* example above. As the authors pointed out, it is unlikely that any associations would be as readily identifiable where there are multiple genes involved (and interactions thereof) with lower penetrance involved in determining a phenotype, and it is likely that this represents a "best case" scenario *(26)*. As the technologies for WGA become more refined and accessible, and experience is gained in generating and analysing the data, it will be interesting to follow progress in this area, although it is likely that a bipartite approach of CGA and WGA will prove most useful in the future.

3.3 Collection Strategies

The rare and unexpected nature of ADRs which occur spontaneously over the entire geographical region where a causative drug is marketed presents researchers with special issues in establishing cohorts for study, based on the (in)ability to identify and recruit cases and controls into any study. With the additional need for appropriate ethical committee approval from all regions where samples will be collected, and the variable pharmacovigilance reporting structures and regulatory requirements within each country, there are unique challenges involved in being able to recruit subjects to study the genetics of ADRs. There are various strategies available.

3.3.1 Use of Clinical Trial Material

If an ADR is detected during the clinical trial process, and DNA collection has been instigated as part of that clinical trial (which is now becoming more routine in many pharmaceutical companies), then the material and clinical data is available to study the genetics related to that ADR and that drug. With pre-specified inclusion and exclusion criteria for the study, such a sample set has the advantages of being homogenous and well controlled in terms of drugs, dosages, concurrent medication, indications, and other possible confounders, as well as having control samples available for study.

Depending on the timing of the research, the discovery of an association between a gene (or genes) and an ADR may not have any utility for the particular drug in question. For example, it may not be possible to develop and use as a predictive test a genetic association that is discovered late in development and which does not have a sufficiently strong predictive value to identify at-risk patients. Other considerations must also be taken into account at this stage, such as the risk:benefit profile of the drug versus the ADR and thus the viability of a personalised medicine approach, the status of backup compounds under development within a company, as well as portfolio considerations for the company. The utility of this approach may ultimately lie in increasing the understanding of mechanisms of specific ADRs, with the potential to impact on future drug development. Hence GlaxoSmithKline's investment in the DNA collections that allowed exploration of the association between *UGT1A1* and tranilast, which could subsequently be applied to explain hyperbilirubinaemia observed in the development of other drugs.

Even if DNA collection was not included as an original component of the clinical trial protocol, it is possible to retrospectively approach case and control subjects who participated in a clinical study where a safety signal was observed, and request a sample after the study has been completed. This approach has been used successfully by Sun *et al.*, who returned to subjects enrolled in the DIAMOND studies in order to study TdP induced by dofetilide, a class III antiarrhythmic agent used for the conversion to and maintenance of normal sinus rhythm in patients with highly symptomatic atrial fibrillation/flutter *(45)*. A missense mutation in the hERG channel (R1047L) was detected in 2 out of 7 cases, versus 5 out of 98 controls, and subsequent functional characterisation showed slower activation kinetics of the variant channel, potentially leading to a 15% prolongation of the action potential.

Even using this collection strategy, the authors noted that the numbers were limited because of difficulties in locating and obtaining consent from many patients. In addition, retrospective sample collection has the added expense required to re-instate a clinical study, re-open study centres, perform ethical committee submissions, etc., thus making routine defensive banking of DNA samples during clinical studies a much more pragmatic solution.

3.3.2 Retrospective Collections Identified Through Pharmacovigilance Reporting Systems

For samples from ADR cases that were not collected during the clinical trial, or for those that occur when the drug has been marketed, retrospective identification and collection is the only strategy available.

All European countries have their own procedures for spontaneous ADR reporting and tracking which are augmented by reports from pharmaceutical companies. It is possible to perform a retrospective inspection of these pharmacovigilance databases to identify relevant ADR cases and to use this as a potential route to re-contact individual subjects for a DNA sample. Although feasible, this approach has many challenges that need to be considered when assessing the utility of this strategy.

Normally, ADR reporting is voluntary and can often be regarded as a time-consuming burden by the reporting physician. In some countries, such as Sweden, it is not mandatory that the contact information for the reporting physician be provided. This results in an under reporting of ADRs and the loss of many potential cases to follow up. Where reporter information is available, follow up requires that physicians are still contactable and that they are willing to invest time and effort to re-trace specific cases. Even if physicians are contactable, and willing to participate, many subjects may be lost to follow-up, or themselves unwilling to participate in such an initiative.

With possible attrition at so many points, it is clear that retrospective collection can be a time-consuming and relatively inefficient way to collect cases. Nevertheless, this approach has shown some limited success. Ford *et al.* used the yellow card reporting system to identify cases of terodiline-induced cardiotoxicity reported to the Medical Control Agency (MCA) in the UK *(46)*. Twenty-eight cases were identified, of which 26 were followed up by the MCA by contact with general practitioners, which took place 3–4 years after the initial case reports. From these 26 cases only 6 samples were obtained. When looking at the causes of attrition, 2 patients were reported to have died, 6 were lost to followup, and no reply was received from 12 GPs. No controls were collected and population study data was used instead. The results of the analysis showed that possession of a variant allele of the CYP2C19 phase I drug metabolising enzyme (the *CYP2C19*2* allele) appeared to contribute to adverse cardiac reactions to terodiline. Although the validity of these results may be questioned, since there is no evidence that either terodiline or its enantiomers undergo metabolism by CYP2C19, and may indeed be a false positive result given the small sample sets and unmatched controls, the study does highlight the feasibility of a spontaneous adverse drug reaction reporting system to obtain blood samples from patients with relatively rare ADRs.

A more ambitious effort based on this strategy is presently underway in Europe. EUDRAGENE is a European collaboration, funded with support from the European Union, aimed at establishing an ADR case-control DNA collection using the existing spontaneous reporting systems available within participating countries *(47)*. In a survey of European countries, it was found that no one individual country would generate a sufficient number of cases of any ADR within a reasonable time frame, thus necessitating this collaborative cross-community program. These efforts have been aided by the harmonisation of national pharmacovigilance reporting systems through the European Medicines Evaluation Agency, which is compiling a Europe-wide database of ADR reports *(48)*. The aim of this collaborative effort is to make the resulting collections available for use by both academic and industrial researchers, on the proviso that all resultant genotype data is submitted to the main database for use by subsequent researchers, hence providing a potentially powerful resource to expedite research in this field.

At present, there is no equivalent US-wide collection of ADR cases. This is partly because, in the US, there is no reporting structure equivalent to that available within Europe. This, along with the fact that there is no single ethics committee or institutional review board capable of giving approval for the whole region, means that pharmacovigiliance collections within the USA are more problematic. Whilst there are a number of US-based initiatives ongoing (see below), these are more often based on clinical registries rather than being US-wide collections. Alternative sources of ADR reports could be through US health care provider and insurance company databases; and given the size of the American market and the number of prescriptions written in the US, an appropriate collection strategy would have great utility in this field.

3.3.3 Real-Time Collection of Post-Marketing Cases

The possibility of collecting post-marketing ADR cases in real time, i.e., as and when they are reported, takes the above strategy one step further. By reducing the time lag between case reporting and contact, it is hoped that there will be less attrition due to reporting physicians and cases being lost to follow-up. To date, however, there are no successful examples of this approach. The main issue appears to be the time-consuming process of approaching each country individually to obtain ethical approval that will allow collection across the entire country, as well as the differing ADR reporting structures and local regulations that need to be considered for each country. In countries where there is a central ethical committee capable of providing consent for the entire country, such as the UK MREC, this is relatively simple. For other countries where there is no single EC/IRB that is capable of approval for a whole country, the challenges faced by either getting approval from each separate EC/IRB in advance or approaching the relevant body as and when a case arises has, so far, proven prohibitive. Furthermore, the ability to identify and confirm "pure" cases without confounders can be difficult, and actual numbers can also be very low. In summary, practical and logistical issues mean that returns are likely to be poor in respect to the effort required, and as such this route has not been a fruitful source of material for our company.

3.3.4 Registries Developed Through Dedicated Clinical Centres

Initiatives to recruit cases both retrospectively and in real time from dedicated clinical centres are also underway. With experienced clinicians leading each centre, this approach has the advantage of ensuring an appropriate and accurate clinical review of each case, with the aim of minimising noise within the sample set by ensuring that subjects fall within clear criteria for a drug-induced ADR. Furthermore, because of the nature of these centres, they often have databases of patients established over a period of time, from which relevant cases and controls can be identified retrospectively. The UK and US Drug-Induced Liver Injury Networks (DILIGEN and DILIN, respectively) are examples where this approach is currently being used. US DILIN aims to establish a registry of fully characterised patients who have experienced drug-induced liver injury (DILI), and to develop a systematic classification system *(49)*. The research will involve collection of epidemiological data, clinical data, and biological samples (blood, DNA, urine, and liver tissue) from affected patients and matched controls. The programme consists of a retrospective study aiming to recruit 50–100 samples (and matched controls) from DILI caused by each of four different drugs: isoniazid, phenytoin, clavulanic acid/amoxicillin (augmentin), and valproic acid, as well as a prospective study following DILI cases presenting from any drug. This combination of patient material collection and the opportunity for multifactorial characterisation should provide a powerful tool with which to explore any genetic component involved in susceptibility to DILI as well as a resource for biomarker development.

3.4 Control Cohorts

Strategies for the collection of appropriate controls are as important as the collection of cases. Ideally, the control population should represent the "at-risk" population as closely as possible, whilst not presenting with the specific ADR of interest. Theoretically, the more representative the control population is of the affected population, then the higher is the probability of detecting true associations, whilst reducing the number of cases required to detect the association. However, all of the issues associated with identifying and collecting postmarketing ADR cases also apply to identifying and recruiting controls, with the additional problems of appropriate matching for drug treatment, underlying disease, exposure, and concurrent medications in a post-marketing setting.

Whilst the use of similarly treated but unaffected controls remains the ideal, some researchers have recommended the use of population control samples. By using such a sufficiently large collection of a representative population, it is possible to circumvent the need for a tightly matched control set. Although any at-risk alleles will also be present in the population control group, if the control group is appropriately large and the risk allele(s) appropriately rare in the population (which is almost certainly the case for ADRs), then they will likely be represented at such a low frequency that statistical associations will still be identified, given the over-representation of the risk allele in the case group. Obviously, this lack of tight matching means that, while the power to detect genetic associations is not reduced, the potential for false positives is increased, as is the number of controls required. This should be taken into account in the research strategy.

The power to detect genetic associations can be increased by the use of up to 3–4 controls per case. However, because confounding may occur, it is important that these controls should be collected using a sampling method that does not introduce a systematic bias in genotype frequencies. In particular, matching, as far as possible, should be performed for age, gender, residency, clinical history, self-reported race, and ethnicity (according to FDA guidelines).

Although establishment of such a control set is potentially resource intensive and expensive, it would have general benefits across the scientific community. This has been recognised by the Wellcome Trust, who have established a 3000-subject control set which is available for general use by researchers (given adherence to specific regulations) *(50)*. As long as controls are selected based on the above criteria, then this could provide one solution to provision of controls for ADR case-control studies.

3.5 Uptake of Predictive Biomarkers: Use in the Clinic

It is now 50 years since Motulsky published his landmark paper on adverse drug reactions and genetics, and over subsequent decades several biomarkers have been discovered that now have established associations with ADRs

(*(51, 52);* Table 7.4). Despite this long record of genetic association and potential predictive value, very few, if any, of these genetic tests are in routine use in clinical practice to guide therapy and predict patients at risk of ADRs. So what factors are preventing the uptake of these biomarkers to avoid ADRs in the clinic?

3.5.1 Scientific and Technical Issues

Lack of a clear correlation between ADRs and genetic variation is perceived as one of the major barriers to clinical uptake of PGx tests *(53)*. Even one of the most well-established genetic associations, that of thiopurine methyltransferase (TPMT) and the side effects of 6-mercaptopurine (6-MP) and azathiopurine (AZA) therapy, is now known to have a complex mechanism and is subject to conflicting data correlating genotype with phenotype that affects its interpretation and use in the clinic.

ADRs resulting from treatment with 6-MP or AZA affect 2–4% of individuals and manifest as bone marrow supression with leucopenia and neutropenia. Activation of 6-MP and AZA occurs through a multistep pathway to yield 6-thioguanine (6-TG) metabolites, which are responisible for the cytotoxic side effects of these drugs, and these pathways compete with the deactivation of the drugs via TPMT *(54, 55)*. Hence, individuals with low TPMT levels are prone to the cytotoxic side effects of the drug because of accumulation of the 6-TG metabolites; whereas those with high (normal) TPMT levels are relatively free from ADRs (but prone to nonresponse).

Table 7.4 Valid genetic/genomic biomarkers in the context of FDA-approved drug labels (Adapted from *[50]*)

Biomarker	Use	Test	Prototypic Drug
2.1 Genetic biomarkers; all contexts			
CYP2C19	Drug exposure	3	Voriconazole
CYP2C9	Drug exposure	3	Celecoxib, Warfarin
CYP2D6	Drug exposure	3	Atomoxetine
NAT variants	Drug exposure	3	Rifampin, isoniazid, pyrazinamide
TPMT variants	Myelotoxicity	2	Azathiopurine
UGT1A1 variants	Neutropenia	2	Irinotecan
2.2 Genomic biomarkers; safety contexts only			
Dihydropyrimidine Dehydrogenase (DPD) deficiency	Stomatitis, diarrhea, neutropenia, neurotoxicity	3	Capecitabine
Glucose-phosphate Dehydrogenase (G6PD) deficiency	Hemolysis	3	Rasburicase
Protein C deficiencies	Tissue necrosis	2	Warfarin

Test: 1 = test required, 2 = test recommended, 3 = information only

Approximately 90% of Caucasians are homozygous for the wild-type TPMT alleles, whilst 9–10% are heterozygous and 0.3% are homozygous for mutant alleles. To date 21 variant TPMT alleles have been identified that are associated with decreased activity, compared with the *TPMT*1* wild-type allele; although it is reported that more than 95% of defective TPMT activity can be explained by the three most frequent mutant alleles, *TPMT*2*, **3A*, and **3C* *(56)*. Several studies have shown excellent concordance between TPMT status and ADR phenotype, with one study showing that all homozygous-deficient TPMT patients required reductions in their doses of 6-MP to eliminate toxicity and maintain efficacy, compared to 35% of heterozygotes and only 7% of wild-type subjects *(57, 58, 59, 60)*. Other studies have, however, not proven so convincing, suggesting that other factors are also involved in determining adverse response *(61)*, and that, in fact, only 30–50% of ADRs may be predicted by TPMT status *(62)*. Furthermore, it has been estimated that the genetic tests currently available detect only approximately 90% of nonfunctional alleles and would thus misclassify a proportion of TPMT poor metabolisers.

In summary, the example of TPMT as a biomarker to prevent ADRs is one of the simplest, best established, and most often referenced in safety genetics. Clinical diagnostic genotyping is available for TPMT status, and the drug label has been revised to include information about the increased risk of ADRs in genetically determined TPMT poor metabolisers. Despite this, there is considerable complexity around the scientific basis and the interpretation of the test, and the conflicting data in this example is perceived as a barrier to the use of the genotype test in the clinic. Hence, uptake of the test is low, with no routine use in four EU countries surveyed, even when the test is available free of charge *(53)*.

3.5.2 Cost

Many studies have now been performed on the cost-effectiveness of genetic biomarkers to predict patients at risk of ADRs, and both TPMT and HLA-B57 testing have been shown to be cost-effective tests for the prevention of ADRs in acute lymphoblastic leukemia (ALL) therapy and abacavir therapy, respectively *(63, 18)*. Nevertheless, recent studies have shown that physicians' perceptions are often that these tests are not cost–effective; and there is evidence that even when the tests are provided free of charge, uptake may still be low *(53)*. The solution to this issue is likely to be increased education and training of the prescribing physicians, rather than decreased costs.

3.5.3 Knowledge

One of the major barriers to the uptake of current and future biomarkers to predict patients at risk of ADRs may be the perceived complexity of the test versus the knowledge base of the clinicians who decide whether to utilise it. An ideal biomarker for patient selection would have a 100% PPV or NPV. In practice, PPV and

NPV for tests available for ADR prediction show a range of values, even for the same drug, and may also vary according to the population studied and tested, as highlighted previously with the HLA/abacavir data *(18)*.

The data around associations between genotype and ADRs, and the absence of a single predictive genetic biomarker with a sufficiently high PPV and NPV, as highlighted with the TPMT and HLA examples previously, are perhaps the main reasons behind the slow implementation and uptake of genetic safety biomarkers. For the majority of examples available to date, it seems that a single genotype will not provide the required predictive power to be used in clinical decision making. The emerging data suggest that any genetic biomarker will probably require integration of a number of genotypes, along with other additional clinical markers and susceptibility factors, in order to develop an algorithm sufficiently sensitive to be of value in the prediction of ADRs. For irinotecan there is exploratory data to support this, with polymorphisms in *UGT1A7*, *UGT1A9*, and the drug transporter genes *ABCB1*, *ABCC2*, and *ABCG2* also appearing to influence exposure to the pharmacologically active metabolites *(64, 65)*.

Clinicians will need to be educated that it is not reasonable to have expectations that any genetically-based predictive test will be 100% effective in predicting ADRs *(55)*; indeed, certainty within all fields of clinical medicine is rare, and very few predictive tests are 100% sensitive in predicting ADRs. Furthermore, it is likely that there will be some education of primary care physicians needed in how to interpret and apply the results of these tests, as well as how to understand and interpret the pharmacogenetic information on the drug label. A survey carried out across four countries in the EU found that clinicians trained before the 1990s (who make up the majority of physicians practicing today) have little knowledge of genetics *(53)*. As a consequence, primary care physicians may not carry out pre-treatment pharmacogenetic testing, even if it was made mandatory, because they are not aware of the benefits of such tests, and are unable to properly interpret the data. It is apparent that, as well as efforts in developing the science, there should also be equivalent efforts in educating those who will be in the front line of using the outcomes.

4 Conclusions: Delivering the Promises

There are major drivers to improve drug safety, and any advances that can be made in this area will be of major benefit to patients, health care providers, regulatory authorities, pharmaceutical companies, and their shareholders alike. In order to achieve this goal all possible areas are being explored, and there is increasing evidence to indicate that susceptibility to ADRS is, to some extent, genetically driven. With the increasing public, regulatory and commercial pressure, and improvements in knowledge and technologies, the genetics of ADRs is gaining increased attention. The previous chapter has highlighted some of the benefits to be gained from studying this area and has also indicated some of the specific challenges that are faced.

Whilst previous work in this area has generally, by necessity, been restricted to candidate gene analysis performed on sub-optimal sample sets, there is a growing recognition that in order for genetics to be fully exploited, more robust study designs, including replication sets, are required to ensure that the results are more conclusive. With sample availability a major issue, larger collaborative efforts are likely to be more fruitful, and efforts such as EUDRAGENE, US DILIN, and UK DILIGEN seem to offer the best chance of generating more definitive results. Advances in technologies and analysis methods also mean that alternative approaches, such as whole genome analysis, are becoming increasingly feasible. As more experience is gained with handling and analysing data from these studies, and as they are applied to the emerging cohort collections, it is likely that there will be major advances in this field within the foreseeable future.

The ability to develop and market safer drugs is being increasingly recognised as a common unifying goal for a number of parties. In recognition of this, and the specific challenges involved in studying this area, there is a greater drive towards pre-competitive collaborative efforts in this area. Efforts such as the Serious Adverse Event Consortium (SAEC), a US FDA-instigated cross-pharmaceutical/academic consortium with the aim of studying the genetics of ADRs, are also beginning to emerge. Whilst still in its formation stage, this consortium has already recognised the need for precompetitive international collaboration by attempting to facilitate integration of initiatives such as EUDRAGENE, US DILIN, and UK DILIN in order to advance this field. With such momentum behind these initiatives, the challenges in this area will be addressed, and these collaborative efforts seem to offer the best chance of success. It will be interesting to monitor how such consortia can form and operate, what information is generated, and how it is utilised.

What is also increasingly apparent is that studying genetics in isolation will not, in the majority of cases, provide the clarity that is required to move this field forward. Genetics is likely to be only one piece of the jigsaw that will need to be integrated with other data to generate the full picture of susceptibility to, and understanding the mechanisms of, drug safety. These data will include that generated experimentally, and will require integration with clinical, epidemiological, and demographic information in order to develop algorithms to predict ADRs. Efforts to increase the expectations and knowledge base of prescribing physicians are essential and will also aid progress in this area.

This is a fast developing area with high interest and high stakes, and it is likely that there will be substantial advances in the field over the coming years. It will be interesting to review this field again in five years to see what has become of the potential and drive that is present today.

Acknowledgements I would like to thank Dr. Ruth March for her input into this chapter, and Dr. Simon Smith and Professor Ann Daly for their critical reviews and comments.

References

1. Pirmohamed M, James S, Meakin S, Green C, Scott AK, Walley TJ, Farrar KB, Kevin Park BK, Breckenridge AM (2004) Adverse drug reactions as cause of admission to hospital: prospective analysis of 18 820 patients. BMJ 329:15–19.
2. Jefferys DB, Leakey D, Lewis JA, Payne S, Rawlins MD (1998) New active substances authorized in the United Kingdom between 1972 and 1994. Br J Clin Pharmcol 45: 151–156.
3. http://www.fda.gov/bbs/topics/news/2004/NEW01122.html.
4. http://money.cnn.com/2004/09/30/news/fortune500/merck/?cnn=yes.
5. http://www.adrugrecall.com/news/baycol-bayer.html.
6. http://en.wikipedia.org/wiki/TGN1412.
7. Howard Rl, Avery AJ, Slavenburg S, Royal S, Pipe P, Lucassen P, Pirmohamed M (2006) Which drugs cause preventable admissions to hospital? A systematic review. Br J Clin Pharmacol 63:136–147.
8. http://www.findarticles.com/p/articles/mi_m0ISW/is_2001_June/ai_75178713.
9. Pirmohamed M, Park BK (2001) Genetic susceptibility to adverse drug reactions. TIPS 22:298–305.
10. Rothenberg ML, Meropol NJ, Poplin EA (2001) Mortaility associated with irinotecan plus bolus flouracil/leucovorin: summary findings of an independent panel. J Clin Oncol 19:3801–3807.
11. Humerickhouse R, Lohrbach K, Li L, Bosron WF, Dolan ME (2000) Characterization of CPT-11 hydrolysis by human liver carboxylesterase isoforms hCE-1 and hCE-2. Cancer Res 60:1189–1192.
12. Fisher MB, VandenBranden M, Findlay K, Burchell B, Thummel KE, Hall SD, Wrighton SA (2000) Tissue distribution and interindividual variation in human UDP-glucuronosyltransferase activity: relationship between UGT1A1 promoter genotype and variability in a liver bank. Pharmacogenetics 10:727–739.
13. McLeod Hl, Watters JW (2004) Irinotecan pharmacogenetics: is it time to intervene. J Clin Oncol 22:1356–1359.
14. Innocenti F, Undevia SD, Iyer L, Chen PX, Das S, Kocherginsky M, Karrison T, Janisch L, Ramirez J, Rudin CM, Vokes EE, Ratain MJ (2004) Genetic variants in the UDP-glucuronosyltransferase 1A1 gene predict the risk of severe neutropenia of irinotecan. J Clin Oncol 22:1382–8.
15. Haga SB, Thummel KE, Burke W (2006) Adding pharmacogenetics information to drug labels: lessons learned. Pharmacogenet Genom 16:847–854.
16. Mallal S, Nolan D, Witt C, Masel G, Martin AM, Moore C, Sayer D, Castley A, Mamotte C, Maxwell D, James I, Christiansen FT (2002) Association between presence of HLA-B*5701, HLA-DR7, and HLA-DQ3 and hypersensitivity to HIV-1 reverse-transcriptase inhibitor abacavir. Lancet 359:727–732.
17. Hetherington S, Hughes AR, Mosteller M, Shortino D, Baker KL, Spreen W, Lai E, Davies K, Handley A, Dow DJ, Fling ME, Stocum M, Bowman C, Thurmond LM, Roses AD (2002) Genetic variations in HLA-B region and hypersensitivity reactions to abacavir. Lancet 359:1121–22.
18. Hughes DA, Javier V, Ward CC, Alfirevic A, Park KB, Pirmohamed M (2004) Cost-effectiveness analysis of HLA-B*5701 genotyping in preventing abacavir hypersensitivity. Pharmacogenetics 14:335–342.
19. March R (2006) Challenges and opportunities of pharmacogenetics in drug development. Personalised Medicine 3:195–206.
20. Piquette RK (1999) Torsade de pointes induced by cisapride/clarithromycin interaction. Ann Pharmacother 33:22–26.
21. Paulussen ADC, Gilissen RAHJ, Armstrong M, Doevendans PA, Verhasselt P, Smeets HJM, Schulze-Bahr E, Haverkamp W, Breithardt G, Cohen N, Aerssens J (2004) Genetic variations

of KCNQ1, KCNH2, SCN5A, KCNE1, and KCNE2 in drug-induced long QT syndrome patients. J Mol Med 82:182–188.
22. Carr DF, Alfirevic A, Tugwood JD, Barratt BJ, Sherwood J, Smith J, Pirmohamed M, Park KB (2006) Molecular and genetic association of interleukin-6 in tacrine-induced hepatotoxicity. Gastroenterology (In press).
23. http://www.fda.gov/cber/gdlns/iche14qtc.htm.
24. Pauli-Magnus C, Meier PJ (2005) Hepatocellular transporters and cholestasis. J Clin Gastroenterol 39(supp 2):S103–S110.
25. Shah R (2006) Can pharmacogenetics help rescue drugs withdrawn from the market? Pharmacogenomics 7:889–908.
26. Roses AD (2004) Pharmacogenetics and drug development: the path to safer and more effective drugs. Nat Rev Genet 5:645–656.
27. Marshall A (1997) Getting the right drug into the right patient. Nat Biotechnol 15: 1249–1252.
28. Palareti G, Leali N, Coccheri S, Poggi M, Manotti C, D'Angelo A, Pengo V, Erba N, Moia M, Ciavarella N, Devoto G, Berrettini M, Musolesi S (1996) Bleeding complications of oral anticoagulant treatment: an inception-cohort prospective collaborative study (ISOCAT). Lancet 348:423–428.
29. Fanikos J, Grasso-Correnti N, Shah R, Kucher N, Goldhaber SZ (2005) Major bleeding complications in a specialized anticoagulation service. Am J Cardiol 96:595–8.
30. Wadelius M, Chen LY, Eriksson N, Bumpstead S, Ghori J, Wadelius C, Bentley D, McGinnis R, Deloukas P (2007) Association of warfarin dose with genes involved in its action and metabolism. Hum Genet 121:23–34.
31. Reynolds KK, Bukavekas BL (2007) Current status of applied pharmacogenetics in clinical practice. Personalised Medicine 2007; 4:221–225.
32. Aithal GP, Day CP, Leathart JBS, Daly AK (2000) Relationship of polymorphism in CYP2C9 to genetic susceptibility to diclofenac-induced hepatitis. Pharmacogenetics 10:511–518.
33. Long QT database initiative of the Working Group on Arrhythmias of the European Society of Cardiology. http://pc4.fsm.it:81/cardmoc/.
34. Splawski I, Shen J, Timothy KW, Lehmann MH, Priori S, Robinson JL, Moss AJ, Schwartz PJ, Towbin JA, Vincent GM, Keating MT (2000) Spectrum of mutations in long-QT syndrome genes KvLQT1, HERG, SCN5A, KCNE1 and KCNE2. Circulation 102:1178–1185.
35. Mohler PJ, Schott J-J, Gramolini AO, Dilly KW, Guatimosim S, duBell WH, Song LS, Haurogne K, Kyndt F, Ali ME, Rogers TB, Lederer WJ, Escande D, Le Marec H, Bennett V (2003) Ankyrin-B mutation causes type 4 long-QT cardiac arrhythmia and sudden cardiac death. Nature 421:634–639.
36. Priori SG, Napolitano C, Schwartz PJ (1999) Low penetrance in the long QT syndrome. Clinical impact. Circulation 99:529–533.
37. Redfern WS, Carlsson L, Davis AS, Lynch WG, MacKenzie I, Palethorpe S, Siegl PKS, Strang I, Sullivan AT, Wallis R, Camm AJ, Hammond TG (2003) Relationships between preclinical cardiac electrophysiology, clinical QT interval prolongation and torsade de pointes for a broad range of drugs: evidence for a provisional safety margin in drug development. Cardiovasc Res 58:32–45.
38. Fenichel RR, Malik M, Antzelevitch C, Sanguinetti M, Roden DM, Priori SG, Ruskin JN, Lipicky RJ, Louis R, Cantilenar LR (2004) Drug-induced torsades de pointes and implications for drug development. J Cardiovasc Electrophysiol 15:475–494.
39. Abbott GW, Sesti F, Splawski I, Buck ME, Lehmann MH, Timothy KW, Keating MT, Goldstein SA (1999) MiRP1 forms IKr potassium channels with HERG and is associated with cardiac arrhythmia. Cell 97:175–187.
40. Sesti F, Abbott GW, Wei J, Murray KT, Saksena S, Schwartz PJ, Priori SG, Roden DM, George AL Jr, Goldstein SA (2000) A common polymorphism associated with antibiotic-induced cardiac arrhythmia. Proc Natl Acad Sci USA 97:10613–10618.
41. Yang P, Kanki H, Drolet B, Yang T, Wei J, Viswanathan PC, Hohnloser SH, Shimizu W, Schwartz PJ, Stanton M, Murray KT, Norris K, George AL Jr, Roden DM (2002) Allelic

variants in long-QT disease genes in patients with drug-associated torsades de pointes. Circulation 105:1943–1948.
42. Chevalier P, Rodriguez C, Bontemps L, Miquel M, Kirkorian G, Rousson R, Potet F, Schott JJ, Baro I, Touboul P (2001) Non-invasive testing of acquired long QT syndrome: evidence for multiple arrhythmogenic substrates. Cardiovasc Res 50:386–398.
43. Danoff TM, Campbell A, McCarthy LC, Lewis KF, Repasch MH, Saunders AM, Spurr NK, Purvis IJ, Roses AD, Xu CF (2004) A Gilbert's syndrome UGT1A1 variant confers susceptibility to tranilast-induced hyperbilirubinemia. Pharmacogenomics J 4:49–53.
44. Xu C-F, Lewis KF, Yeo AJ, McCarthy LC, Maguire MF, Anwar Z, Danoff TM, Roses AD, Purvis IJ (2004) Identification of a pharmacogenetic effect by linkage disequilibrium mapping. Pharmacogenomics J 4:374–378.
45. Sun Z, Milos PM, Thompson JF, Lloyd DB, Mank-Seymour A, Richmond J, Cordes JS, Zhou J (2004) Role of a KCNH2 polymorphism (R1047 L) in dofetilide-induced torsades de pointes. J Mol Cell Cardiol 37:1031–9.
46. Ford GA, Wood SM, Daly AK (2000) CYP2D6 and CYP2C19 genotypes of patients with terodiline cardiotoxicity identified through the yellow card system. Br J Clin Pharmacol 50:77–80.
47. Molokhia M, McKeigue P (2006) EUDRAGENE: European collaboration to establish a case-control DNA collection for studying the genetic basis of adverse drug reactions. Pharmacogenomics 7:633–639.
48. www.eudravigilance.org/human/evGateway01.asp.
49. http://dilin.dcri.duke.edu/about/index.html.
50. http://www.wtccc.org.uk/.
51. Motulsky AG (1957) Drug reactions, enzymes and biochemicalgenetics. JAMA 165:835–837.
52. http://www.fda.gov/cder/genomics/genomic_biomarkers_table.htm.
53. Zika E, Gurwitz D, Ibarreta D (2006) Pharmacogenetics and pharmacogenomics: state-of-the-art and potential socio-economic impact in the EU. Institute for Prospective Technological Studies.
54. Lennard L (1992) The clinical pharmacology of 6-mercaptopurine. Eur J Clin Pharmacol 43:329–339.
55. Wang L, Weinshilboum R (2006) Thiopurine S-methyltransferase pharmacogenetics: insights, challenges and future directions. Oncogene 25:1629–1638.
56. McLeod HL, Krynetski EY, Relling MV, Evans WE (2000) Genetic polymorphism of thiopurine methyltransferase and its clinical relevance for childhood acute lymphoblastic leukemia. Leukemia 14:567–572.
57. Relling MV, Hancock ML, Rivera GK, Sandlund JT, Ribeiro RC, Krynetski EY, Pui C-H, Evans WE (1999) Mercaptopurine therapy intolerance and heterozygosity at the thiopurine S-methyltransferase gene locus. J Natl Cancer Inst 91:2001–2008.
58. Evans WE, Horner M, Chu YQ, Oellerich M (1991) Altered mercaptopurine metabolism, toxic effects and dosage requirement in a thiopurine methyltransferase deficient child with acute lymphoblastic leukemia. J Pediatr 119:985–89.
59. Schutz E, Gummert J, Mohr F, Oellerich M (1993) Azathiopurine-induced myelosuppression in thiopurine methyltransferase deficient heart transplant recipients. Lancet 341:436.
60. Lennard L, Welch JC, Lilleyman JS (1997) Thiopurine drugs in the treatment of childhood leukemia: the influence of inherited thiopurine methyltransferase activity on drug metabolism and cytotoxicity. Br J Clin Pharmacol 44:455–61.
61. Cunliffe RN, Scott BB (2002) Monitoring for drug side-effects in inflammatory bowel disease. Aliment Pharmacol Ther 16:647–662.
62. Winter J, Walker A, Shapiro D, Gaffney D, Spooner RJ, Mills PR (2004) Cost effectiveness of thiopurine methyl transferase genotype screening in patients about to commence azathioprine therapy for treatment of inflammatory bowel disease. Aliment Pharmacol Ther 20:593–599.
63. van den Akker-van Marle ME, Gurwitz D, Detmar SB, Enzing CM, Hopkins MM, Gutierrez de Mesa E, Ibarreta D (2006) Cost-effectiveness of pharmacogenomics in clinical practice: a

case study of thiopurine methyltransferase genotyping in acute lymphoblastic leukemia in Europe. Pharmacogenomics 7:783–92.
64. Carlini LE, Meropol NJ, Bever J, Andria ML, Hill T, Gold P, Rogatko R, Wang H, Blanchard RL (2005) UGT1A7 and UGT1A9 polymorphisms predict response and toxicity in colorectal cancer patients treated with capecitabine/irinotecan. Clin Cancer Res 11:1226–1236.
65. Smith NF, Figg WD, Sparreboom A (2006) Pharmacogenetics of irinotecan metabolism and transport: an update. Toxicol In Vitro 20:163–75.
66. Morgan MY, Rehef R, Shah RR, Oates NS, Smith RL, Sherlock S (1984) Impaired oxidation of debrisoquine in patients with perhexiline liver injury. Gut 25:1057–1064.
67. Ando Y, Saka H, Ando M, Sawa T, Muro K, Ueoka H, Yokohama A, Saitoh S, Shimokata K, Hasegawa Y (2000) Polymorphisms of UDP-glucuronosyltransferase gene and irinotecan toxocity: a pharmacogenetic analysis. Cancer Res 60:6921–6926.
68. Hetherington S, Hughes AR, Mosteller M, Shortino D, Baker KL, Spreen W, Lai E, Davies K, Handley A, Dow DJ, Fling ME, Stocum M, Bowman C, Thurmond LM, Roses AD (2002) Genetic variations in HLA-B region and hypersensitivity reactions to abacavir. Lancet 359:1121–1122.
69. Pirmohamed M, Lin K, Chadwick D, Park BK (2001) TNF-alpha promoter region gene polymorphisms in carbamazepine-hypersensitive patients. Neurology 56:890–6.

Chapter 8
Strategies and Resources for Marker Selection and Genotyping in Genetic Association Studies

Nicole Soranzo, Dong-Jing Fu, and Qingqin S. Li

Contents

Abstract The release of millions of polymorphisms by recently completed, large-scale sequencing and genotyping efforts has provided us with unprecedented resources for carrying out genetic association analyses of drug response and disease predisposition. This chapter provides a guide to some general principles and available resources for the analysis of human genetic variation in genetic association studies. We first describe some principles of association studies and discuss the utility of different experimental designs in clinical practice. We then describe current repositories of human genetic variation and bioinformatics tools that have been developed for the efficient retrieval and evaluation of these genetic variants in the context of human genome annotation and disease. Finally, we survey pros and cons of current genotyping methodologies and available commercial products for genetic association studies.

Keywords bioinformatics, genome-wide, candidate gene, genotyping, genetic association, common disease

Nicole Soranzo
Wellcome Trust Sanger Institute, Cambridge, UK
ns6@sanger.ac.uk

N. Cohen (ed.) *Pharmacogenomics and Personalized Medicine*,

Glossary

Allele. Alternative forms of a DNA variant occupying a given locus (position) on a chromosome. DNA variants can entail a substitution of a nucleotide base with a different base (SNP), an insertion or deletion of one or more nucleotides (indel polymorphism) or a variation in the number of repeat variants.

Functional SNP. SNPs that have an a priori probability of affecting gene function through mRNA transcription, protein levels or structure, etc. SNPs are classified based on their localization in coding regions (synonymous and nonsynonymous), intron-exon boundaries, gene promoters, or regulators of transcription such as enhancer or silencer elements. For a more detailed description of effects, refer to Chapter 10.

Haplotype. A unique combination of alleles at different loci on the same chromosome.

Linkage disequilibrium (LD). The nonrandom association of alleles at two or more loci. Linkage disequilibrium describes a situation in which some combinations of alleles or genetic markers occur more or less frequently in a population than would be expected from a random formation of haplotypes from alleles based on their frequencies.

Minor allele frequency. The ratio of chromosomes in the population carrying the less common variant at a given locus, to those with the more common variant. Usually one refers to SNPs with a minor allele frequency of >5% as common SNPs, and to SNPs with a minor allele frequency of ≤5% as rare SNPs; 1%, 2%, or 10% thresholds are also used. Note that a variant that may be common in a population, for instance in a European sample, may be rare in a different population, such as an Asian or an African American sample.

Single nucleotide polymorphism (SNP). A DNA sequence variation occurring when a single nucleotide (A, T, C or G) at a genomic location differs between chromosomes in an individual or among individuals in a population. For example, two sequenced DNA fragments from different individuals, AAGCCTA to AAGCTTA, contain a difference in a single nucleotide. In this case we say that there are two alleles C and T. Almost all ommon SNPs have only two alleles.

Tag SNPs (tSNPs or tagging SNPs). Representative SNPs in a region of the genome with high linkage disequilibrium. Tag SNPs define optimal SNP sets that allow identifying common genetic variations in a chromosomal region of interest without genotyping every SNP in the region.

1 Introduction

Genetic association studies measure the correlation between variations in human genes ("genetic polymorphisms") and phenotypes of interest. The sequencing of the human genome *(1, 2)* and the release of a comprehensive map of genetic variation for human populations (the HapMap *(3)*) have provided us with the tools to implement genetic association analyses of drug response and disease predisposition routinely. The aim of this chapter is to describe strategies and resources for identifying relevant genetic variations and for carrying out pharmacogenomics studies from a practical standpoint, while study design and analysis are discussed in detail in Chapter 9. In particular, we will describe: (i) general principles and resources for genetic association studies; (ii) bioinformatic tools for the retrieval of data on genes and genetic variants; and (iii) genotyping methodologies and available commercial products for genetic association studies.

2 Strategies for Genetic Association Studies of Disease and Drug Response

The choice of study design, and hence genotyping strategy, depends on many factors. Some are practical, such as economical cost and DNA sample availability. Others are related to the overall purpose of the study, for example whether the study is designed to test a specific hypothesis (e.g., a drug mechanism of action) or rather to generate a new hypothesis (e.g., to identify novel drug targets for a disease of interest).

2.1 *Study Designs*

Candidate polymorphism. Candidate polymorphism studies entail genotyping one or few polymorphisms in a limited number of genes. This approach may apply in cases where there is a strong hypothesis for the role of the polymorphism in disease causation, or strong evidence for a functional genetic variant that is relevant to disease (the phenotype of interest). In these cases, we can test directly the hypothesis that such variant is causal (C, in Fig. 8.1) to the disease phenotype by comparing the frequency of the genetic variant in a group of patients and controls. Candidate polymorphism studies in pharmacogenomics have mostly been directed towards testing the effect of functional alleles in genes affecting the drug pharmacokinetics, in particular drug metabolizing enzymes and transporters (DMETs), but also in genes affecting drug pharmacodynamics (targets) *(4, 5)*.

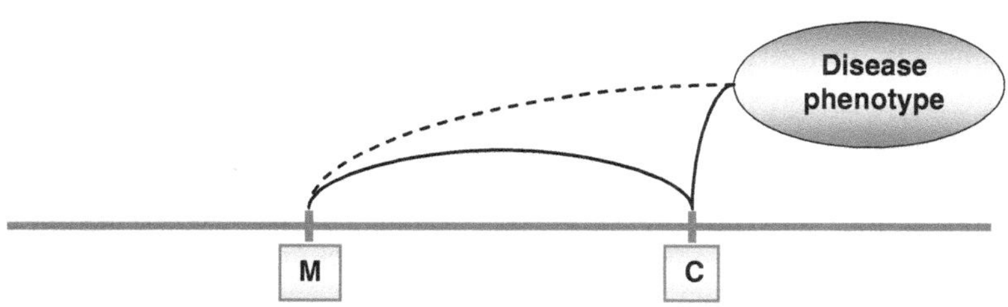

Fig. 8.1 Schematic representation of the principle of genetic association studies The marker locus M is typed in a case-control study, and the association with the disease phenotype (DP) is assessed using statistical methods. The association between the variant that is causal to the disease phenotype (C) and the disease phenotype itself is not observed directly, but can be inferred indirectly if the statistical association between M and C (r^2) is sufficiently high

Candidate gene. A candidate gene study may involve studying one to thousands of genes in a single experiment, with a relatively small number of SNPs *(5–50)* genotyped within each gene. A gene is generally defined to include coding sequence, un-translated sequence and flanking regions, and possibly splice or known regulatory elements; and may be either a positional candidate that results from a prior linkage study or a functional candidate identified based on its known or presumed role in the phenotype of interest. When the causal variant to the phenotype is not known, we can seek to identify it indirectly by genotyping one or more marker variants (M) in a genomic region where we suspect C may be found. In this scenario, the effect of C can be detected if M and C have a sufficiently high statistical association to drive a significant association between M and the disease phenotype. Such indirect approaches exploit linkage disequilibrium (see later) for searching novel disease variants.

Candidate gene approaches represent the bulk of the genetic association studies published to date and have led to the identification of a number of clinically important genetic variants. One clinically relevant example is the discovery of genetic variants in *VKORC1* and *GGCX* (together with the drug metabolism enzyme *CYP2C9)* explaining one third of the variance in the dosing of warfarin *(6, 7)*. Warfarin is a widely used anticoagulant, where incorrect dosage carries a high risk of either severe bleeding or failure to prevent thromboembolism.

Genome-wide. Genome-wide studies entail assessing genetic associations between a disease or drug response phenotype and genotypes at 100,000 to 1 M well-chosen polymorphisms in a single experiment. An advantage of genome-wide over candidate gene studies is that they do not rely on a priori *hypotheses* for the role of a specific gene or biological function. This raises the possibility of identifying novel disease genes, thus improving knowledge of the underlying causative mechanisms. At the time of writing a handful of genome-wide association studies have been published *(8–17)*, with many large-scale collaborative efforts due to release genetic association data for major diseases in thousands of cases and controls within the next few months. To date, however, no genome-wide scan of drug response has been published. A possible reason for this lies in the relative difficulty of evaluating drug response retrospectively, which has delayed collecting sufficiently large patient populations with homogeneous drug response phenotypes.

Fine mapping. A fine mapping study is carried out to obtain in-depth assessment of a region of interest, such as a region containing a signal of positive association with a disease trait or a genetic linkage peak. Fine mapping studies generally entail genotyping several hundred polymorphisms over large genomic regions (up to 10 Mb in length) that may span several genes. Resequencing may be applied to obtain in-depth characterization of all genetic variants present in the region.

Resequencing. The ever-decreasing cost of DNA sequencing suggests that in the near future extensive resequencing of genomic regions, and ultimately of entire genomes, might become the strategy of choice for comparing patient groups. Deep resequencing of patient populations will allow a comprehensive evaluation of the contribution of both rare and common genetic variants. Current efforts are seeking to reduce the cost of sequencing an entire human genome to less than US$1000.

2.2 The HapMap Project

The HapMap project represents a fundamental milestone for human genetic research *(3)*, established in 2002 with the goal of generating the first map of linkage disequilibrium for the human genome. Linkage disequilibrium, or LD, is a property of genomes whereby some combinations of alleles or genetic markers occur more or less frequently in a population than would be expected by chance. The main purpose of the HapMap project was to provide a tool for selecting and assessing genetic variants for association studies of common disease. The data generated however has also provided unprecedented insight into human genome structure and evolution *(3)*.

HapMap focuses on three reference human populations: 30 father-mother-child trios of northern European descent (CEPH from Utah, symbol CEU); 30 trios of African descent (Yoruba from Ibadan, Nigeria, YRI) and 90 unrelated individuals of Asian descent, including 44 unrelated individuals from Tokyo, Japan (JPT) and 45 unrelated individuals of Han Chinese ancestry from Beijing, China (CHB). The first phase of the project was completed in October 2005, with ~1.1 Million SNPs genotyped in the 269 samples, corresponding to an average SNP density of 1 SNP genotyped for every 5 kb of human genome. Phase I also performed exhaustive SNP discovery in ten representative 500-kb regions (ENCODE) by resequencing 48 unrelated DNA samples from a multiethnic panel (16 Yoruba, 8 Japanese, 8 Han Chinese and 16 CEPH); all the SNPs found within these regions, and known SNPs in dbSNP, were later genotyped in the same 269 HapMap individuals. This resequencing/genotyping effort allowed a first assessment of how well the HapMap resource represents unknown variants in the human genome *(3)*. Phase II was also completed in October 2005, with the release of an additional 3.9 Million SNPs in the same 269 individuals (average SNP spacing ~1 SNP/Kb). The current release of HapMap (#21a, January 2007, Table 8.1) contains data from HapMap phase I+II and major predefined SNP genotyping panels (Illumina Infinium 100k and 300k, Affymetrix non-synonymous SNPs and high-resolution extended Major Histocompatibility Complex (MHC) locus SNPs *(18)*. In addition, HapMap also contains data for two types of structural variants: i) segmental duplications from High-Depth Celera Reads *(19–21)* and ii) structural variation datasets including CNV regions determined in HapMap samples *(22)*, CNV datasets *(23–26)*, and deletions *(27–29)*. A third unofficial effort phase currently ongoing will type the same SNPs in additional world-wide population samples.

Table 8.1 Content of HapMap at time of writing (release #21a, January 2007) for the three HapMap reference populations: CEPHs of European origin (CEU), Beijing Chinese and Tokyo Japanese (CHB+JPT) and Yoruban African (YRI)

	Populations		
SNP type	CEU	CHB+JPT	YRI
Total Non-Redundant	3,904,218	3,936,482	3,846,092
Total QC+ SNPs	4,871,127	4,881,441	4,774,448
Total Genotyped SNPs	**6,838,923**	**6,799,238**	**6,798,546**

The data is fully accessible and downloadable from the HapMap genome browser (link in Table 8.3), which can be searched by gene, feature ID, or chromosomal region. The browser can be used for visualizing and downloading SNP frequencies, linkage disequilibrium plots and phased haplotypes. The individual genotype data can be downloaded for import into several tag SNP design programs. The browser also implements a modified version of HaploView for easy retrieval of tag SNPs for regions of interest. Details of HapMap contents and usage are given in several excellent publications *(3, 30, 31)* and the project website, and will not be discussed further.

2.3 Tagging SNP Approaches and Software for Tag SNP Selection

Tagging SNP approaches take advantage of linkage disequilibrium to identify sets of SNPs (called "tagging SNPs" or "tag SNPs") that exhaustively capture genetic variation in a gene or genomic region of interest *(32)*. The purpose is to improve genotyping efficiency in association studies. Figure 8.2 depicts a hypothetical genomic region with nine segregating sites (SNPs). Although 2^9 possible combinations of these nine sites (also called "haplotypes") are in theory possible, only five are found in this given population sample, owing to linkage disequilibrium. In this simplified example, the sites identified with the same font formatting are in high linkage disequilibrium. This implies that among the sites identified by the same formatting, the allele status of one site can be used to predict univocally the allele status at each of the other sites. In this simplified example, by genotyping well-chosen subsets of four SNPs, one can capture the five chromosomes as exhaustively as if the entire nine sites were genotyped.

A widely used measure of linkage disequilibrium that is relevant to genetic association studies is r^2, a summary statistic that measures the statistical association between pairs of alleles. r^2 is sensitive to the population frequency differences among pairs of alleles *(33)*; it varies between 0 (no association between two alleles) and 1 (complete association). r^2 provides a summary statistic for how well genetic variation in a gene or region of interest is captured by a set of tagging SNPs. Generally, tag SNPs are selected to capture each common variant in the gene with a minimum r^2 of 0.85. This is assumed to represent a good trade-off between genotyping efficiency and statistical power.

Several statistical algorithms for SNP selection have been developed to deal with variation of linkage disequilibrium among different regions of the genome. We will here briefly outline some common tagging methods and programs (Table 8.2), while we direct the reader to several papers describing exhaustive evaluations of these methods and their relative merits *(34–37)*. Briefly, available methods can be classified into two general categories:

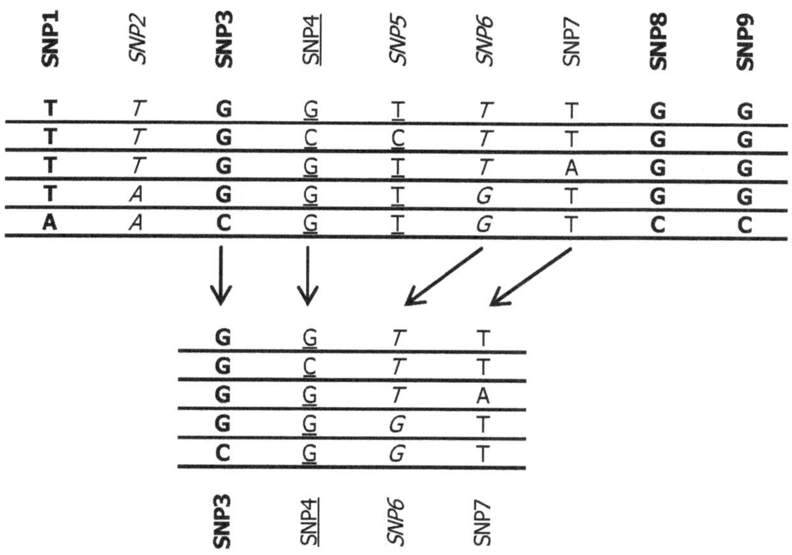

Fig. 8.2 Schematic representation of tagging SNPs. Alleles at nine segregating SNPs (SNP1-9) are arranged in five different haplotypes (chromosomes) in a population. SNPs with the same color are co-inherited in this population. A reduced SNP set made of one SNP per each font type can be selected to fully represent the nine SNPs. In this simplified scenario, SNP3 has equivalent tagging properties to SNP1, SNP8 and SNP9; SNP7 does not have an equivalent tag SNP (i.e., it represents a "singleton" or "untaggable" SNP).

- Methods that rely on the determination of haplotypes prior for calculation of optimal tag SNPs sets. These are often referred to as haplotype-block based, and are implemented by commonly used programs such as htSNP, Hapblock, tagSNPs and TagIt. A main initial limitation to these approaches has been the computational burden required for reconstructing haplotypes in the case of many SNPs, but these limitations have been eased with the implementation of more efficient Partition Ligation EM (PLEM) algorithms for haplotype reconstruction *(38)*.
- Haplotype-free methods rely on calculation of the pairwise statistic r^2, a measure of linkage disequilibrium that measures the statistical association among alleles *(33)*. Among the more widely used programs using pairwise r^2 are LDSelect *(39)* and Tagger *(40)*. In general, because they do not require haplotype inference, these methods can be more straightforward to use for nonexpert users.

Alternative methods for tag-SNP selection are based on clustering algorithms *(41)* or multivariate linear regression *(42)*; others allow users to specify variable thresholds for markers based on their genomic regions or SNP information *(43)*. This feature is useful when wishing to prioritize genomic regions that have a higher a priori probability of containing disease markers. Comparative evaluations of different tagging

Table 8.2 Software for linkage disequilibrium analysis and tag SNP selection

Software name	Principle and description	Platform	Reads HapMap data?	Can constrain chosen SNP sets?	Website	Reference
Haploview	Similar to Tagger, but limited to a maximum of 3-marker tests	Web-based, MS/DOS, Linux	Yes	Yes	www.broad.mit.edu/mpg/haploview/	*(155)*
LDSelect	Pairwise r^2	Perl	No	Yes	http://droog.gs.washington.edu/ldSelect.html	*(39)*
Tagger	Block-based	Web-based, Unix	Yes	Yes	http://www.broad.mit.edu/mpg/tagger/	*(40)*
TagIt	Haplotye-based or pairwise r^2	MatLab	No	Yes	http://web.genome.duke.edu/tagit/Tagit_v3_13.zip	*(156)*
TagSNPs	Block-based		Yes	Yes	http://www-rcf.usc.edu/~stram/tagsnpsv1.zip	*(157)*
htSNP2		Stata	No		http://www-gene.cimr.cam.ac.uk/clayton/software/stata/htSNP2.pkg	*(35)*
BNTagger	Bayesian					*(41)*
HapBlock	Block-based		Yes	Yes	http://www-hto.usc.edu/msms/HapBlock/	*(158)*
Hclust.R		R-project			http://www.wpic.pitt.edu/WPICCompGen/hclust.htm	*(159)*
MLS-Tagging	Multivariate linear regression (MLR)	Linux	No	Yes	http://alla.cs.gsu.edu/~software/tagging/	*(42)*
WCLUSTAG	Hierarchical clustering	Web-based, MS/DOS, Linux	Yes	Yes (allows the user to specify variable tagging thresholds for different SNPs)	http://bioinfo.hku.hk/wclustag/	*(43)*
CLUSTAG	Hierarchical clustering	Web-based, MS/DOS, Linux	No		http://bioinfo.hku.hk/clustag/	*(160)*

methods and their tagging space have shown that, in general, haplotype-based methods are more efficient than pairwise methods when the haplotype phase can be correctly inferred. Pairwise r^2 methods, on the contrary, are less sensitive to genotyping errors and uncertainty in haplotype phase *(40, 44, 45)*.

The use of the HapMap resource in clinical practice suffers from two main caveats. The first is that HapMap was created to target common genetic variation. The term "common" is generally used for variants that are found at frequencies greater than 5% in a given population, although other thresholds (1% or 10%) are also used. On the contrary, rare variants are not exhaustively represented in HapMap nor captured by tagging methods. This makes sense in terms of the proposed use of HapMap, since current genetic association studies are underpowered in the case of rare variants with small effects *(3, 40, 45)*. Efforts will need to be directed towards characterizing rare variants in patient populations, likely through resequencing. A second area of concern is whether the reference HapMap populations are good proxies for the populations investigated in clinical trials, as tagging properties of SNPs are sensitive to differences in the underlying linkage disequilibrium patterns among these two sets of populations. Several studies have addressed this issue, either comparing linkage disequilibrium patterns between HapMap and non-HapMap populations *(46–48)*, or by explicitly simulating the loss in power arising from applying tag SNPs selected in HapMap to a different population sample *(40, 44, 45, 49)*. Results so far have been encouraging confirming that the HapMap is a suitable resource for the evaluation of common variation in populations of similar ancestry. The same does not apply to rare variants, which will require evaluation in the populations under study.

3 Resources for Selecting Genes and Genetic Variants in Genetic Association Studies

For a researcher wishing to carry out a genetic association study using a candidate gene approach, the first task is to identify a list of genes that are relevant to the phenotype of interest, and secondly to select representative genetic variants within them. Candidate gene lists seek to capture current knowledge of the genetics underlying the trait of interest. For instance, a candidate gene study of drug efficacy may include known drug targets, or genes involved in drug metabolism, absorption, or transport. A study of drug safety, where the drug has an adverse effect that affects thrombovascular events, might try to capture genes in the blood clotting pathways, platelet synthesis and degradation, and so on. In candidate gene studies, a rate-limiting step is the systematic evaluation of current medical and biological knowledge. Several centralized data repositories and shared bioinformatic tools are now available for the storage, annotation and retrieval of genetic and phenotypic data. Some of these tools will be presented in this section; more are listed in Table 8.3.

Table 8.3 List of web resources

Repository	Description	URL	Reference
Gene and disease databases			
Online Mendelian Inheritance in Man (OMIM)	Catalog of human genes and genetic disorders	http://www.ncbi.nlm.nih.gov/entrez/query.fcgi?db=OMIM	*(52)*
Genetic Association Database (GAD)	Archive of human genetic association studies of complex diseases and disorders	http://geneticassociationdb.nih.gov	*(53)*
CAESAR	A computational system to select candidate genes for complex human traits	http://visionlab.bio.unc.edu/caesar/	*(54)*
Disease Gene Prediction	A database of human genes with their probability of being involved in a hereditary disease	http://cgg.ebi.ac.uk/services/dgp	*(55)*
Genecards	An integrated database of human genes that includes automatically-mined genomic, proteomic and transcriptomic information, as well as orthologies, disease relationships, SNPs, gene expression, gene function	http://genecards.weizmann.ac.il	*(161)*
The Pharmacogenetics and Pharmacogenomics Knowledge Base (PharmGKB)	Reference database for pharmacogenomics variants and datasets	www.pharmgkb.org/	*(162)*
Human Genome Epidemiology Network (HuGENet)	Global collaboration for assessing genome variation in human health	http://www.cdc.gov/genomics/hugenet/default.htm	*(163)*
HUGO nomenclature database	Repository of approved gene nomenclature	http://www.gene.ucl.ac.uk/nomenclature/	*(164)*
Pathway resources			
Pathguide	Complete listing of all Pathguide resources	http://www.pathguide.org/	*(51)*
The Pharmacogenetics and Pharmacogenomics Knowledge Base (PharmGKB)	Curated knowledge about the relationships among drugs, diseases and genes, including their variations and gene products	http://www.pharmgkb.org/	*(162)*

Ariadne Genomics Pathway Studio/MedScan	Software for visualization and analysis of biological pathways	http://www.ariadnegenomics.com/products/pathway-studio/medscan/	*(165)*
Biomolecular Object Network Databank (BOND)	Tool for cross-database searches of available sequence, interaction, complex and pathway information	http://bond.unleashedinformatics.com/	*(166)*
Ingenuity Pathways Analysis (IPA)	Knowledge base of biological networks, drugs and diseases	http://www.ingenuity.com/	–
Database of Interacting Proteins (DIP)	Online database of protein-protein interactions	http://dip.doe-mbi.ucla.edu/	*(167)*
Search Tool for the Retrieval of Interacting Genes/Proteins (STRING)	A database of known and predicted protein-protein interactions.	http://string.embl.de/	*(168)*
Reactome KnowledgeBase	A curated knowledgebase of biological pathways	http://www.reactome.org/	*(169)*
Human Protein Reference Database (HPRD)	A centralized platform for depicting and integrating information on domain architecture, post-translational modifications, interaction networks and disease association	http://www.hprd.org/	*(170)*
Kyoto Encyclopedia of Genes and Genomes (KEGG)	Collection of manually drawn pathway maps on molecular interactions and reaction networks	www.genome.jp/kegg/pathway.html	*(171)*
Biocarta	A collection of pathway charts	http://www.biocarta.com/	–
Tools for literature data retrieval and annotation			
PubMed	Freely accessible online database of biomedical journal citations and abstracts	http://www.ncbi.nlm.nih.gov/entrez/query.fcgi?db=PubMed	–
PubGene	Tool for retrieval of information on genes and proteins	http://www.pubgene.org/	*(57)*
Genes2Diseases (G2D)	Algorithms to scan human genome region for genes related to an inherited disease	http://www.ogic.ca/projects/g2d_2	*(59)*
OSIRIS	Tool for the retrieval of articles from MEDLINE related to human sequence variants	http://ibi.imim.es/osirisform.html	*(172)*

(continued)

Table 8.3 (continued)

Repository	Description	URL	Reference
EBIMed	Web application for Information Retrieval and Extraction from Medline and analysis for associations between UniProt protein/gene names, GO annotations, drugs and species	http://www.ebi.ac.uk/Rebholz-srv/ebimed	*(173, 174)*
GoPubMed	Tool for retrieval and analysis of PubMed data using gene ontology	http://www.gopubmed.org	*(175)*
MeshPubMed	Tool for retrieval and analysis of PubMed data based on MeSH	http://www.meshpubmed.org/	–
MedMiner	Text mining tool for biomedical information	http://discover.nci.nih.gov/textmining	*(176)*
PubFinder	A tool for finding thematically related literature by scanning PubMed abstracts for discriminating keywords	http://www.glycosciences.de/tools/PubFinder	*(177)*
XplorMed	Tool for exploring a set of abstracts derived from a MEDLINE search	http://www.ogic.ca/projects/xplormed	*(178)*
iProLINK	Tool for facilitating text mining in the area of literature-based database curation, named entity recognition and protein ontology development	http://pir.georgetown.edu/iprolink	*(179)*
PreBIND	Tool for locating biomolecular interaction information in the literature	http://prebind.bind.ca	*(180)*
Arrowsmith	Tool for linking documents, disciplines, investigators and databases	http://arrowsmith.psych.uic.edu	*(181)*
BITOLA	Interactive literature-based biomedical discovery support system	http://www.mf.uni-lj.si/bitola	*(182)*
ProLinks	A collection of inference methods used to predict functional linkages between proteins	http://dip.doe-mbi.ucla.edu/pronav	*(183)*
Human genome browsers and SNP repositories			
Perlegen Genome Browser	Access to Perlegen data	http://genome.perlegen.com/browser/index.html	*(65)*
dbSNP	Reference database of sequence variants	http://www.ncbi.nlm.nih.gov/SNP/	*(66)*

ENSEMBL	Reference database of sequence variants	http://www.ensembl.org	*(68)*
The HapMap Project Genome Browser	Access to HapMap data	http://www.hapmap.org/	*(184)*
Decode Genotyping	Access to Decode genotyping resources	http://www.decode.com/genotyping/	–
SNP500Cancer	Repository of genetic variation in cancer genes	http://snp500cancer.nci.nih.gov	*(185, 186)*
GeneSNPs	Web resource integrating gene, sequence and polymorphism data into individually annotated gene models	http://www.genome.utah.edu/genesnps/	–
GenomeVariation Server	Tool for rapid access to human genotype data found in dbSNP and to provide tools for analysis of genotype data	http://gvs.gs.washington.edu/GVS/	–
HGVbase	A curated summary of human DNA variation and phenotypes	http://hgvbase.cgb.ki.se/	*(187)*
Human Gene Mutation Database	Database of human gene mutations	http://www.hgmd.cf.ac.uk/ac/index.php	*(188)*
Seattle SNPs	Repository of association data for candidate genes and pathways for inflammatory response	http://pga.gs.washington.edu/	–
UCSC Genome Browser		http://genome.ucsc.edu	*(189)*
Wellcome Trust Case Control Consortium	Genome wide association data for common diseases	http://www.wtccc.org.uk	*Link to poster*
dbGaP (Database of Genotype and Phenotype	Database of genotype-phenotype correlation studies	http://www.ncbi.nlm.nih.gov/entrez/query.fcgi?db=gap	–
Whole Genome Association Resource	Repository of clinical phenotypes and whole genome genotype data	http://www.ncbi.nlm.nih.gov/WGA/	–
Functional annotation of SNPs			
PolyMAPr	Interdisciplinary resource for the evaluation of pathways regulating drug activity	http://pharmacogenomics.wustl.edu	*(70)*
TAMAL	Tool for functional SNP identification	http://neoref.ils.unc.edu/tamal	*(71)*
PupaSNP	Tool for functional SNP selection	http://pupasuite.bioinfo.cipf.es/	*(72)*

(continued)

Table 8.3 (continued)

Repository	Description	URL	Reference
PolyPhen	Prediction of effect of amino acid substitution on protein structure and function	http://genetics.bwh.harvard.edu/pph/data/index.html	*(73)*
LS-SNP	Annotated database of SNPs	http://alto.compbio.ucsf.edu/LS-SNP/	*(74)*
SNPs3D	Molecular functional effects of nonsynonymous SNPs based on structure and sequence analysis	http://www.snps3d.org/	*(75)*
ESEfinder	Tool for annotation of exonic splicing enhancers	http://rulai.cshl.edu/cgi-bin/tools/ESE3/esefinder.cgi?process=home	*(76)*
SNP@Domain	Tool for functional SNP selection	http://snpnavigator.net	*(77)*
SNPper	Tool for retrieval of known SNPs by position or by association with a gene	http://snpper.chip.org	*(190)*
Alternative Splicing Database	A database of alternative splice events and the resultant isoform splice patterns of genes from human and other model species	http://www.ebi.ac.uk/asd/index.html	*(191)*

3.1 Pathway Repositories

Pathway resources allow the visualization and retrieval of information on interactions among genes, proteins and compounds *(50)*. There are currently hundreds of different such repositories focusing on different aspects of organismal biology, so we will not attempt their description. A comprehensive, updated resource list is available at Pathguide *(51)*, where the repositories can be ranked by their popularity, in order to obtain an approximate indication of their usage. The main areas of focus are protein-protein interactions, signaling and metabolic pathways and transcription and gene regulatory networks. Protein-compound interactions may be useful resources for identifying genes relevant to drug response. Pathway diagrams are particularly useful for visualization of cellular processes and interactions among genes. Some resources allow direct download of gene lists (e.g., IPA, HPRD and STRING), a feature that is useful for compiling gene lists for large-scale association studies. Among these repositories, some are assembled through manual curation of literature studies while others rely on bioinformatic annotation of genes. Because manually curated repositories describe interactions that are experimentally validated in published studies, they have a higher a priori likelihood of describing real interactions. On the other hand, automatic annotation can result in false positives (i.e., not all predicted interactions will be true). The utility of such databases extends to the data analysis, where such databases are used for rapidly gaining insights into complex biological interactions underlying the observed genetic associations.

The Ingenuity Pathways Analysis (IPA), accessible only through commercial license, is currently the largest knowledge base of biological networks. It is based on Ingenuity Pathways Knowledge Base, a repository that houses millions of expert relationships between proteins, genes, complexes, cells, tissues, drugs and diseases manually curated from the scientific literature. It contains several categories of data, including information on protein, gene, protein complex, cell, cellular component, tissue, organ, small molecule and disease relationships; chemical and drug information, including clinical candidates and FDA-approved drugs and pathway interactions extracted from the literature. The data is easily searched by gene, disease, function, or drug, thanks to cross referencing of entries through internal ontology, synonym and homonym mapping, representation of biological context and systematic capture of canonical pathway relationships.

The Kyoto Encyclopedia of Genes and Genomes (KEGG) provides a comprehensive, open access resource to information on pathway maps for biological processes, functional hierarchies of biological systems, gene catalogs, and ortholog relations in complete genomes and chemical compounds, drugs, glycans, and reactions, each of these categories accessible through separate search interfaces. In addition, it provides a tool for functional annotation of genes into pathways through comparison against the manually curated KEGG GENES database. The KEGG pathway resource contains 278 pathways classified into six main categories: metabolism (144 entries), genetic information processing (15 entries), environmental information processing (18 entries), cellular processes (33 entries), human diseases (23 entries) and drug development (45 entries). KEGG DRUG, a part of the KEGG

LIGAND database, contains chemical structures of all approved drugs in Japan and the U.S., together with additional information such as therapeutic categories and target molecules.

3.2 Databases of Human Diseases

Candidate gene lists typically seek to capture findings from existing genetic association studies. While the reference source for such information remains the published literature, several curation efforts are seeking to organize the findings in specialized databases. Bearing in mind that any curation effort suffers the risk of falling behind the current literature records, these resources can be a useful starting point for gene list curation.

The Online Mendelian Inheritance in Man (OMIM) is a catalog of human genes and genetic disorders of the National Center for Biotechnology Information (NCBI). The database contains manually curated textual information and references to published studies. It also contains links to MEDLINE and sequence records in the Entrez system and to additional related resources at NCBI and elsewhere *(52)*. OMIM gene records may contain a narrative section (allelic variants) summarizing important genetic variants within a gene, their putative functional consequence, or the relevant findings from genetic association studies. OMIM can be searched using different terms fields including MIM number, chromosome, allelic variant, references, clinical synopsis, gene map disorder and many others. The MIM records are prefixed with different symbols for different classes of records: the prefix * indicates a gene with known sequence; + indicates genes with known sequence and phenotype; # indicates phenotype description with known molecular basis; % indicates Mendelian phenotype or locus with unknown molecular basis; no symbol indicates any other category, mainly phenotypes with a suspected Mendelian basis.

OMIM is a text-based database focusing mainly on Mendelian diseases (some information on common diseases is currently being incorporated). The Genetic Association Database (GAD) *(53)* was created to archive information on genetic association studies of complex diseases and disorders. In 2006 GAD increased its content from 8,000+ records to the current 28,338 records as a result of the integration of a major contribution of records of published genetic association studies compiled from PubMed by the National Office of Public Health Genomics (NOPHG) at the Centers for Disease Control and Prevention (CDC). The data is organized in a tabular format that facilitates searching the database. GAD records are manually curated from published studies and seek to capture information for several relevant searchable keys. These include gene identifiers, disease class, disease subphenotype and endophenotype, study information (e.g., sample size, study population), author-described alleles, rs IDs, p-value and significance of the association (YES/NO) and environmental factor/gene-gene interaction. The breakdown of information into data fields facilitates searching, although the completeness of such information depends on the different database curators and varies widely among different records.

Many other specialized disease resources are available on the web (Table 8.3). Increasingly, computerized algorithms are being produced for the automatic annotation of disease databases *(54, 55)*.

3.3 Software for Literature Data Mining

Literature mining tools are bound to assume an increasingly important role in allowing sifting though a rapidly increasing body of scientific evidence. The most commonly used resources for literature mining include information retrieval tools such as PubMed, MedMiner, and many others (see Table 8.3 and note 56). Key components of most complex literature mining systems are entity recognition methods for identifying the genes, proteins and other entities that are mentioned in the literature. More complex methods are being developed for extracting biomedical facts from sequence context text and will probably soon become mainstream tools for the annotation and analysis of large-scale experimental data sets.

Three distinct entities and their relationships are useful for text mining of disease association data, each with intrinsic advantages and limitations: gene/mRNA/protein, disease and genetic variants. *Gene/mRNA/protein* molecular entities are captured by many biological databases and are relatively easy to search for, especially when synonyms are also captured in the database. One problem arises when different laboratories refer to the same molecule with different names. Text mining's ability to correctly recognize such entities as one is limited, unless the algorithms are trained to take the context information into consideration. In the case of the *disease* entity, such complications should be reduced by current ontology efforts aimed at standardizing the disease classification (for instance, the Medline MeSH Heading classification). As with the molecular entity, the *genetic variants* entity suffers from similar ambiguities: while dbSNP RefSNP ID provides a centralized catalog for polymorphisms deposited into dbSNP, classification of variant identifiers from published studies is lagging behind. Consistent efforts are needed to build a synonyms list for genetic variants, and to encourage the scientific community to adopt such standard nomenclature. For instance, the requirement of most journals that novel variants are assigned rs IDs prior to publications is a step in this direction.

With the three entities defined, the goal of the relationship inference is to infer gene-disease/phenotype, disease/phenotype-variants, and gene-variants relationships. PubGene *(57)* has implemented exactly this type of text mining functionality to facilitate retrieving a list of variants starting from MeSH Heading terms or Gene Ontology terms and associating these variants with the gene entities. This is a good starting point, although one that still requires careful review of the outcomes.

A challenge for the future will be to use such resources for making discoveries through integrating relationships at multiple levels. By combining facts that have been extracted from several papers, text mining methods can both discover global trends and generate new hypotheses that are based on the existing literature. An important application of this will be to use literature mining tools to prioritize candidate genes with potential roles in inherited diseases for further study. Some of these systems are already available. G2D *(58, 59)* combines the MeSH annotation in Medline with the Gene Ontology annotation of entries in the NCBIRefseq database to infer logical chains of connections from disease names, through chemicals and drugs, to molecular functions. Combined with functional annotations that are inferred from sequence similarity, this allows the genes within a mapped region to be ranked on the basis of a score that represents their likelihood of being associated with the disease in question. A second system, BITOLA, relies instead on pure text mining to find candidate genes that are indirectly connected to a given disease and subsequently filters these on the basis of chromosomal mapping data about the disease *(60)*.

Several proof of principle studies suggest potential applications of data mining and integration software to generate new knowledge *(61)*. Software for data mining has been used for different purposes: for integrating genetic linkage mapping data with data from the literature to suggest candidate genes for inherited diseases *(58)*, *(59)*; for linking genotypes to phenotypes by comparing species profiles of genes and literature-derived keywords *(62)*; or for identifying novel candidate disease genes through linking literature-based molecular networks and genetic linkage mapping *(63)* or through combining tissue-expression data with disease-tissue relationships extracted from the literature *(64)*.

To realize the full discovery potential of literature mining, integration with other data types will be fundamental. Protein networks are well suited for unifying large-scale experimental data with knowledge that has been extracted from the biomedical literature.

3.4 Databases of Genetic Variants and Genome Browsers

SNPs and other types of genetic variations are stored in databases accessed through genome browsers. dbSNP and Ensembl are the main public repositories for the SNPs identified from public and private SNP discovery efforts *(65)*. Within the entries, SNPs from the HapMap currently represent the bulk of validated SNPs with known allele frequency information and genotype data. In addition, both databases contain SNPs validated at differing levels of accuracy: 1) by frequency—the SNP has been genotyped in at least one study population and the frequency of the alleles is known; 2) by cluster—at least two laboratories have reported the SNP and at least one of the reports is via a noncomputational approach; or 3) double-hit—all alleles are observed in at least two chromosomes. SNPs inferred from computational analysis of sequence data, and with no experimental validation, are also included. This SNP category has the highest probability of containing SNPs that represent false predictions.

dbSNP. The Single Nucleotide Polymorphism database (dbSNP) is a public domain archive for a broad collection of genetic polymorphisms, including single-base nucleotide changes (SNPs), small-scale single-/multi-base insertions or deletions (INDELs or DIPs) and retroposable element insertion and microsatellite repeat variations (also called short tandem repeats or STRs) *(66)*. For our discussion here, the term "SNP" is generalized to include all different classes of genetic polymorphisms. As a result of the commitment from the International HapMap Project and growing interest from commercial entities and academic institutes, in the past 4+ years the SNP content of dbSNP has increased dramatically. When comparing the dbSNP build 106 (released in August 2002) with build 126 (May 2006), the number of submitted SNPs has increased 5.7 fold while the number of rsSNPs has increased 4.2 fold and the rsSNP in genes has increased 3 fold. With the advancement of high throughput genotyping assays, the number of validated SNPs has increased by ~11 fold (Fig. 8.3).

dbSNP records are of two different types *(67)*. Submitted dbSNP entries are identified by unique ss IDs, and include flanking sequence context of the polymorphism, the assay leading to the observations of sequence variation and the allele frequency of the polymorphism (by population or individual if known). As a SNP can be defined on either strand of the DNA sequence, the strand for the first submitted SNP is defined arbitrarily as the forward strand. Computationally derived dbSNP entries include reference SNP clusters and other annotations. During the dbSNP build cycle, the flanking sequence of each newly submitted SNP is aligned to the genomic contig. The ss numbers mapped to the same position of the contig are defined as a "reference SNP cluster" and are provided with a unique RefSNP ID (rs#). By convention, the

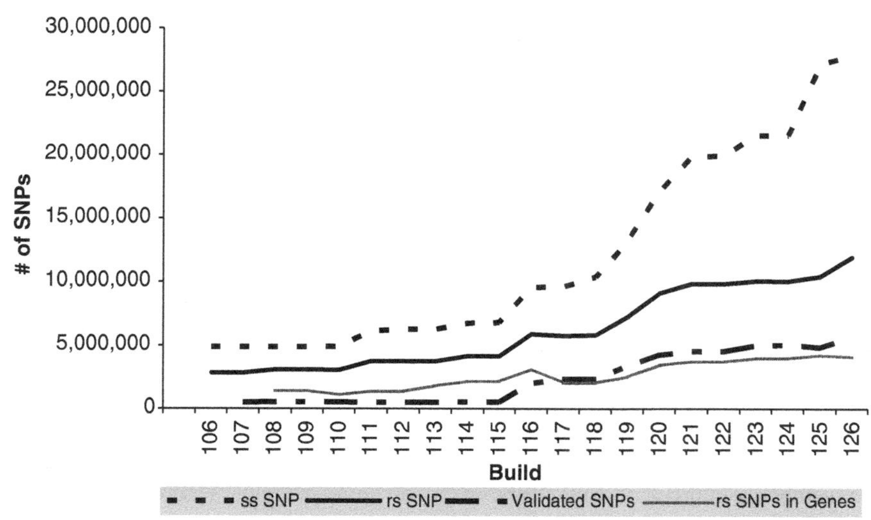

Fig. 8.3 Growth of dbSNP from dbSNP build 106 (August 2002) to build 126 (May 2006) ssSNP = data submissions (redundant); rsSNP = non-redundant SNP entries

cluster examplar is the member of a cluster with the longest flanking sequence and can be in either the forward or the reverse strand, while dbSNP preserves the orientation of the refSNP across the dbSNP build.

The content of dbSNP is annotated in reference to NCBI RefSeq sequence collections, genome assembly (both the reference genome and the alternative Celera genome), Entrez Gene and other Entrez databases. The annotation of sequence variants against gene features is helpful for selecting functional classes of SNPs. These include: 1) locus region—variants within 2 Kb 5' (upstream) or 500 bp 3' (downstream) of a gene; 2) coding-synonymous—the variant allele does not cause a change in the amino acid; 3) coding-nonsynonymous—the variant causes a change in the encoded amino acid; 4) mRNA-UTR—in the untranslated portion of the transcript; 5) intron; and 6) splice-site—in the first two or last two bases of the introns.

Ensembl. Ensembl is a joint project between the EMBL-EBI and the Sanger Institute, aimed at developing an automatic annotation system for prokaryote and eukaryote genomes (33 genomes as of 2007) *(68)*. Ensembl imports data from dbSNP; in addition, it computes SNPs from resequencing data using the ssahaSNP SNP calling algorithm, merging them with dbSNP content *(68)*. While dbSNP references the manually curated RefSeq gene set, Ensembl references the gene set created via an automatic gene build pipeline. Because of these different annotation systems, Ensembl is more likely to capture novel transcripts that may not be curated by RefSeq. However, this comes at the cost of some erroneous prediction of exons/transcripts. Because annotation of coding SNPs is transcript dependent, this may affect the accuracy of such SNP predictions. Another occasional problem in Ensembl is the assignment of transcripts to clusters of genes in nearby locations.

Ensembl annotates alleles to the (+)/(–) strand of the reference human genome, a more straightforward approach than the forward/reverse system used by dbSNP. Another advantage of Ensembl over dbSNP is that it makes its data and software sources publicly available. This allows custom data analysis via the Perl language application programming interfaces (APIs) available on the Ensembl interface together with extensive documentation and the remote databases hosted. This option is increasingly utilized as the database dumps become too large to download.

The most efficient way to visualize SNPs in the genome is via a genome browser: NCBI, Ensembl, and UCSC all have their own implementation of a genome browser, where SNPs are displayed side-by-side in tracks with other useful biological information such as transcript variants, protein domains, evolutionary sequence conservation and other features. SNP annotations are generally consistent between databases. Some problems, however, may arise for SNPs that are mapped to positions in the genome where the genome assembly has not been finalized, or for SNPs in regions where reference human genome maps differ. This has caused for instance a number of SNPs to be excluded from the latest HapMap release due to mapping inconsistencies in Build 35 relative to Build 36. Finally, annotation of splice site and regulatory elements is algorithm-dependent and may vary between databases, particularly as experimental validation of these variants is limited.

3.5 Tools for the Functional Annotation of Genetic Variants

Even though HapMap is an excellent resource for designing genetic association studies, it covers only approximately 40% of the reported genetic variation in the human genome. For this reason, in candidate gene studies one often seeks to supplement tagging SNP approaches with additional "preferred" SNPs, in particular SNPs that have a high a priori probability of being functional. Such SNPs may be amino-acid altering SNPs or SNPs that are predicted to alter gene expression, alternative splicing, or protein folding or turnover (see Chapter 10 for an in-depth discussion of different types of variants). Such genetic polymorphisms can be identified with the aid of specialized bioinformatics resources *(69–75)*.

A common goal of these resources are to improve the efficiency of public SNP database mining and polymorphism annotation by ensuring accurate annotations for genes and polymorphisms, eliminating inter- and intra-database redundancy, integrating data from multiple public sources with data generated locally and prioritizing the variants for further study. Available resources include platforms such as TAMAL *(71)*, PupaSNP *(72)*, PolyPhen *(73)*, LS-SNP *(74)*, SNPs3D *(75)*, Esefinder *(76)*, SNP@Domain *(77)* and PolyMAPr *(70)* (Table 8.3). These web resources are input with gene names, SNP identifiers, or nucleotide sequences. SNP identified through linking to public SNP databases (dbSNP, CGAP, JSNP, etc.) or local SNP discovery efforts are mapped to the annotated gene sequences and are compared against either local databases or specialized algorithms. The functional effects of nonsynonymous coding-region SNPs (cSNPs) and any variants that might alter exon splicing enhancer (ESE) sites, putative transcription factor binding sites, or intron-exon splice sites are then predicted. The output files are accessible though the relative browser interfaces.

The SNP Function Portal *(69)* is designed to be a clearing house for all public domain SNP functional annotation data as well as in-house functional annotations derived from different data sources. It contains SNP functional annotations in six major categories (genomic elements, transcription regulation, protein function, pathway, disease and population genetics). One interesting function is that it allows searching the HapMap Phase II data and known genes for genetically related SNPs to genetic markers of interest, a function that should greatly facilitate knowledge discovery in genome-wide SNP scanning experiments.

3.6 Repositories of Genotype and Phenotype Data

Genotype browsers allow access to genotype data for SNPs and other variants, as well as information on the linkage disequilibrium relationship between SNPs and the haplotype block structure in the region. The major repository of genotype data is the HapMap project, described before. The first comprehensive study of common genetic variation in human populations, however, was produced by a private initiative. Perlegen Sciences genotyped over 1.5 million unique genetic variants in

71 individuals of European American, African American, or Han Chinese ancestry, with an average distance between adjacent SNPs of 1,871 base pairs. The results of this study are accessible through the Perlegen Sciences genotype browser (Table 8.3). Genotype data for non-HapMap and Perlegen populations are collected in dbSNP, which can be used for assessing allele frequency of variants not included in the HapMap and Perlegen efforts (in particular, rare variants).

The Whole Genome Association website at the National Center for Biotechnology Information (NCBI) represents the reference database for association studies. It was created to manage data submission, storage, and access to clinical phenotypes and whole-genome genotype data. The database will serve as the main repository for several ongoing programs, including the Genetic Association Information Network (GAIN), the Genes and Environment Initiative (GEI), the National Heart Lung and Blood Institute, and NINDS DNA and Cell Line Repository at Cornell. Studies within each program will be regulated through different funding mechanisms and access restrictions. NCBI and NIH are committed to make this data widely available to the research community via the Database of Genotype and Phenotype (dbGaP), while protecting the privacy of the participants as defined by consent agreements for individual projects.

dbGaP will allow open access to studies, study documents, phenotypic variables and selected genotype-phenotype analyses. Access to deidentified phenotypes and genotypes for individual study subjects, pedigrees and other precomputed univariate genotype-phenotype associations would need to be authorized by the Data Access Committee (DAC).

To date, there is no standard in data management for storage of the large volume of individual genotype or phenotype data and relevant study designs, unlike the MIAMI standard for gene expression studies. It is clear that the exponential release of genotype data by whole genome association studies and other high-throughput genotyping efforts represents a challenge in terms of data storage and sharing, particularly if one considers the need to store both genotype and phenotype data. Researchers have to manage and analyze datasets consisting of hundreds of millions or even a few billion SNP genotypes. Database scalability, therefore, is becoming a major issue. At the moment, several commercial entities are attempting to address data management and analytic capability issues through their software products (Biocomputing Platform's BC|SNPmax, Decode Genetics, and Rosetta Biosoftware) or through custom-made LIMS systems. As for sequencing databases, it is likely that flat file format databases will replace relational databases for genotype/phenotype data storage.

3.7 An Integrated Pharmacogenetics and Pharmacogenomics Knowledge Base (PharmGKB)

Ultimately, it will be desirable to create a single, publicly accessible integrated knowledge base for pharmacogenomics. The Pharmacogenetics and Pharmaco-genomics

Knowledge Base (PharmGKB) *(78, 79)* has been created by investigators of the NIH Pharmacogenetics Research Network (PGRN) with the goal of becoming the reference information source for the interaction of genetic variability and drug response. PharmGKB collects and organizes information on five levels: (1) primary genotyping data that are important for drugs' PK or PD; (2) phenotype measures of drug response at the molecular, cellular, and organismal level and their correlations with genotypic data; (3) curation of major findings of the published literature for gene-drug interactions; (4) information about drug response pathways (both PK and PD); and (5) additional curation of very important pharmacogenes (VIP genes) that are critical for understanding pharmacogenomics, including information on variant genes, drugs, diseases and pathways and phenotypes of drug response *(78, 79)*.

Currently PharmGKB contains information about genetic variation in more than 200 genes important for PK or PD and their variants, and includes information on more than 300 diseases and 400 drugs. It contains more than 1.2 million individual SNPs measured in at least 13,000 subjects, corresponding to multiple loci in the human genome. PharmGKB has established novel displays of drug response pathways, and specific pages summarizing data about VIP genes that may facilitate research design and data analysis. Finally, more than 1,500 articles in pharmacogenetics can be accessed through PharmGKB. PharmGKB has the potential to become a key resource for pharmacogenomics research, provided that it maintains its mandate of exhaustively integrating, aggregating and annotating important data sets for pharmacogenomics.

4 DNA Genotyping Resources

4.1 Genotyping Technologies and Applications

Genotyping technologies which enable large-scale genetic analysis even at the whole genome level have advanced significantly over the years *(80–102)*. The principle of genotyping is to discriminate different alleles at a locus. The allelic discrimination is generally done by allele-specific hybridization, primer extension/minisequencing, allele-specific ligation, or allele-specific cleavage (Table 8.4). The readouts of these reactions are typically fluorescence, luminescence, or mass spectrometry. The details of genotyping methodologies have been reviewed elsewhere, *(103–108)* and therefore will not be the focus here. This section provides a summary of available genotyping technologies, and points to consider when choosing a method, a service provider, and off-the-shelf products. The choice of genotyping method depends on the scope of the study (candidate gene or whole genome association), whether an exploratory/hypothesis generation study or a study to support clinical trials, the number of samples and the number of markers.

Table 8.4 Summary of genotyping methodologies

Technology	Advantages, limitations and throughput sweet spot	Commercial examples
TaqMan, real time PCR, molecular beacons	• Closed tube; probe amplification and detection in single step. Many off-the-shelf assays available • Specificity may be limited by cross-hybridization; limited multiplexing capability; requires PCR • Genotype several to several hundred of SNPs on up to several hundred samples	ABI TaqMan assays
Invader assay	• Closed tube; probe amplification and detection in single step; no PCR required, isothermal reaction • Limited multiplexing capability; requires very pure probes to avoid false positive • Genotype several to several hundred of SNPs on up to several hundred swamples	Third Wave
LDR and OLA	• High degree of multiplexing; high level of specificity and sensitivity; capable of detecting small insertion and deletion • Require PCR prior to or after ligation • Suitable to genotype up to several thousand SNPs on several thousand samples depending on the platform	• ABI SNPlex: a variation of OLA, 48-plex run on ABI sequencers) • Illumina GoldenGate Assay: a variation of OLA, up to 1,536-plex)
Primer extension, mini-sequencing	• High level of sensitivity and specificity; high degree of multiplexing on some platforms; capable of detecting small insertion and deletion; amendable for MALDI-TOF mass spectrometry etection, thus does not require labeling • Some platforms require PCR • Suitable to genotype several SNP to genome-wide scan depending on the platform	• Illumina Infinium Assay: a variation of primer extension, custom array to whole genome product • Luminex: xMap up to 100-plex, also suitable for OLA • Sequenom: MALDI-TOF readout, up to 36-plex
Padlock probes, rolling circle amplification	• High level of sensitivity and specificity; high degree of multiplexing; does not require PCR prior to allele specific discrimination; capable of detecting small insertion and deletion • Requires long oligonucleotide probes • Suitable to genotype several thousand to tens of thousands SNP	• Affymetrix/ParAllele molecular inversion probes: a variation of the technology, up to 25,000-plex
Hybridization microarray	• High degree of multiplexing • Specificity may be limited by cross-hybridization; requires PCR • Suitable to genotype several thousands SNP to genome-wide scan	• Affymetrix: custom array to whole genome chip • Perlegen: custom array to whole genome product

LDR: ligase detection reaction; OLA oligonucleotide ligation assay

4.2 Candidate Gene or Candidate Region Genotyping

As mentioned earlier in this chapter, the candidate gene or candidate region approach allows scientists to analyze genes or regions of interest. The genes and regions are from biological understanding, prior linkage, or association studies. SNP markers (tagging SNPs) are selected to maximize the representation of SNPs or their potential functions. One may choose to analyze several candidate genes or several thousand genes, whereas the number of SNPs ranges from several dozens to tens of thousands. Table 8.4 lists selected genotyping platforms, their advantages and limitations, throughput and commercial examples. The cost of genotyping has dropped considerably over the years, ranging from $2 per genotype for a "small-scale study" (thousands of genotypes) to 1-2 cents per genotype for a "large-scale study" (hundreds of millions of genotypes). Assay conversion rate is typically 80–90% cross platforms. Quality control filters are usually applied to genotyping data prior to association analysis, such as call rate (at least over 80%, typically higher than 95%), Mendelian errors for trio samples (typically less than 1%), reproducibility for duplicated samples (usually at least 99%) and Hardy-Weinberg P-value (typically >0.001 for the control population) *(3)*. Genotyping accuracy is usually 99% or higher for all genotyping methods. The highest quality genotyping is usually obtained from genomic DNA extracted from blood. The quantity of DNA needed per genotype is usually in low nanogram levels for the medium throughput technologies and much less for a whole genome scan. Many technologies can successfully genotype large number of SNPs on DNA isolated from formalin fixed and frozen tissue samples, FTA cards, buccal cells and-whole genome amplified DNA. Genotyping technologies evolve quickly, making it attractive resource-wise and cost-wise to contract out genotyping projects rather than bring a system in-house. There are many genotyping service providers available; *(109–124)* several of them are GLP (Good Laboratory Practices [125]) or ISO9000 *(126)*-certified laboratories; *(112, 115–117, 127)* and a small number of the providers are CLIA (the Clinical Laboratory Improvement Amendments [128])-certified or capable of validating assays under CLIA-compliance *(112, 116, 129–131)*. Some points to consider for choosing a genotyping vendor are the scope of the project, the number of samples and SNPs, the turn-around time and the cost.

4.3 Whole Genome Genotyping Arrays

To date, there are 11 million human SNPs identified and about half of them are validated in dbSNP *(132)*. Although it is not yet technically possible to genotype all 11 million SNPs, it is feasible to perform a whole genome scan by genotyping 100,000 to 500,000 SNPs per sample *(8, 15, 82, 89, 90, 93, 96, 101, 133–136)*. The cost of an individual whole genome genotyping array has dropped to as low as $250 per sample on reagent and chip cost for an Affymetrix 500K-panel. It is not practical to select different sets of SNPs for each study, thus commercial products with a fixed panel of SNPs are widely adopted. Affymetrix 100K and 500K markers are selected primarily on technical quality and are quasi-randomly distributed across the genome *(96)*. In contrast, SNPs in the 300K and higher Illumina panels were selected using tagging approaches by leveraging HapMap CEPH genotyping data; these SNP panels seek to capture the majority of unmeasured common SNPs in the entire genome *(89, 90)*. Although there are substantial differences in genotyping methodologies, marker selection strategies, and number of markers assayed, the above three whole-genome scan panels (Affymetrix 100K, 500K, and Illumina 300K) offer similar levels of genome coverage when evaluated against HapMap phase II data *(137)*. SNPs are the most common genetic variants; however, during the last few years, structural variants such as copy number variants (CNVs) have attracted much attention. CNVs are defined as DNA segments that are 1 kb or larger in size, present at variable copy number in comparison with a reference genome *(22)*. CNVs are quite common in the human genome and can have dramatic phenotypic consequences as a result of altering gene dosage, disrupting coding sequences, or perturbing long-range gene regulation *(138, 139)*. Recently, Affymetrix has released the SNP Array 5.0, a single microarray featuring all SNPs from the original two-chip 500K array and 420,000 additional nonpolymorphic probes for CNVs. Illumina has released a 550K panel that includes tagging SNPs on non-European populations; 4,300 SNPs in CNV regions of the genome; 7,800 nonsynonymous SNPs; 1,800 tag SNPs in MHC; 177 mitochondrial SNPs; and 11 Y-chromosome SNPs, in addition to the 300K panel. Both Affymetrix and Illumina have recently announced a plan to market a 1-million-SNP panel in the near future. Illumina's 1M panel will include additional SNPs in coding regions of the genome, SNPs and probes in CNV regions, Caucasian and Asian tagging SNPs, African tagging SNPs, evenly spaced SNPs, and ADME/MHC SNPs on top of the 550K panel. Affymetrix has not disclosed publicly the content of its 1-million-SNP array.

4.4 Predefined SNP Panels

In addition to predefined whole-genome scan products, there are smaller sets of polymorphisms of particular interest made commercially available for genetic or pharmacogenetic applications. These include coding SNPs panels, ADME SNPs, MHC SNPs, disease-related SNPs, and admixture-mapping panels (Table 8.5). There are several specialty pharmacogenetic tests available; some of them are CLIA-certified tests that are marketed directly to the consumer, such as *CYP2C9* and *VKORC1* genotyping for warfarin dosing *(112, 127, 129–131)*, *HLA-DQB1* genotyping to predicate the probability of developing agranulocytosis in response to clozapine, *(112)* the FAMILION® test (analysis of *KCNQ1, KCNH2, SCN5A, KCNE1,* and *KCNE2* genes related to cardiac channelopathies, including Long QT Syndrome and Brugada Syndrome), *(112)* and drug metabolizing enzyme genotyping by several vendors *(111, 112, 115, 116, 127, 129, 131)*.

Table 8.5 Predefined polymorphism panels

Product	Description
Affymetrix 10K cSNP Kit	10,000 validated (double-hit) nonsynonymous public SNPs
Affymetrix 20K cSNP Kit	Additional 10K on top of the original 10K cSNP kit
Affymetrix Immune and Inflammation 9K SNP Kit	Selected informative markers for 1,000 genes thought to be involved in the inflammation response and genetics of immunobiology
Affymetrix Human MALD 3K SNP Kit	Designed for admixture mapping
Affymetrix DMET panel	A set of 1228 polymorphisms on 169 ADME genes and drug transporters (47 phase I CYP enzyme genes, 79 phase II ADME genes, and 49 transporter genes); is being validated in CLIA certified lab
Roche AmpliChip CYP450 Test	FDA-approved in vitro diagnostic test (510K) on 27 CYP2D6 alleles and 3 CYP2C19 alleles
Illumina Cancer SNP Panel	1421 SNP loci chosen from the NCI SNP500 Cancer Database
Illumina HumanNS-12	11,000 non-synonymous SNPs across the genome and tag SNP across the Major Histocompatibility Complex (MHC) region
Illumina MHC panel set	MHC Exon-Centric Panel: >1200 SNPs within 10Kb of coding regions in the MHC
	MHC Mapping Panel: >1250 SNPs with average spacing of 3.8Kb

4.5 GLP and CLIA Assays

Large scale genomic and pharmacogenomic studies are generally carried out in "research" mode, without the documentation trail that is required in FDA submissions. When applying pharmacogenomics to drug development, it is important to consider whether a study needs to be done in a GLP- or ISO 9000- or CLIA-compliant environment. In practice, a pharmacogenomics study for hypothesis generation is typically performed under non-GLP or non-CLIA condition, although the sample collection in a clinical trial is routinely carried out following GLP- or Good Clinical Practice *(140)*. (GCP)-regulation. It is beneficial to carry out exploratory genotyping for clinical studies in a GLP-compliant laboratory On the other hand, assay validation under GLP is time-consuming and labor intensive, so it is probably not necessary to validate each individual assay under GLP conditions. If a pharmacogenomics study will be validated and employed to support registration of a clinical endpoint, it warrants performing genotyping and validating individual assays under GLP-conditions. If a pharmacogenomics test is intended to guide patient treatment, such as selection of medications and dosing, the test needs to be FDA-approved (510K) or validated and performed under CLIA conditions for a homebrew test.

4.6 *Needs for SNP/Mutation Discovery and Whole-Genome Resequencing*

The HapMap project and available whole genome scan panels are designed on the hypothesis that common diseases are caused by common variants, with an aim to identify causal variants with tag SNPs. The recent publications on whole-genome associations may reveal the coverage of the whole-genome scan panels and their potential impact *(8, 11, 15, 134–136, 141)*. Some of the significant findings reported are identified by only a single SNP, *(8, 15, 141)* suggesting that the current whole-genome scan marker sets provide incomplete genome coverage *(142, 143)*. It is likely that in the future, whole-genome studies will employ even larger numbers of SNPs, including additional population-specific SNPs and low frequency SNPs. A recent analysis of the HapMap ENCODE data suggested that current whole-genome scan panels provide lower coverage of genic SNPs than nongenic SNPs, especially in Caucasians *(144)*. The report suggested that gene-centric genome-wide association studies could be more efficient for detecting causal variants than existing whole genome panels. In addition, the report estimated that more than 50% of important nonsynonymous SNPs have yet to be discovered. Thus the identification of low allele frequency nonsynonymous SNPs is desired, since most of the common SNPs have already been discovered. A practical approach for causal variant discovery might be to combine whole-genome scans with SNP/mutation discovery through resequencing of candidate coding regions. There are existing and emerging technologies available to carry out high-throughput SNP/mutation discovery, such as ParAllele's mismatch repair detection *(145–147)*, Sequenom's MALDI-TOF mass spectrometry analysis *(148, 149)*, Affymetrix's re-sequencing by microarray hybridization, Transgenomic's DHPLC denaturing high performance liquid chromatography mutation detection, *(150)* conventional sequencing, or whole-genome resequencing platforms by 454 *(151, 152)* and Solexa *(153, 154)*.

Acknowledgments The authors would like to thank Dr. Reyna Favis for her technical insight.

References

1. Venter JC, Adams MD, Myers EW et al (2001) The sequence of the human genome. Science 291(5507):1304–51.
2. Lander ES, Linton LM, Birren B et al (2001) Initial sequencing and analysis of the human genome. Nature 409(6822):860–921.
3. The International HapMap Consortium (2005) A haplotype map of the human genome. Nature 437(7063):1299–320.
4. Goldstein DB, Tate SK, Sisodiya SM (2003) Pharmacogenetics goes genomic. Nat Rev Genet 4(12):937–47.
5. Tate SK, Depondt C, Sisodiya SM et al (2005) Genetic predictors of the maximum doses patients receive during clinical use of the anti-epileptic drugs carbamazepine and phenytoin. Proc Natl Acad Sci U S A 102(15):5507–12.

6. Wadelius M, Chen LY, Downes K et al (2005) Common VKORC1 and GGCX polymorphisms associated with warfarin dose. Pharmacogenomics J 5(4):262–70.
7. Rieder MJ, Reiner AP, Gage BF et al (2005) Effect of VKORC1 haplotypes on transcriptional regulation and warfarin dose. N Engl J Med 352(22):2285–93.
8. Sladek R, Rocheleau G, Rung J et al (2007) A genome-wide association study identifies novel risk loci for type 2 diabetes. Nature 445(7130):881–5.
9. Edwards AO, Ritter R 3rd, Abel KJ, Manning A, Panhuysen C, Farrer LA (2005) Complement factor H polymorphism and age-related macular degeneration. Science 308(5720):421–4.
10. Kiessling A, Ehrhart-Bornstein M (2006) Transcription factor 7-like 2 (TCFL2)—a novel factor involved in pathogenesis of type 2 diabetes. Comment on: Grant et al (2006) Nat Genet, Published online 15 January 2006. Horm Metab Res 38(2):137–8.
11. Herbert A, Gerry NP, McQueen MB et al (2006) A common genetic variant is associated with adult and childhood obesity. Science 312(5771):279–83.
12. Amundadottir LT, Sulem P, Gudmundsson J et al (2006) A common variant associated with prostate cancer in European and African populations. Nat Genet 38(6):652–8.
13. Gudmundsson J, Sulem P, Manolescu A et al (2007) Genome-wide association study identifies a second prostate cancer susceptibility variant at 8q24. Nat Genet 39(5):579–80.
14. Horvath A, Boikos S, Giatzakis C et al (2006) A genome-wide scan identifies mutations in the gene encoding phosphodiesterase 11A4 (PDE11A) in individuals with adrenocortical hyperplasia. Nat Genet 38(7):794–800.
15. Duerr RH, Taylor KD, Brant SR et al (2006) A genome-wide association study identifies IL23R as an inflammatory bowel disease gene. Science 314(5804):1461–3.
16. Helgason A, Palsson S, Thorleifsson G et al (2007) Refining the impact of TCF7L2 gene variants on type 2 diabetes and adaptive evolution. Nat Genet 39(2):218–25.
17. Helgadottir A, Manolescu A, Helgason A et al (2006) A variant of the gene encoding leukotriene A4 hydrolase confers ethnicity-specific risk of myocardial infarction. Nat Genet 38(1):68–74.
18. de Bakker PI, McVean G, Sabeti PC et al (2006) A high-resolution HLA and SNP haplotype map for disease association studies in the extended human MHC. Nat Genet 38(10):1166–72.
19. She X, Jiang Z, Clark RA et al (2004) Shotgun sequence assembly and recent segmental duplications within the human genome. Nature 431(7011):927–30.
20. Bailey JA, Yavor AM, Viggiano L et al (2002) Human-specific duplication and mosaic transcripts: the recent paralogous structure of chromosome 22. Am J Hum Genet 70(1):83–100.
21. Bailey JA, Yavor AM, Massa HF, Trask BJ, Eichler EE. (2001) Segmental duplications: organization and impact within the current human genome project assembly. Genome Res 11(6): 1005–17.
22. Redon R, Ishikawa S, Fitch KR et al (2006) Global variation in copy number in the human genome. Nature 444(7118):444–54.
23. Iafrate AJ, Feuk L, Rivera MN et al (2004) Detection of large-scale variation in the human genome. Nat Genet 36(9):949–51.
24. Sebat J, Lakshmi B, Troge J et al (2004) Large-scale copy number polymorphism in the human genome. Science 305(5683):525–8.
25. Sharp AJ, Locke DP, McGrath SD et al (2005) Segmental duplications and copy-number variation in the human genome. Am J Hum Genet 77(1):78–88.
26. Tuzun E, Sharp AJ, Bailey JA et al (2005) Fine-scale structural variation of the human genome. Nat Genet 37(7):727–32.
27. Hinds DA, Kloek AP, Jen M, Chen X, Frazer KA (2006) Common deletions and SNPs are in linkage disequilibrium in the human genome. Nat Genet 38(1):82–5.
28. Conrad DF, Andrews TD, Carter NP, Hurles ME, Pritchard JK (2006) A high-resolution survey of deletion polymorphism in the human genome. Nat Genet 38(1):75–81.
29. McCarroll SA, Hadnott TN, Perry GH et al (2006) Common deletion polymorphisms in the human genome. Nat Genet 38(1):86–92.
30. Barnes MR (2006) Navigating the HapMap. Brief Bioinform 7(3):211–24.

31. Thorisson GA, Smith AV, Krishnan L, Stein LD (2005) The International HapMap Project web site. Genome Res 15(11):1592–3.
32. Johnson GC, Esposito L, Barratt BJ et al (2001) Haplotype tagging for the identification of common disease genes. Nat Genet 29(2):233–7.
33. Pritchard JK, Przeworski M (2001) Linkage disequilibrium in humans: models and data. Am J Hum Genet 69(1):1–14.
34. Stram DO (2005) Software for tag single nucleotide polymorphism selection. Hum Genomics 2(2):144–51.
35. Lowe CE, Cooper JD, Chapman JM et al (2004) Cost-effective analysis of candidate genes using htSNPs: a staged approach. Genes Immun 5(4):301–5.
36. Halldorsson BV, Istrail S, De La Vega FM (2004) Optimal selection of SNP markers for disease association studies. Hum Hered 58(3–4):190–202.
37. Stram DO (2004) Tag SNP selection for association studies. Genet Epidemiol 27(4):365–74.
38. Qin ZS, Niu T, Liu JS (2002) Partition-ligation-expectation-maximization algorithm for haplotype inference with single-nucleotide polymorphisms. Am J Hum Genet 71(5):1242–7.
39. Carlson CS, Eberle MA, Rieder MJ, Yi Q, Kruglyak L, Nickerson DA (2004) Selecting a maximally informative set of single-nucleotide polymorphisms for association analyses using linkage disequilibrium. Am J Hum Genet 74(1):106–20.
40. de Bakker PI, Yelensky R, Pe'er I, Gabriel SB, Daly MJ, Altshuler D (2005) Efficiency and power in genetic association studies. Nat Genet 37(11):1217–23.
41. Lee PH, Shatkay H (2006) BNTagger: improved tagging SNP selection using Bayesian networks. Bioinformatics 22(14):e211–9.
42. He J, Zelikovsky A (2006) MLR-tagging: informative SNP selection for unphased genotypes based on multiple linear regression. Bioinformatics 22(20):2558–61.
43. Sham PC, Ao SI, Kwan JS et al (2007) Combining functional and linkage disequilibrium information in the selection of tag SNPs. Bioinformatics 23(1):129–31.
44. Ke X, Miretti MM, Broxholme J et al (2005) A comparison of tagging methods and their tagging space. Hum Mol Genet 14(18):2757–67.
45. Zeggini E, Rayner W, Morris AP et al (2005) An evaluation of HapMap sample size and tagging SNP performance in large-scale empirical and simulated data sets. Nat Genet 37(12):1320–2.
46. Gonzalez-Neira A, Ke X, Lao O et al (2006) The portability of tagSNPs across populations: a worldwide survey. Genome Res 16(3):323–30.
47. Taylor JA, Xu ZL, Kaplan NL, Morris RW (2006) How well do HapMap haplotypes identify common haplotypes of genes? A comparison with haplotypes of 334 genes resequenced in the environmental genome project. Cancer Epidemiol Biomarkers Prev 15(1):133–7.
48. Ribas G, Gonzalez-Neira A, Salas A et al (2006) Evaluating HapMap SNP data transferability in a large-scale genotyping project involving 175 cancer-associated genes. Hum Genet 118(6):669–79.
49. Ahmadi KR, Weale ME, Xue ZY et al (2005) A single-nucleotide polymorphism tagging set for human drug metabolism and transport. Nat Genet 37(1):84–9.
50. Soranzo N (2004) Genetic association studies: web-based resources for effective screening and assessment of candidate genes and pathways. Hum Genomics 1(4):307–9.
51. Bader GD, Cary MP, Sander C (2006) Pathguide: a pathway resource list. Nucl Acids Res 34(suppl_1):D504–6.
52. McKusick VA: Mendelian Inheritance in Man. A Catalog of Human Genes and Genetic Disorders. Baltimore: Johns Hopkins University Press, 1998 (12th edition). and Online Mendelian Inheritance in Man, OMIM (TM). McKusick-Nathans Institute of Genetic Medicine, Johns Hopkins University (Baltimore, MD) and National Center for Biotechnology Information, National Library of Medicine (Bethesda, MD), {date of download}. World Wide Web URL: http://www.ncbi.nlm.nih.gov/omim.
53. Becker KG, Barnes KC, Bright TJ, Wang SA (2004) The genetic association database. Nat Genet 36(5):431–2.
54. Gaulton KJ, Mohlke KL, Vision TJ (2007) A computational system to select candidate genes for complex human traits. Bioinformatics 23(9):1132–40.

55. Lopez-Bigas N, Ouzounis CA (2004) Genome-wide identification of genes likely to be involved in human genetic disease. Nucl Acids Res 32(10):3108–14.
56. Jensen LJ, Saric J, Bork P (2006) Literature mining for the biologist: from information retrieval to biological discovery. Nat Rev Genet 7(2):119–29.
57. Jenssen TK, Laegreid A, Komorowski J, Hovig E (2001) A literature network of human genes for high-throughput analysis of gene expression. Nat Genet 28(1):21–8.
58. Perez-Iratxeta C, Wjst M, Bork P, Andrade MA (2005) G2D: a tool for mining genes associated with disease. BMC Genet 6:45.
59. Perez-Iratxeta C, Bork P, Andrade MA (2002) Association of genes to genetically inherited diseases using data mining. Nat Genet 31(3):316–9.
60. Hristovski D, Peterlin B, Mitchell JA, Humphrey SM (2005) Using literature-based discovery to identify disease candidate genes. Int J Med Informat 74(2–4):289–98.
61. Swanson DR (1986) Fish oil, Raynaud's syndrome, and undiscovered public knowledge. Perspect Biol Med 30(1):7–18.
62. Korbel JO, Doerks T, Jensen LJ et al (2005) Systematic association of genes to phenotypes by genome and literature mining. PLoS Biol 3(5):e134.
63. Krauthammer M, Kaufmann CA, Gilliam TC, Rzhetsky A (2004) Molecular triangulation: bridging linkage and molecular-network information for identifying candidate genes in Alzheimer's disease. Proc Natl Acad Sci U S A 101(42):15148–53.
64. Tiffin N, Kelso JF, Powell AR, Pan H, Bajic VB, Hide WA (2005) Integration of text- and data-mining using ontologies successfully selects disease gene candidates. Nucleic Acids Res 33(5):1544–52.
65. Hinds DA, Stuve LL, Nilsen GB et al (2005) Whole-genome patterns of common DNA variation in three human populations. Science 307(5712):1072–9.
66. Sherry ST, Ward MH, Kholodov M et al (2001) dbSNP: the NCBI database of genetic variation. Nucleic Acids Res 29(1):308–11.
67. Kitts A, Sherry S (2006) The single nucleotide polymorphism database (dbSNP) of nucleotide sequence variation. The NCBI Handbook <javascript:BVShow('handbook')> Part 1. The Databases <javascript:BVShow('handbook.part.1')> Updated: July 17, 2007 <http://www.ncbi.nlm.nih.gov/books/bv.fcgi?rid=handbook.chapter.ch5>.
68. Hubbard TJ, Aken BL, Beal K et al (2007) Ensembl 2007. Nucleic Acids Res 35(Database issue):D610–7.
69. Wang P, Dai M, Xuan W et al (2006) SNP Function Portal: a web database for exploring the function implication of SNP alleles. Bioinformatics 22(14):e523–9.
70. Freimuth RR, Stormo GD, McLeod HL (2005) PolyMAPr: Programs for polymorphism database mining, annotation, and functional analysis. Hum Mutat 25(2):110–7.
71. Hemminger BM, Saelim B, Sullivan PF (2006) TAMAL: an integrated approach to choosing SNPs for genetic studies of human complex traits. Bioinformatics 22(5):626–7.
72. Conde L, Vaquerizas JM, Santoyo J et al (2004) PupaSNP Finder: a web tool for finding SNPs with putative effect at transcriptional level. Nucleic Acids Res 32(Web Server issue):W242–8.
73. Ramensky V, Bork P, Sunyaev S (2002) Human non-synonymous SNPs: server and survey. Nucleic Acids Res 30(17):3894–900.
74. Karchin R, Diekhans M, Kelly L et al (2005) LS-SNP: large-scale annotation of coding non-synonymous SNPs based on multiple information sources. Bioinformatics 21(12):2814–20.
75. Yue P, Melamud E, Moult J (2006) SNPs3D: candidate gene and SNP selection for association studies. BMC Bioinformatics 7:166.
76. Cartegni L, Wang J, Zhu Z, Zhang MQ, Krainer AR (2003) ESEfinder: A web resource to identify exonic splicing enhancers. Nucleic Acids Res 31(13):3568–71.
77. Han A, Kang HJ, Cho Y, Lee S, Kim YJ, Gong S (2006) SNP@Domain: a web resource of single nucleotide polymorphisms (SNPs) within protein domain structures and sequences. Nucl Acids Res 34(suppl_2):W642–4.
78. Giacomini KM, Brett CM, Altman RB et al (2007) The pharmacogenetics research network: from SNP discovery to clinical drug response. Clin Pharmacol Ther 81(3):328–45.
79. Altman RB (2007) PharmGKB: a logical home for knowledge relating genotype to drug response phenotype. Nat Genet 39(4):426.

80. Ahmadian A, Ehn M, Hober S (2006) Pyrosequencing: history, biochemistry and future. Clin Chim Acta 363(1–2):83–94.
81. Bell PA, Chaturvedi S, Gelfand CA et al (2002) SNPstream UHT: ultra-high throughput SNP genotyping for pharmacogenomics and drug discovery. Biotechniques Suppl:70–2, 4, 6–7.
82. Bierut LJ, Madden PAF, Breslau N et al (2007) Novel genes identified in a high-density genome wide association study for nicotine dependence. Hum Mol Genet 16(1):24–35.
83. van den Boom D, Beaulieu M, Oeth P et al (2004) MALDI-TOF MS: a platform technology for genetic discovery. Int J Mass Spectrometry 238(2):173–88.
84. De la Vega FM, Lazaruk KD, Rhodes MD, Wenz MH (2005) Assessment of two flexible and compatible SNP genotyping platforms: TaqMan SNP genotyping assays and the SNPlex genotyping system. Mutat Res 573(1–2):111–35.
85. Dunbar SA (2006) Applications of Luminex xMAP technology for rapid, high-throughput multiplexed nucleic acid detection. Clin Chim Acta 363(1–2):71–82.
86. Fan JB, Gunderson KL, Bibikova M et al (2006) Illumina universal bead arrays. Methods Enzymol 410:57–73.
87. Favis R, Gerry NP, Cheng YW, Barany F (2005) Applications of the universal DNA microarray in molecular medicine. Methods Mol Med 114:25–58.
88. Gibson NJ (2006) The use of real-time PCR methods in DNA sequence variation analysis. Clin Chim Acta 363(1–2):32–47.
89. Gunderson KL, Kuhn KM, Steemers FJ, Ng P, Murray SS, Shen R (2006) Whole-genome genotyping of haplotype tag single nucleotide polymorphisms. Pharmacogenomics 7(4):641–8.
90. Gunderson KL, Steemers FJ, Ren H et al (2006) Whole-genome genotyping. Methods Enzymol 410:359–76.
91. Hardenbol P, Baner J, Jain M et al (2003) Multiplexed genotyping with sequence-tagged molecular inversion probes. Nat Biotechnol 21(6):673–8.
92. Hardenbol P, Yu F, Belmont J et al (2005) Highly multiplexed molecular inversion probe genotyping: over 10,000 targeted SNPs genotyped in a single tube assay. Genome Res 15(2):269–75.
93. Hinds DA, Stuve LL, Nilsen GB et al (2005) Whole-genome patterns of common DNA variation in three human populations. Science 307(5712):1072–9.
94. Keen-Kim D, Grody WW, Richards CS (2006) Microelectronic array system for molecular diagnostic genotyping: Nanogen NanoChip 400 and molecular biology workstation. Expert Rev Mol Diagn 6(3):287–94.
95. Kennedy GC, Matsuzaki H, Dong S et al (2003) Large-scale genotyping of complex DNA. Nat Biotechnol 21(10):1233–7.
96. Matsuzaki H, Dong S, Loi H et al (2004) Genotyping over 100,000 SNPs on a pair of oligonucleotide arrays. Nat Methods 1(2):109–11.
97. Mein CA, Barratt BJ, Dunn MG et al (2000) Evaluation of single nucleotide polymorphism typing with invader on PCR amplicons and its automation. Genome Res 10(3):330–43.
98. Moorhead M, Hardenbol P, Siddiqui F et al (2006) Optimal genotype determination in highly multiplexed SNP data. Eur J Hum Genet 14(2):207–15.
99. Patil N, Berno AJ, Hinds DA et al (2001) Blocks of limited haplotype diversity revealed by high-resolution scanning of human chromosome 21. Science 294(5547):1719–23.
100. Ragoussis J, Elvidge G (2006) Affymetrix GeneChip system: moving from research to the clinic. Expert Rev Mol Diagn 6(2):145–52.
101. Steemers FJ, Gunderson KL (2007) Whole genome genotyping technologies on the BeadArray platform. Biotechnol J 2(1):41–9.
102. Tobler AR, Short S, Andersen MR et al (2005) The SNPlex genotyping system: a flexible and scalable platform for SNP genotyping. J Biomol Tech 16(4):398–406.
103. Gut IG (2001) Automation in genotyping of single nucleotide polymorphisms. Hum Mutat 17(6):475–92.
104. Kwok PY (2000) High-throughput genotyping assay approaches. Pharmacogenomics 1(1):95–100.

105. Kwok PY (2001) Methods for genotyping single nucleotide polymorphisms. Annu Rev Genomics Hum Genet 2:235–58.
106. Tsuchihashi Z, Dracopoli NC (2002) Progress in high throughput SNP genotyping methods. Pharmacogenomics J 2(2):103–10.
107. Sobrino B, Brion M, Carracedo A (2005) SNPs in forensic genetics: a review on SNP typing methodologies. Forensic Sci Int 154(2–3):181–94.
108. Hirschhorn JN, Daly MJ (2005) Genome-wide association studies for common diseases and complex traits. Nat Rev Genet 6(2):95–108.
109. http://www.acgtinc.com/
110. http://www.affymetrix.com/
111. http://www.bioserve.com/
112. http://www.cogenics.com/
113. http://www.decode.com/
114. http://www.ellipsisbio.com/
115. http://www.epidauros.com/cms/en/index.html
116. http://www.expressionanalysis.com/
117. http://www.genizon.com/
118. http://www.illumina.com/
119. http://www.jurilab.com/
120. http://www.marligen.com/
121. http://www.polymorphicdna.com/
122. http://www.sequenom.com/
123. http://www.seqwright.com/
124. www.perlegen.com
125. http://www.fda.gov/ora/compliance_ref/bimo/GLP/qna.htm
126. http://www.iso.org/iso/en/iso9000–14000/index.html
127. http://www.gentris.com/
128. http://www.fda.gov/cdrh/clia/
129. http://www.genelex.com/
130. http://www.genomas.net/
131. http://www.tmbioscience.com/
132. http://www.ncbi.nlm.nih.gov/projects/SNP/index.html
133. Low YL, Wedren S, Liu J (2006) High-throughput genomic technology in research and clinical management of breast cancer. Evolving landscape of genetic epidemiological studies. Breast Cancer Res 8(3):209.
134. Papassotiropoulos A, Stephan DA, Huentelman MJ et al (2006) Common kibra alleles are associated with human memory performance. Science 314(5798):475–8.
135. Schymick JC, Scholz SW, Fung HC et al (2007) Genome-wide genotyping in amyotrophic lateral sclerosis and neurologically normal controls: first stage analysis and public release of data. Lancet Neurol 6(4):322–8.
136. Yang Z, Camp NJ, Sun H et al (2006) A variant of the HTRA1 gene increases susceptibility to age-related macular degeneration. Science 314(5801):992–3.
137. Pe'er I, de Bakker PI, Maller J, Yelensky R, Altshuler D, Daly MJ (2006) Evaluating and improving power in whole-genome association studies using fixed marker sets. Nat Genet 38(6):663–7.
138. Feuk L, Marshall CR, Wintle RF, Scherer SW (2006) Structural variants: changing the landscape of chromosomes and design of disease studies. Hum Mol Genet 15 Spec No 1:R57–66.
139. Stranger BE, Forrest MS, Dunning M et al (2007) Relative impact of nucleotide and copy number variation on gene expression phenotypes. Science 315(5813):848–53.
140. http://www.fda.gov/oc/gcp/
141. Lencz T, Morgan TV, Athanasiou M et al (2007) Converging evidence for a pseudoautosomal cytokine receptor gene locus in schizophrenia. Mol Psychiatry 12(6):572–80. Epub.
142. Cardon LR (2006) Genetics. Delivering new disease genes. Science 314(5804):1403–5.

143. Freimer NB, Sabatti C (2007) Human genetics: variants in common diseases. Nature 445(7130):828–30.
144. Jorgenson E, Witte JS (2006) A gene-centric approach to genome-wide association studies. Nat Rev Genet 7(11):885–91.
145. Faham M, Baharloo S, Tomitaka S, DeYoung J, Freimer NB (2001) Mismatch repair detection (MRD): high-throughput scanning for DNA variations. Hum Mol Genet 10(16):1657–64.
146. Fakhrai-Rad H, Zheng J, Willis TD et al (2004) SNP discovery in pooled samples with mismatch repair detection. Genome Res 14(7):1404–12.
147. http://www.affymetrix.com/technology/mrd_technology.affx.
148. Stanssens P, Zabeau M, Meersseman G et al (2004) High-throughput MALDI-TOF discovery of genomic sequence polymorphisms. Genome Res 14(1):126–33.
149. Ragoussis J, Elvidge GP, Kaur K, Colella S (2006) Matrix-assisted laser desorption/ionisation, time-of-flight mass spectrometry in genomics research. PLoS Genet 2(7):e100.
150. Qiu P, Shandilya H, D'Alessio JM, O'Connor K, Durocher J, Gerard GF (2004) Mutation detection using Surveyor nuclease. Biotechniques 36(4):702–7.
151. Margulies M, Egholm M, Altman WE et al (2005) Genome sequencing in microfabricated high-density picolitre reactors. Nature 437(7057):376–80.
152. http://www.454.com/
153. Bentley DR (2006) Whole-genome re-sequencing. Curr Opin Genet Dev 16(6):545–52.
154. www.solexa.com.
155. Barrett JC, Fry B, Maller J, Daly MJ (2005) Haploview: analysis and visualization of LD and haplotype maps. Bioinformatics 21(2):263–5.
156. Weale ME, Depondt C, Macdonald SJ et al (2003) Selection and evaluation of tagging SNPs in the neuronal-sodium-channel gene SCN1A: implications for linkage-disequilibrium gene mapping. Am J Hum Genet 73(3):551–65.
157. Stram DO, Haiman CA, Hirschhorn JN et al (2003) Choosing haplotype-tagging SNPS based on unphased genotype data using a preliminary sample of unrelated subjects with an example from the Multiethnic Cohort Study. Hum Hered 55(1):27–36.
158. Zhang K, Qin Z, Chen T, Liu JS, Waterman MS, Sun F (2005) HapBlock: haplotype block partitioning and tag SNP selection software using a set of dynamic programming algorithms. Bioinformatics 21(1):131–4.
159. Rinaldo A, Bacanu SA, Devlin B, Sonpar V, Wasserman L, Roeder K (2005) Characterization of multilocus linkage disequilibrium. Genet Epidemiol 28(3):193–206.
160. Ao SI, Yip K, Ng M et al (2005) CLUSTAG: hierarchical clustering and graph methods for selecting tag SNPs. Bioinformatics 21(8):1735–6.
161. Rebhan M, Chalifa-Caspi V, Prilusky J, Lancet D (1997) GeneCards: integrating information about genes, proteins and diseases. Trends Genet 13(4):163.
162. Klein TE, Chang JT, Cho MK et al (2001) Integrating genotype and phenotype information: an overview of the PharmGKB project. Pharmacogenetics Research Network and Knowledge Base. Pharmacogenomics J 1(3):167–70.
163. Lin BK, Clyne M, Walsh M et al (2006) Tracking the epidemiology of human genes in the literature: the HuGE Published Literature database. Am J Epidemiol 164(1):1–4.
164. Wain HM, Lush MJ, Ducluzeau F, Khodiyar VK, Povey S (2004) Genew: the Human Gene Nomenclature Database, 2004 updates. Nucleic Acids Res 32(Database issue):D255–7.
165. Novichkova S, Egorov S, Daraselia N (2003) MedScan, a natural language processing engine for MEDLINE abstracts. Bioinformatics 19(13):1699–706.
166. Alfarano C, Andrade CE, Anthony K et al (2005) The Biomolecular Interaction Network Database and related tools 2005 update. Nucleic Acids Res 33(Database issue): D418–24.
167. Salwinski L, Miller CS, Smith AJ, Pettit FK, Bowie JU, Eisenberg D (2004) The Database of Interacting Proteins: 2004 update. Nucl Acids Res 32(suppl_1):D449–51.
168. Mering CV, Huynen M, Jaeggi D, Schmidt S, Bork P, Snel B (2003) STRING: a database of predicted functional associations between proteins. Nucl Acids Res 31(1):258–61.

169. Joshi-Tope G, Gillespie M, Vastrik I et al (2005) Reactome: a knowledgebase of biological pathways. Nucleic Acids Res 33(Database issue):D428–32.
170. Peri S, Navarro JD, Amanchy R et al (2003) Development of human protein reference database as an initial platform for approaching systems biology in humans. Genome Res 13(10):2363–71.
171. Kanehisa M, Goto S, Hattori M et al (2006) From genomics to chemical genomics: new developments in KEGG. Nucleic Acids Res 34(Database issue):D354–7.
172. Bonis J, Furlong LI, Sanz F (2006) OSIRIS: a tool for retrieving literature about sequence variants. Bioinformatics 22(20):2567–9.
173. Rebholz-Schuhmann D, Kirsch H, Arregui M, Gaudan S, Riethoven M, Stoehr P (2007) EBIMed—text crunching to gather facts for proteins from Medline. Bioinformatics 23(2): e237–44.
174. Rebholz-Schuhmann D, Kirsch H, Arregui M, Gaudan S, Rynbeek M, Stoehr P (2006) Protein annotation by EBIMed. Nat Biotechnol 24(8):902–3.
175. Doms A, Schroeder M (2005) GoPubMed: exploring PubMed with the Gene Ontology. Nucleic Acids Res 33(Web Server issue):W783–6.
176. Tanabe L, Scherf U, Smith LH, Lee JK, Hunter L, Weinstein JN (1999) MedMiner: an internet text-mining tool for biomedical information, with application to gene expression profiling. Biotechniques 27(6):1210–4, 1216–7.
177. Goetz T, von der Lieth CW (2005) PubFinder: a tool for improving retrieval rate of relevant PubMed abstracts. Nucleic Acids Res 33(Web Server issue):W774–8.
178. Perez-Iratxeta C, Bork P, Andrade MA (2001) XplorMed: a tool for exploring MEDLINE abstracts. Trends Biochem Sci 26(9):573–5.
179. Hu ZZ, Mani I, Hermoso V, Liu H, Wu CH (2004) iProLINK: an integrated protein resource for literature mining. Comput Biol Chem 28(5–6):409–16.
180. Donaldson I, Martin J, de Bruijn B et al (2003) PreBIND and Textomy—mining the biomedical literature for protein-protein interactions using a support vector machine. BMC Bioinformatics 4:11.
181. Smalheiser NR, Swanson DR (1998) Using ARROWSMITH: a computer-assisted approach to formulating and assessing scientific hypotheses. Comput Methods Programs Biomed 57(3):149–53.
182. Hristovski D, Peterlin B, Mitchell JA, Humphrey SM (2005) Using literature-based discovery to identify disease candidate genes. Int J Med Inform 74(2–4):289–98.
183. Bowers PM, Pellegrini M, Thompson MJ, Fierro J, Yeates TO, Eisenberg D (2004) Prolinks: a database of protein functional linkages derived from coevolution. Genome Biol 5(5):R35.
184. The International HapMap Consortium. A haplotype map of the human genome. Nature 437(7063):1299–320.
185. Packer BR, Yeager M, Staats B et al (2004) SNP500Cancer: a public resource for sequence validation and assay development for genetic variation in candidate genes. Nucleic Acids Res 32(Database issue):D528–32.
186. Packer BR, Yeager M, Burdett L et al (2006) SNP500Cancer: a public resource for sequence validation, assay development, and frequency analysis for genetic variation in candidate genes. Nucleic Acids Res 34(Database issue):D617–21.
187. Fredman D, Munns G, Rios D et al (2004) HGVbase: a curated resource describing human DNA variation and phenotype relationships. Nucleic Acids Res 32(Database issue):D516–9.
188. Stenson PD, Ball EV, Mort M et al (2003) Human Gene Mutation Database (HGMD): 2003 update. Hum Mutat 21(6):577–81.
189. Kent WJ, Sugnet CW, Furey TS et al (2002) The Human Genome Browser at UCSC. Genome Res 12(6):996–1006.
190. Riva A, Kohane IS (2004) A SNP-centric database for the investigation of the human genome. BMC Bioinformatics 5:33.
191. Stamm S, Riethoven JJ, Le Texier V et al (2006) ASD: a bioinformatics resource on alternative splicing. Nucleic Acids Res 34(Database issue):D46–55.

Chapter 9
Study Design and Statistical Issues in Pharmacogenetics Research

From Candidate Genes to Genome-Wide Screens

Nicholas J. Schork, Nathalie Malo, and Eric J. Topol

Contents

Abstract Pharmacogenetics research focuses on the identification of inherited DNA sequence variations that influence an individual's response to therapeutic agents. Discovering such variations is nontrivial and may require enormous and potentially unrealistic sample sizes for appropriately therapeutic-response powered studies, unless one has sufficient a priori knowledge about genomic regions likely to harbor relevant variations. In addition, once relevant variations have been identified, it is important to evaluate their clinical utility, especially with respect to the appropriate therapeutic agents. In this very basic review we consider strategies for identifying genetic variations that influence response to therapeutic agents. We also consider strategies for evaluating the use of these genetic variations in the design and conduct of clinical trials assessing the utility of these variations in guiding therapeutic decisions.

Keywords Genetic mapping, haplotype, clinical trial, Single Nucleotide Polymorphism

1 Introduction

The availability of very high throughput DNA analysis technologies and the development of databases harboring information about the genomic positions of DNA sequence variations have provided geneticists with efficient and powerful tools for identifying

Nicholas J. Schork
Scripps Genomic Medicinethe Scripps Research Institute, La Jolla, CA
nschork@scripps.edu

N. Cohen (ed.) *Pharmacogenomics and Personalized Medicine*,

inherited DNA sequence variations that contribute to phenotypic expression and variability. In fact, it is now possible to test literally hundreds of thousands, if not a million or so, polymorphic markers for association with a particular phenotype in a single study (see Tables 9.1, 9.2, and 9.3). If an association between a particular genetic variation and a phenotype of interest (such as a disease) is found among the subjects studied, then one could infer that either the variation in question causally influences the phenotype, or there are such causal variations in the vicinity of the variation-exhibiting association (i.e., the associated variation is simply acting as a "surrogate" marker for the presence of the causal variations). Studies of this kind can focus on particular sets of variations having some a priori biological appeal as variations that could influence a particular phenotype, or focus on as many variations as possible in the absence of such a priori knowledge in what has been termed a genome-wide association (GWA) study.

Although there are many issues plaguing genetic association studies, they have been applied to virtually all diseases of contemporary public health importance (Tables 9.1, 9.2, and 9.3). The results of these studies have been of great interest not only to biomedical researchers, but also to researchers seeking to devise effective treatments for these diseases, since knowledge of a gene or genes harboring variations that cause or contribute to a disease may lead to insights into appropriate therapeutic pathways and drug targets. In addition, clinical and therapeutic researchers have also adopted genetic association analysis strategies in the identification of inherited DNA sequence variations that influence responses to particular treatments and therapies. If an association between a genetic variation and a response to a prevention strategy, treatment, or cure for a disease can be found, then clinicians can prescribe the prevention strategy, therapy, or intervention to those people most likely to respond due to their genetic makeup. This pharmacogenetic research paradigm has begun to generate a lot of interest and attention, but is also not without problems for various reasons.

In this short review, we consider contemporary genetic strategies that exploit the association study paradigm for identifying genes and genetic variations that influence the response to particular treatments or therapies. We start by offering a description of some important distinctions that will help put into perspective some of the material to be discussed in greater detail later in the chapter. We next describe basic genetic strategies for identifying inherited DNA sequence variations that influence particular phenotypes, and consider their shortcomings, especially with respect to their applicability in pharmacogenetics research. We then consider the immediate clinical research utility of genetic variations identified as either likely to influence disease susceptibility or treatment response, by focusing on the design of more efficient and less expensive clinical trials of appropriate prevention and treatment strategies. We end with a basic discussion of the future of pharmacogenetics research and some of the hurdles that need to be overcome if it is to have an impact in shaping what many consider to be the endgame of clinical research and practice: individualized or personalized medicine.

Table 9.1 Recent genome-wide association (GWA) studies investigating the genetic determinants of disease

Ref	Disease	Population	# Markers	Cases	Controls	# Sig. Markers	Criteria
(49)	Alzheimer's	NR	502,627	1086	1086	1	5×10^{-34}
(50)	Asthma	UK & German	317,000	994	1,243	34	5% FDR
(51)	Atrial Fibrillation	Icelandic	316,515	550	4,476	3	1.6×10^{-7}
(52)	Bipolar Disorder	European	500,568	2,000	3,000	1	5×10^{-7}
(53)	Breast Ca	European	528,173	1,145	1,142	6	1×10^{-5}
(54)	Breast Ca	UK	266,722	408	400	1,162	0.05
(55)	Celiac	UK	310,605	778	1,422	56	1×10^{-4}
(56)	CAD	German	272,602	870/772	1,644	NR	NR
(52)	CAD	European	500,568	2,000	3,000	1	5×10^{-7}
(57)	CHD	Canadian	100,000	322	312	2,586	0.025
(58)	Colorectal Ca	Canadian	99,632	1,257	1,336	1,143	NR
(59)	Colorectal Ca	UK	550,163	930	960	27,673	0.05
(52)	Crohn's	European	500,568	2,000	3,000	9	5×10^{-7}
(60)	Crohn's	American	317,503	988	1,007	27	1×10^{-5}
(61)	Crohn's	Belgium & France	317,497	547	928	3	1×10^{-6}
(62)	Crohn's	N. Germany	19,779	735	368	72	0.01
(63)	Crohn's	German	NR	645/676	1,190	1	2×10^{-7}
(64)	Diabetic Nephropathy	Japanese	56,648	94	94	402	0.01
(65)	Esophageal Ca	Chinease	11,555	50	50	39	4.9×10^{-6}
(66)	Gallstone Disease	German	382,492	280	360	235	5×10^{-4}
(52)	Hypertension	European	500,568	2,000	3,000	0	5×10^{-7}
(67)	Inflammatory Bowel	European	308,332	567	571	3	5.1×10^{-9}
(68)	Macular Degeneration	White, not Hisp	116,204	96	50	2	4.8×10^{-7}
(69)	Myocardial Infarction	Icelandic	305,953	1,607	6,728	3	1×10^{-6}
(70)	Myocardial Infarction	Japanese	65,671	94	658	12–18	1×10^{-4}
(71)	Parkinson	US	408,000	267	270	26	4.9×10^{-4}
(72)	Parkinson	US	198,345	443	443	1,862	0.01
(73)	Prostate Ca	Icelandic	316,515	1,453	3,064	4	1×10^{-11}
(74)	Prostate Ca	European	550,000	1,172	1,157	5	1×10^{-4}
(75)	Restless Legs Syndrome	Augsburg	236,758	1,644	401	4	1×10^{-6}
(52)	Rheumatoid Arthritis	European	500,568	2,000	3,000	2	5×10^{-7}
(76)	Schizophrenia	NR	500,000	178	144	4,346	0.01
(77)	Systemic Sclerosis	Choctaw Indians	400*	20	76	17	0.05
(78)	T1D	European	534,071	563	1,146	392	8.6×10^{-8}
(52)	T1D	European	500,568	2,000	3,000	5	5×10^{-7}
(79)	T1D	Great Britain	6,500	2,029	1,755	10	3.2×10^{-4}
(52)	T2D	European	500,568	2,000	3,000	3	5×10^{-7}
(80)	T2D	UK	393,453	1,924	2,938	30	1×10^{-5}

(continued)

Table 9.1 (continued)

Ref	Disease	Population	# Markers	Cases	Controls	# Sig. Markers	Criteria
(81)	T2D	Finnish	317,503	1,161	1,174	41	1×10^{-4}
(82)	T2D	Icelandic	313,179	1,399	5,275	46	5×10^{-5}
(83)	T2D Mellitus	French	392,935	1,363	1,363	71	1×10^{-4}
(84)	T2D& Trigliceride L.	Finland & Sweden	500,568	1,022	1,075	3	1×10^{-10}

Key: NR = not reported; *note that microsatellite markers were used for this study (otherwise SNPs were used); **note that the phenotype was quantitative for this study (otherwise studies are case-control); CAD = Coronary Artery Disease; CHD = Coronary Heart Disease; T1D = Type 1 Diabetes; T2D = Type 2 Diabetes.

Table 9.2 Recent family-based genome-wide association (GWA) studies investigating the genetic determinants of disease

Ref	Disease	Population	# Markers	Subjects	Criteria
(85)	Alcoholism/Schizophrenia	COGA data	15,878	1,614	0.01
(86)	Alcoholism&Smoking	COGA data	4,720	1,614	1×10^{-5}
(87)	Blood Serotonin	Hutterites (South Dakota)	658*	1,623	0.01
(88)	Hypertension	All ethnicities	387*	13,524	0.01
(89)	SL Countertransport	CEPH data	7746*	62	1×10^{-6}

*microsatellites (otherwise markers are SNPs)

2 Important Concepts and Distinctions

2.1 Genetics, Genomics, Discovery, and Function

There are at least two important distinctions to keep in mind when evaluating genetics studies. These distinctions are between genetics and genomics, and between gene discovery and gene effect characterization. Genetics research involves hereditary factors and builds off concepts such as Mendel's laws, polymorphism, recombination, Hardy-Weinberg and linkage equilibrium, and related phenomena associated with the transmission of DNA from parents to offspring and from generation to generation. Genomics research involves the study of genomes and focuses on the content, organization, and role of genomes in mediating molecular physiologic phenomena. Although very interrelated, genetics and genomics are therefore not synonymous. Thus, pharmacogenetics research investigates inherited DNA sequence-based factors mediating response to drugs, whereas pharmacogenomics research considers how genomic phenomena such as the organization of genes, transcriptional machinery, and the structure of encoded proteins, etc., influence drug response.

Table 9.3 Recent DNA pooling-based genome-wide association (GWA) studies investigating the genetic determinants of disease

Ref	Disease	Population	# Markers	Cases	Controls	# Sig. Markers	Criteria
(90)	Addiction	Euro/Afro-American	639,401	420	320	6,666	0.05
(91)	Alzheimer's	UK & US	17,343	1,808	2,062	Meta-Analysis	
(92)	Bipolar Disorder	European	550,000	461	563	37	0.05
(93)	Diabetic Nephropathy	Irish	6000*	200	200	2	3×10^{-6}
(94)	End-Stage Renal	NR	115,352	105	102	3	NR
(95)	Human Narcolepsy	Japanese	23,244*	95	95	2,686	NR
(96)	Hypertension	Japanese	18,977*	385	385	95	0.05
(97)	Knee Osteoarthristis	UK	25,494	335	335	11	0.0001
(98)	Lung Ca	Italian	100,000	50	50	38	0.05
(99)	MS	North Portugal	3,974*	200	200	46	0.05
(100)	MS	Portuguese	4,661*	188	188	78	0.01
(101)	MS	Polish	4,219*	200	200	287	0.05
(102)	MS	Italian	4,192*	224	231	142	0.01
(103)	MS	N. Irish	2,537*	200	200	70	0.01
(104)	MS	Icelandic	4,804*	200	200	169	0.05
(105)	MS	Hungarian	5,532*	88	128	150	0.05
(106)	MS	Finnish	108	195	205	108	0.05
(107)	MS	Belgian	4,875*	204	198	217	0.025
(108)	Nicotine Dependence	Raleigh-Durham	520,000	134	320	88,937	0.005
(109)	Nicotine Dependence	US & Australian	2,427,354	482	466	35	0.0001
(110)	Rheumatoid Arthritis	Japanese	27,039*	940	940	2847	0.05

Key: NR = not reported; *note that microsatellite markers were used for this study (otherwise SNPs were used); MS = multiple sclerosis.

2.2 *Genetics vs. Genomics*

The distinction between gene discovery and gene effect characterization, although a bit more obvious than the distinction between genetics and genomics, is equally important and enlightening. Gene discovery strategies seek to identify genes and genetic variants that influence a particular phenotype in the absence of a priori knowledge about such genes. Meiotic or linkage mapping and linkage disequilibrium or association mapping are two gene discovery strategies that exploit genetics principles (1–3). Gene expression analysis and homology/synteny mapping with model organisms are more genomics-oriented gene discovery strategies, as they go beyond the mere use of the principles of heredity to discover genes and rather rely on the molecular, physiologic, and evolutionary phenomena shaping genomes to assist in gene discovery.

2.3 Gene Discovery vs. Gene Effect Characterization

Gene effect characterization strategies are those that consider what genes and genetic variations actually do in a molecular, physiologic, or general biological sense once they have been "discovered." There are many ways to characterize the effect of a gene or genetic variation, however. One can characterize its physiologic significance by asking, e.g., what tissues the gene is expressed in and/or what biochemical pathway or genetic network the genetic variation may disrupt. One could also assess the significance of a gene or variation in the population at large by asking questions such as, "What fraction of a disease would be eliminated if deleterious variations were removed?" or, "Do variations in a gene, deleterious or not, differ in frequency across different populations?" Finally, one could consider the clinical significance of a gene by considering the utility of phenotype-altering variations in those genes as diagnostic or prognostic markers. This chapter focuses on discovering genetic variations that influence phenotypes, such as drug response, via genetics approaches, as well as the clinical "effect" or significance of genetic variations that might influence disease and treatment-related outcomes.

3 Genetic Strategies for Discovering Genes

3.1 Genetic Mapping

Genetic approaches to gene discovery involve identifying genomic loci that harbor DNA sequence variations that appear to cosegregate (i.e., are inherited together with) a particular phenotype, most often a disease. The offending variations do not necessarily have to be causally associated with a disease, but rather simply reside on the same chromosome or chromosomal segment with variations that causally influence the phenotype. The reason that one can expect variations at noncausal loci to cosegregate with variations that are, in fact, causal has to do with the fact that genetic variations at adjacent genomic loci are not inherited independently; rather, individuals inherit chromosomal segments that harbor variations, and the size of those chromosomal segments is dictated by where recombination events (and other more rare phenomena such as mutations and gene conversion events) occur in relevant meioses leading up to the formation of the gametes (i.e., egg and sperm) which are combined during fertilization and the formation of zygotes. Thus, individuals inherit a "patchwork" of chromosomal segments from maternal and paternal chromosomes.

Note that due to meiotic/recombination events occurring over the course of many generations, the size of any one "ancestral" chromosomal segment harboring a variant that causes a phenotype (i.e., a segment of an individual's chromosome harboring the first appearance of a mutation that causes a phenotype) will be reduced in size over those generations. Figure 9.1 depicts this phenomenon and provides the essential framework for genetic mapping. Essentially, the founder chromosome in Figure 9.1 harbored the variations 123-T-C-DEL-T-A-INS-132-G-G at 10 adjacent loci, with the "A" allele or hypothetical variant at the 6th locus being a variant that is the first appearance of a phenotype-causing variant. As time passes and generations elapse, that part of the chromosome harboring the phenotype-causing variant that contains variations flanking that phenotype-causing variant that were on the original chromosome harboring it is reduced in size due to recombination events. However, genetic descendents of the founder individual have some probability of being transmitted genetic material from this founder, and hence could have inherited the phenotype-causing variant and some of the chromosomal material harboring variations at loci flanking this phenotype-causing variant. Thus, in Figure 9.1, the five descendents of the founder have all inherited the phenotype-causing variant as well as additional flanking variants, such that each has inherited the haplotype DEL-T-A-INS-132. In this manner, if individuals possessing the phenotype of interest were genotyped at any of these five loci, they would be observed to possess the same alleles or variants, suggesting that the phenotype-causing variant was observed to be either carried by them after genotyping a relevant locus (in the case of the "A" variant) or on the same chromosome with the phenotype-causing variant and hence near the locus that they were genotyped on (in the case of the "DEL," "T," "INS," and/or "132" variants).

3.2 Linkage Disequilibrium

Variations at neighboring loci that appear to cosegregate together from generation to generation are said to be in "linkage disequilibrium" (LD) with each other (if the probability of observing one variant is independent of the probability of observing another, then the variations are in "linkage equilibrium"). There are many factors that influence LD strength, including the number of generations that have elapsed since the alleles or variants were introduced into the population (a surrogate for the number of meiotic or recombination events that have taken place since the introduction of the variation into the population), mutation rates (since any variation may mutate to another variation and hence disrupt the cosegregation of the original founder chromosome variations), recombination rates (which are known to differ throughout different chromosomes), and mating patterns in the population (e.g., individuals producing more offspring are more likely to have the variations they posses—in whatever combinations—appear more frequently in ensuing generations and hence the population at large).

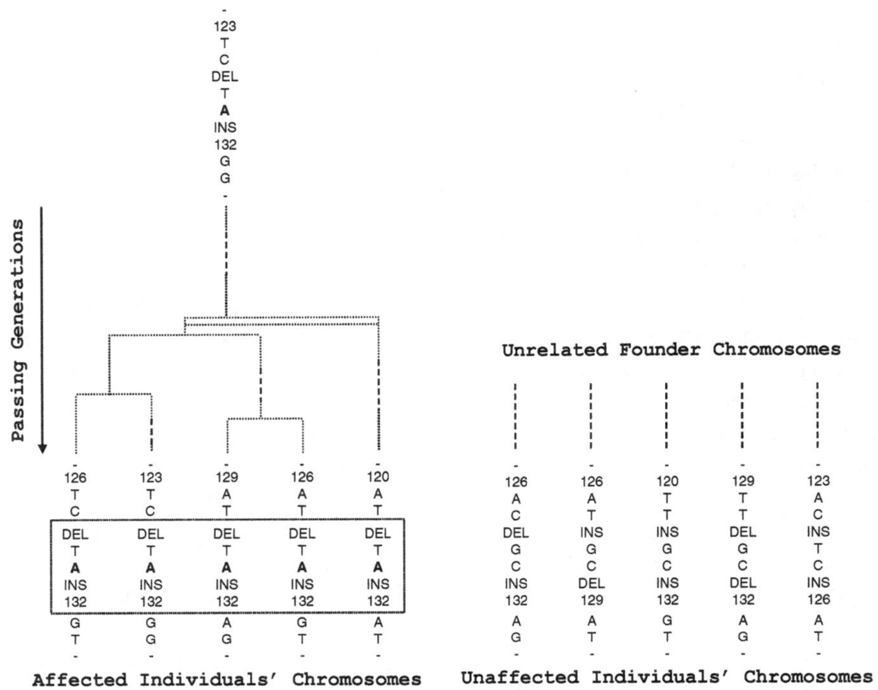

Fig. 9.1 Diagrammatic representation of the transmission of chromosomal segments from generation to generation. Rectangular lists of letters/numbers represent individual chromosomes and each set of letters/numbers corresponding to alleles at adjacent loci whose positions relative to one another correspond to their row positions. Numbers represent repeat lengths at microsatellie loci, DEL/INS represents deletion or insertion variations, A, C, T, and G represent different nucleotides at single nucleotide polymorphic (SNP) loci. The individual chromosome on the upper left represents a chromosome from an original ("founder") individual who carried the highlighted "A" allele at the 6th locus, which causes a disease. Descendents of this individual who are transmitted this allele, and hence are susceptible to disease, are also likely to carry neighboring alleles from the founder chromosome as well. Due to recombination events occurring in relevant meiosis within the passing generations, individuals harboring the mutation may only share a small segment of the original ancestral chromosomal material from the founder, especially if the genealogical links separating these individuals from the founder and amongst themselves are complex (denoted by the shaded lines). However, some alleles at neighboring loci surrounding the position of the susceptibility allele may be preserved from the founder chromosome, as denoted by the box surrounding the hypothetical alleles possessed by five individuals carrying the susceptibility "A" allele in the latest generation. Individuals without the susceptibility will not show this same pattern (as denoted by the five individual chromosomes on the left). Thus, linkage disequilibrium between the "A" allele and the DEL, T, INS, and 132 alleles at the loci surrounding its position would mark haplotypes defined by this pattern alleles as those also carrying the susceptibility allele

The exploitation of LD for genetic mapping is thus straightforward in theory, but complicated in practice. For example, one could, e.g., genotype individuals with and without a certain phenotype at loci dispersed throughout the genome and see which variations individuals with the phenotype have in greater frequency than those without the phenotype of interest. The loci that have alleles that are more frequent among individuals with the phenotype are the most likely phenotypically-relevant loci. However, in testing large numbers of loci for association one must account for multiple comparisons or multiple testing to avoid false positive associations. Although there has been a great deal of debate about the appropriate threshold for declaring significance, there is no real consensus (see, e.g., *[4, 5]*). This is evidenced by the fact that researchers pursuing GWA studies have exploited different statistical criteria in studies to identify loci that are potentially associated with a phenotype or that will at least be further assessed (see Tables 9.1–9.4). In addition, the number of loci likely to be contributing to a particular phenotype might be quite large, such that the contribution of any one of these loci might be quite small, making it difficult to achieve the appropriate power to detect their effects without very large sample sizes (*[6, 7]*; Tables 9.1–9.3). Finally, if one wants to pursue a comprehensive GWA association study, one may have to genotype individuals on as many as 500,000 to 1,000,000 loci (Tables 9.1–9.3). Efficient and cost-effective genotyping technologies are therefore required, as is an appropriate choice of loci to genotype, as there may be some 10,000,000 total polymorphic sites in the human genome. The recent results by the International HapMap Project consortium provide insight into the appropriate loci to consider based on LD patterns in the genome *(8, 9)*.

Since recombination is fundamental to genetic mapping strategies for gene discovery, researchers have considered different study designs for genetic mapping. Traditional linkage analysis approaches involve consideration and identification of the chromosomal segments that are shared among individuals with a phenotype among families of 2–4 generations *(1)*. Since only 2–4 generations' worth of recombination is not likely to reduce the size of original parental generation

Table 9.4 Recent (2006+) candidate gene association studies involving pharmacologically-related outcomes

Gene	SNPs or RS#	Drug	Effect size	p-value	N	Reference
MMP1	rs5854,	Aseptic failure	3.27, 1.76	0.001	312	*(111)*
VDR	rs10735810	"		0.007		
COMT	NR	Neuroleptic	NR		411	*(112)*
CDA	Ala70Thr	Gemcitabine	12–25%	<.0001	256	*(113)*
RRFC-1	His27Arg	Methotrexate	OR = 3.32	0.021	174	*(114)*
APOE	E2/3/4	Warfarin dose	11 mg	0.014	111	*(115)*
HTR2C	−759 C/T	Antipsychotics	>5%	0.03	84	*(116)*
NTRK2	RS10780691	Alcohol	NR	0.0059	516	*(117)*
LEPR	Q223R	Olanzapine rx	2.55 kg/m2	0.049	37	*(118)*
LEP	2548G/A	"		NR		
SLCO1B1	T521C	Simvastatin	221%	<.001	32	*(119)*
CB2	Q63R	Alcohol	OR = 1.25	0.007	NR	*(120)*

Key: NR = not reported, RA = rheumatoid arthritis, NRT = nicotine replacement therapy

chromosomes to a high degree, the segment sizes typically identified in linkage studies are quite large (e.g., 20–30 "megabases" or millions of base pairs), making it difficult to know the precise location of offending phenotypically-relevant variations *(1, 10)*. Classical linkage disequilibrium studies usually consider the segments shared among individuals separated by many *(5–12)* generations *(10)* for which genealogical information might be known *(10–12)*. The size of the shared segments among individuals with a particular phenotype might extend between 500 kilobases and 2 megabases). Modern genetic association analyses typically forego insight into the exact relationships between individuals and instead interrogate enough markers to identify shared segments of haplotype-induced associations that encompass only 1–100 kilobases making it easier but not necessarily trivial to identify offending phenotypically-relevant variations (*[6]*; Table 9.1). Some researchers have adopted hybrid approaches in which general associations are sought among individuals within and across different families (Table 9.2).

3.3 Admixture Mapping

There are a number of variations of the genetic mapping paradigm. Admixture mapping involves the study of individuals known to be descendents of (reasonably) close ancestors that emanate from two genetically distinct populations that differ in the frequency of a phenotype or disease. The intuition behind admixture mapping is similar in spirit to the intuition behind studies involving crosses between two inbred strains, in that the chromosomal segments that an admixed individual has will be easier to identify, as they will most likely be marked by their derivation from one of the two populations based on observed patterns of genetic variation in those populations *(13)*. In this manner individuals that possess the phenotype known to be of greater frequency in one of the two parental populations will share chromosomal segments marked by variations that are also known to be of greater frequency in that parental population (see *(14)* for an example).

As a possible prelude to potential admixture mapping studies, many investigators have tested associations between broad (even self-reported) racial category, individual ancestry, and degree of admixture and phenotypes of interest *(15–17)*. If an association is found, then one can infer the existence of genetic variations with reasonable frequency within one of the ancestral populations or racial groups. Although of great interest, such studies have proven controversial with respect to drug response, as is evidenced by the case of the drug BiDil *(18–20)*.

3.4 DNA Pooling

One very cost-effective way of pursuing association studies, whether genome-wide or candidate gene-based, is to take advantage of DNA pooling. DNA pooling involves literally taking the DNA (importantly, in equal aliquots) from each subject and combining it to form a "pool" of DNA. Allele frequencies at each locus are then estimated by assessing the amplification of each allele in the pool. By forming a case pool and a control pool, one can contrast allele frequencies to identify associations. Thus, one can do with two genotyping assays what would have normally been done with assays equal to the number of subjects in the study. There are many technical problems that plague DNA pooling-based association studies *(21)*. Despite this, there have been a number of such studies, as evidenced by Table 9.3.

4 Drug Response Phenotypes, Replication, and Functional Effect Characterization

4.1 Phenotypes and Study Design

Applications of genetic association mapping-based approaches to gene discovery have largely focused on disease phenotypes. For example, although there have been a number of candidate gene association studies investigating the relationship of particular genetic variations to a wide variety of drug response phenotypes (see, e.g., the references in *(22)* and *(23)* as well as Table 9.4 for more recent studies with very recent interest focusing on drugs used to treat neuropsychiatric conditions; *[24, 25]*), there have been no large-scale GWA studies of a drug response phenotype. There are many reasons for this, not the least of which is the availability of large enough samples, as well as the availability of replication samples. It is accepted that in order to make compelling claims about an association, not only is an appropriately powered initial study necessary, but so also are samples to replicate the findings *(26)*. In fact, one very popular design that has been used with great success in genetic mapping studies, especially GWA studies, is a multistage design, whereby loci exhibiting associations with a phenotype at prespecified strengths in an initial analysis stage are tested in subsequent stages with different samples *(27)*.

4.2 Functional Characterization

In the event that an association is found and is replicated, questions as to the biological significance of the association will inevitably arise. The functional consequences of DNA sequence variations are not always obvious and may require a great deal of laboratory and model organism work to assess. In addition, what is of great interest in the context of recently published GWA studies investigating genetic determinants of disease phenotypes is that the variations that have emerged as strongly associated with many diseases have no obvious function and in many instances do not reside within or near known genes *(28)*. The recently published initial findings of the ENCODE project *(29)*—a project whose goal is to identify and characterize the biologically active or functional components of the human genome—are consistent with this, in the sense that the ENCODE researchers found that many of the functional elements within the human genome could not have been anticipated with conventional assays or beliefs about what DNA sequence patterns (e.g., evolutionary conservation levels) were indicative of functionality.

Although assessing the biological function of particular genetic variations is essential for some research activities—such as designing appropriate therapeutics that would counteract the deleterious effects of that variation—such an assessment may not be necessary (at least not initially) in other contexts. For example, if a genetic variation of unknown function discriminates between responders and nonresponders to a particular compound, then one could use knowledge of that variation to simply decide on who should or should not get treated with that particular compound. Thus, the clinical diagnostic and/or pharmacogenetic utility of genetic associations have an immediacy that a clinical drug development utility may not.

4.3 Drug Target Polymorphism Screening

One important question in the study of genetic variations that influence individual responses to therapeutics is just when such a study should take place. Genetic association studies are pursued when one is interested in a particular phenotype and has observed variation in that phenotype. In the context of therapeutics, one might observe that some individuals respond better or worse to a particular compound and hence might want to identify genetic variations that explain this phenomenon via association studies, as discussed. However, drug targets are often specific genes or proteins (e.g., receptors), such that knowledge of how much variation these genes and proteins exhibit in the population could be incorporated into the very early stages of the drug development cycle. Thus, before proceeding to large-scale clinical trials of a compound only to learn that it may be important to consider the role of genetic variations in the target in mediating the response to that compound, it may make sense to assess (at least) how polymorphic the target is and to assess the potential influence of identified variations on the compound's activities. This concept is certainly true in the early stage analysis of the pharmacokinetic properties of a particular compound, as it is known that variations in relevant drug metabolizing enzymes could help guide dosing studies. As a case in point, the target of the drug clopidogrel, which is the receptor gene P2Y12, was found to have naturally occurring variations within it that influence clopidogrel's activity on the basis of association studies involving participants in a large clinical trial *(30)*. However, when the P2Y12 receptor was chosen as a target, it may have made sense to assess evidence for sequence polymorphism within it that could influence the drug's activity, so that researchers could either design the drug around those variations or anticipate limiting the drug's testing (see Section 5 below) and general use to individuals with the appropriate genomic profile.

5 Clinical Effect Characterization and Genotype-Informed Clinical Trials

5.1 Targeted Clinical Trials

It is now widely recognized that if compounds or therapeutics work on only a subset of all individuals, then clearly the identification of those individuals is important. However, equally important (if not more so) is proving that the compound or therapeutic is clearly better for that subset of individuals than other compounds or therapeutics. Proving the efficacy of a compound involves designing and implementing appropriate clinical trials, and proving the efficacy of a compound for a subset of all possible individuals involves designing and implementing targeted or restricted clinical trials. Such trials are receiving a great deal of attention in the wake of the identification of targeted therapeutics for cancer, such as Herceptin *(31)*, and can be conceived of in at least two different ways.

The first strategy or motivation for targeted clinical trials involves simply limiting the conduct of the trial to individuals with a certain characteristic (e.g., individuals possessing a tumor with HER-2 positivity in order to receive Herceptin therapy). Individuals with this characteristic would be randomized to a control or test compound, and the efficacy of the compound evaluated. This strategy could potentially enrich the sample used in the clinical trial for individuals likely to benefit from the drug, thereby increasing the power of the study, and lower the required sample size *(32–33)*. The second strategy involves testing for pharmacogenetic effects associated with the compound by contrasting the utility of the compound among individuals with and without a given characteristic. Thus, for an example involving Herceptin, individuals with HER-2 positive tumors would be randomized to a control and Herceptin group, and a third group of individuals that do not have HER-2 positive tumors would be treated with Herceptin. In this way, one could not only assess the benefit of the treatment among individuals with HER-2 positive tumors, but also determine if Herceptin is more efficacious among individuals with HER-2 positive tumors than those without HER-2 positive tumors.

In the context of GWA and candidate gene association study results involving disease phenotypes, it might make sense to consider clinical trials that target individuals carrying variations associated with particular disease endpoints. If the associations suggest that individuals carrying certain variations are more susceptible to a particular disease or disease-related outcome, then restricting the trial to individuals possessing those variations would enrich the sample for individuals likely to benefit from a relevant preventive strategy or compound. Testing for the pharmacogenetic effect of the genetic variations is more complicated, since the design of a relevant trial would require individuals both with and without the genetic variations, but this has been discussed in the literature *(34–36)*.

5.2 A Hypothetical Example of a Genotype-Restricted or Targeted Clinical Trial

Lipitor is a lipid-lowering drug that is known to prevent heart attacks *(37–39)*. It has been shown through extremely large clinical trials that individuals not taking Lipitor have heart attacks at a rate of 3%, whereas individuals taking Lipitor have heart attacks at a rate of 2% (see, e.g., [37–39]). To detect this (one-sided) difference in a clinical trial examining Lipitor efficacy with 80% power and a type I error rate of 5% using a standard z-test to assess the difference between two independent rates or proportions measuring the heart attack rate over a defined period of time, one would need to randomize 3013 subjects to Lipitor and 3013 subjects to a placebo, for a total sample size of 6026 subjects. A two-sided test would require a total of 3826 individuals taking and not taking Lipitor, for a total sample size of 7652 subjects.

In two recently published GWA studies, it was found that individuals carrying two copies of a particular variant or allele near the CDKN2A/B locus are expected to have 1.64 times the rate of heart attacks compared to noncarriers of this variant *(40–41)*. This suggests that, in contrast to the general population not taking Lipitor, individuals with two copies of the CDKN2A/B variant will have a $0.03 \times 1.64 = 0.049$ rate of heart attacks relative to noncarriers of this variant. If Lipitor actually reduces the rate of heart attack by 0.33 as suggested, then individuals on Lipitor who carry two copies of the CDKN2A/B susceptibility allele will have a rate of heart attacks of $0.66 \times 0.049 = 0.033$. In order to detect the difference between the heart attack rate of 0.049 among carriers of two copies of the CDKN2A/B alleles versus a 0.033 rate among noncarriers in a clinical trial examining Lipitor efficacy with 80% power and a type I error rate of 5%, one would need to randomize 1899 subjects to Lipitor and 1899 subjects to placebo, for a total of 3798 subjects. A two-sided test would require $2410 \times 2 = 4820$ total subjects. Thus, one would require a trial with only 3798/6026 or nearly 40% of the total number of subjects needed for a nontargeted trial. The savings would be much greater if a trial assessing Lipitor efficacy on early onset heart attacks was restricted to individuals carrying two copies of the CDKN2A/B susceptibility allele, as it has been shown that such individuals have ~2.02 times the rate of early-onset heart attacks as noncarriers (*[40–41]*; only 1468 subjects assigned to Lipitor and 1468 subjects assigned to a placebo, for a total of 2936 subjects would be needed; a two-sided test would require 3726 total subjects).

Genotype-targeted clinical trials have the obvious need of identifying individuals possesing the relevant characteristics. Thus, in the context of the Lipitor example, there would arise the issue of the cost of screening and genotyping people in order to identify those individuals who carry two copies of the susceptibility allele. If the homozygous genotype for the CDK2NA/B susceptibility allele occurs in 0.21 (21%) of the population at large as reported *(69)*, then one would have to sample and genotype, based on the negative binomial distribution, 7143 (+/–184) individuals, on average, in order to identify 1899 individuals who carry two copies of the susceptibility allele.

5.3 The Sensitivity and Specificity of Genotype Screening Tests

The utility of genotype-based screening for the design of clinical trials depends on how much additional information (concerning, e.g., susceptibility to an outcome or response to a particular compound) can be obtained via the use of genotypic information over and above information gleaned from nongenetic risk factors and indicators, such as family history or blood-based tests. Thus, if the specificity and sensitivity of genotype-based diagnostics and screening tools is poor, their clinical utility is in doubt. However, it is quite likely that responses to particular compounds, as well as susceptibilities to the diseases and outcomes these compounds are meant to combat, are mediated by many genes *(42)*. Thus, multilocus and/or multiparameter diagnostics and screening tools will likely be a reality in clinical settings and will have the ability to achieve the appropriate and necessary sensitivity and specificity *(43)*.

6 Discussion

The human genome project and related DNA sequencing and genotyping initiatives have created an enormous set of expectations about what one can expect in the future. There is no doubt that first and foremost on the minds of the biomedical researchers is the potential that genetics and genomics research has to reshape the way in which clinical and public health practices are pursued *(44–46)*. However, the enthusiasm over genetics and genomics research needs to be tempered by many technological, biological, and practical scientific realities. For example, although candidate gene and GWA association studies have indeed produced compelling insights into the genetic basis of many common chronic diseases, the clinical utility of these insights is in doubt, as the variations identified through these studies individually explain only a small fraction of disease risk. In addition, the application of genetic association study strategies to pharmacogenetics settings is problematic, in that these strategies require appropriate replication and functional characterization standards in order to be accepted by the scientific community. Despite this, genetic association studies hold great promise for pharmacogenetics research, if for no other reason than the fact that DNA sequence variants associated with particular diseases can be used to screen and select subjects for pharmacogenetic clinical trials.

In this light, there are a number of very positive directions adopted by the pharmacogenetics research community and a few directions that could be emphasized more. For example the development of databases, such as the Pharmacogenetics Knowledge Base *(47)*; PharmGKB, http://www.pharmgkb.org/), which contain information on genetic associations involving drug responses, and the establishment of consortia dealing with the identification of individuals exhibiting adverse responses to treatments *(48)* will clearly help congeal and spark further genetics research. However, more clinical researchers should consider the influence of individual ancestry and genetic background on treatment efficacy as a prelude to the identification of specific DNA sequence variations that might influence treatment response. In addition, it would make sense for drug developers to assess and consider variations in specific drug targets at the time the drugs are being developed and not after the drug is released or tested in a large trial.

Probably one of the biggest factors, if not the biggest, that would help propel forward genetic studies involving responses to particular treatments would be the recognition by pharmaceutical companies that genetically-mediated responses to therapeutics of all sorts, as well as the scientific motivation for personalized medicine initiatives as a whole, truly represent ubiquitous, nonignorable biological realities, and not simply complementary approaches or potential alternatives to the traditional frameworks within which drugs and preventive strategies are developed.

Acknowledgements Aspects of the research represented in this chapter were supported in part by grants from the following institutions: The National Heart Lung and Blood Institute Family Blood Pressure Program [FBPP; U01 HL064777–06]; The National Institute on Aging Longevity Consortium [U19 AG023122–01]; the National Institute of Mental Health Consortium on the Genetics of Schizophrenia [COGS; 5 R01 HLMH065571–02]; the National Institutes of Health [R01s: HL074730–02 and HL070137–01]; and Scripps Genomic Medicine. The authors would like to thank Dr. Jennifer Wessel for help in assembling some of the material for this chapter.

References

1. Ott J (1999) Analysis of human genetic linkage. Johns Hopkins University Press, Baltimore.
2. Thomas DC (2004) Statistical methods in genetic epidemiology. Oxford University Press, Oxford.
3. Khoury MJ, Beaty TH, Cohen BH (1993) Fundamentals of genetic epidemiology. Oxford University Press, Oxford.
4. Storey JD, Tibshirani R (2003) Statistical significance for genomewide studies. Proc Natl Acad Sci U S A 100(16):9440–9445.
5. Dudbridge F, Gusnanto A, Koeleman BP (2006) Detecting multiple associations in genome-wide studies. Hum Genomics 2(5):310–317.
6. Lawrence RW, Evans DM, Cardon LR (2005) Prospects and pitfalls in whole genome association studies. Philos Trans R Soc Lond B Biol Sci 360(1460):1589–1595.
7. Carlson CS, Eberle MA, Kruglyak L, Nickerson DA (2004) Mapping complex disease loci in whole-genome association studies. Nature 429(6990):446–452.
8. International HapMap Consortium (2005) A haplotype map of the human genome. Nature 437(7063):1299–1320.
9. Xu Z, Kaplan NL, Taylor JA (2007) Tag SNP selection for candidate gene association studies using HapMap and gene resequencing data. Eur J Hum Genet [Epub ahead of print].
10. Houwen RH, Baharloo S, Blankenship K, Raeymaekers P, Juyn J, Sandkuijl LA, Freimer NB (1994) Genome screening by searching for shared segments: mapping a gene for benign recurrent intrahepatic cholestasis. Nat Genet 8(4):380–386.
11. Jorde LB (1995) Linkage disequilibrium as a gene-mapping tool. Am J Hum Genet 56(1):11–14.
12. de la Chapelle A, Wright FA (1998) Linkage disequilibrium mapping in isolated populations: the example of Finland revisited. Proc Natl Acad Sci U S A 95(21):12416–12423.
13. Nievergelt CM, Schork NJ (2005) Admixture mapping as a gene discovery approach for complex human traits and diseases. Curr Hypertens Rep 7(1):31–37.

14. Freedman ML, Haiman CA, Patterson N, McDonald GJ, Tandon A, Waliszewska A, Penney K, Steen RG, Ardlie K, John EM, Oakley- Girvan I, Whittemore AS, Cooney KA, Ingles SA, Altshuler D, Henderson BE, Reich D (2006) Admixture mapping identifies 8q24 as a prostate cancer risk locus in African-American men. Proc Natl Acad Sci U S A 103(38):14068–14073.
15. Shaffer JR, Kammerer CM, Reich D, McDonald G, Patterson N, Goodpaster B, Bauer DC, Li J, Newman AB, Cauley JA, Harris TB, Tylavsky F, Ferrell RE, Zmuda JM (2007) Genetic markers for ancestry are correlated with body composition traits in older African Americans. Osteoporos Int 18(6):733–741.
16. Salari K, Choudhry S, Tang H, Naqvi M, Lind D, Avila PC, Coyle NE, Ung N, Nazario S, Casal J, Torres- Palacios A, Clark S, Phong A, Gomez I, Matallana H, Perez- Stable EJ, Shriver MD, Kwok PY, Sheppard D, Rodriguez- Cintron W, Risch NJ, Burchard EG, Ziv E (2005) Genetic admixture and asthma-related phenotypes in Mexican American and Puerto Rican asthmatics. Genet Epidemiol 29(1):76–86.
17. Bonilla C, Shriver MD, Parra EJ, Jones A, Fernandez JR (2004) Ancestral proportions and their association with skin pigmentation and bone mineral density in Puerto Rican women from New York City. Hum Genet 115(1):57–68.
18. Taylor AL, Cohn JN, Worcel M, Franciosa JA (2002) A-HeFT Investigators. African-American Heart Failure Trial. The African-American Heart Failure Trial: background, rationale and significance. J Natl Med Assoc 94(9):762–769.
19. Flack JM (2007) Editorial commentary on fixed combination isosorbide dinitrate/hydralazine for nitric-oxide-enhancing therapy in heart failure. Expert Opin Pharmacother 8(3):275–277.
20. Hoover EL (2007) There is no scientific rationale for race-based research. J Natl Med Assoc 99(6):690–692.
21. Sham P, Bader JS, Craig I, O'Donovan M, Owen M (2002) DNA pooling: a tool for large-scale association studies. Nat Rev Genet 3(11):862–871.
22. Evans WE, McLeod HL (2003) Pharmacogenomics—drug disposition, drug targets, and side effects. N Engl J Med 348(6):538–549.
23. Thomas FJ, McLeod HL, Watters JW (2004) Pharmacogenomics: the influence of genomic variation on drug response. Curr Top Med Chem 4(13):1399–1409.
24. McMahon FJ, Buervenich S, Charney D, Lipsky R, Rush AJ, Wilson AF, Sorant AJ, Papanicolaou GJ, Laje G, Fava M, Trivedi MH, Wisniewski SR, Manji H (2006) Variation in the gene encoding the serotonin 2A receptor is associated with outcome of antidepressant treatment. Am J Hum Genet 78(5):804–814.
25. Perlis RH, Purcell S, Fava M, Fagerness J, Rush AJ, Trivedi MH, Smoller JW (2007) Association between treatment-emergent suicidal ideation with citalopram and polymorphisms near cyclic adenosine monophosphate response element binding protein in the STAR*D study. Arch Gen Psychiatry 64(6):689–697.
26. NCI-NHGRI Working Group on Replication in Association Studies, Chanock SJ, Manolio T, Boehnke M, Boerwinkle E, Hunter DJ, Thomas G, Hirschhorn JN, Abecasis G, Altshuler D, Bailey- Wilson JE, Brooks LD, Cardon LR, Daly M, Donnelly P, Fraumeni JF Jr, Freimer NB, Gerhard DS, Gunter C, Guttmacher AE, Guyer MS, Harris EL, Hoh J, Hoover R, Kong CA, Merikangas KR, Morton CC, Palmer LJ, Phimister EG, Rice JP, Roberts J, Rotimi C, Tucker MA, Vogan KJ, Wacholder S, Wijsman EM, Winn DM, Collins FS (2007) Replicating genotype-phenotype associations. Nature 447(7145):655–660.
27. Elston RC, Lin DY, Zheng G (2007) Multistage sampling for genetic studies Annu Rev Genomics Hum Genet [Epub ahead of print].
28. Topol EJ, Murray SS, Frazer KA (2007) The genomics gold rush. JAMA 298(2):218–221.
29. ENCODE Project Consortium (2007) Identification and analysis of functional elements in 1% of the human genome by the ENCODE pilot project. Nature 447(7146):799–816.
30. Ziegler S, Schillinger M, Funk M, Felber K, Exner M, Mlekusch W, Sabeti S, Amighi J, Minar E, Brunner M, Muller M, Mannhalter C (2005) Association of a functional polymorphism in the clopidogrel target receptor gene, P2Y12, and the risk for ischemic cerebrovascular events in patients with peripheral artery disease. Stroke 36(7):1394–1399.

31. Emens LA (2005) Trastuzumab: targeted therapy for the management of HER-2/neu-overexpressing metastatic breast cancer. Am J Ther 12(3):243–253.
32. Simon R, Maitournam A (2004) Evaluating the efficiency of targeted designs for randomized clinical trials. Clin Cancer Res 10(20):6759–6763. Erratum in: Clin Cancer Res 2006 May 15;12(10):3229.
33. Maitournam A, Simon R (2005) On the efficiency of targeted clinical trials. Stat Med 24(3):329–339.
34. Elston RC, Idury RM, Cardon LR, Lichter JB (1999) The study of candidate genes in drug trials: sample size considerations. Stat Med 18(6):741–751.
35. Cardon LR, Idury RM, Harris TJ, Witte JS, Elston RC (2000) Testing drug response in the presence of genetic information: sampling issues for clinical trials. Pharmacogenetics 10(6):503–510.
36. Trepicchio WL, Essayan D, Hall ST, Schechter G, Tezak Z, Wang SJ, Weinreich D, Simon R (2006) Designing prospective clinical pharmacogenomic (PG) trials: meeting report on drug development strategies to enhance therapeutic decision making. Pharmacogenomics J 6(2):89–94.
37. Baigent C, Keech A, Kearney PM, Blackwell L, Buck G, Pollicino C, Kirby A, Sourjina T, Peto R, Collins R, Simes R (2005) Cholesterol Treatment Trialists' (CTT) Collaborators. Efficacy and safety of cholesterol-lowering treatment: prospective meta-analysis of data from 90,056 participants in 14 randomised trials of statins. Lancet 366(9493):1267–1278. Erratum in: Lancet 2005 Oct 15–21;366(9494):1358.
38. Law MR, Wald NJ, Rudnicka AR (2003) Quantifying effect of statins on low density lipoprotein cholesterol, ischaemic heart disease, and stroke: systematic review and meta-analysis. BMJ 326(7404):1423.
38. Mukherjee D, Topol EJ (2003) Pharmacogenomics in cardiovascular diseases Curr Probl Cardiol 28(5):317–347.
40. McPherson R, Pertsemlidis A, Kavaslar N, Stewart A, Roberts R, Cox DR, Hinds DA, Pennacchio LA, Tybjaerg- Hansen A, Folsom AR, Boerwinkle E, Hobbs HH, Cohen JC (2007) A common allele on chromosome 9 associated with coronary heart disease. Science 316(5830):1488–1491.
41. Helgadottir A, Thorleifsson G, Manolescu A, Gretarsdottir S, Blondal T, Jonasdottir A, Jonasdottir A, Sigurdsson A, Baker A, Palsson A, Masson G, Gudbjartsson DF, Magnusson KP, Andersen K, Levey AI, Backman VM, Matthiasdottir S, Jonsdottir T, Palsson S, Einarsdottir H, Gunnarsdottir S, Gylfason A, Vaccarino V, Hooper WC, Reilly MP, Granger CB, Austin H, Rader DJ, Shah SH, Quyyumi AA, Gulcher JR, Thorgeirsson G, Thorsteinsdottir U, Kong A, Stefansson K (2007) A common variant on chromosome 9p21 affects the risk of myocardial infarction. Science 316(5830):1491–1493.
42. Yang Q, Khoury MJ, Friedman J, Little J, Flanders WD (2005) How many genes underlie the occurrence of common complex diseases in the population? Int J Epidemiol 34(5):1129–1137.
43. Yang Q, Khoury MJ, Botto L, Friedman JM, Flanders WD (2003) Improving the prediction of complex diseases by testing for multiple disease-susceptibility genes. Am J Hum Genet 72(3):636–649. Erratum in: Am J Hum Genet 2004 Feb;74(2):372.
44. Collins FS, McKusick VA (2001) Implications of the Human Genome Project for medical science. JAMA 285(5):540–544.
45. Collins FS, Green ED, Guttmacher AE, Guyer MS (2003) US National Human Genome Research Institute. A vision for the future of genomics research. Nature 422(6934):835–847.
46. Willard HF, Angrist M, Ginsburg GS (2005) Genomic medicine: genetic variation and its impact on the future of health care. Philos Trans R Soc Lond B Biol Sci 360(1460): 1543–1550.
47. Giacomini KM, Brett CM, Altman RB, Benowitz NL, Dolan ME, Flockhart DA, Johnson JA, Hayes DF, Klein T, Krauss RM, Kroetz DL, McLeod HL, Nguyen AT, Ratain MJ, Relling MV, Reus V, Roden DM, Schaefer CA, Shuldiner AR, Skaar T, Tantisira K, Tyndale RF, Wang L, Weinshilboum RM, Weiss ST, Zineh I (2007) Pharmacogenetics Research Network.

The pharmacogenetics research network: from SNP discovery to clinical drug response. Clin Pharmacol Ther 81(3):328–345.
48. Giacomini KM, Krauss RM, Roden DM, Eichelbaum M, Hayden MR, Nakamura Y (2007) When good drugs go bad. Nature 446(7139):975–977.
49. Coon KD et al (2007) A high-density whole-genome association study reveals that APOE is the major susceptibility gene for sporadic late-onset Alzheimer's disease. J Clin Psychiatry 68(4):613–618.
50. Moffatt MF, Kabesch M, Liang L, Dixon AL, Strachan D, Heath S, Depner M, von Berg A, Bufe A, Rietschel E, Heinzmann A, Simma B, Frischer T, Willis- Owen SA, Wong KC, Illig T, Vogelberg C, Weiland SK, von Mutius E, Abecasis GR, Farrall M, Gut IG, Lathrop GM, Cookson WO (2007) Genetic variants regulating ORMDL3 expression contribute to the risk of childhood asthma. Nature 448(7152):470–473.
51. Gudbjartsson DF et al (2007) Variants conferring risk of atrial fibrillation on chromosome 4q25. Nature 448(7151):353–357.
52. Wellcome Trust Case Control Consortium (2007) Genome-wide association study of 14,000 cases of seven common diseases and 3,000 shared controls. Nature 447(7145):661–678.
53. Hunter DJ et al (2007) A genome-wide association study identifies alleles in FGFR2 associated with risk of sporadic postmenopausal breast cancer. Nat Genet 39(7):870–874. Epub 2007 May 27.
54. Easton DF, Pooley KA, Dunning AM, Pharoah PD, Thompson D, Ballinger DG, Struewing JP, Morrison J, Field H, Luben R, Wareham N, Ahmed S, Healey CS, Bowman R; SEARCH collaborators, Meyer KB, Haiman CA, Kolonel LK, Henderson BE, Le Marchand L, Brennan P, Sangrajrang S, Gaborieau V, Odefrey F, Shen CY, Wu PE, Wang HC, Eccles D, Evans DG, Peto J, Fletcher O, Johnson N, Seal S, Stratton MR, Rahman N, Chenevix- Trench G, Bojesen SE, Nordestgaard BG, Axelsson CK, Garcia- Closas M, Brinton L, Chanock S, Lissowska J, Peplonska B, Nevanlinna H, Fagerholm R, Eerola H, Kang D, Yoo KY, Noh DY, Ahn SH, Hunter DJ, Hankinson SE, Cox DG, Hall P, Wedren S, Liu J, Low YL, Bogdanova N, Schurmann P, Dork T, Tollenaar RA, Jacobi CE, Devilee P, Klijn JG, Sigurdson AJ, Doody MM, Alexander BH, Zhang J, Cox A, Brock IW, Mac Pherson G, Reed MW, Couch FJ, Goode EL, Olson JE, Meijers- Heijboer H, van den Ouweland A, Uitterlinden A, Rivadeneira F, Milne RL, Ribas G, Gonzalez- Neira A, Benitez J, Hopper JL, McCredie M, Southey M, Giles GG, Schroen C, Justenhoven C, Brauch H, Hamann U, Ko YD, Spurdle AB, Beesley J, Chen X; kCon Fab; AOCS Management Group, Mannermaa A, Kosma VM, Kataja V, Hartikainen J, Day NE, Cox DR, Ponder BA (2007) Genome-wide association study identifies novel breast cancer susceptibility loci. Nature 447(7148):1087–1093.
55. Van Heel et al (2007) A genome-wide association study for celiac disease identifies risk variants in the region harboring IL2 and IL21. Nat Genet 39(7):827–829. Epub 2007 Jun 10.
56. Samani NJ et al (2007) Genomewide association analysis of coronary artery disease. N Engl J Med. 357(5):443–453. Epub 2007 Jul 18.
57. McPherson R, Pertsemlidis A, Kavaslar N, Stewart A, Roberts R, Cox DR, Hinds DA, Pennacchio LA, Tybjaerg- Hansen A, Folsom AR, Boerwinkle E, Hobbs HH, Cohen JC (2007) A common allele on chromosome 9 associated with coronary heart disease. Science 316(5830):1488–1491.
58. Zanke BW et al (2007) Genome-wide association scan identifies a colorectal cancer susceptibility locus on chromosome 8q24. Nat Genet 39(8):989–994. Epub 2007 Jul 8.
59. Tomlinson I et al (2003) A genome-wide association scan of tag SNPs identifies a susceptibility variant for colorectal cancer at 8q24.21. Nat Genet 39(8):984–988. Epub 2007 Jul 8.
60. Rioux JD et al (2007) Genome-wide association study identifies new susceptibility loci for Crohn disease and implicates autophagy in disease pathogenesis. Nat Genet 39(5):596–604.
61. Libioulle C et al (2007) Novel Crohn disease locus identified by genome-wide association maps to a gene desert on 5p13.1 and modulates expression of PTGER4. PLoS Genet 3(4):e58.
62. Hampe J et al (2007) A genome-wide association scan of nonsynonymous SNPs identifies a susceptibility variant for Crohn disease in ATG16L1. Nat Genet 39(2):207–211.

63. Cummings JR et al (2007) Confirmation of the role of ATG16L1 as a Crohn's disease susceptibility gene. Inflamm Bowel Dis 13(8):941–946.
64. Tanaka N et al (2003) Association of solute carrier family 12 (sodium/chloride) member 3 with diabetic nephropathy, identified by genome-wide analyses of single nucleotide polymorphisms. Diabetes 52(11):2848–2853.
65. Hu N et al (2005) Genome-wide association study in esophageal cancer using GeneChip mapping 10K array. Cancer Res 65(7):2542–2546.
66. Buch S, Schafmayer C, Volzke H, Becker C, Franke A, von Eller- Eberstein H, Kluck C, Bassmann I, Brosch M, Lammert F, Miquel JF, Nervi F, Wittig M, Rosskopf D, Timm B, Holl C, Seeger M, Elsharawy A, Lu T, Egberts J, Fandrich F, Folsch UR, Krawczak M, Schreiber S, Nurnberg P, Tepel J, Hampe J (2007) A genome-wide association scan identifies the hepatic cholesterol transporter ABCG8 as a susceptibility factor for human gallstone disease. Nat Genet 39(8):995–999.
67. Duerr RH et al (2006) A genome-wide association study identifies IL23R as an inflammatory bowel disease gene. Science 314(5804):1461–1463.
68. Klein RJ et al (2005) Complement factor H polymorphism in age-related macular degeneration. Science 308(5720):385–389.
69. Helgadottir A, Thorleifsson G, Manolescu A, Gretarsdottir S, Blondal T, Jonasdottir A, Jonasdottir A, Sigurdsson A, Baker A, Palsson A, Masson G, Gudbjartsson DF, Magnusson KP, Andersen K, Levey AI, Backman VM, Matthiasdottir S, Jonsdottir T, Palsson S, Einarsdottir H, Gunnarsdottir S, Gylfason A, Vaccarino V, Hooper WC, Reilly MP, Granger CB, Austin H, Rader DJ, Shah SH, Quyyumi AA, Gulcher JR, Thorgeirsson G, Thorsteinsdottir U, Kong A, Stefansson K (2007) A common variant on chromosome 9p21 affects the risk of myocardial infarction. Science 316(5830):1491–1493.
70. Ozaki K et al (2002) Functional SNPs in the lymphotoxin-alpha gene that are associated with susceptibility to myocardial infarction. Nat Genet 32(4):650–654.
71. Fung HC et al (2007) Genome-wide genotyping in Parkinson's disease and neurologically normal controls: first stage analysis and public release of data. Lancet Neurol 5(11):911–916.
72. Maraganore DM (2005) High-resolution whole-genome association study of Parkinson disease. Am J Hum Genet 77(5):685–693.
73. Gundmundsson J et al (2007) Genome-wide association study identifies a second prostate cancer susceptibility variant at 8q24. Nat Genet 39(5):631–637.
74. Yeager M et al (2007) Genome-wide association study of prostate cancer identifies a second risk locus at 8q24. Nat Genet 39(5):645–649.
75. Winkelmann J et al (2007) Genome-wide association study of restless legs syndrome identifies common variants in three genomic regions. Nat Genet 39(8):1000–1006. Epub 2007 Jul 18.
76. Lencz et al (2007) Converging evidence for a pseudoautosomal cytokine receptor gene locus in schizophrenia. Mol Psychiatry 12(6):572–580.
77. Zhou X et al (2003) Genome-wide association study for regions of systemic sclerosis susceptibility in a Choctaw Indian population with high disease prevalence. Arthritis Rheum 48(9):2585–2592.
78. Hakonarson H et al. A genome-wide association study identifies KIAA0350 as a type 1 diabetes gene. Nature 2007 Jul 15 (to appear).
79. Smyth DJ et al (2006) A genome-wide association study of nonsynonymous SNPs identifies a type 1 diabetes locus in the interferon-induced helicase (IFIH1) region. Nat Genet 38(6):617–619.
80. Zeggini E et al (2007) Replication of genome-wide association signals in UK samples reveals risk loci for type 2 diabetes. Science 316(5829):1336–1341. Epub 2007 Apr 26. Erratum in: Science 317(5841):1035–6.
81. Scott LJ et al. (2007) A genome-wide association study of type 2 diabetes in Finns detects multiple susceptibility variants. Science 316(5829):1341–1345. Epub 2007 Apr 26.

82. Steinthorsdottir V, Thorleifsson G, Reynisdottir I, Benediktsson R, Jonsdottir T, Walters GB, Styrkarsdottir U, Gretarsdottir S, Emilsson V, Ghosh S, Baker A, Snorradottir S, Bjarnason H, Ng MC, Hansen T, Bagger Y, Wilensky RL, Reilly MP, Adeyemo A, Chen Y, Zhou J, Gudnason V, Chen G, Huang H, Lashley K, Doumatey A, So WY, Ma RC, Andersen G, Borch- Johnsen K, Jorgensen T, van Vliet- Ostaptchouk JV, Hofker MH, Wijmenga C, Christiansen C, Rader DJ, Rotimi C, Gurney M, Chan JC, Pedersen O, Sigurdsson G, Gulcher JR, Thorsteinsdottir U, Kong A, Stefansson K (2007) A variant in CDKAL1 influences insulin response and risk of type 2 diabetes. Nat Genet 39(6):770–775.
83. Sladek R et al (2007) A genome-wide association study identifies novel risk loci for type 2 diabetes. Nature 445(7130):881–885.
84. Saxena R et al (2007) Genome-wide association analysis identifies loci for type 2 diabetes and triglyceride levels. Science 316(5829):1331–1336. Epub 2007 Apr 26.
85. Namkung J et al (2005) Whole-genome association studies of alcoholism with loci linked to schizophrenia susceptibility. BMC Genet 6(Suppl 1):S9.
86. Ye Y et al (2007) A genome-wide tree- and forest-based association analysis of comorbidity of alcoholism and smoking. BMC Genet 6(Suppl 1):S135.
87. Weiss LA et al (2004) Genome-wide association study identifies ITGB3 as a QTL for whole blood serotonin. Eur J Hum Genet 12(11):949–954.
88. Gu CC et al (2007) An investigation of genome-wide associations of hypertension with microsatellite markers in the family blood pressure program (FBPP). Hum Genet 121(5):577–590.
89. Schork NJ et al (2002) Genomic association/linkage of sodium lithium countertransport in CEPH pedigrees. Hypertension 40(5):619–628.
90. Liu QR et al (2006) Addiction molecular genetics: 639,401 SNP whole genome association identifies many cell adhesion genes. Am J Med Genet B Neuropsychiatr Genet 141(8):918–925.
91. Grupe A et al (2007) Evidence for novel susceptibility genes for late-onset Alzheimer's disease from a genome-wide association study of putative functional variants. Hum Mol Genet 16(8):865–873.
92. Baum AE et al (2007) A genome-wide association study implicates diacylglycerol kinase eta (DGKH) and several other genes in the etiology of bipolar disorder. Mol Psychiatry 13(2):197–207. Epub 2007 May 8.
93. McKnight AJ et al (2006) A genome-wide DNA microsatellite association screen to identify chromosomal regions harboring candidate genes in diabetic nephropathy. J Am Soc Nephrol 17(3):831–836.
94. Hanson RL et al (2007) Identification of PVT1 as a candidate gene for end-stage renal disease in type 2 diabetes using a pooling-based genome-wide single nucleotide polymorphism association study. Diabetes 56(4):975–983.
95. Kawashima M et al (2006) Genomewide association analysis of human narcolepsy and a new resistance gene. Am J Hum Genet 79(2):252–263.
96. Yatsu et al (2007) High-resolution mapping for essential hypertension using microsatellite markers. Hypertension 49(3):446–452.
97. Spector TD et al (2006) Association between a variation in LRCH1 and knee osteoarthritis: a genome-wide single-nucleotide polymorphism association study using DNA pooling. Arthritis Rheum 54(2):524–532.
98. Spinola et al (2007) Genome-wide single nucleotide polymorphism analysis of lung cancer risk detects the KLF6 gene. Cancer Lett 251(2):311–316.
99. Martins Silva B et al (2003) A whole genome association study in multiple sclerosis patients from north Portugal. J Neuroimmunol 143(1–2):116–119.
100. Santos M et al (2003) A whole genome screen for association with multiple sclerosis in Portuguese patients. J Neuroimmunol 143(1–2):112–115.
101. Bielecki B et al (2003) A whole genome screen for association in Polish multiple sclerosis patients. J Neuroimmunol 143(1–2):107–111.

102. Liguori M et al (2003) A whole genome screen for linkage disequilibrium in multiple sclerosis performed in a continental Italian population. J Neuroimmunol 143(1–2):97–100.
103. Heggarty S et al (2003) A genome wide scan for association with multiple sclerosis in a N. Irish case control population. J Neuroimmunol 143(1–2):93–96.
104. Jonasdottir A et al (2003) A whole genome association study in Icelandic multiple sclerosis patients with 4804 markers. J Neuroimmunol 143(1–2):88–92.
105. Rajda C et al (2003) A genome-wide screen for association in Hungarian multiple sclerosis. J Neuroimmunol 143(1–2):84–87.
106. Laaksonen M et al (2003) A whole genome association study in Finnish multiple sclerosis patients with 3669 markers. J Neuroimmunol 143(1–2):70–73.
107. Goris A et al (2003) New candidate loci for multiple sclerosis susceptibility revealed by a whole genome association screen in a Belgian population. J Neuroimmunol 143(1–2): 65–69.
108. Uhl GR et al (2007) Molecular genetics of nicotine dependence and abstinence: whole genome association using 520,000 SNPs. BMC Genet 8:10.
109. Bierut LJ et al (2007) Novel genes identified in a high-density genome-wide association study for nicotine dependence. Hum Mol Genet 16(1):24–35.
110. Tamiya G et al (2005) Whole genome association study of rheumatoid arthritis using 27,039 microsatellites. Hum Mol Genet 14(16):2305–2321.
111. Malik MH, Jury F, Bayat A, Ollier WE, Kay PR (2007) Genetic susceptibility to total hip arthroplasty failure: a preliminary study on the influence of matrix metalloproteinase 1, interleukin 6 polymorphisms and vitamin D receptor. Ann Rheum Dis 66(8): 1116–1120. Epub 2007 Mar 15.
112. Molero P, Ortuño F, Zalacain M, Patiño-García A (2007) Clinical involvement of catechol-O-methyltransferase polymorphisms in schizophrenia spectrum disorders: influence on the severity of psychotic symptoms and on the response to neuroleptic treatment. Pharmacogenomics J 7(6):418–426. Epub 2007 Mar 13.
113. Sugiyama E, Kaniwa N, Kim SR, Kikura- Hanajiri R, Hasegawa R, Maekawa K, Saito Y, Ozawa S, Sawada J, Kamatani N, Furuse J, Ishii H, Yoshida T, Ueno H, Okusaka T, Saijo N (2007) Pharmacokinetics of gemcitabine in Japanese cancer patients: the impact of a cytidine deaminase polymorphism. J Clin Oncol 25(1):32–42.
114. Drozdzik M, Rudas T, Pawlik A, Gornik W, Kurzawski M, Herczynska M (2007) Reduced folate carrier-1 80G>A polymorphism affects methotrexate treatment outcome in rheumatoid arthritis. Pharmacogenomics J 7(6):404–407. Epub 2007 Feb 27.
115. Kimmel SE, Christie J, Kealey C, Chen Z, Price M, Thorn CF, Brensinger CM, Newcomb CW, Whitehead AS (2007) Apolipoprotein E genotype and warfarin dosing among Caucasians and African Americans. Pharmacogenomics J 8(1):53–60. Epub 2007 Feb 27.
116. Ryu S, Cho EY, Park T, Oh S, Jang WS, Kim SK, Lee D, Hong KS (2007) –759 C/T polymorphism of 5-HT2C receptor gene and early phase weight gain associated with antipsychotic drug treatment. Prog Neuropsychopharmacol Biol Psychiatry 31(3):673–677. Epub 2007 Jan 12.
117. Xu K, Anderson TR, Neyer KM, Lamparella N, Jenkins G, Zhou Z, Yuan Q, Virkkunen M, Lipsky RH (2007) Nucleotide sequence variation within the human tyrosine kinase B neurotrophin receptor gene: association with antisocial alcohol dependence. Pharmacogenomics J 7(6):368–379. Epub 2007 Jan 2.
118. Ellingrod VL, Bishop JR, Moline J, Lin YC, Miller del D (2007) Leptin and leptin receptor gene polymorphisms and increases in body mass index (BMI) from olanzapine treatment in persons with schizophrenia. Psychopharmacol Bull 40(1):57–62.
119. Pasanen MK, Neuvonen M, Neuvonen PJ, Niemi M (2006) SLCO1B1 polymorphism markedly affects the pharmacokinetics of simvastatin acid. Pharmacogenet Genomics 16(12):873–879.
120. Ishiguro H, Iwasaki S, Teasenfitz L, Higuchi S, Horiuchi Y, Saito T, Arinami T, Onaivi ES (2006) Involvement of cannabinoid CB2 receptor in alcohol preference in mice and alcoholism in humans. Pharmacogenomics J 7(6):380–385. Epub 2006 Dec 26.

Chapter 10
Holy SNP, Batman!

Reyna Favis

Contents

Abstract The interaction between genetic variation and environment is widely acknowledged as the underlying explanation for differences in drug response among individuals, as well as the stratifying force behind disease phenotypes. When DNA variation is found to associate with a phenotype, the investigator's first inclination is to try to explain the finding. The SNP(s) identified (or others in LD) are generally thought to cause either a change in amino acid sequence that alters protein structure/function or a change in gene product expression that is due to altered affinity between *cis*- and *trans*-acting factors in the promoter. There is currently an underappreciation for the multifarious interactions that exist between SNPs and the cellular machinery and how this may impact drug response and disease genetics. The purpose of this chapter is to dispel the common view that so-called functional SNPs will be recognizable either by their ability to alter the sequences of *cis*-acting sites or by their ability to change the amino acid sequences of proteins. Other interactions of functional consequence will also be presented for consideration.

Keywords SNP, variation, pharmacogenomics, DNA structure

Reyna Favis
Johnson and Johnson Pharmaceutical Research and Development, L.L.C., 1000 Route 202, Raritan, NJ 08869
rfavis@prdus.jnj.com

N. Cohen (ed.) *Pharmacogenomics and Personalized Medicine*,

1 Introduction

The current content of dbSNP, a database of human genetic variation maintained by NCBI, is over 9 million unique SNPs. A selection of these SNPs is used to populate genotyping platforms that are capable of looking for associations with phenotypes across the whole genome. The SNPs are chosen in an attempt to create a picket fence that is more or less evenly spaced and covers the entire genome. Candidate gene association studies that take advantage of tagging SNPs also tend to select variation with the objective of covering as much genic real estate as possible. Because of these designs for whole genome and candidate gene association studies, SNPs that are found to associate with a phenotype can be located in both coding and noncoding sequences. Similar to association studies, linkage studies can also identify SNPs in both coding and noncoding regions that appear to be inherited in conjunction with the trait of interest.

Interpreting the functional significance of associating SNPs is no easy task. While nonsense mutations and certain types of missense mutations are largely amenable to interpretation and can contribute to a cogent explanation for what may underlie a phenotype of interest, most types of variation are not so straightforward. As will be discussed below, many missense and almost all noncoding SNPs can be a challenge to functionally classify. Given the open design of whole genome and, to a lesser extent, candidate gene analyses, there is no guarantee that the SNP(s) emerging from a study as the likely suspect(s) will localize to a coding sequence and be a type of variation that is easy to interpret.

To increase the clinical utility of an association, it is imperative that the finding has explanatory power. Purely correlative biomarkers have limitations in that they do not necessarily facilitate a biological understanding of the phenotype. Stopping short of a more complete understanding of the correlation can prevent or delay development of needed drugs or diagnostics. In some cases, researchers will be lucky, and an unclassified variation found to associate with a phenotype will be obviously related to a functional effect. In other cases, an associating SNP will be in linkage disequilibrium with a SNP that can clearly account for an alteration in phenotype. However, these scenarios will not always be the case, and it is more likely that interpretation will be far more complex.

The purpose of this chapter is to help to integrate various fields in biology to facilitate a more system-wide view of the effect of genetic variation. In general, interpreting variation will come down to changes in state (i.e., altered function) and/or changes in level (i.e., altered expression). The information presented below highlights cellular and developmental processes and structural states, as well as insights from evolution, to help explain how genetic variation can affect changes in function and expression. The various sections below discuss nonsynonymous and synonymous variation in the coding region of genes, as well as the impact of variation in noncoding regions that are both proximal to and quite distant from the genes influenced. For both coding and noncoding sequences, both *cis* (e.g., promoters, enhancers, locus control regions) and *trans* (e.g., micro RNAs) effects are considered. Also included are structural conformations of DNA and specific regulatory elements that have been associated with disease and that can be affected by variation. These structures will not be easy to recognize using conventional methods. Finally, maternal effect will be discussed to present an example of variation that has unquestionable influence over phenotype, but is rarely considered. If available, online resources are provided to facilitate SNP interpretation efforts for the specific scenarios described. Where possible, examples from published work are supplied to substantiate the biological reality of the scenario. Throughout, compelling stories from the literature will be related to describe how investigators triumphed despite the presence of elusive and obscure variation that resisted easy classification. The objective of this chapter is to encourage the reader to depart from the conventional and to consider more esoteric explanations for functional effect when similarly challenged.

2 Interpreting Variation in Coding Sequences

2.1 Missense Variation

The biological consequences of SNPs that create nonsense mutations or alter splice junctions are relatively easy to interpret. Obviously, these types of alterations are expected to radically change or impede protein function. Missense mutations, on the other hand, are frequently difficult to interpret. Although in vitro assays are available to facilitate interpretation in some cases, this is usually not the fastest or most economical route to understanding the likely consequences of variation. To obtain an overview of publicly available online tools to clarify the significance of SNPs, the reader should refer to Chapter 8, Strategies and resources for marker selection and genotyping in genetic association studies. While these online methods are convenient, it is difficult to assess the true success rate for these tools when categorizing SNPs as functional or neutral. The example of interpreting variation in *BRCA1* is described below, in order to provide a specific test case to assess the general basis for the methodology that is widely applied to assigning functional consequence to missense variation.

BRCA1 is among the most intensely studied genes in the human genome and over 12,000 entries for gene variants have been submitted to the Breast Cancer Information Core (BIC; http://research.nhgri.nih.gov/projects/bic). In an effort to understand the significance of variation discovered for this gene, Abkevich et al. *(1)* combined the insight provided by comparing the chemical distances among amino acids and the 20/20 hindsight provided by evolutionary comparisons among gene sequences from distantly related organisms. The investigators first analyzed a limited number of missense variants that were already classified in order to understand the range of values expected using this system of analysis. Evidence for a functional effect for these variants had been previously established through a combination of segregation analysis, functional assay, and association study. Next, Abkevich et al. assessed unclassified variants in *BRCA1* that were probably either deleterious or were neutral or of little clinical significance. Overall, 314 distinct missense variants from full sequences belonging to 20,000 individuals were assessed.

For both classified and unclassified *BRCA1* variants, one criterion of assessment was the degree of sequence conservation across multiple diverse organisms. Sequences were chosen from organisms where an equal number of sequences per clade were available and where all segments of the protein were equally represented. Amino acid sequences from human, chimpanzee, mouse, dog, chicken, xenopus, and puffer fish were aligned using a parsimony-based method. The method was used to calculate the minimum number of missense substitutions required to create the observed alignment and took into account the underlying phylogenetic tree *(2)*. It was found that the position of deleterious missense mutations was strongly biased towards coinciding with invariant amino acids in the multiple sequence alignment. Neutral missense variants, on the other hand, aligned with residues where multiple substitutions were tolerated during the evolution of *BRCA1*.

The second criterion for missense classification was the physicochemical similarity between the variant amino acid and the residues found in the corresponding position in the multiple sequence alignment. For this assessment, the Grantham chemical difference matrix *(3)* was used as the basis for comparisons. This chemical difference matrix takes into account residue side chain composition, polarity and volume. Similar pairs of amino acids have scores between 5 and 60, while disparate pairs have scores of greater than 100. Using the data from the Human Genome Mutation Database (http://www.hgmd.cf.ac.uk), it was found that amino acid substitutions underlying disease phenotypes have an average chemical difference of 93.4. For the 21 known deleterious *BRCA1* mutations, the average chemical difference score was 122.0, while the score was 64.8 for the missense variants that had been previously classified as neutral or of little clinical significance.

When analyzing the unclassified variants, the authors applied the following criteria to identify potentially deleterious mutations: 1) the highest pairwise chemical difference score between the amino acid position from the aligned orthologous sequences corresponding to the human variant of interest is ≤ 61; and 2) the chemical difference score for the human variant of interest is ≥ 3x the highest pairwise chemical difference score in the alignment at that position. Similarly, variants that are likely to be neutral or of little clinical significance were identified using the following criteria: 1) the chemical difference score for the human missense variant is < 61; and 2) the chemical difference score for the human variant should be less than one third of the highest chemical difference score of an interspecific genetic variation at that position.

As an additional check for functional significance, the authors also queried their dataset for the presence of homozygotes and transheterozygotes for the alleles of interest. This test was based on the assumption that it would be extremely unlikely for the same individual to carry two deleterious mutations. For suspected deleterious alleles, neither class of genotype was evident in the data; in contrast, alleles suspected to be either neutral or of little clinical significance could be found to co-occur with alleles that were deemed deleterious.

To summarize the results from Abkevich et al., of the 314 unique missense variants identified, 106 could be classified as neutral or not likely of clinical significance and 71 could be classified as deleterious, using both functional tests and a combination of physicochemical and evolutionary conservation analyses. The remaining 137 unclassified missense variants still lacked classification, indicating that additional insight into the stratification of variation is still required.

Recently, Chan et al. *(4)* compared computational algorithms designed to characterize missense variants. Methods using evolutionary conservation alone, amino acid change alone, and a combination of conservation and amino acid change were used to assess the consequences of 254 missense variants in five genes (*CDKN2A*, *MLH1*, *MSH2*, *MECP2*, and *TYR*). The classifications made by algorithms based solely on evolutionary conservation (BLOSUM62 matrix score *5, [6]*) or both phylogeny and structure (SIFT *(7)* http://blocks.fhcrc.org/sift/SIFT.html; PolyPhen *(8)* http://genetics.bwh.harvard.edu/pph; A-GVGD *(9, 10)* http://agvgd.iarc.fr/agvgd_input.php) were compared to classifications made for the variants in curated locus-specific mutation databases and published functional data. The authors found that the methods using both phylogeny and structure to distinguish neutral from deleterious amino acid changes did not improve results significantly over using evolutionary conservation alone: the overall predictive value for all genes averaged 76.9% for the methods using both phylogeny and structure, versus 78.0% for the method using evolutionary conservation. However, the positive predictive value increased to almost 90% when the amino acid of interest did not vary in the multiple species sequence alignment, or when three or four methods agreed that the variant was deleterious.

In an effort to classify *BRCA1* missense variants using an integrative approach, Phelan et al. *(11)* used the methodology implemented by Abkevich et al. in combination with an in vitro transcriptional activation assay, a determination of co-occurrence with other deleterious mutations, a pedigree analysis, previously published results using an algorithm that predicts structure/function consequences for variation *(12)*, and a protease-based assay *(13)*. Of 17 missense variants *(11, 14)*, eight variants were in full agreement across all approaches where data was available and could be classified with relative confidence. The remainder had either equivocal results in the in vitro transcriptional activation assay or had shown some degree of contradiction across the tests for which data could be compared. It was concluded that no single method could be used alone to reliably classify *BRCA1* missense variants and that a combination of several efforts was necessary to better make this prediction.

In conclusion, the application of multiple in silico and in vivo tests is the best approach to reliably assign functional consequence to unclassified variants. When limited to computational methods, multiple in silico approaches should be used to look for consensus.

2.2 Synonymous Variation

Synonymous SNPs do not change the amino acid in the affected codon, and hence are not generally considered of clinical significance. The exception to this assessment is if the base change is thought to impact exon/intron splicing. An interesting finding for *MDR*1 has cast into doubt the view that synonymous SNPs are of little functional importance. As described below, a functional consequence that has nothing to do with splicing has now been ascribed to this type of polymorphism.

A synonymous SNP in exon 26 (C3435T) of *MDR*1 has been associated with both altered and reduced P-glycoprotein activity *(15–19)*. Kimchi-Sarfaty et al. *(20)* considered three possible scenarios to explain this effect: 1) C3435T is in linkage disequilibrium with the causative SNP(s) for the phenotype; 2) the change in sequence causes mRNA secondary structure differences for the two alleles and influences splicing, processing, or translational control and regulation; and 3) the change in sequence influences protein activity or function.

To determine which of the hypotheses explained the phenotypic effects of the C3435T variant, Kimchi-Sarfaty et al. *(20)* transfected several different cell lines with constructs bearing one of the following: wild-type *MDR*1, each individual *MDR*1 polymorphism (C1236T, G2377T and C3435T), combinations of pairs of polymorphisms, or all three variants. To test the drug transport function of each of the cell lines, fluorescent-activated cell sorting was used to assess the intracellular accumulation or efflux of various fluorescently labeled compounds. Through these experiments, the presence of the C3435T polymorphism in the context of double or triple haplotypes was linked to differences in the effectiveness of P-glycoprotein inhibitors. This finding eliminated the possibility that the true causative SNP was in linkage disequilibrium with C3435T. Comparisons of mRNA and protein levels between wild-type cells and the cells bearing the 3-variant haplotype showed comparable levels of both types of gene products. This result eliminated the possibility that mRNA secondary structure was influencing the amount of *MDR*1 gene product. To test the final hypothesis that C3435T was affecting protein activity or function, Kimchi-Sarfaty et al. assessed whether a conformational difference between the wild-type and the 3-variant haplotype could be detected. Using both a conformation-sensitive monoclonal antibody and digestion with trypsin, it was shown that a difference in tertiary structure existed between these two forms of *MDR*1. The investigators deduced that the use of certain codons, where the abundance of the cognate tRNA may be low, might influence the translation rate and thus affect the folding of the protein. This supposition was shown to have merit when a 3-variant haplotype that replaced C3435T with C3435A was tested for drug transport function. Similarly to C3435T, C3435A also creates an unpreferred codon for isoleucine in the sequence, but the A allele codon is used even less frequently in human sequences. In line with the relative synonymous codon usage for these two alleles, it was found that C3435A showed even larger decreases in inhibitor effects than the T allele.

Based on the above findings, nonsynonymous SNPs should not be immediately dismissed as only indirect evidence for the presence of a causative SNP. Clearly, nonsynonymous SNPs may be affecting protein structure, and this should be considered when interpreting association data. A convenient source for the frequency of use for various codons in humans can be found in Kliman et al. *(21)*. In addition, this report also provides information on the correlations of codon frequencies (within amino acid) with gene expression in 12 human tissues. While the authors make the point that local base compositional bias is the primary influence on codon usage in mammals, the aim of their investigation was to explore the more subtle influences of natural selection on human codon usage by focusing on usage in human-infecting viruses. One specific finding of this study was that the arginine codon AGG and the leucine codon TTG were selectively disfavored in both humans and human-infecting viruses. The usage of these codons could not be explained by local base composition; and in humans, AGG and TTG rose in frequency as all other C- and G-ending codons decreased in frequency. These two codons were the only C- or G-ending codons with usages that negatively correlated with gene expression in humans. SNPs creating these intriguing codons, as well as infrequently used codons, are obvious candidates for inducing functional effects in the corresponding protein.

3 Interpreting Variation in Noncoding Sequences

3.1 Variation in cis-Acting Sequences

In 2003, the National Human Genome Research Institute (NHGRI) launched a public research consortium named ENCODE, the Encyclopedia of DNA Elements (http://www.genome.gov/10005107). The purpose of this consortium is to identify all functional elements in the human genome sequence. The data from this effort that are linked to the genomic sequence can be accessed on the University of California, Santa Cruz browser (http://genome.ucsc.edu/ENCODE/). The current aims of the consortium are to compare existing analysis methods to determine where the gaps exist in capabilities and then to determine which approaches should be scaled up to manage the high throughput identification of all functional elements in the human genome. The data produced by this effort will be an invaluable source for interpreting the consequences of variation found in regulatory sequences. Until the full data from this consortium are available, it will be necessary to rely upon existing information and algorithms. A number of online tools can be found on http://www3.oup.co.uk/nar/database/subcat/1/4, a site maintained by the journal *Nucleic Acids Research* to provide access to the databases described in the first issue published by this journal every year. While specific tools are mentioned below, the reader is encouraged to explore other available online resources. Additional information on specific uses for online tools to interpret regulatory

SNPs can be found in Chapter 5, The HAP MAP, SNP Selection and Genotyping Methods. The information below provides insight into the functional consequences of variation in both proximal and distal regulatory sites.

3.1.1 Local Control

3.1.1.1 Promoter Elements

The most obvious type of variation in the promoter that has a functional consequence is a sequence change in an identified *cis*-acting element that causes either an increase or decrease in the binding affinity of *trans*-acting factors. Changing the residence time of bound proteins on the promoter alters the rate of transcription. A less obvious consequence of variation in the promoter region is the creation of a new promoter element. One such gain-of-function regulatory SNP was described by De Gobbi et al. *(22)* during an investigation aimed at identifying the genetic lesion underlying a particularly severe form of α thalassemia, called HbH disease. The authors first eliminated alternate explanations for reduced α-globin expression, which is diagnostic of this disorder. Analyses confirmed that no deletions, chromosomal rearrangements, DNA methylation, or unclassified sequence variants in the regulatory elements of the major and minor α-like genes were detected. De Gobbi et al. next narrowed down the region of interest through linkage and association studies, and then cloned the implicated ~213 kb region into a BAC construct. Deep sequencing revealed an unwieldy 283 SNPs and/or sequence differences in the clone. To try to resolve which SNP(s) were involved in α-globin down-regulation, the authors constructed a tiled array representing all regions of nonrepetitive DNA in the locus and compared expression in normal and HbH individuals. Analysis revealed a major new peak of RNA transcription localizing to the α-globin region. Quantitative RT-PCR showed that expression from this region was in excess of 1000-fold higher in HbH RNA than in wild-type; and the expression of the α^{D} gene, directly downstream of this region, was decreased approximately 80-fold in HbH RNA compared to wild-type. The region associated with the high expression peak in the array contained 17 SNPs, and 10 of these could be eliminated from consideration because they had been previously observed in nonthalassemic individuals. Of the remaining 7 SNPs, only one SNP was found to segregate with thalassemia in affected families, showed complete association with HbH, and could not be found in nonthalassemic individuals. The sequence created by the presence of the C allele of this SNP resembled the binding site for the GATA-1 transcription factor. De Gobbi et al. confirmed binding by GATA-1 through chromatin immunoprecipitation and electromobility gel super shift using an antibody directed against GATA-1. It was found that the new binding site created by the C allele nucleated the assembly of a pentameric erythroid complex. It was theorized that the erythroid transcription complex preferentially interacted with this new site, outcompeting the endogenous α-globin promoters and leading to down-regulation of α-globin genes. Interestingly, the authors pointed out that conventional wisdom dictated that regions containing putative *cis*-acting elements should be the focus of investigations aimed at explaining down-regulation of gene expression. Because promoter deletion analysis had previously demonstrated that the identified region of interest could be eliminated with no effect on α-globin expression (and hence was not likely to contain a *cis*-acting element), the region containing this gain-of-function regulatory SNP would likely have been eliminated from consideration under normal circumstances.

3.1.1.2 Methylation

There are two classes of mammalian promoters: TATA box-enriched promoters and CpG-rich promoters. The TATA box promoters are associated with tissue-specific expression; CpG-rich promoters, on the other hand, account for all housekeeping and widely expressed genes, as well as 40% of genes with a tissue-specific or limited expression *(23)*. In the mammalian genome, the CpG-rich promoters are the predominant type of promoter *(24)*. Methylation of promoter CpG islands plays an important role in regulating gene expression. These sites recruit protein complexes that include histone deacetylases, which covalently modify histones to create a more closed chromatin conformation and thereby contribute to down-regulation of transcription *(25)*. Aberrant methylation patterns are well documented in cancer *(26)*, and it has been suggested that methylation profiles would serve as useful markers for early detection of this disease *(27)*. Methylation has also been implicated in the etiology of the autoimmune diseases scleroderma *(28)* and lupus erythrematosis *(29)*, in atherosclerosis *(30)*, and in mixed genetic/epigenetic models of autism *(31)*, bipolar disorder, and schizophrenia *(32, 33)*. Given that these sequences play such a dominant role in regulating gene expression and have been implicated in human disease, it is noteworthy that a recent study has identified close to 35,000 putative CpG islands in the human genome and over 133,000 SNPs that map to these sequences *(34)*. Clearly, gene regulation by methylation will be influenced by any changes in the CpG sequence, and variation in these motifs is a ripe area for investigation.

3.1.1.3 Untranslated Regions

Untranslated regions in 5' and 3' ends of mRNAs (5' and 3' UTRs) are involved in many posttranscriptional events that control mRNA localization, stability, and translational efficiency (see *(35)* for a review). The biological activity of control elements in these untranslated regions relies both on the primary sequence, as well as on secondary structure produced by folding these control elements in the RNA.

Iron metabolism is an instructive example of regulation using UTRs (reviewed in *[36]*). Under conditions of low iron abundance, *trans*-acting iron regulatory proteins are induced to bind iron response elements in the 5' UTRs of several genes involved in the metabolism of iron. Binding to the 5' UTRs of these genes suppresses translation initiation. Meanwhile, these same proteins bind to the 3' UTRs of transferrin receptor mRNAs to bring about selective stabilization of these messages. Under conditions of iron overload, the binding affinity of the *trans*-acting iron regulatory proteins is reduced, allowing translation of iron metabolizing genes and degradation of transferrin receptor mRNA. Variation in the iron response elements has been linked to at least one hereditary disorder, called hereditary hyperferritinemia-cataract syndrome. Variation in other 3' UTRs has been associated with complex disease; cancers, psychiatric, neurological, cardiovascular, and metabolic diseases have all been implicated (for review see [37]).

To facilitate the analysis of untranslated sequences uncovered during association studies, one online resource is UTResource (http://bighost.area.ba.cnr.it/BIG/UTRHome/) *(38)*. This site contains curated, nonredundant sequences of 5' and 3' UTRs from eukaryotic mRNAs.

3.1.2 Action at a Distance

3.1.2.1 Enhancers and Silencers

Elements acting in *cis* that function in a proximal fashion tend to control expression of a single gene with a transcription start point located within 1 kb of the control element. In some cases, *cis*-acting elements can exert long-range control over a much larger chromosomal region, and there is increasing evidence for coordinate regulation of gene clusters. Enhancers and silencers tend to operate at a distance to increase or decrease (respectively) the rate of transcription. These elements may operate at a distance of 50 kb or more, either upstream or downstream of the promoter they control. Genes located in the vicinity may compete for the action of these distal elements through various assemblies of *trans*-acting factors and controlled looping actions that bring into proximity these distal elements with proximal promoter elements.

Variation in enhancers has been investigated and associated with diseases in humans. For example, in chronic obstructive pulmonary disease (COPD), a SNP in a predicted enhancer region of the *CCL*1 gene was significantly associated with acute exacerbations in COPD *(39)*. In diabetes, a SNP in the beta-cell specific enhancer in the *IPF*1 gene was found to increase susceptibility to type 2 diabetes among African American individuals, but not in Caucasians *(40)*. An enhancer SNP at the *GLUT*1 locus was found to be associated with susceptibility to diabetic nephropathy in type 1 diabetes *(41)*. Cancer also has its examples. Thymidylate synthase (*TS*) intra-tumoural expression is thought to be a prognostic marker, predicting the outcome of 5-fluorouracil (5-FU)-based chemotherapy in colorectal cancer patients. An upstream enhancer affecting the *TS* gene contains a tandem repeat that can be present in two or three copies, as well as a SNP site. Individuals who were homozygous for three tandem repeats and who possessed the G allele of the SNP demonstrated increased levels of *TS* gene expression compared to other genotypes for this locus *(42)*.

An excellent resource for experimentally validated human noncoding fragments with gene enhancer activity is the VISTA Enhancer Browser (http://enhancer.lbl.gov/)

(43). Enhancer activity is assessed in transgenic mice, and sequence selection for testing is based on conservation across other vertebrate species. Using this tool, it is possible to retrieve elements near single genes of interest, search for enhancers that target reporter gene expression to a particular tissue, or download entire collections of enhancers with a defined tissue specificity or conservation depth.

3.1.2.2 Nuclear Matrix Dynamics and Locus Control Regions

The nucleus is generally only thought of as an organelle whose sole function is to house DNA. Far from being only a protective environment to shield DNA from nucleases, the nucleus also provides structural support for the numerous processes conducted in this dynamic environment, including transcription, DNA replication, repair, and mRNA processing and transport. Supporting these processes requires controlled interactions between protein components of the nuclear matrix (recently reviewed in *[44, 45]*) and DNA sequences.

In cells of higher eukaryotes, the DNA is arranged in loops of 50–100 kb in length that are held in this conformation through AT-rich DNA segments referred to as matrix attached regions (MARs). While heterochromatin is highly condensed and usually found in the peripheral area of the nucleus, the loops of euchromatic DNA are more central and dispersed.

Locus control regions (LCRs) are genetic regulatory elements that confer tissue-specific and physiological levels of expression on the genes to which they are linked. LCRs are responsible for establishing and maintaining an open functional domain in the chromatin and tend to be situated at a distance from the genes they influence. In contrast to LCRs, other types of regulatory elements that can also act at a distance (e.g., enhancers and silencers) or act in a proximal fashion (e.g., promoter elements) are strongly influenced by the chromatin environment in which they are situated. This is known as position effect. When an LCR is integrated into a genome in the context of a transgene, the linked gene is able to express at wild-type levels independent of the position of integration *(46)*. One of the most intensely studied LCRs is associated with β-globin expression.

The β-globin LCR is located about 15 kb upstream of the first of five developmentally regulated globin genes contained in the locus and consists of four DNase I hypersensitive sites. These sites are rendered hypersensitive to enzymatic digestion when nuclear matrix proteins bind these elements *(47, 48)* during transcription and create an open chromatin conformation. Variation in one of the hypersensitive sites mapping to the β-globin LCR has been shown to associate with β-thalassemia in individuals lacking coding sequence mutations in both Indian *(49)* and Thai *(50)* populations.

From this example, it is clear that variation in regions quite distant from coding sequences can still affect linked genes. Because there is still quite a bit of controversy over the exact composition and organization of the nuclear matrix, it is unclear to what extent variation associated with sequences that contact the nuclear matrix contribute to phenotype. However, when confronted with an associating SNP that is seemingly in the middle of nowhere with respect to mapped genes, one might consider the possibility that the region may be involved with long-range interactions characteristic of LCRs and MARs. A convenient repository of sequences associated with MARs can be found at http://smartdb.bioinf.med.uni-goettingen.de/ *(51)* and should serve as a useful comparison for context sequence surrounding SNPs of interest.

3.2 Variation Affecting Structure

In contrast to the regulatory elements described above, functional elements creating a distinct secondary structure that contribute to gene regulation will not necessarily have defined canonical or consensus sequences. The important product from these sequences is solely the structure fashioned from folding the primary sequence, and structure can frequently be achieved using divergent primary sequences. In these cases, conservation across species may not be a useful indicator of functional significance and may even be misleading. While there is less available in the literature to point to the connection between variation in the sites that create these structures and phenotypic consequences, connections to disease and/or responses to drugs will be mentioned below, where possible. An online resource to support DNA structure identification is http://ndbserver.rutgers.edu/, a repository of three-dimensional structural information about nucleic acids *(52)*.

3.2.1 Z-DNA

DNA is usually depicted as a right-handed helix with 10.2 bases per helical turn and a helix diameter of 23.7 Å. This structure is known as B-DNA. Alternate forms of DNA exist and have been documented in vivo. One such unusual structure is Z-DNA *(53, 54)*, which is a left-handed helix comprised of alternating purine-pyrimidine sequences that is much narrower than B-DNA (only 18.4 Å) and has a much flatter major groove compared to the B form. Evidence for the existence of Z-DNA in vivo came when it was recognized that patients suffering from systemic lupus erythrematosis produced antibodies that bound preferentially to Z-DNA compared to B-DNA *(55–59)*. Another piece of evidence indicating an in vivo role for Z-DNA is that the RNA editing enzyme, ADAR1, bound to Z-DNA in a highly specific manner, withstanding challenge from a 10,000-fold excess B-DNA competitor *(60–62)*. More recently, reports of Z-DNA responsive promoters have indicated a role in regulating transcription *(63–66)*. The hypothesis of how the presence of Z-DNA promoted transcription hinges on the observation that Z-DNA cannot be incorporated into nucleosomes *(67)* and thus leaves an open chromatin conformation that is inviting to certain transcription factors. It is thought that during transcriptional activation, the mammalian SWI/SNF complex remodels the chromatin by destabilizing the histone-DNA interactions and in so doing, releases negative superhelicity, which in turn provides the energy for Z-DNA formation *(63)*.

The formation of Z-DNA maintains an open chromatin conformation at the affected promoter and facilitates assembly of the transcriptional machinery.

It has recently been demonstrated that E3L, a poxvirus virulence factor, binds Z-DNA *(68)*. In the absence of the Z-DNA binding region on the protein, mice infected with a normally lethal dose of poxvirus survived. It was determined that E3L promotes virus reproduction by facilitating transcription of antiapoptotic genes, thus preventing apoptosis of infected host cells and providing a safe haven for virus replication.

In order to identify potential Z-DNA sites in the genome, sequence files up to 1 MB can be submitted to the online tool ZHUNT (http://gac-web.cgrb.oregonstate.edu/zDNA/) *(69, 70)*. The search algorithm for this program has been optimized to search large sequences for the potential occurrence of Z-DNA, taking into account sequence type, length, and cooperativity for a given stretch of potential Z-DNA-forming nucleotides.

3.2.2 Quadruplex

Quadruplex conformation is an alternative DNA structure that can occur when repetitive bases align the two strands of DNA in a structure resembling a chair. Hurley and colleagues have identified a G-quadruplex structure in the promoter of the oncogene *cMYC (71, 72)*. When this quadruplex is stabilized by the binding of specific cellular proteins, transcription of *cMYC* is inhibited *(73)*. If the sequence of the regulatory region is altered by mutating a single G to an A, the quadruplex is destabilized and a tremendous increase in *cMYC* expression ensues, resulting in uncontrolled cell proliferation *(71)*. Hurley et al. hypothesized that stabilization of the G-quadruplex would stem the tide of *cMYC* overexpression and stop the uncontrolled cell proliferation. Towards that end, a small molecule was used to stabilize this promoter structure and, without *cMYC*'s constant push towards proliferation, the cancer cells underwent apoptosis *(74)*.

3.2.3 Triple Helix

Triple helices, also known as H-DNA, form at DNA regions containing mirror repeat symmetry. One half of the repeat can dissociate into a single strand (using the energy provided by supercoiling DNA when RNA polymerase processes through a template during transcription) and swivel its backbone parallel to the purine-rich strand still in duplex to create a three-stranded helix *(75, 76)*. The unpaired complementary strand formerly associated with the migrating strand remains single-stranded.

Triple helix formations have been found to be a source of genetic instability, inducing double-stranded breaks near H-DNA loci. In particular, the *cMYC* promoter contains an endogenous triple helix forming sequence and it is thought that this region may be a contributing factor to *cMYC* translocations in diseases such as Burkitt's lymphoma *(77)*.

3.2.4 Cruciform

Another DNA structure that induces genetic instability and chromosomal breaks is called cruciform. The cruciform conformation requires a palindromic double-stranded sequence that separates and then base pairs in an intrastrand fashion to form a four-way junction consisting of two long duplex DNA arms and two comparatively short hairpin arms. Similar to H-DNA, this structure is also stabilized through negative supercoiling. Similar to Z-DNA, cruciform structures also prevent nucleosome formation and maintain an open chromatin conformation.

Tyrosine hydroxylase (TH) is the first and rate-limiting enzyme involved in the synthesis of catecholamines. Mutations in the *TH* gene have been associated with disorders involving involuntary jerky movements, Segawa syndrome, and extrapyramidal movement disorder. The *TH* promoter contains a palindromic sequence referred to as the dyad symmetry element (DSE1). Kim et al. *(78)* found that the presence of palindromic sequence in the *TH* promoter is conserved in the human, rat, and bovine gene and that DSE1 assumes an imperfect cruciform conformation in supercoiled DNA. Footprint experiments showed that nuclear factors bound to this formation with a significantly higher affinity than to the same sequence in linear duplex conformation. Deletion of either arm of the palindrome prevented the formation of a cruciform structure and markedly reduced the expression of a reporter gene. Together, these results suggest that the cruciform element is likely a target for *trans*-acting factors that influence the expression level of the *TH* gene.

4 MicroRNAs

MicroRNAs (miRNAs) *(79, 80)* are small noncoding RNAs that regulate gene expression by binding to imperfect complementary sequences in the 3' untranslated regions of messenger RNAs (mRNAs) queued for translation *(81)*. The end result is a reduction in the stability and/or translation of the targeted mRNAs. miRNAs are single-stranded RNAs that are 20 to 24 nucleotides in length and are derived from larger endogenous transcripts from which ~80 nucleotides can be processed to form hairpin structures. These RNA hairpins are processed by RNase III-type enzymes and rendered single-stranded by a helicase. The resulting short, single-stranded RNA product is eventually incorporated into a ribonucleoprotein complex known as miRISC (miRNA-containing RNA-induced silencing complex).

The genomic locations of miRNAs have been extensively explored *(79, 80, 82–87)*. miRNAs can be found either scattered throughout the genome as isolated entities or grouped in clusters. When clustered, they are arranged and expressed in a manner that suggests that the miRNAs are treated as a multi-cistronic primary transcript in the cell. The majority of miRNAs are found in defined transcription units. When located in the introns of pre-mRNAs, their orientation is aligned with the direction of transcription of the host gene, and thus they appear to rely on their host gene for expression. miRNAs can also be found in non-protein-coding RNAs in either exons or introns.

It is estimated that miRNAs regulate at least 20–30% of all genes *(81, 88–90)*. A registry of miRNAs curated from the literature has been established by the Sanger Institute (http://microrna.sanger.ac.uk/) *(91, 92)*, and there are currently close to 500 entries for human sequences. Since miRNAs have been implicated in such crucial biological processes as differentiation, apoptosis, and proliferation *(79)*, it is no surprise that alterations in miRNAs have been implicated in human disease.

The main mechanism underlying the contribution of miRNAs to human cancer development and progression appears to be aberrant gene expression, resulting from genomic amplifications and deletions that change the copy number of regions containing miRNAs *(93)*. However, there is also evidence of germline and somatic mutations in both miRNA genes and in the targeted regions of mRNAs that may have functional significance in human cancers. In chronic lymphocytic leukemia (CLL), Calin and colleagues identified a germline mutation in the miR-16–1-miR-15a primary precursor that diminished microRNA expression both in vitro and in vivo and was associated with deletion of the normal allele *(94)*. Overall, this study found germline or somatic mutations in 5 of 42 sequenced microRNAs in 11 of 75 patients with CLL, with no evidence of these mutations in 160 subjects without cancer. In a study involving papillary thyroid carcinoma (PTC), He and collaborators found a dramatic loss of *cKIT* transcript and Kit protein, which associated in 5 of 10 cases with a germline single-nucleotide change in the two recognition sequences in *cKIT* for miR-221, -222, and -146 *(95)*.

miRNAs have also been shown to affect processes in the central nervous system (CNS). Using a custom microarray, Krichevsky and colleagues demonstrated that miRNAs are extensively regulated during brain development *(96)*. A direct link to human CNS disease can be found in Tourette's syndrome, a genetically influenced developmental neuropsychiatric disorder characterized by chronic vocal and motor tics. Abelson et al. identified a sequence variant in the binding site for hsa-miR-189 in the gene Slit and Trk-like 1 (*SLITRK1*) *(97)*. Interestingly, both miRNA and gene showed an overlapping expression pattern in a region of the brain previously implicated in Tourette's syndrome; additionally, only the wild-type *SLITRK1*, but not the mutant, enhanced dendritic growth in primary neuronal cultures *(97)*. While this example concerns a frameshift mutation and not a true SNP, it is not unreasonable to predict that variation of the single nucleotide variety may also be described in the near future for this and other CNS-related disorders.

Although suggestive, the examples above are unlikely to be followed up by many reports of common variants in miRNAs and their binding sites that impact gene expression. In general, genetic polymorphisms in miRNAs and their target genes are under strong negative selection *(98)* and are likely to be present as low frequency variants in human populations. However, when variations are present in these sequences, it is likely that they are deleterious, and these variants should be seriously considered as candidate polymorphisms that contribute to human disease *(98)*. Since variation in miRNA processing enzymes has been observed (e.g., human homologs of both *Dicer* and *Drosha* contain several nonsynonymous SNPs), such enzymes may also be of interest as additional targets for disease association.

5 Maternal Effect

In developmental biology, maternal effect is a well-known contributor to phenotype. In the classical context, it is thought of as the cytoplasmic determinant in eggs (produced by the mother, and therefore governed by the mother's genotype) that specify the body pattern of the developing embryo. In a more general sense, maternal effects are phenotypic effects that parents have on phenotypes of their offspring that are unrelated to the offspring's own genotype.

The impact of maternal genotype is well illustrated in a recent study involving CNS development in the mouse. Serotonin is commonly thought of as a neuromodulator/neurotransmitter; however, a role for mammalian brain development and maturation is also being ascribed to this substance. Because serotonin biosynthesis has thus far not been detected in mouse embryos or extra-embryonic structures, Côté et al. *(99)* investigated the role of maternal serotonin in CNS morphogenesis in the embryo. A mouse line deficient in peripheral serotonin biosynthesis was generated by targeted disruption of the tryptophan hydroxylase 1 (*tph1*) gene, which is responsible for the synthesis of peripheral serotonin. Null mutants produce levels of circulating serotonin that are 3–15% of their wild-type counterparts. Wild-type female mice or females that were homozygous or heterozygous for the *tph1* knockout were mated with *tph1* wild-type, heterozygous, or null males in all combinations. 80–90% of pups born to *tph1*-null mothers showed abnormalities in the development of the brain (e.g., the head takes on a flattened morphology and there is reduced mitosis in the structure that develops into the cerebral cortex) and other tissues, irrespective of whether the embryos' genotypes were *tph1* +/– or –/–. Thus, the phenotype of the embryos depends on the genotype of the mothers and not on that of the embryo.

In humans, diabetes is one example of a disease with genetic determinants that has been shown to produce measurable phenotypes in offspring due to the maternal effect. Recently, a whole-genome association study has uncovered several risk loci for type 2 diabetes *(100)* that explain a substantial portion of disease risk, thus emphasizing the genetic component of this disease. It has been known for some time that postnatal neurobehavioral abnormalities can be observed in the offspring of diabetic mothers *(101–103)*. For example, although the IQ scores of children born to well-controlled diabetic mothers are generally similar to those of control children, these children perform less well than controls in fine and gross motor functions. They also seem to have a higher rate of inattention and/or hyperactivity compared to controls *(101, 103)* and a deficit in explicit memory performance, as assessed by their ability to recall multistep event sequences after a delay is imposed *(102)*. It is thought that neurological developmental abnormalities are the result of exposure to multiple risk factors in the prenatal environment, including chronic hypoxia, hyperglycemia/reactive hypoglycemia, and iron deficiency.

While maternal effect is rarely considered and can be difficult to pursue in disease genetics studies, it is obvious that there is an effect. This area should perhaps be contemplated as a future research direction, in order to improve our understanding of certain diseases.

6 Concluding Remarks

It is clear that numerous cellular processes shaped by evolution *(104)* both affect and are affected by genetic variation. It is hoped that the information presented in this chapter will help to spur integrative thinking about the interactions between cellular, developmental, structural, and evolutionary mechanisms and genetic variation.

References

1. Abkevich V, Zharkikh A, Deffenbaugh AM, et al. (2004) Analysis of missense variation in human BRCA1 in the context of interspecific sequence variation. J Med Genet 41:492–507.
2. Fitch WM, Markowitz E (1970) An improved method for determining codon variability in a gene and its application to the rate of fixation of mutations in evolution. Biochem Genet 4:579–593.
3. Grantham R (1974) Amino acid difference formula to help explain protein evolution. Science 185:862–864.
4. Chan PA, Duraisamy S, Miller PJ, et al. (2007) Interpreting missense variants: comparing computational methods in human disease genes CDKN2A, MLH1, MSH2, MECP2, and tyrosinase (TYR). Hum Mutat.
5. Henikoff S, Henikoff JG (1992) Amino acid substitution matrices from protein blocks. Proc Natl Acad Sci U S A 89:10915–10919.
6. Cargill M, Altshuler D, Ireland J, et al. (1999) Characterization of single–nucleotide polymorphisms in coding regions of human genes. Nat Genet 22:231–238.
7. Ng PC, Henikoff S (2006) Predicting the effects of amino Acid substitutions on protein function. Annu Rev Genomics Hum Genet 7:61–80.
8. Ramensky V, Bork P, Sunyaev S (2002) Human non-synonymous SNPs: server and survey. Nucleic Acids Res 30:3894–3900.
9. Tavtigian SV, Deffenbaugh AM, Yin L, et al. (2006) Comprehensive statistical study of 452 BRCA1 missense substitutions with classification of eight recurrent substitutions as neutral. J Med Genet 43:295–305.
10. Mathe E, Olivier M, Kato S, Ishioka C, Hainaut P, Tavtigian SV (2006) Computational approaches for predicting the biological effect of p53 missense mutations: a comparison of three sequence analysis based methods. Nucleic Acids Res 34:1317–1325.
11. Phelan CM, Dapic V, Tice B, et al. (2005) Classification of BRCA1 Missense Variants of Unknown Clinical Significance. J Med Genet 42:138–146.
12. Mirkovic N, Marti-Renom MA, Weber BL, Sali A, Monteiro AN (2004) Structure-based assessment of missense mutations in human BRCA1: implications for breast and ovarian cancer predisposition. Cancer Res 64:3790–3797.
13. Williams RS, Chasman DI, Hau DD, Hui B, Lau AY, Glover JN (2003) Detection of protein folding defects caused by BRCA1-BRCT truncation and missense mutations. J Biol Chem 278:53007–53016.
14. Carvalho MA, Monteiro AN (2007) Correction: Functional Analysis of BRCA1 M1628V Variant. J Med Genet. 44:e78.
15. Hoffmeyer S, Burk O, von Richter O, et al. (2000) Functional polymorphisms of the human multidrug-resistance gene: multiple sequence variations and correlation of one allele with P-glycoprotein expression and activity in vivo. Proc Natl Acad Sci U S A 97:3473–3478.
16. Drescher S, Schaeffeler E, Hitzl M, et al. (2002) MDR1 gene polymorphisms and disposition of the P-glycoprotein substrate fexofenadine. Br J Clin Pharmacol 53:526–534.

17. Goto M, Masuda S, Saito H, et al. (2002) C3435T polymorphism in the MDR1 gene affects the enterocyte expression level of CYP3A4 rather than Pgp in recipients of living-donor liver transplantation. Pharmacogenetics 12:451–457.
18. Ambudkar SV, Kimchi-Sarfaty C, Sauna ZE, Gottesman MM (2003) P-glycoprotein: from genomics to mechanism. Oncogene 22:7468–7485.
19. Salama NN, Yang Z, Bui T, Ho RJ (2006) MDR1 haplotypes significantly minimize intracellular uptake and transcellular P-gp substrate transport in recombinant LLC-PK1 cells. J Pharm Sci 95:2293–2308.
20. Kimchi-Sarfaty C, Oh JM, Kim I-W, et al. (2007) A "Silent" Polymorphism in the MDR1 Gene Changes Substrate Specificity. Science 315:525–528.
21. Kliman RM, Bernal CA (2005) Unusual usage of AGG and TTG codons in humans and their viruses. Gene 352:92–99.
22. De Gobbi M, Viprakasit V, Hughes JR, et al. (2006) A regulatory SNP causes a human genetic disease by creating a new transcriptional promoter. Science 312:1215–1217.
23. Larsen F, Gundersen G, Lopez R, Prydz H (1992) CpG islands as gene markers in the human genome. Genomics 13:1095–1107.
24. Carninci P, Sandelin A, Lenhard B, et al. (2006) Genome-wide analysis of mammalian promoter architecture and evolution. Nat Genet 38:626–635.
25. Wade PA, Gegonne A, Jones PL, Ballestar E, Aubry F, Wolffe AP (1999) Mi-2 complex couples DNA methylation to chromatin remodelling and histone deacetylation. Nat Genet 23:62–66.
26. Baylin SB (2005) DNA methylation and gene silencing in cancer. Nat Clin Pract Oncol 2 Suppl 1:S4–11.
27. Ehrich M, Field JK, Liloglou T, et al. (2006) Cytosine methylation profiles as a molecular marker in non-small cell lung cancer. Cancer Res 66:10911–10918.
28. Wang Y, Fan PS, Kahaleh B (2006) Association between enhanced type I collagen expression and epigenetic repression of the FLI1 gene in scleroderma fibroblasts. Arthritis Rheum 54:2271–2279.
29. Sekigawa I, Kawasaki M, Ogasawara H, et al. (2006) DNA methylation: its contribution to systemic lupus erythematosus. Clin Exp Med 6:99–106.
30. Post WS, Goldschmidt-Clermont PJ, Wilhide CC, et al. (1999) Methylation of the estrogen receptor gene is associated with aging and atherosclerosis in the cardiovascular system. Cardiovasc Res 43:985–991.
31. Jiang YH, Sahoo T, Michaelis RC, et al. (2004) A mixed epigenetic/genetic model for oligogenic inheritance of autism with a limited role for UBE3A. Am J Med Genet A 131:1–10.
32. Abdolmaleky HM, Cheng KH, Faraone SV, et al. (2006) Hypomethylation of MB-COMT promoter is a major risk factor for schizophrenia and bipolar disorder. Hum Mol Genet 15:3132–3145.
33. Dempster EL, Mill J, Craig IW, Collier DA (2006) The quantification of COMT mRNA in post mortem cerebellum tissue: diagnosis, genotype, methylation and expression. BMC Med Genet 7:10.
34. Zhao Z, Zhang F (2006) Sequence context analysis of 8.2 million single nucleotide polymorphisms in the human genome. Gene 366:316–324.
35. Pesole G, Mignone F, Gissi C, Grillo G, Licciulli F, Liuni S (2001) Structural and functional features of eukaryotic mRNA untranslated regions. Gene 276:73–81.
36. Mikulits W, Schranzhofer M, Beug H, Mullner EW (1999) Post-transcriptional control via iron-responsive elements: the impact of aberrations in hereditary disease. Mutat Res 437:219–230.
37. Chen JM, Ferec C, Cooper DN (2006) A systematic analysis of disease-associated variants in the 3' regulatory regions of human protein-coding genes II: the importance of mRNA secondary structure in assessing the functionality of 3' UTR variants. Hum Genet 120:301–333.
38. Mignone F, Grillo G, Licciulli F, et al. (2005) UTRdb and UTRsite: a collection of sequences and regulatory motifs of the untranslated regions of eukaryotic mRNAs. Nucleic Acids Res 33:D141–146.

39. Takabatake N, Shibata Y, Abe S, et al. (2006) A single nucleotide polymorphism in the CCL1 gene predicts acute exacerbations in chronic obstructive pulmonary disease. Am J Respir Crit Care Med 174:875–885.
40. Karim MA, Wang X, Hale TC, Elbein SC (2005) Insulin Promoter Factor 1 variation is associated with type 2 diabetes in African Americans. BMC Med Genet 6:37.
41. Ng DP, Canani L, Araki S, et al. (2002) Minor effect of GLUT1 polymorphisms on susceptibility to diabetic nephropathy in type 1 diabetes. Diabetes 51:2264–2269.
42. Morganti M, Ciantelli M, Giglioni B, et al. (2005) Relationships between promoter polymorphisms in the thymidylate synthase gene and mRNA levels in colorectal cancers. Eur J Cancer 41:2176–2183.
43. Visel A, Minovitsky S, Dubchak I, Pennacchio LA (2007) VISTA Enhancer Browser–a database of tissue-specific human enhancers. Nucleic Acids Res 35:D88–92.
44. Boyka Anachkova VDGR (2005) Nuclear matrix support of DNA replication. Journal of Cellular Biochemistry 96:951–961.
45. Kimiko M. Tsutsui KS, Ken Tsutsui (2005) Dynamic view of the nuclear matrix. Acta Med Okayama 59:113–120.
46. Milot E, Fraser P, Grosveld F (1996) Position effects and genetic disease. Trends Genet 12:123–126.
47. Zhang SB, Qian RL (2002) The interaction between the human beta-globin locus control region and nuclear matrix. Cell Res 12:411–416.
48. Ostermeier GC, Liu Z, Martins RP, et al. (2003) Nuclear matrix association of the human beta-globin locus utilizing a novel approach to quantitative real-time PCR. Nucleic Acids Res 31:3257–3266.
49. Kukreti R, C BR, Das SK, et al. (2002) Study of the single nucleotide polymorphism (SNP) at the palindromic sequence of hypersensitive site (HS)4 of the human beta-globin locus control region (LCR) in Indian population. Am J Hematol 69:77–79.
50. Sriroongrueng W, Schleiemacher E, Panich V, et al. (1997) Analysis of beta-thalassemia mutations and beta-locus control region hypersensitive sites 2, 3 and 4 in southern Thailand. Southeast Asian J Trop Med Public Health 28 (Suppl 3):120–127.
51. Liebich I, Bode J, Frisch M, Wingender E (2002) S/MARt DB: a database on scaffold/matrix attached regions. Nucleic Acids Res 30:372–374.
52. Berman HM, Olson WK, Beveridge DL, et al. (1992) The nucleic acid database. A comprehensive relational database of three-dimensional structures of nucleic acids. Biophys J 63:751–759.
53. Wang AJ, Quigley GJ, Kolpak FJ, van der Marel G, van Boom JH, Rich A (1981) Left-handed double helical DNA: variations in the backbone conformation. Science 211:171–176.
54. Crawford JL, Kolpak FJ, Wang AH, et al. (1980) The tetramer d(CpGpCpG) crystallizes as a left-handed double helix. Proc Natl Acad Sci U S A 77:4016–4020.
55. Lafer EM, Moller A, Nordheim A, Stollar BD, Rich A (1981) Antibodies specific for left-handed Z-DNA. Proc Natl Acad Sci U S A 78:3546–3550.
56. Krishna P, Fritzler MJ, Van de Sande JH (1993) Interactions of anti-DNA antibodies with Z-DNA. Clin Exp Immunol 92:51–57.
57. Alam K, Ali R (1992) Human autoantibody binding to multiple conformations of DNA. Biochem Int 26:597–605.
58. Thomas TJ, Meryhew NL, Messner RP (1990) Enhanced binding of lupus sera to the polyamine-induced left-handed Z-DNA form of polynucleotides. Arthritis Rheum 33:356–365.
59. Thomas TJ, Meryhew NL, Messner RP (1988) DNA sequence and conformation specificity of lupus autoantibodies. Preferential binding to the left-handed Z-DNA form of synthetic polynucleotides. Arthritis Rheum 31:367–377.
60. Herbert A, Lowenhaupt K, Spitzner J, Rich A (1995) Chicken double-stranded RNA adenosine deaminase has apparent specificity for Z-DNA. Proc Natl Acad Sci U S A 92:7550–7554.
61. Herbert AG, Spitzner JR, Lowenhaupt K, Rich A (1993) Z-DNA binding protein from chicken blood nuclei. Proc Natl Acad Sci U S A 90:3339–3342.

62. Schwartz T, Rould MA, Lowenhaupt K, Herbert A, Rich A (1999) Crystal structure of the Zalpha domain of the human editing enzyme ADAR1 bound to left-handed Z-DNA. Science 284:1841–1845.
63. Oh DB, Kim YG, Rich A (2002) Z-DNA-binding proteins can act as potent effectors of gene expression in vivo. Proc Natl Acad Sci U S A 99:16666–16671.
64. Liu R, Liu H, Chen X, Kirby M, Brown PO, Zhao K (2001) Regulation of CSF1 promoter by the SWI/SNF-like BAF complex. Cell 106:309–318.
65. Liu H, Mulholland N, Fu H, Zhao K (2006) Cooperative activity of BRG1 and Z-DNA formation in chromatin remodeling. Mol Cell Biol 26:2550–2559.
66. Champ PC, Maurice S, Vargason JM, Camp T, Ho PS (2004) Distributions of Z-DNA and nuclear factor I in human chromosome 22: a model for coupled transcriptional regulation. Nucleic Acids Res 32:6501–6510.
67. Garner MM, Felsenfeld G (1987) Effect of Z-DNA on nucleosome placement. J Mol Biol 196:581–590.
68. Kwon JA, Rich A (2005) Biological function of the vaccinia virus Z-DNA-binding protein E3L: gene transactivation and antiapoptotic activity in HeLa cells. Proc Natl Acad Sci U S A 102:12759–12764.
69. Schroth GP, Chou PJ, Ho PS (1992) Mapping Z-DNA in the human genome. Computer-aided mapping reveals a nonrandom distribution of potential Z-DNA-forming sequences in human genes. J Biol Chem 267:11846–11855.
70. Ho PS, Ellison MJ, Quigley GJ, Rich A (1986) A computer aided thermodynamic approach for predicting the formation of Z-DNA in naturally occurring sequences. Embo J 5:2737–2744.
71. Siddiqui-Jain A, Grand CL, Bearss DJ, Hurley LH (2002) Direct evidence for a G-quadruplex in a promoter region and its targeting with a small molecule to repress c-MYC transcription. Proc Natl Acad Sci U S A 99:11593–11598.
72. Rangan A, Fedoroff OY, Hurley LH (2001) Induction of duplex to G-quadruplex transition in the c-myc promoter region by a small molecule. J Biol Chem 276:4640–4646.
73. Hurley LH (2001) Secondary DNA structures as molecular targets for cancer therapeutics. Biochem Soc Trans 29:692–696.
74. Grand CL, Han H, Munoz RM, et al. (2002) The cationic porphyrin TMPyP4 down-regulates c-MYC and human telomerase reverse transcriptase expression and inhibits tumor growth in vivo. Mol Cancer Ther 1:565–573.
75. Htun H, Dahlberg JE (1988) Single strands, triple strands, and kinks in H-DNA. Science 241:1791–1796.
76. Voloshin ON, Mirkin SM, Lyamichev VI, Belotserkovskii BP, Frank-Kamenetskii MD (1988) Chemical probing of homopurine-homopyrimidine mirror repeats in supercoiled DNA. Nature 333:475–476.
77. Wang G, Vasquez KM (2004) Naturally occurring H-DNA-forming sequences are mutagenic in mammalian cells. Proc Natl Acad Sci U S A 101:13448–13453.
78. Kim EL, Peng H, Esparza FM, Maltchenko SZ, Stachowiak MK (1998) Cruciform-extruding regulatory element controls cell-specific activity of the tyrosine hydroxylase gene promoter. Nucleic Acids Res 26:1793–1800.
79. Bartel DP (2004) MicroRNAs: Genomics, Biogenesis, Mechanism, and Function. Cell 116:281–297.
80. Kim VN, Nam J-W (2006) Genomics of microRNA. Trends in Genetics 22:165–173.
81. Michalak P (2006) RNA world - the dark matter of evolutionary genomics. J Evol Biol 19:1768–1774.
82. Lagos-Quintana M, Rauhut R, Lendeckel W, Tuschl T (2001) Identification of novel genes coding for small expressed RNAs. Science 294:853–858.
83. Lau NC, Lim LP, Weinstein EG, Bartel DP (2001) An abundant class of tiny RNAs with probable regulatory roles in Caenorhabditis elegans. Science 294:858–862.
84. Lim LP, Glasner ME, Yekta S, Burge CB, Bartel DP (2003) Vertebrate microRNA genes. Science 299:1540.

85. Lim LP, Lau NC, Weinstein EG, et al. (2003) The microRNAs of Caenorhabditis elegans. Genes Dev 17:991–1008.
86. Mourelatos Z, Dostie J, Paushkin S, et al. (2002) miRNPs: a novel class of ribonucleoproteins containing numerous microRNAs. Genes Dev 16:720–728.
87. Rodriguez A, Griffiths-Jones S, Ashurst JL, Bradley A (2004) Identification of mammalian microRNA host genes and transcription units. Genome Res 14:1902–1910.
88. Krek A, Grun D, Poy MN, et al. (2005) Combinatorial microRNA target predictions. Nat Genet 37:495–500.
89. Lewis BP, Burge CB, Bartel DP (2005) Conserved seed pairing, often flanked by adenosines, indicates that thousands of human genes are microRNA targets. Cell 120:15–20.
90. Xie X, Lu J, Kulbokas EJ, et al. (2005) Systematic discovery of regulatory motifs in human promoters and 3' UTRs by comparison of several mammals. Nature 434:338–345.
91. Griffiths-Jones S (2004) The microRNA Registry. Nucl Acids Res 32:D109–111.
92. Griffiths-Jones S, Grocock RJ, van Dongen S, Bateman A, Enright AJ (2006) miRBase: microRNA sequences, targets and gene nomenclature. Nucleic Acids Res 34:D140–144.
93. Calin GA, Croce CM (2006) MicroRNA signatures in human cancers. Nat Rev Cancer 6:857–866.
94. Calin GA, Ferracin M, Cimmino A, et al. (2005) A MicroRNA signature associated with prognosis and progression in chronic lymphocytic leukemia. N Engl J Med 353:1793–1801.
95. He H, Jazdzewski K, Li W, et al. (2005) The role of microRNA genes in papillary thyroid carcinoma. Proc Natl Acad Sci U S A 102:19075–19080.
96. Krichevsky AM, King KS, Donahue CP, Khrapko K, Kosik KS (2003) A microRNA array reveals extensive regulation of microRNAs during brain development. RNA 9:1274–1281.
97. Abelson JF, Kwan KY, O'Roak BJ, et al. (2005) Sequence variants in SLITRK1 are associated with Tourette's syndrome. Science 310:317–320.
98. Chen K, Rajewsky N (2006) Natural selection on human microRNA binding sites inferred from SNP data. Nat Genet 38:1452–1456.
99. Cote F, Fligny C, Bayard E, et al. (2007) Maternal serotonin is crucial for murine embryonic development. PNAS 104:329–334.
100. Sladek R, Rocheleau G, Rung J, et al. (2007) A genome-wide association study identifies novel risk loci for type 2 diabetes. Nature 445:881–885.
101. Ornoy A (2005) Growth and neurodevelopmental outcome of children born to mothers with pregestational and gestational diabetes. Pediatr Endocrinol Rev 3:104–113.
102. DeBoer T, Wewerka S, Bauer PJ, Georgieff MK, Nelson CA (2005) Explicit memory performance in infants of diabetic mothers at 1 year of age. Dev Med Child Neurol 47:525–531.
103. Ornoy A, Ratzon N, Greenbaum C, Wolf A, Dulitzky M (2001) School-age children born to diabetic mothers and to mothers with gestational diabetes exhibit a high rate of inattention and fine and gross motor impairment. J Pediatr Endocrinol Metab 14 (Suppl 1):681–689.
104. Shakespeare W. "There are more things in heaven and earth, Horatio, Than are dreamt of in your philosophy." In: Hamlet Act 1 Scene V abt 1601.

Chapter 11
Predictive Biomarker Classifiers in the Design of Pivotal Clinical Trials

Richard Simon

Contents

Abstract In this chapter we distinguish the use of predictive biomarkers from surrogate endpoint biomarkers. We also distinguish the use of predictive biomarkers for selecting patients for pivotal clinical trials of a new drug from the use of predictive biomarkers for optimizing the utilization of an existing drug. We summarize the key steps in the development of predictive biomarker classifiers for use in new drug development. We discuss the design of targeted clinical trials in which a predictive biomarker classifier is used to restrict entry, and present results comparing the efficiency of targeted trials relative to standard randomized pivotal trials. We also discuss alternative designs in which the predictive biomarker classifier is not used to restrict entry of patients but is used to prospectively define an analysis plan for evaluating the new drug in classifier negative and positive patients. The development of predictive biomarker classifiers can be subjective, but pivotal trials should test hypotheses about the effectiveness of a new drug in subsets defined in a completely prespecified manner by a predictive classifier, and should not contain any subjective components. The data used to develop the predictive classifier should be distinct from the data used to evaluate a new drug in subsets determined by the classifier. The purpose of the pivotal trial is to evaluate the new drug in patient groups defined prospectively by the predictive classifier, not to refine or reevaluate the classifier or its components. New drug development should move from a correlative science mode to a predictive medicine mode.

Richard Simon
Biometric Research Branch, National Cancer Institute Bethesda, MD
rsimon@nih.gov

N. Cohen (ed.) *Pharmacogenomics and Personalized Medicine*,

Keywords Predictive biomarker, clinical trial design, gene expression, supervised classification, targeted clinical trial

1 What is a Predictive Biomarker?

A "biomarker" is any measurement made on a biological system. Biomarkers are used for very different purposes, and this often leads to confusion in discussions of biomarker development, use, and validation. In its most common usage, a biomarker is a measurement that tracks disease pace: increasing as disease progresses, holding constant as a disease stabilizes, and decreasing as disease regresses. There are many uses for such endpoint biomarkers in developmental studies for establishing proof of concept, dose selection, and identification of patients most suitable for inclusion in pivotal trials. In some cases there is also interest in using an endpoint biomarker in pivotal trials as a surrogate for clinical outcome. The standards for validation of a surrogate endpoint are stringent, however. It is not sufficient to demonstrate that the biomarker value is correlated with clinical outcome. It is necessary to show that treatment that impacts the biomarker value, also impacts clinical outcome. This requires analysis of a series of randomized clinical trials, showing that the differences in biomarker change between the randomized treatment groups are concordant with the differences in clinical outcome *(1–3)*. These standards are stringent because of the key role of the pivotal trial endpoint in claims. There are well known examples where biomarkers of disease pace were not valid surrogate endpoints of clinical outcome. Because of the stringency of the requirements for establishing a biomarker as a valid surrogate endpoint, it is often best to perform pivotal totals using standard measures of clinical outcomes as endpoints.

Biomarkers can be pretreatment measurements used to characterize the patient's disease in order to determine whether the patient is a good candidate for a treatment. These are called *predictive biomarkers*. The term *predictive* denotes predicting the outcome to a specific treatment. This is in contrast to *prognostic* biomarkers, which are correlated with the outcome of untreated patients or with the survival of heterogeneously treated patients. Most prognostic factor studies are based on convenience samples of patients for whom tissue is available. The studies are often not focused on a particular medical decision facing physicians, and hence the resulting prognostic factors identified have no therapeutic relevance and are not widely used. The greatest advantage of using tissue specimens derived from patients in a clinical trial is that it tends to restrict the study to a medical context from which therapeutically relevant biomarkers can be developed. The fact that patients in clinical trials are uniformly staged and adequately followed is an important bonus.

2 Development of Predictive Biomarker Classifiers

In this chapter we will focus on the use of predictive biomarker classifiers in the design of pivotal clinical trials. The term *classifier* indicates that the biomarker can be used to classify patients. We will generally be interested in classifying patients as either good candidates for the new drug or not good candidates, i.e., binary classifiers. If we were advising patients about their likelihood of benefit from a treatment, and probability of benefit or an index might be more informative than a binary classifier. The development of such a predictor would, however, require much more extensive data than generally available prior to performing the pivotal trial(s). We shall restrict ourselves here to binary classifiers that can be used to select patients for inclusion or exclusion from the pivotal trials.

Predictive binary classifiers can be of many types. The simplest might reflect, for example, the presence or absence of a point mutation in the EGFR gene, or amplification of the HER2 gene. At the other extreme, the binary classifier may be based on the expression levels of a large number of genes. In such cases, the component genes are generally selected for their correlation with response or patient outcome. The component genes do not themselves constitute the classifier. The individual gene expression levels must be combined in some mathematically determined manner.

There are two kinds of gene expression-based classifiers that are frequently used. The first is based on a weighted average of expression of the selected genes. A training set of data is used consisting of pretreatment expression levels for patients treated with the drug. The signature genes that are differentially expressed between the responders and nonresponders are identified. A weighted average of the expression levels for the signature genes is adopted as a predictive index. Many of the commonly used classifier types are based on such weighted averages. These include Golub's weighted voting classifier *(4)*, the compound covariate predictor *(5)*, Fisher's linear discriminant and diagonal linear discriminant analysis *(6)*, support vector machine with inner product kernel *(7)*, naive Bayes classifier *(8)*, and perceptrons *(9)*. The methods differ in how they define the weights. Using the training data to define the weights and threshold results in a completely specified binary classifier. The predictive accuracy of the binary classifier must be evaluated on a separate set of data. Using the same data to develop a classifier and evaluate its accuracy results in very misleading results unless special methods of complete cross-validation methods are used *(10)*. Unfortunately, cross-validation methods are used improperly in many cases *(11)*.

The second kind of binary classifier widely used for gene expression data is a nonparametric distance-based method, such as nearest neighbor, k-nearest neighbor, nearest centroid, and shrunken centroid classifiers *(6, 12)*. These methods also use signature genes selected on the basis of the correlation of their expression levels with response or outcome. A distance metric is adopted for measuring the similarity or dissimilarity between expression profiles with regard to the signature genes. Usually Euclidean distance or correlation distance is used. If a new patient is to be classified, one finds the training sample to which the new patient profile is most similar (smallest distance). That training sample is called the "nearest neighbor" of the profile of the new patient. If that nearest neighbor was a responder, then the new patient is predicted to be a responder; if the nearest neighbor was a nonresponder, then the new patient is predicted to be a nonresponder. The k-nearest neighbor algorithm is similar, except a majority vote of the classes of the k closest profiles to that of a new patient is used for prediction. Nearest centroid and shrunken centroid methods are similar. The comments made in the previous paragraph about the use of independent data to evaluate prediction accuracy apply equally to these nonparametric distance-based classifiers.

Although many other types of binary classifiers have been developed, and strong claims for them are often made by their developers, independent evaluations have generally concluded that other more complex methods rarely outperform weighted average-based methods or nonparametric distance-based methods. For any training set of data it is recommended here to develop weighted average-based or nonparametric distance based classifiers and use either complete cross-validation or a separate test set of data to evaluate the prediction accuracy of these methods. The BRB-Array Tools Software *(13)* provides a convenient integrated environment for identifying signature genes, developing weighted average- and nonparametric distance-based classifiers, and validly evaluating prediction accuracy. The software is available at http://linus.nci.nih./gov/brb. Additional details about the development of predictive biomarker classifiers based on gene expression data are available *(14–16)*.

3 Use of Predictive Biomarkers in the Design of Pivotal Trials

The objective of a pivotal clinical trial is to evaluate whether a new drug, given in a defined manner, has a medical utility in specified patient population groups. The role of a predictive biomarker classifier is to specify a population of patients. The process of biomarker classifier development may be exploratory and subjective, but the use of the classifier in the pivotal trial must not be. If the data from a pivotal trial is to be used to develop or refine a biomarker classifier, then treatment hypotheses involving that classifier should be tested in a separate pivotal trial. One exception is the adaptive trial of Friedlin and Simon *(17)*, where some data from a pivotal trial is used to develop a classifier, and that data is excluded from the data for that same pivotal trial that is used to test a treatment hypothesis in the subset of patients defined as positive by that classifier.

Figure 11.1 depicts the process of developing a predictive biomarker classifier and using it to restrict eligibility to a pivotal trial. The purpose of the study is to evaluate the new treatment regimen in classifier positive patients, not to validate the predictiveness of the classifier. If the treatment is shown to be effective and there is a reproducible assay for classifier positivity, then there is a medical usefulness in the treatment in classifier positive patients, even if the treatment hasn't been tested in classifier negative patients. In cases where the classifier is biologically based on the target of the drug, it may not be ethically appropriate to treat classifier negative patients. Whether the trial design shown in Figure 11.1 is sufficient for licensing the classifier itself is somewhat more complex and depends on the regulatory agency, specific regulatory language, and agency interpretations.

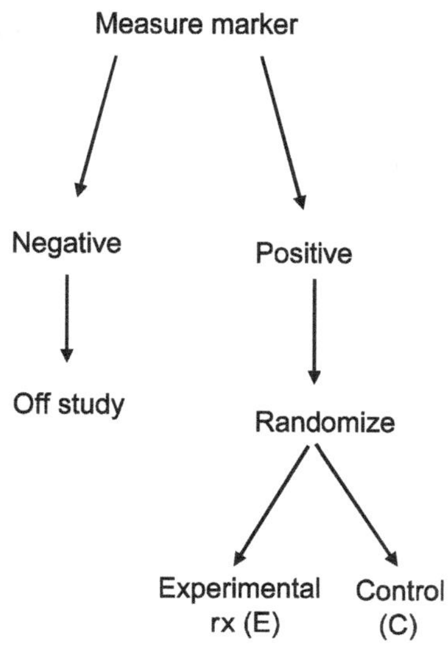

Fig. 11.1 Enrichment design

4 Efficiency of Targeted Designs

Simon and Maitournam *(18–20)* evaluated the efficiency of the targeted design shown in Figure 11.1 relative to the conventional broad randomization design, in which the classifier is not used to restrict entry. One measure of relative efficiency is the number of randomized patients required for the targeted design relative to the conventional design. A second measure of efficiency is the number of patients required for screening in the targeted design relative to the number required to randomize for the standard design. If n_T randomized patients are required for the targeted design, and γ_+ is the fraction of patients who are classifier positive, then approximately n_T/γ_+ patients are required to be screened for the targeted design. For example, suppose half as many patients are required for randomization with the targeted design as compared to the standard design, but only 25% of the patients are classifier positive. Then twice as many patients will be required for screening for the targeted design as for randomization with the standard design.

Relative efficiency of the targeted and standard designs depends on the specificity of benefit of the new treatment for classifier positive patients and the prevalence of the classifier positivity. The specificity of the treatment benefit can itself be broken down into the specificity of the treatment benefit for the biological state measured by the assay, and the measurement accuracy of the assay. For example, the biological state may be an amplification of a gene, and it is possible that the treatment benefit for a classifier negative patient results both from some treatment benefit in patients without the amplification and from the false negative assays for gene amplification. Usually there will not be separate estimates for these components of treatment specificity, and hence no real value in considering them separately in planning a pivotal trial. Here we will use the composite effect.

Simon and Maitournam*(18, 21)* showed that for binary endpoint trials, the ratio of the number of patients required for randomization in the standard trial compared to that in the targeted trial is approximately:

$$n_s / n_T \approx \left(\frac{1}{\gamma_+ + (1-\gamma_+)\delta_- / \delta_+} \right)^2 f, \qquad (1)$$

where γ_+ denotes the proportion classifier positive, and δ_-/δ_+ is the ratio of the treatment effect for classifier negative patients to the treatment effect for classifier positive patients. The parameter f is generally close to 1 unless the control response ratio is very low. In cases where the benefit of the new treatment is limited to classifier positive patients, $\delta_- = 0$ and the formula simplifies to f / γ_+^2. If the treatment is half as effective in classifier negative patients as classifier positive patients, then the formula simplifies to $4f/(\gamma_+ + 1)^2$. Table 11.1 shows the ratio of the number of randomized patients using the formula with $f = 1$.

Since the number of patients required to screen for the targeted trial is n_T / γ_+, the screened ratio of efficiency is:

$$n_s / screened_T \approx \frac{\gamma_+ f}{\left(\gamma_+ + (1-\gamma_+)\ \delta_- / \delta_+\right)^2}. \qquad (2)$$

If $\delta_- = 0$, this equals f/γ_+. If the treatment is half as effective for classifier negative patients as for classifier positive patients, then *(2)* equals $4\gamma_+ f/(\gamma_+ + 1)^2$. The screened ratio approximate efficiency for these two cases is also illustrated in Table 11.1.

When the proportion of classifier positive patients is less than one-half, the number of patients required for randomization in the targeted design is much

Table 11.1 Efficiency of targeted design

	$\delta_- / \delta_+ = 0$		$\delta_- / \delta_+ = .5$	
Proportion classifier positive	Randomized for standard design / Randomized for targeted design	Randomized for standard design / screened for targeted design	Randomized for standard design / Randomized for targeted design	Randomized for standard design / screened for targeted design
.5	4	2	1.8	0.89
.4	6.25	2.5	2.0	0.82
.3	11.1	3	2.4	0.71
.2	25	5	2.8	0.56
.1	100	10	3.3	0.33

smaller than for the standard design, at least by a factor of two, regardless of whether the treatment effect is completely specific for classifier positive patients or whether the classification negative patients benefit half as much as the positive patients. In the former case, however, the targeted design also requires many fewer patients to screen than are required for randomization with the standard design. If, however, the treatment effect for classifier negative patients is half that for the classifier positive patients, then the targeted design may require more patients to screen than are required for randomization with the standard design. Hence, this targeted design is most appropriate when the treatment benefit is expected to be quite specific for classifier positive patients. When the proportion of patients who are classifier positive exceeds 50%, the efficiency advantages of the targeted trial are reduced.

A web-based interactive program for planning targeted clinical trials is available at http://linus.nci.nih.gov/brb. It provides a comparison of the targeted design to the standard design with regard to the number of randomized and screened patients. It uses more accurate formulas than the approximations utilized above, and also provides a comparison for studies in which there is a time-to-event endpoint, such as survival or progression-free survival. Figure 11.2 shows a screen shot of the web page of input dialog for the time-to-event calculation. For the example shown, the median survival for the control group is 1 year, and 25% of the patients are classifier positive. For power calculations it is postulated that the new treatment reduces the hazard of death by 50% for the classifier positive patients and is ineffective for the classifier negative patients. A screen shot of the output of the program is shown in Figure 11.3. With an accrual of 100 patients per year and a follow-up period of two years after the end of accrual, a targeted trial of 4.27 years would randomize 107 target positive patients and achieve a power of 0.90. In contrast, an untargeted trial of 4.27 years of accrual would randomize 427 patients but have a statistical power of only 0.45, because the overall treatment effect is so diluted by the lack of treatment effect in the 75% of patients who are classifier negative. In this setting the targeted trial is very advantageous. If however, the treatment reduced the hazard of death by 20% for classifier negative patients, then the statistical power of the untargeted design after 4.27 years of accrual is 0.925, very similar to that of the targeted design (results not shown). In that circumstance, the targeted design is not advantageous. The targeted design is most valuable when the treatment benefit is limited to target positive patients and the assay for measuring the classifier is quite accurate.

5 Stratified Designs

Simon and Wang *(22)* have described clinical trial designs in which both classifier negative and classifier positive patients are randomized and the classifier is measured. In this case, it is important to have a predefined analysis plan for using the classifier information. It is not sufficient to merely "stratify" the randomization

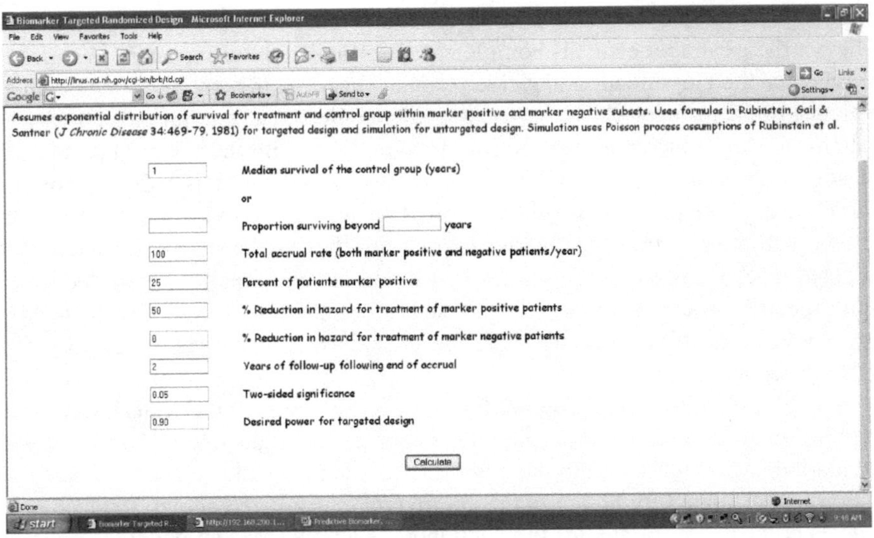

Fig. 11.2 Input screen for planning targeted design

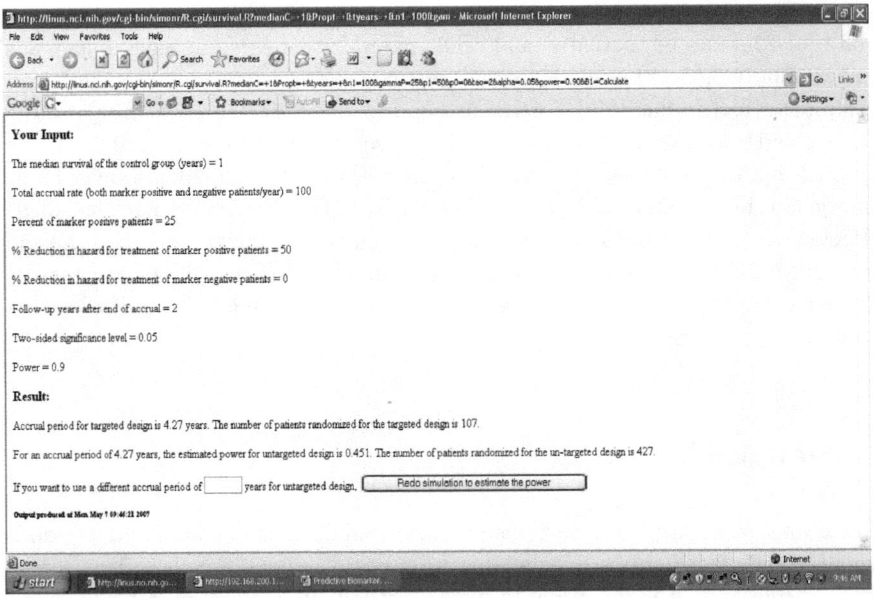

Fig. 11.3 Output of web-based program for planning targeted design

process by the classifier. Simon and Wang propose dividing the usual 5% type I error into a portion $\alpha_{overall}$ for comparing the treatment groups overall for all randomized patients, and a portion $.05-\alpha_{overall}$ for comparing the treatment groups in the predefined subset of patients who are classifier positive. The subset test would only be performed if the overall test is not significant at the reduced threshold $\alpha_{overall}$. A web-based interactive program for planning stratified clinical trials of this type is also available at http://linus.nci.nih.gov/brb.

References

1. Torri V, Simon R, Russek-Cohen E, Midthune D, Freidman M (1992) Relationship of response and survival in advanced ovarian cancer patients treated with chemotherapy. J Natl Cancer I 84:407.
2. Burzykowski T, Molenberghs G, Buyse M, Geys H, Renard D (2001) Validation of surrogate endpoints in multiple randomized clinical trials with failure time end points. J Roy Stat Soc C-App 50(4):405.
3. Korn EL, Albert PS, McShane LM (2004) Assessing surrogates as trial endpoints using mixed models. Stat Med 24:163–82.
4. Golub TR, Slonim DK, Tamayo P et al (1999) Molecular classification of cancer: class discovery and class prediction by gene expression modeling. Science 286:531–7.
5. Radmacher MD, McShane LM, Simon R (2002) A paradigm for class prediction using gene expression profiles. J Comput Biol 9:505–11.
6. Simon RM, Korn EL, McShane LM, Radmacher MD, Wright GW, Zhao Y (2003) Design and analysis of DNA microarray investigations. Springer, New York.
7. Ramaswamy S, Tamayo P, Rifkin R et al (2001) Multiclass cancer diagnosis using tumor gene expression signatures. Proc Natl Acad Sci U S A 98(26):15149–54.
8. Hand DJ, Yu K (2001) Idiot's Bayes—not so stupid after all? Int Stat Rev 69(3):385–98.
9. Khan J, Wei JS, Ringner M et al (2001) Classification and diagnostic prediction of cancers using gene expression profiling and artificial neural networks. Nat Med 7(6):673–9.
10. Simon R, Radmacher MD, Dobbin K, McShane LM (2003) Pitfalls in the analysis of DNA microarray data: class prediction methods. J Natl Cancer I 95:14–8.
11. Dupuy A, Simon R (2007) Critical review of published microarray studies for cancer outcome and guidelines on statistical analysis and reporting. (Submitted for publication) 99:147–57.
12. Tibshirani R, Hastie T, Narasimhan B, Chu G (2002) Diagnosis of multiple cancer types by shrunken centroids of gene expression. Proc Natl Acad Sci U S A 99(10):6567–72.
13. Simon R, Lam A, Li MC, Ngan M, Menenzes S, Zhao Y (2007) Analysis of gene expression data using BRB-ArrayTools. Cancer Informat 2:11–7.
14. Simon R (2003) Using DNA microarrays for diagnostic and prognostic prediction. Expert Rev Mol Diagn 3(5):587–95.
15. Simon R (2003) Diagnostic and prognostic prediction using gene expression profiles in high dimensional microarray data. Brit J Cancer 89:1599–604.
16. Simon R (2005) A roadmap for developing and validating therapeutically relevant genomic classifiers. J Clin Oncol 23:7332–41.
17. Freidlin B, Simon R (2005) Adaptive signature design: an adaptive clinical trial design for generating and prospectively testing a gene expression signature for sensitive patients. Clin Cancer Res 11:7872–8.
18. Simon R, Maitournam A (2004) Evaluating the efficiency of targeted designs for randomized clinical trials. Clin Cancer Res 10:6759–63.
19. Simon R, Maitournam A (2006) Correction & Supplement: Evaluating the efficiency of targeted designs for randomized clinical trials. Clin Cancer Res 12:3229.

20. Maitournam A, Simon R (2005) On the efficiency of targeted clinical trials. Stat Med 24:329–39.
21. Simon R, Maitnourim A (2006) Evaluating the efficiency of targeted designs for randomized clinical trials: Supplement and Correction. Clin Cancer Res 12:3229.
22. Simon R, Wang SJ (2006) Use of genomic signatures in therapeutics development. Pharmacogenomics J 6:1667–173.

Chapter 12
Translation of Biomarkers into Clinical Utility

William L. Trepicchio and George Mulligan

Contents

Abstract Biomarkers are an integral part of a successful clinical drug development strategy and the associated commercialization of drug development programs. Biomarkers are used as necessary and as they are available to optimize drug development in early and late stage clinical trials. Achieving the full value of biomarkers hinges on the ability to successfully translate them for clinical use. Translation involves validation of the biomarker assay, as well as qualification of the biomarker with its intended clinical endpoint. Biomarkers must be planned and developed in a timely fashion, in order to meet the needs of clinical drug development and product approval as appropriate. Biomarkers come in many flavors, based on their intended use during early or late stage clinical development. Pharmacodynamic biomarkers and disease-related biomarkers may be used in early clinical development to optimize go/no-go decisions and to aid in appropriate dose and/or schedule selection. Disease-related biomarkers and pharmacogenomic biomarkers may be used to optimize later clinical development by facilitating the recognition of more homogeneous patient populations. Furthermore, biomarker research may be performed during clinical trials to optimize the development of future products or to identify markers that can enhance the commercial value of current products post-launch. The implementation of biomarkers into clinical development strategies should lead to more efficient drug development and improve the benefit-to-risk ratio for patients.

William L. Trepicchio
Millennium Pharmacenticals, Cambride, MA
william.Trepicchio@mpi.com

N. Cohen (ed.) *Pharmacogenomics and Personalized Medicine*,

Keywords biomarkers, pharmacodynamics, pharmacogenomics, translational research, clinical trials

1 Introduction

1.1 Biomarker Classification

A biomarker associated with clinical development is a quantitative measurement including, but not limited to, an image, a protein, a nucleic acid sequence, a small molecule, or a physiologic or pathologic assay *(1)*. The measurement of a biomarker in clinical trials can employ any relevant technology. Rapid development of genomic technologies has advanced the concept of multimarker analysis, which in theory can increase the power and accuracy of biomarkers.

There are many types of biomarkers and they have been classified in different ways based on their clinical utility. A helpful classification is found in Table 12.1. This is not a complete list. Furthermore, absolute divisions between biomarkers cannot always be drawn. For example, pharmacodynamic (PD) biomarkers and disease biomarkers (DB) can also be pharmacogenomic (PGx) biomarkers, depending on their intended use.

For clinical and regulatory decision making purposes during drug development, it is essential to establish biomarkers that are precise, accurate, specific, and sensitive enough for their intended purpose. This "fit-for-purpose" approach involves validation of the biomarker assay as well as linkage of the biomarker to relevant biological and clinical endpoints. Linkage involves a graded evidentiary process, termed qualification *(2, 3)*. The degree of evidence required for qualification is based on the intended use of the biomarker. For example, biomarkers used for internal decision making purposes require less evidence of linkage than biomarkers used as surrogate clinical endpoints. During early development, the biomarkers must be rigorous enough for use, in order for them to stop a program. During later

Table 12.1 Biomarker classification

Biomarkers Related to Drug Action and Metabolism

- Pharmacodynamic biomarkers (PD)
- Pharmacogenomic biomarkers (PGx)
  - Biomarkers that measure genomic variations in a target or target related pathway in normal or disease tissue, thus allowing one to monitor or predict drug response
  - Biomarkers that measure genomic variation associated with toxicity
  - Biomarkers monitoring or predicting variation in drug metabolism

Biomarkers Related to Disease (Disease-related Biomarker—DB)

- Correlative to clinical endpoints
- Monitor or predict disease progression, improvement, severity, or complications
- Predict disease susceptibility

development, biomarkers, particularly ones that may lead to a diagnostic test, must be sufficiently qualified to pass regulatory evaluation. Surrogate endpoints are a subtype of DB that are the most rigorous disease-related biomarkers because they may substitute for clinical endpoints. However, surrogate endpoints are only occasionally available and have long development timelines.

2 Biomarker Use during Clinical Drug Development

Biomarkers may be employed in all stages of clinical drug development *(3, 4)*. Table 12.2 gives an over view of the use. This is discussed in detail below.

2.1 Pharmacodynamic Biomarkers (PD)

The biomarker for drug activity, or a pharmacodynamic marker, may be a clinical measurement which is evident from the mechanism of action of the drug *(5)*. This biomarker should be an in vivo measure of target function. The term "proof of mechanism" is used by some to describe this observation of target function. PD markers indicate which doses of drug and associated plasma levels are biologically active in vivo. These PD markers guide the search for which doses of drug are associated with therapeutic activity and improvement of disease-related endpoints. A reproducible, quantitative, and stable measure is characteristic of a PD which will provide the foundation for dose finding in patients.

The development of a pharmacodynamic biomarker should be highly feasible, based upon knowledge of the pathway in which the target resides. A literature review may reveal the existence of assays that might be useful as markers (e.g., phosphoERK inhibition as a indication of receptor tyrosine kinase blockade) *(6)*. If none is clearly available, then development of such a marker should be given a high priority 1 to 2 years before starting human studies.

Table 12.2 Use of biomarkers to optimize clinical drug development

Phase	Type of Marker
1	PD, (DB), PGx
2	
A	PD, DB, PGx
B	DB, PGx
3	DB, PGx
4	DB, PGx

2.2 *Disease-related Biomarkers (DB)*

DB refers to a broad range of markers of human disease. Therefore, in Table 12.1 the disease-related biomarker category may include genomic as well as many other different types of biomarkers, as described above. In early clinical development, biomarkers related to disease endpoints are necessary if early go/no-go decisions are to be made by the end of phase 2A.

The development of a DB may or may not be feasible, depending on the disease being studied. Therefore, established biomarkers for disease processes will be simpler to use, since they are more likely to have been previously evaluated and validated. PSA for prostate cancer is an example of a preexisting marker. In other instances, the PD marker may serve also as a DB marker. Occasionally, knowing how the drug is likely to modify the disease process will allow creative approaches for measurement. For example, a drug causes increased thermogenesis and is being tested as an antiobesity therapy *(7)*. A PD marker is a measurement of thermogenesis by indirect calorimetry in patients. However, increased thermogenesis causes weight loss by increasing calorie output. Increased calorie output is directly related to weight loss and is a DB biomarker.

Alternatively, it is possible that novel targets will require the establishment of new disease biomarkers. Such disease-related biomarkers may also be useful in later clinical development including late phase 2 and beyond (Table 12.1).

2.3 *Pharmacogenomic Biomarkers (PGx)*

Pharmacogenomics is a branch of science that attempts to explain variability of drug response and to search for the genetic basis of such variation at the individual and population levels *(8)*. It encompasses a range of biomarkers focused on drug targets and pathways and/or drug metabolism. Two seminal developments have highlighted the extensive genetic variation between individuals and within specific disease types. The first development was the sequencing of the human genome, and the second is the widespread use of DNA microarrays to quantify both gene expression and DNA variants across the genome. Some of this variation, in concert with environmental influences, can alter disease processes as well as give rise to differences in response to drugs. There may be genetic variation related to a disease or drug therapy that makes an individual more or less responsive to drug therapy. Pharmacogenomic readouts about specific effects of a disease or drug therapy include DNA genotyping, transcriptional profiling, and proteomic analysis *(9–11)*. Recent examples include her2/neu protein overexpression in breast cancer, response to trastuzumab (Herceptin) and EGFR mutations in non-small cell lung cancer, and response to EGFR antagonists such as gefitinib (Iressa) *(12–13)*.

Pharmacogenomics has been preceded by pharmacogenetics. Pharmacogenetics is defined as the study of inherited variations in drug effects *(14)*. The term pharmacogenomics reflects the evolution of pharmacogenetics into the study of the entire spectrum of genes (at the DNA, RNA, and protein level) that determine drug response, including the assessment of diversity of the human genome sequence and its clinical consequences. Pharmacogenetics can impact clinical development in a variety of ways to:

1. provide explanatory information on PK outliers that can lead to a "more informative drug label;"
2. provide correlative data to ADR's for more informed go/no-go decision making;
3. modify clinical trial design to:
   - address the problem of over- or under-representation of poor or ultra-rapid metabolizers in Phase I studies;
   - increase statistical power of early clinical trials that aim to compare PK data for poor and ultra-rapid metabolizers;
   - allow differential dosing for poor and ultra-rapid metabolizers.

An example of a pharmacogenetic biomarker is a genetic variant in the drug metabolizing enzyme, cytochrome p450 2D6 gene (CYP2D6). This variant causes inactivation of the CYP2D6 gene, leading to a poor metabolizer phenotype. Individuals who are homozygous for this variant and receive drugs predominantly metabolized by CYP2D6 have higher drug concentrations, which may lead to toxic side effects *(15)*.

It is noteworthy that up to 50% of variability in drug activity may relate to alterations in drug metabolism. Biomarkers relating to common variants of drug metabolizing enzymes may be used to delineate different patient populations during clinical drug development *(16)*.

3 Biomarker Translation

The translation of biomarkers for use in clinical drug development requires a strategic assessment of the biomarker need, if any, for each phase of development, and the appropriate selection, validation, and qualification of the type of biomarker that will achieve the objective *(17)*. Strategic planning for biomarkers assesses whether a clinical measurement is sufficient, whether an existing biomarker can do the job, or whether a biomarker must be discovered and a method for its measurement developed, validated, and qualified. For biomarker use in Ph1 and Ph2A, biomarkers must be discovered, validated, and qualified preclinically. The specific steps for this biomarker translation for an oncology drug candidate are outlined below using a hypothetical case study.

3.1 Strategic Assessment of Biomarker Needs

The biomarker needs for the development of a novel compound should be assessed early in the development life cycle, in many instances prior to lead selection. As part of the strategic biomarker assessment, a number of questions should be asked:

1. What are the current and future clinical development needs and limitations to effectively move a compound into the clinic and towards registration?
2. Are there any currently existing biomarkers that would facilitate these needs? If not, can biomarkers be discovered and validated in time to meet the clinical timelines?
3. What technologies (i.e., transcriptional profiling, whole genome SNP screening, proteomics, imaging) would be used to facilitate the discovery and use of biomarkers?
4. Are the right personnel and technologies available to perform these tasks?

Based on the answers to these questions, a research plan incorporating assay development, validation, and qualification for the biomarkers for all phases of development is established. This plan must be consistent with the needs and timelines of the clinical development plan.

3.2 *Preclinical Development (Prior to First-in-Man Studies)*

3.2.1 Mechanisms of Action and Pathophysiology Studies for Indication Selection

A challenge for the efficient development of a targeted oncology drug is the appropriate cancer indication selection. To facilitate indication selection, knowledge of the drug target and disease pathway in the context of target inhibition is essential. Preclinically, it is important to develop a thorough understanding of the mechanism of action (MOA) of the compound on the target and the target pathway, as well as an understanding of the pathophysiology of the target and pathway in relationship to the disease indication. A series of in vitro cell culture experiments and in vivo animal studies are initiated to carefully evaluate the mechanism of action of the compound and the linkage of the target and pathway to disease pathophysiology. This information is important for several reasons. First, it is critical for the development of PD, efficacy, and disease biomarkers. Second, in conjunction with future clinical outcome data, it can assist in second generation compound development and in issues management. Finally, it will be an essential component of regulatory filings.

As part of the identification and validation of the target and linkage of the target to disease pathophysiology, evaluation of human cell lines and primary tumor tissue determines that a somatic mutation in the drug target results in constitutive activation of the target through autophosphorylation. Further preclinical studies with mutated constructs confirm that this constitutive activation can lead to cellular transformation. Such findings in the BCR/Abl translocation in human chronic myelogenous leukemia (CML) facilitated the development of imatinib (Gleevec) *(18)*. In our hypothetical scenario, no data in the literature has previously described this mutation and its relationship to disease, therefore, an epidemiological study is devised to assess the frequency and distribution of this mutation in a broader cancer patient population and to determine if this mutation is a prognostic marker of disease.

Tumor material and patient outcome data is obtained from a variety of tumor types. These studies indicate that 40% of colorectal cancers exhibit this mutation. These data also suggest that patients with this mutation have inferior outcomes when compared to patients without the mutation. Mutations are also detected at lower frequency in other cancers. This information can guide the selection of colorectal cancer patients as a population to study early in the development of the compound. The high frequency of the mutation in this population would allow for relatively fast screening and entry of patients into randomized clinical trials. This strategy would allow for the most efficient development of the compound. Alternative tumor types harboring the mutation could be subsequently studied once proof of concept was established in colorectal cancer patients.

Given the prevalence of the mutation, it is decided that the compound will first be developed in the general colorectal cancer patient population and the mutation will be retrospectively correlated in Ph1/2 studies with response rates. This will allow risk/benefit to be assessed in the wild-type population. Based on the outcome of early efficacy studies, a decision can be made whether to test the drug in Ph3 in the general colorectal cancer population or only in the 40% of patients harboring the mutation. In the latter scenario, the presence of the mutation would serve as an entry requirement.

3.2.2 Pharmacodynamic Marker Development

For early clinical development, it is determined that a PD marker will be required to assess the optimal dose and schedule selection for this compound. In addition, since this is an unprecedented target, it is important to determine mechanistically that the compound is binding and inhibiting the target, as would be anticipated from in vitro and in vivo preclinical studies. As part of preclinical MOA studies, the autophosphorylation site on the target is proposed as a suitable PD marker. The compound should block this autophosphorylation, resulting in the inactivation of the target and reduction of the transformed phenotype. However, measuring changes in the phosphorylation state of this receptor has never been examined in humans. Issues such as intra- and inter-patient variability must be assessed. Therefore, studies are conducted to assess the clinical feasibility of this type of PD marker. Using in vitro cell culture assays as well as mouse xenograft studies, the appropriate reagents, controls, and conditions for assessing phosphorylation changes in this target in humans are developed. In addition, the target phosphorylation sites are assayed in cancer biopsies, including samples of colorectal cancer metasteses to the liver. Results from these studies are used internally to validate the assay and for future Ph1 protocol development.

3.2.3 Pharmacogenetic Biomarker

In vitro and in vivo studies to identify the mechanism of absorption, distribution, metabolism, and excretion (ADME) of the compound are conducted. The ADME studies have determined that the compound is partially metabolized by CYP2D6. This information is used to develop plans for assaying CYP2D6 polymorphisms in the Ph1/2 programs. Information obtained from Ph1/2 studies will be used to help explain PK variability if it is observed. It may also be used to insure that at least some patients containing slow or fast metabolizing phenotypes are enrolled in the Ph1 studies. If PK variability is extensive and correlates to slow or fast genotypes, future trials could be planned whereby such patients are excluded or stratified in the analysis.

3.2.4 Drug Sensitivity Markers

Clinical response rates in colorectal cancer are traditionally low. Observing statistically significant differences between treatment groups in small studies is difficult. Even when drugs are developed to specific molecular subpopulations, response rates never approach 100% *(19)*. Therefore, it would be desirable to have markers of efficacy that could be used to stratify patients during later clinical trials and increase the power of the studies. This would allow smaller clinical studies to be performed. However, identification of biomarkers that predict response to therapy prior to first-in-man clinical trials is challenging because response or nonresponse is an outcome that can be assessed only *after* treatment of patients with the drug.

A recent approach to the identification of genomic markers predictive of tumor sensitivity to drug treatment prior to first-in-man studies has been proposed *(20)*. In this approach, cell lines sensitive and resistant to the novel compound are identified and a series of global expression profiling studies are conducted to characterize the mechanistic reasons for response. An mRNA signature is identified that defines drug sensitivity in vitro. This signature is further validated in vivo using mouse xenografts. The signature is also assessed in primary human colorectal tumor tissue by expression profiling to assess the prevalence of the signature in the colorectal cancer population. Following these experiments, the measurement of this signature is incorporated into planned Ph2 studies to qualify the signature with patient outcome data. If successful, the signature can be used in planned Ph3 studies.

In addition to the identification of sensitive tumor signatures, molecular profiling studies can also serve to identify tumors that are potentially resistant to treatment. Such tumors may respond to other drugs or drug combinations. Recently, an approach was described to utilize large scale genomic datasets generated from cell lines treated with various common drugs, to identify drug or drug combinations that can reverse a resistant tumor genotype *(21)*. Such approaches can serve during drug development to identify potentially novel drug combinations that will provide the greatest treatment benefit.

An alternative or complementary approach is to evaluate the target under development for somatic mutations resulting in variability of response to treatment. Such mutations have been identified in the EGFR receptor and mediate the response to EGFR antagonists *(1)*. To understand if the novel target has drug sensitive mutations besides the activating mutations that lead to constitutive activation (as done in the earlier epidemiology study), the target sequence is evaluated in publicly available sequence databases. Only a few rare polymorphisms are identified with no functional consequence. However, sequencing of colorectal tumor material identifies two classes of somatic mutations clustering in two loop domains of the receptor within the compound binding site. To further evaluate the importance of these mutations, constructs containing the gene with various mutations introduced are prepared and transfected into cells to look at dose response relationships of the compound on the transfected constructs. It is determined that these somatic mutations have functional consequences in vitro. Class 1 is characterized by a decrease in the concentration of compound required to inhibit cellular growth by 50% (IC50), while class 2 is characterized by an increase. Further analysis of these classes indicates that a conformational change in the receptor results in a higher (class 1) or lower (class 2) binding potential for the compound.

The frequency of the mutations in the desired clinical indication are now required to be assessed in a larger patient population to determine if this will be a rare or frequent clinical observation. If class 1 is a relatively rare mutation, it can be managed during clinical development through patient selection or stratification, using the mutation as an efficacy biomarker. The patient's tumor material can be sequenced or genotyped for the mutation. If class 2 is a frequent mutation, selection of a backup compound with more desirable binding characteristics relative to the somatic mutations may be necessary. The mutation frequencies are further assessed statistically in a larger colorectal cancer patient population to further validate the biomarker. The mutation rate for class 1 is determined to be 15% of the intended treatment population. Class 2 mutations are found to be <5% of the population, deemed to be insignificant for drug development purposes, and are not pursued further at this point. This finding needs to be prospectively validated with clinical outcome data in a treated patient population in order for this information to be used to power the Ph 2/3 clinical studies. In addition, enrolled patients could be genotyped for the mutations and stratified according to the mutations as an efficacy endpoint. Examination of the mutation frequency in other cancer indications is also now warranted and will be pursued prior to starting clinical trials in those populations.

3.3 Early Clinical Development

3.3.1 Disease Biomarker Assay Development

A clinically feasible assay to identify the 40% of colorectal cancer patients carrying the mutated constitutively activated receptor is identified. It is determined that constitutive activation of the receptor correlates with protein overexpression as measured by the immunohistochemistry (IHC) of the tumor tissue. A reliable IHC test is developed and transferred to hospital labs to be used for enrollment of patients into the Ph1/2 trials. Primary tumor material will also be obtained for sequencing to confirm IHC studies.

3.3.2 Pharmacodynamic Studies in Ph1/2

The PD assay described above is incorporated into early Ph1/2 studies in colorectal cancer patients to assist in dose and schedule selection and validate the mechanism of action. The PD assay is configured as a Western blot. Prior to Ph1, the assay performance criteria are established and an appropriate lab to conduct the clinical assays is identified. The quantitative PD data obtained is evaluated for performance and accuracy and associated with the pharmacokinetic (PK) data to model future dose and schedule selection.

3.3.3 Pharmacogenetics

One role of pharmacogenetic profiling in early clinical trials is to ensure a representative population by inclusion of poor and ultrarapid metabolizers, who may be underrepresented or overrepresented in a randomly selected patient population. To achieve this, patients would have to be genotyped prior to enrollment in the study and then invited into the study in proportions equal to their population representation. Alternatively, it may be useful to *oversample* certain groups of metabolizers, so that sufficient statistical power is available to detect differences between groups. For example, if one phenotype is present at a low frequency, e.g., in 2 to 5% of the population, a company could screen the subjects to readjust the balance between the phenotype (e.g., include 20 poor metabolizers and 20 extreme metabolizers). In an alternative approach, the company could conduct two separate studies, essentially studying extensive metabolizers in a first trial at one dose, and then studying poor metabolizers in a second trial at a different dose.

3.3.4 Drug Sensitivity Biomarker Assessment

Phase 1 studies define a tolerable dose with PD activity. Based upon the epidemiological and preclinical data, colorectal cancer was the first cancer further evaluated in Ph1/2. Primary tumor tissue is collected from patients enrolled in the Ph1/2 studies and genotyped to clinically validate the class 1 efficacy mutations. Mutation status is correlated with clinical outcome data in the 100 patient Ph2 study. 10% of patients enrolled in the trial harbor the class 1 mutations, and the majority were either complete or partial responders to the compound. Tumor tissue from nonresponders did not harbor the class 1 mutations. 10% of patients without the mutations also responded to treatment. This information validates the preclinical findings and will be used to stratify patients in a pivotal Ph3 study.

Validation of the gene efficacy signature is also built into the Ph2 studies. Primary colorectal tumor tissue is obtained and sufficient RNA of suitable quality extracted. Results are correlated with patient response, time to progression, and survival. The preclinical studies estimated a test accuracy of 80%, but Ph2 data indicates only 60% accuracy in correlation to various treatment endpoints. This test will not be used for Ph3 studies.

3.4 Late Clinical Development

3.4.1 Efficacy Biomarker for Enrollment Criteria

Primary tumor tissue is assayed by IHC for overexpression of the drug target. This biomarker is used to enroll stage III/IV colorectal cancer patients who have failed two or more lines of previous therapy. This IHC test will be required to be codeveloped along with the drug.

Primary tumor tissue is obtained and assayed for the presence of class 1 mutations in the TK receptor. A clinically feasible assay is then established that can be conducted by an outside contract lab under GLP conditions. Incorporation of this patient selection biomarker into the trial design results in an increase in the power of the study without increasing the trial size.

The compound is originally developed in colorectal cancer patients who have failed previous therapies. However, the sensitivity and specificity of the patient selection biomarker is significant enough, and the clinical benefit of the drug in the selected population medically meaningful enough, to move this compound into frontline treatment of patients carrying the mutations. Regulatory authorities agree to allow the label of the drug to include frontline treatment in mutation positive patients as well as in all 2nd or 3rd line refractory patients, regardless of their mutation status.

3.4.2 Toxicity Markers

The drug is administered as an IV infusion, and during early Ph1/2 development a small subset of patients is observed to develop an idiosyncratic hypersensitivity reaction following reinfusion of the compound. It is hypothesized that this could be related to genetic variation in HLA genes similar to hypersensitivity reactions observed with the anti-HIV nucleoside reverse transcriptase inhibitor, abacavir (Ziagen) *(22)*. To further investigate the hypersensitivity reaction, DNA is collected from all patients to genotype for germline MHC class I polymorphisms. These studies from Ph3 and postmarketing studies show that haplotype mapping confirms a strong genetic association between the 57.1 ancestral haplotype and definite hypersensitivity to the compound, and help explain the observed adverse drug reaction. Further in vitro research indicates that the compound or its metabolites haptenates endogenous peptides presenting “altered self” in the context of the rare MHC haplotype.

This information can be used in regulatory updates, in 2nd-generation compound development, and to provide a plausible mechanistic explanation for this ADR.

4 Conclusions

Biomarkers are becoming an increasingly valuable tool for the efficient development of novel drug compounds. They have multiple uses during the drug development life cycle, but to be effectively utilized they must be sufficiently validated and qualified. One role of translational medicine is to insure that biomarkers are adequately identified early enough in the development process to have utility, and that they are "fit-for-purpose." Bringing together multiple stakeholders in the drug discovery process from discovery scientists, to assay development specialists, to clinical physician-scientists, will insure the appropriate translation from bench to bedside. This should lead to more efficient drug development, with the benefit of reduced drug costs as well as optimization of the benefit/risk ratio for patients most in need of these novel therapies.

References

1. Biomarkers Definitions Working Group (2001) Biomarkers and surrogate endpoints: preferred definitions and conceptual framework. Clin Pharmac Ther 69: 89–95.
2. Wagner JA, Williams SA, Webster CJ (2007) Biomarkers and surrogate end points for fit-for-purpose development and regulatory evaluation of new drugs. Clin Pharmacol Ther 81:104–7.
3. Trepicchio WL, Essayan D, Hall ST, Schechter G, Tezak Z, Wang SJ, Weinreich D, Simon R (2006) Designing prospective clinical pharmacogenomic (PG) trials: meeting report on drug development strategies to enhance therapeutic decision making. Pharmacogenomics J 6:89–94.
4. Trepicchio WL, Williams GA, Essayan D, Hall ST, Harty LC, Shaw PM, Spear BB, Wang SJ, Watson ML (2004) Pharmacogenomic data submissions to the FDA: clinical case studies. Pharmacogenomics 5:519–24.
5. Kwon, Y (2001) Handbook of essential pharmacokinetics, pharmacodynamics, and drug metabolism for industrial scientists. New York, Kluwer Academic/Plenum.
6. Sarker D, Workman P (2007) Pharmacodynamic biomarkers for molecular cancer therapeutics. Adv Cancer Res 96:213–68.
7. Sarac F, Pehlivan M, Celebi G, Saygili F, Yilmaz C, Kabalak T (2006) Effects of sibutramine on thermogenesis in obese patients assessed via immersion calorimetry. Adv Ther 23:1016–29.
8. Mendrick DL (2007) Current trends and strategic directions in the use of pharmacogenomics to identify translational biomarkers. Curr Opin Drug Discov Devel 10:37–42.
9. Hardiman G (2006) Microarrays technologies 2006: an overview. Pharmacogenomics 7:1153–8.
10. Tao F, Lazarev A (2007) Clinical proteomics: opportunities for diagnostics, pharmaceuticals and the clinical laboratory. Expert Rev Proteomic 4:9–11.
11. Giacomini KM, Brett CM, Altman RB, Benowitz NL, Dolan ME, Flockhart DA, Johnson JA, Hayes DF, Klein T, Krauss RM, Kroetz DL, McLeod HL, Nguyen AT, Ratain MJ, Relling MV,

Reus V, Roden DM, Schaefer CA, Shuldiner AR, Skaar T, Tantisira K, Tyndale RF, Wang L, Weinshilboum RM, Weiss ST, Zineh I (2007) The pharmacogenetics research network: from SNP discovery to clinical drug response. Clin Pharmacol Ther 81:328–45.
12. Bartlett JM (2005) Pharmacodiagnostic testing in breast cancer: focus on HER2 and trastuzumab therapy. Am J Pharmacogenomic 5:303–15.
13. Sequist LV, Bell DW, Lynch TJ, Haber DA (2007) Molecular predictors of response to epidermal growth factor receptor antagonists in non-small-cell lung cancer. J Clin Oncol 25(5):587–95.
14. Kalow W, Werner DM (1995) In: Scriver CR, Beaudet AL, Sly WS, Valle D (eds) Pharmacogenetics in the metabolic basis of inherited disease, 7th ed. New York, McGraw-Hill, pp 293–326.
15. Kirchheiner J, Seeringer A (2007) Clinical implications of pharmacogenetics of cytochrome P450 drug metabolizing enzymes. Biochim Biophys Acta 1770(3):489–94.
16. Lazarou J, Pomeranz BH, Corey PN (1998) Incidence of adverse drug reactions in hospitalized patients: a meta-analysis of prospective studies. JAMA 279(15):1200–1205.
17. Burczynski ME, Oestreicher JL, Cahilly MJ, Mounts DP, Whitley MZ, Speicher LA, Trepicchio WL (2005) Clinical pharmacogenomics and transcriptional profiling in early phase oncology clinical trials. Curr Mol Med 5(1):83–102.
18. Druker BJ (2002) Perspectives on the development of a molecularly targeted agent. Cancer Cell 1:31–6.
19. Vogel CL, Cobleigh MA, Tripathy D, Gutheil JC, Harris LN, Fehrenbacher L, Slamon DJ, Murphy M, Novotny WF, Burchmore M, Shak S, Stewart SJ (2001) First-line Herceptin monotherapy in metastatic breast cancer. Oncology 61(Suppl 2):37–42.
20. Bild AH, Potti A, Nevins JR (2006) Linking oncogenic pathways with therapeutic opportunities. Nat Rev Cancer 6:735–41.
21. Lamb J (2007) The connectivity map: a new tool for biomedical research. Nat Rev Cancer 7:54–60.
22. Martin A, Nolan D, Almeida CA, Rauch A, Mallal S (2006) Predicting and diagnosing abacavir and nevirapine drug hypersensitivity: from bedside to bench and back again. Pharmacogenomics 7:15–23.

Chapter 13
Pharmacogenomic Study Feasibility Assessment and Pharmaceutical Business Decision-Making

Monique Franc and Theresa Frangiosa

Contents

Abstract With the relatively short history of pharmacogenomics being applied in the context of the pharmaceutical industry, many questions and concerns (some legitimate, some not so legitimate) arise regarding the appropriate implementation of this technology to deliver the greatest value. Questions on how to make a decision about whether to embark on a given pharmacogenomic study, concerns around generating potentially uninterpretable results in a regulated environment, and uncertainty regarding the true business value and implications of this research are not uncommon. This chapter offers recommendations for a systematic approach to assessing the feasibility and the added value of pharmacogenomic studies in clinical trials. Specifically, the Multi-Attribute Decision Analysis (MADA) approach is described and tailored to the application of pharmacogenomics in industry. Particular attention is given to one attribute of the MADA, namely *Commercial Value and Risk.* A sensitivity analysis for assessing this attribute is presented by highlighting the potential impact of pharmacogenomic biomarkers on basic forecast factors. Since feasibility assessments must be tailored on a case by case basis, it is not realistic to offer a specific set of instructions that will apply to every possible situation. A number of examples are used to draw attention to some of the key points to consider. The overall intent is to help improve the probability of success of pharmacogenomics in the industry and to highlight the importance of education and cooperation among experts from a range of divergent functional areas.

Monique Franc
Johnson and Johnson Pharmaceutical, Research and Development, L.L.C.,
1000 Route 202, Raritan, NJ 08869
mfranc@prdus.jnj.com

N. Cohen (ed.) *Pharmacogenomics and Personalized Medicine*,

Keywords Pharmacogenomics, clinical trials, pharmaceutical industry, commercial, study feasibility, business decision-making, multi-attribute decision analysis (MADA), sensitivity analysis

1 Introduction

Many concerns have been raised as reasons not to pursue pharmacogenomic research in pharmaceutical development. Most notable is the apprehension that drugs would be "niched" to only a subset of the originally intended patient population and that this reduction in market share would lead to lost product sales. The loss of the blockbuster at the hands of pharmacogenomics is a key fear expressed by some marketers. Another concern is that pharmacogenomics would introduce regulatory risk to drug development programs owing to the potential uncertainty associated with the interpretability of the data. In addition, there continues to be skepticism about whether pharmacogenomics will ever result in tangible improvements to the drug development process and to the delivery of new products and patient care.

In an article by Stan Bernard, MD, MBA, entitled *The Five Myths of Pharmacogenomics (1),* the author notes that although there are commercial risks associated with the implementation of some pharmacogenomic strategies (like the loss of patients who are at risk for adverse events, and the loss of low/non-responders), there are also tremendous benefits, including earlier market introductions with faster approvals, recruitment of patients from less effective drugs, increased use in diagnosed but untreated patients, expansion of treatment to new subgroup/diseases, earlier/preventative use, enhanced patient compliance, and potential for higher pricing and reimbursement for best-in-class drugs. Whether the market share gains will outweigh the market share losses remains to be seen. Decisions about which pharmacogenomic studies to undertake in the context of the pharmaceutical industry are complex. Since the industry operates in a strictly regulated environment—i.e., regulated by health authorities such as the U.S. Food and Drug Administration (FDA), the European Medicines Agency (EMEA), and the Japan Ministry of Health, Labor and Welfare (MHLW), among others—and has obligations to stakeholders including patients, physicians, and stockholders, the benefits and risks of pharmacogenomic studies must be thoughtfully weighed, particularly if this research is being conducted within the context of an active drug development program. The pharmaceutical industry has relatively limited experience with this rapidly evolving science and the risks associated with undertaking this research are (or are perceived to be) higher than in the more familiar realm of conventional drug development.

2 Multi-Attribute Decision Analysis (MADA)

There are many factors that are important to ensuring that research studies having high benefit/risk ratios and high probability of success will be prioritized over others. These factors, some of which are interrelated, can be integrated into one overarching feasibility assessment that takes into account both scientific and business interests. One such assessment is the Multi-Attribute Decision Analysis (MADA) *(2, 3)* which captures and integrates, in a formal manner, the decision-making process of experts associated with a given field of interest. The MADA has been utilized in different ways for applications ranging from battlefield air interdiction to ecosystem management *(4, 5)*. As it applies to pharmacogenomics in pharmaceutical development, the MADA captures the decision-making process of experts in the areas of genetics, clinical pharmacology, statistics, commercial/marketing, legal, and regulatory affairs. The MADA is a decision-making method that identifies and integrates objective information (e.g., data, calculated forecasts) and subjective information (e.g., judgments, predictions, estimations, opinions) for a set of predefined attributes. It incorporates both qualitative and quantitative elements and works to clearly represent and to formally and systematically assess the important aspects of a decision-making situation. In general, it is ill-advised to make unstructured and informal assumptions about the feasibility of potential pharmacogenomic studies, but rather to count on the MADA to "do the work" by structuring the communication and integrating all relevant information such that a reasoned and information-driven decision can be reached. The intent of the MADA is to guide a decision in the presence of uncertainty.

In developing a MADA analysis for assessing the feasibility of pharmacogenomic opportunities, pharmaceutical organizations may consider proceeding with the following steps 1) identifying the potential opportunities, 2) selecting key attributes (factors for comparing among opportunities) and assigning weights to the importance of those attributes (relative to the others), 3) qualitatively evaluating the opportunities for each attribute using relevant criteria for evaluation, and 4) assigning quantitative scores to each evaluation. The details of this procedure are elaborated below, although it is recognized that there may be a number of variations to the MADA concept.

Step 1. Identifying Potential Opportunities. The first step in the MADA analysis involves the high-level identification of potential research opportunities. For pharmacogenomics, these opportunities generally will fall under four broad categories of relevance i) efficacy ii) safety iii) pharmacokinetics, and iv) mechanistic/disease. The specific opportunities (i.e., studies or projects) are primarily driven by the existing or anticipated clinical issues associated with a drug (or drug class) and/or by the near- and long-term therapeutic focus of a pharmaceutical organization. Table 13.1 shows some generic examples of potential opportunities for a hypothetical drug. It is recommended that the decision-making body remain as liberal as possible in Step 1 of the MADA analysis. It has been the experience of the authors that potential opportunities that appear improbable at first intuition can often migrate to the top of the priority list after undergoing a formal MADA analysis. An open mind is important at all stages of the MADA, but this is particularly true in the earliest stages.

Step 2. Defining the Multiple Attributes and Criteria for Evaluation. The next step in the MADA involves the defining of the Multiple Attributes. The attributes are the key factors to consider in deciding which opportunities (identified in Step 1) have the most promise and are worth undertaking. The primary attributes that are relevant to pharmacogenomic studies conducted in industry include i) scientific

Table 13.1 Examples of potential pharmacogenomic research opportunities for a hypothetical drug (MADA Step 1)

Category	Pharmacogenomic Opportunity
Efficacy	Identification of responders (defined by primary or secondary efficacy endpoints)
	Identification of extreme (robust) responders
	Identification of refractory patients (extreme non-responders) (non-robust responders)
	Rescue of secondary indication for which there was insufficient efficacy
Safety	Identification of markers for QT prolongation/shortening
	Identification for markers for alanine aminotransferase (ALT) elevations
	Identification of markers for class-effect adverse events (e.g., tardive dyskinesia for antipsychotics)
Pharmacokinetics	Identification of genetic factors that contribute to variability in pharmacokinetics
Mechanistic/Disease	Evidence to support or identify the mode of action
	Evidence to support or identify the isozymes involved in the metabolism of a drug in humans
	Identification of novel drug targets
	Identification of disease sub-types

and technical feasibility, ii) cost and resources, iii) timelines, iv) deliverables added value, and v) commercial and regulatory impact (see Table 13.2). These attributes encompass both scientific and business interests. A weight which reflects the importance of these attributes (relative to the others) can also be applied (see Step 4). For example, if cost/budget is a limitation that cannot be overcome, this attribute would factor heavily into the final decision. However, if cost is no object, but regulatory risks are high (e.g., the drug is nearing registration), then the regulatory risk attribute would be weighted more heavily. The total relative weights for the attributes add up to 100. These weights are predefined, fixed values that are applied equally to all projects undergoing the MADA analysis.

Step 3. Qualitative MADA Evaluation. The next step in the MADA involves a detailed qualitative evaluation of each attribute for each potential opportunity, which is accomplished by entering objective and subjective information for each attribute (Table 13.3). These analyses obviously will vary depending on specific study objectives, but can be guided by the criteria for evaluation presented in Table 13.2. With attributes defined by these criteria, a MADA can provide a thorough qualitative assessment for most pharmacogenomic opportunities.

"Hard numbers" can be applied to some criteria, while informed judgment is necessary for others. Hard numbers could include outputs from i) sophisticated forecasting models to explore "what if" scenarios and the expected impact on existing product forecasts, ii) statistical power calculations for various pharmacogenomic study designs, iii) available funding, and iv) technology options and their associated costs, among others. The subjective input could come from i) a broad review of the landscape, which can heavily influence the understanding of what is feasible, as well as the goals of competitors in a targeted therapeutic area; ii) reviews of the existing peer-reviewed scientific literature; and iii) identification of active or emerging

Table 13.2 Attributes and corresponding criteria for evaluation for a MADA analysis of pharmacogenomic studies (MADA Step 2)

Attribute	Criteria for Evaluation
Scientific/Technical Feasibility	How many samples are available or could become available? Are there sufficient samples for a validation study? What is the power to detect an association (statistical feasibility)? What is the level of scientific understanding of the phenotype (phenotype definition and heterogeneity, multigenic phenotype, pre-existing knowledge of pathway, mechanism, etiology)? What are the confounding factors (co-medication, history, ethnicity, etc.)? What are the available technologies and what are their limitations? What are the alternative approaches that might better address the issue?
Cost and Resources	What will be cost of acquiring and analyzing samples? What are the required human resources (FTEs)? Whare are the potential opportunities for collaboration?
Timelines	At what stage is the product in its lifecycle and is there sufficient time to deliver validated results? What is the potential impact on launch date?
Deliverables and Added Value (short and long-term)	*Clinical*: Optimization of trial design, rescue of compound/indication, etc. *Drug Discovery*: Identification of novel pathways/compounds *Commercial*: Diagnostic, pricing, differentiation from competitors identification of mode of action, information for the label (informative or prescriptive) *Regulatory*: Respond to regulatory questions or concerns, etc. *Other*: Company image, ethical obligations, corporate values, publication, etc.
Commercial and Regulatory Impact	Is the compound in early or late development or is it a marketed compound? Are the samples anonymized? Is the endpoint safety or efficacy related? Will other pre-market, marketed, or follow-up compounds be impacted by any findings?

consortia, competitors' pharmacogenomic activities, academic/hospital center interests, and available technologies that can prompt an organization to think "offensively" or "defensively" as it considers project selection. A sample output of a qualitative MADA analysis for a hypothetical drug is presented in Table 13.3.

Step 4. Quantitative MADA Evaluation. The final step of the MADA involves assigning a quantitative score to each attribute. By assessing the opportunities on their commercial, technical, scientific, and regulatory attributes, a numerical value or "score" that is a composite of risk and benefit can be assigned to each outcome. Table 13.4 shows a representative output of the quantitative component of a MADA, showing the attributes, the weight assigned to each attribute, and the attribute scores for five hypothetical pharmacogenomic studies in a drug development program. The project scores for each attribute are multiplied by the weighting factor and added together to generate a total weighted average score. For example, the weighted total score of 380 for the drug response study in this example was obtained through the following calculation: $[(4 \times 40) + (10 \times 3) + (10 \times 3) + (40 \times 4)]$. In this example, the disease genetics project quantitatively emerges as the best project to pursue. It should be recognized that it may

Table 13.3 Sample output of the qualitative MADA evaluation (MADA Step 3)

Attribute	Project: Efficacy - Identification of Responders
Scientific/Technical Feasibility	Sample size n = 950 (current). Additional samples n = 560 (within 12 months). Statistical power 85% for biomaker discovery phase. Multiple targets/pathways likely, each contributing to the overall effect. More challenging to dissect genetically. Confounding factors affecting efficacy: i) previous and concomitant medications, ii) ethnicity. No strong hypotheses for candidate genes. Some weak candidates available from pre-clinical. Discrete phenotypic endpoint: easy to measure.
Cost and Resources	Funding: $1MM. Genome-wide DNA Chip technology (several platforms available). In-house platform also available, although less coverage. Possibility of additional funding. Human resources: laboratory, data analysis, and project managment available (5 FTEs/year). NME-specific project therefore collaborators/consortia not applicable.
Timelines	Drug is in Late Development: <3 years to registration. Sufficient time for exploratory and validation studies prior to registration if initiated soon.
Deliverables and Added Value (short and long-term)	*Clinical*: Stratification of future trials. Potential rescue strategy if overall efficacy is insufficient. *Drug Discovery:* By-product of study may be the identification of novel pathways. *Commercial*: Differentiation from branded and generic competitors. Possible vehicle for additional exclusivity. *Regulatory*: Demonstrate commitment to novel research. *Other*: Alignment with company commitment to deliver effective therapies. Ethical obligations.
Commercial and Regulatory Impact	Data not anonymized. Likelihood of results resulting in prescriptive labeling is very low. Late development (i.e., <3 years to registration) greater potential risk to compound.

Table 13.4 Sample output of a quantitative MADA evaluation (MADA Step 4)

		Score for Each Potential Study				
Attribute	Weight of Attribute (%)	Drug Response	Adverse Event A	Adverse Event B	Mode of Action	Disease Genetics
Scientific/Technical Feasibility	40	4	4	4	3	4
Cost and Resources	10	3	4	4	3	4
Timelines	10	3	4	4	2	5
Commercial and Regulatory Impact	40	4	2	1	3	4
Weighted average score	100	380	320	280	290	410

Example scores for:

- Scientific feasibility: 5 = highly feasible, 0 = not feasible
- Cost and resources: 5 = inconsequential, 0 = prohibitive
- Timelines: 5 = timed to complete much in advance of requirement for commercialization of product, 0 = cannot be completed in needed timeframe
- Commercial and regulatory impact 5 = highly attractive, 0 = highly unattractive

not always be necessary to select one study to the exclusion of others. There may be significant overlap among studies in terms of the genes and samples to be analyzed, and it is often possible (and advisable) to "piggy-back" studies where possible.

3 Sensitivity Analysis for the Commercial Attribute of the MADA

Of the MADA attributes presented above, further explanations are provided for the Commercial Impact attribute to serve as an example. The score for the Commercial Impact attribute in the MADA can be driven by a classical sensitivity analysis. The purpose of this analysis is to assess the impact of pharmacogenomic findings on sales forecasts for a drug under investigation. It is an intricate process that involves building scenarios, assigning probabilities to those scenarios, and estimating their impact on sales forecast factors and requires the skills of a Commercial expert. In addition to the drug under investigation, sensitivity analyses should also be conducted on any marketed compounds and/or followup compounds in the pipeline that potentially could be affected by these pharmacogenomic findings. For example, it is conceivable that the identification of an efficacy biomarker for Drug X in development could affect sales (either in the positive or negative direction) of the company's already-marketed compound, Drug Y, in the same therapeutic area.

3.1 Forecast Factors

There are several basic sales forecast factors that can be influenced by pharmacogenomic findings:

- **Diagnosis rate** represents the proportion of patients correctly diagnosed with a given disease or disorder. Diagnosis rates vary from disorder to disorder. Disorders such as diabetes or bipolar disorder have historically gone under- or mis-diagnosed. An increase in diagnosis rates can have a significant impact on sales forecasts for both disease diagnostics and for drugs used to treat these diseases (or disease subtypes).
- **Treatment rate** represents the proportion of patients treated with a particular drug for a given indication. Treatment rate can be significantly influenced by available therapies. Generally, more serious disorders (e.g., cancer) will have higher treatment rates, presumably since patients cannot go without therapy (assuming therapy has sufficient benefit to warrant the risks associated with treatment). For less serious conditions (e.g., acid reflux), treatment rates may be lower since the drive to initiate treatment is less strong. A biomarker that could identify subjects who are most likely to benefit from a treatment could potentially increase the proportion of subjects that will be treated, since the drug therapy will be working in these individuals.

- **Market share** is a product's share of the sales of all products with which it competes in a given therapeutic area. Market share can have a very significant impact on sales forecasts. For example, the gain of 1 share point in a $15B market can equal $150M. Any marker that can increase market share even by a small amount would significantly increase sales; the reverse is also true.
- **Compliance** represents the number of days a patient remains on therapy. Compliance is largely dictated by how well a drug works, its side effects, and the recognition of the seriousness of the disorder. For example, drugs for congestive heart failure are taken more days of the year than those to treat mild depression, since, in the former instance, not remaining on the drug could have grave and immediate consequences; whereas in the latter case, not maintaining regular therapy may have more modest and gradual consequences. If a predictive diagnostic can identify patients who are likely to respond, it is likely that patients who respond well will remain on therapy longer. This could potentially increase the average days of therapy for a key product and is particularly relevant for chronic conditions where compliance is often an issue.
- **Dosing assumptions** are the assumptions made about the dose or dose range that is expected to be therapeutically effective in the average intended population. However, the average dose may not always work for every patient. Biomarkers used for dosing can influence sales forecasts, since higher doses can be more expensive (for the patient or payer). For this reason, it is very important to payers that the most appropriate dose be determined prior to product launch. Assuming linear pricing (e.g., 1mg = 1$, 2mg = 2$, 3mg =3$), if patients are receiving higher doses as a result of a pharmacogenomic biomarker, sales will increase, and vice versa. Furthermore, by ensuring appropriate dosing, treatment would be expected to be more efficacious, with potentially fewer side effects, thus improving compliance and consequently sales forecasts.
- **Pricing** is the action of assigning a price that is indicative of the perceived value of the product. Since pricing decisions are made at the time of launch, the best time to define the intended patient population, and price a drug accordingly, is well in advance of the launch. A pharmacogenomic biomarker that helps to define the specific patient population (e.g., patients with overexpression of HER2 necessary for Herceptin® therapy) or that is used to characterize the novelty of the mode of action of a drug could have an influence on pricing and therefore sales forecasts.
- The **assumed launch date** is the anticipated date of launch of the product in the market following registration. To the extent to which regulatory approvals may be fast-tracked with an expedited approval, an organization could potentially gain access to sales six months to a year earlier, leading to further benefits of building on a higher base of sales over the life of the product.

In conducting a sensitivity analysis, the above points should be considered under a variety of relevant scenarios. Examples of such scenarios could be i) labeling requiring the use of a diagnostic test prior to treatment (prescriptive labeling) versus informative labeling, or ii) a label warning versus precautionary information in the label for a known drug side effect. Market share and compliance are key variables that might change under these scenarios. The likelihood of gaining or losing share should be examined thoroughly. Additionally, diagnosis and treatment rate fluctuations can be associated with changes to current treatment paradigms. Further, price and time to launch are relevant for products that have not yet launched (highlighting the benefit of long-range planning). Each project undergoing the commercial feasibility assessment can be evaluated in all of these dimensions. The information that is fed into the sensitivity analysis can be captured in a series of tables containing estimates for various scenarios. Table 13.5 is an example of one such table that contains estimated values for the impact of a biomarker on market share—in this case, as a result of changes in market perception brought about by the biomarker (described below).

3.2 *Impact of a Biomarker on Market Share (An Example)*

"Market perception" refers to how health care providers perceive the efficacy and safety of a drug (whether new or existing). This perception can be influenced by the existence of a biomarker. The adjustment of pre-existing perceptions to the actual reality that the biomarker affords can result in share increases or decreases. Table 13.5 highlights the variables affecting share calls for two different scenarios. In this analysis of the impact of a propensity to side effect A, two potential regulatory outcomes have been envisioned and outlined in the first column. Here, it is assumed that there is a 96% probability that any additional labeling will be informative and a 4% probability that labeling information will result in a restriction to prescribing

Table 13.5 Estimated values for the impact of a biomarker on market share as a result of changes in market perception brought about by a biomarker (example for validated biomarker for hypothetical adverse event A). Base case = 18.0% of market share

		Share calls Impact of Biomarker on Market Perception		
Scenarios	Biomarker Positive/ Negative	Biomarker Worsens Market Perception	Biomarker Does not Change Market Perception	Biomarker Improves Market Perception
		Min/Most Likely/Max	Min/Most Likely/Max	Min/Most Likely/Max
Scenario 1: Prescriptive Labeling (total estimated probability 4%)	Probability of Scenario 1	1%	1%	2%
	Biomarker Positive	2.7 / 6.7 / 8.0	4.0 / 8.0 / 10.7	6.7 / 10.7 / 14.6
	Biomarker Negative	12.0 / 14.6 / 16.6	12.6 / 15.3 / 17.3	13.3 / 16.0 / 18.4
Scenario 2: Informative Labeling (total estimated probability 96%)	Probability of Scenario 2	32%	31%	33%
	Biomarker Positive	11.1 / 12.4 / 15.0	13.7 / 17.7 / 17.8	18.0 / 18.4 / 18.6
	Biomarker Positive	16.4 / 17.7 / 18.0	18.2 / 18.4 / 18.6	18.4 / 18.6 / 18.9

practices (i.e., prescriptive labeling). Three possible outcomes on market perception have been defined: the biomarker will identify patients with a side effect A that is either i) aligned with market perception for the brand (i.e., does not change a health care provider's opinion of the drug), ii) better than those expectations (e.g., allows a health care provider to recognize that the adverse event occurs less frequently than he/she originally perceived), or iii) worse than those perceptions (e.g., emphasizes that the frequency of the adverse event is actually higher than he/she had originally perceived). Probabilities for these potential outcomes on market perception are assigned to each scenario. In this example, it is estimated that there is a 2% probability that a biomarker for side effect A will result in prescriptive labeling that will also improve market perception and thus market share (Table 13.5), and a 33% probability that the biomarker will also result in informative labeling that will improve market perception. The impact of the biomarker on market share (i.e., share calls) was estimated according to three categories: lowest possible share call/most likely share call/highest possible share call (i.e., Min/Most Likely/Max—in the table), and further segregated into shares of responders who tested positive for the biomarker versus those who tested negative. These numerical values are estimates generated from informed knowledge. The use of marketing research to inform thinking around potential changes to market share assumptions is recommended, when possible. The share calls are estimated relative to an existing forecast (i.e., base case) which is 18.0% in this example, which does not discern between responders and nonresponders, since a biomarker does not exist for the base case. If a biomarker was available to predict patients at risk for side effect A (i.e., biomarker-positive patients), for the scenario of prescriptive labeling and worsened market perception, the market share for the biomarker-positive subjects was estimated to range from 2.7% (in the worst case) to 6.7% (in the most likely case) to 8.0% (in the best case). The market share for the population that was biomarker-negative would remain higher, estimated in this instance to range from 12.0% (in the worst case) to 14.6% (in the most likely case) to 16.6% (in the best case). This example focuses on market share; however, the same concept can be applied to other forecast parameters (e.g., compliance rates).

3.3 Commercial Risk of Not Undertaking a Pharmacogenomic Study

It is important to estimate changes to forecast assumptions fairly and without bias. Therefore, an organization should also consider the commercial risk of not embarking on certain pharmacogenomic studies, in the context of key advances being made by competitors in this area. In other words, if a competitor markets a diagnostic to predict responders, or to identify individuals who are predisposed to a certain side effect, what will the availability of a drug-linked diagnostic do to the market share of other agents in that class? The development and communication of a corporate vision for the future of pharmacogenomics and clarity regarding competitor interests, can be important drivers in helping an organization to understand what is at stake by not moving forward with key pharmacogenomic opportunities.

4 Output of a Sensitivity Analysis

Once scenarios are outlined, probabilities are assigned, and changes to forecast assumptions (such as market share and compliance) are estimated for each proposed pharmacogenomic study, a simulation approach such as the Monte Carlo simulation can generate the probabilities of reaching or exceeding the current forecast for a product. The output of this analysis is a comprehensive listing of all potential outcomes (e.g., share increasing / decreasing) arising from various scenarios entered into the sensitivity analysis. Table 13.6 and Figure 13.1 serve to illustrate some ultimate outcomes of a sensitivity analysis for two different drugs. In Table 13.6, three opportunities were evaluated for their ability to at least achieve the base case forecast (last column), with the reality that some scenarios would potentially result in not achieving the existing forecast. The table shows the forecast of peak year revenues for the product with and without a pharmacogenomic component. The base case (no pharmacogenomic component) forecast is $1,006,000,000. For Study 1, the mean forecast with a pharmacogenomic component resulting from all scenario combinations is $1,153,000,000. The bottom 10% of these scenarios resulted in a forecast of $1,007,000,000 (essentially equal to the base case), whereas the top 10% of scenarios resulted in a forecast of $1, 404,000,000. In other words, for Study 1, every scenario results in the capacity to equal or exceed the forecast.

In Figure 13.1, a visual depiction of the output of another sensitivity analysis highlights the fact that many (but not all) scenarios (occurring at greater than $1,186,205,000) result in revenues significantly greater than the base case forecast have a high probability of occurrence. These outputs can be used to assign a score to the Commercial Impact (Risk/Benefit) attribute of the MADA.

There are certainly a number of different methods to assess the commercial feasibility of pharmacogenomic studies conducted in the pharmaceutical industry. The methods described above can be useful in charting a course of proposed pharmacogenomic work. Perhaps less risky opportunities make sense as organizations gain

Table 13.6 Example of an output from a sensitivity analysis: summary of impact on sales for drug X for three potential pharmacogenomic opportunities. Base case compared to mean, bottom 10%, and top 10% of scenarios and probabilities of not achieving the base case

	Peak Year Revenue ($000,000s)				
PGx Opportunities	Base Case (no PGx)	With PGx (Mean)	With PGx (Bottom 10%)	With PGx (Top 10%)	Probability of not Achieving Base Case
Study 1		1,153	1,007	1,404	0%
Study 2	1,006	949	590	1,251	36%
Study 3		967	891	1,023	67%

Numerical Distribution of Sales Potential (year 2009)

Percentile	Forecast values (000s)
0%	$421,830
10%	$695,833
20%	$789,522
30%	$870,921
40%	$1,198,372
50%	$1,211,531
60%	$1,238,491
70%	$1,286,014
80%	$1,336,710
90%	$1,472,813
100%	$1,889,972

Graphical Depiction

Base Case 2009 Sales: $1,186,205,000

2009 Sales Forecast

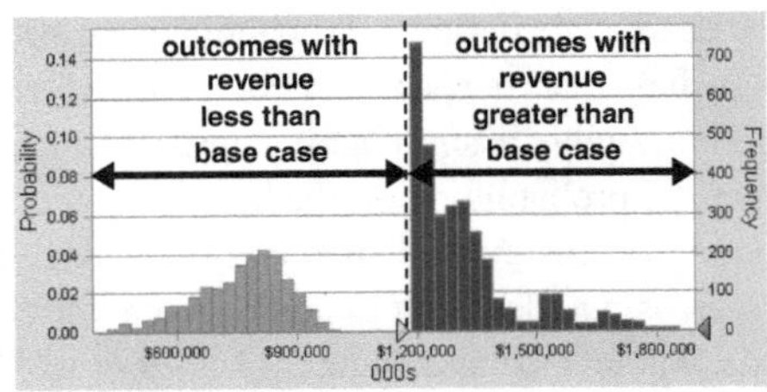

Fig. 13.1 Example of an output from a sensitivity analysis: summary of forecasted impact on sales for a hypothetical pharmacogenomic study

experience in pharmacogenomic work. On the other hand, the fact that biomarker work must be duplicated (i.e., validated) to be considered legitimate allows for some exploration before any impact to a forecast would be realized. Nevertheless, commercial organizations must be comfortable with the impact on their business of the development of drug-linked diagnostics. Because pharmacogenomic work can have a business impact, starting as early as possible in the compound development can allow an organization to strategically drive its business.

5 Conclusion

The fear of the loss of blockbusters, concerns around potential regulatory risks to drug development programs, and skepticism about the true value that pharmacogenomics will bring to the pharmaceutical industry are likely to linger as organizations continue to gain experience with this field and as the regulatory framework for this research continues to grow. In the industry context, the responsibility for pharmacogenomic strategy development cannot lie solely with the pharmacogenomic scientist. It is essential that input come from a range of areas of expertise, including clinical pharmacology, statistics, commercial/marketing, legal, and regulatory affairs, among others. Unfounded, unstructured, and informal assumptions about the feasibility or value of pharmacogenomic studies are reckless and should be avoided. Applying a systematic and integrated approach to assessing feasibility and added value will help to improve the likelihood of success and ultimately contribute to the establishment of pharmacogenomics as a core component of pharmaceutical drug development.

Acknowledgments Special thanks to Joshua Adelson and Steven Peterson for their significant contributions to the development of MADA models as they apply to pharmacogenomic studies in the pharmaceutical industry.

References

1. Bernard S (2003) The five myths of pharmacogenomics. Pharm Exec (October issue).
2. Mollaghasemi M, Pet-Edwards J (1997) Technical briefing: making multiple-objective decisions. IEEE Computer Society Press, Los Altimos, CA.
3. Yoon KP, Hwang C (1995) Multiple attribute decision making: an introduction. Sage Publications, Thousand Oaks, CA.
4. Prato T (1999) Multiple attribute decision analysis for ecosystem management. Ecol Econ 30(2):207–22.
5. Whitney R, Wilson J (1981) Multi-attribute decision analysis approach to the development of a computerized aid to mission planning (MADCAMP) [Master's Thesis].

Chapter 14
Co-Development of Drugs and Pharmacogenomics-Based Diagnostics in Oncology

Jeffrey S. Ross

Contents

Abstract The molecular diagnostic industry continues to grow at a double-digit pace to meet increasing demand for the integration of diagnostic procedures with the selection of therapy, and the development of personalized drugs whose administration is guided by test results. Newly developed anticancer drugs are targeted to tumor-specific gene and protein signatures that may ultimately require co-approval of diagnostic and therapeutic products by the regulatory agencies. At the same time, an increasingly educated public using the Internet and other resources are demanding more and more information about their specific forms of cancer and how they might be arrested or cured with new therapies custom-designed for their individual clinical status. To respond to this demand, major pharmaceutical companies will either partner with diagnostics companies or develop their own in-house capabilities allowing them to efficiently produce more effective and less toxic integrated personalized medicine *"drug and test"* products. For diagnostic laboratories, surgical pathologists, functional imagers, and oncologists, this integration of diagnostics and therapeutics represents a major new opportunity to further advance cancer care as a paradigm of the new medicine based on the use of test results for drug selection, dosage, route of administration, and multidrug combinations.

Keywords cancer, pharmacogenomics, transcriptional profiling, review

---

Jeffrey S. Ross
Department of Pathology and Laboratory Medicine, Albany Medical College, Albany, NY
rossj@mail.amc.edu

N. Cohen (ed.) *Pharmacogenomics and Personalized Medicine*,

1 Introduction

The regulatory approvals in the United States and Europe of trastuzumab (Herceptin®) for the treatment of HER2 overexpressing metastatic breast cancer (Figure 14.1) and imatinib mesylate (Gleevec®) for the treatment of patients with bcr/abl translocation positive chronic myelogenous leukemia and gastrointestinal stromal tumors featuring an activating c-*kit* tyrosine kinase growth factor receptor mutation created a new awareness for anticancer targeted therapy in both the scientific and public communities *(1, 2)*. Major news articles, the world-wide web and public media have highlighted these anticancer drugs that exploit disease-specific genetic defects as the target of their mechanism of action *(3, 4)*. It is anticipated that the integration of molecular oncology and molecular diagnostics will further revolutionize oncology drug discovery and development; customize the selection, dosing, and route of administration of both previously approved traditional agents and new therapeutics in clinical trials; and individualize medical care for the cancer patient *(5–8)*.

2 Targeted Therapies for Cancer

From the regulatory perspective, targeted therapy has been defined as a drug in whose approval label there is a specific reference to a simultaneously or previously approved diagnostic test that must be performed before the patient can be considered eligible to receive that specific drug. The co-approvals of the anti–breast cancer antibody trastuzumab (Herceptin®) and the required tissue-based tests for patient eligibility (Herceptest®, Pathway®, and Pathvysion®) are examples of this strict definition of targeted therapy. However, for many scientists and oncologists, anticancer drugs are considered to be "targeted" when they feature a focused mechanism that specifically acts on a well-defined target or biologic pathway that, when inactivated, causes regression or destruction of the malignant process. Examples of this less rigorous definition of targeted therapy include hormonal-based therapies for breast cancer, small-molecule inhibitors of the epidermal growth factor receptor (EGFR), blockers of invasion and metastasis enabling proteins and enzymes, antiangiogenesis agents, proapoptotic drugs, and proteasome inhibitors. Finally, another definition of targeted therapy involves anticancer antibody therapeutics that seek out and kill malignant cells bearing the target antigen.

3 The Ideal Target

The ideal cancer target (Table 14.1) can be defined as a macromolecule that is crucial to the malignant phenotype and is not significantly expressed in vital organs and tissues; that has biologic relevance that can be reproducibly measured in readily obtained clinical samples; that is definably correlated with clinical outcome; and

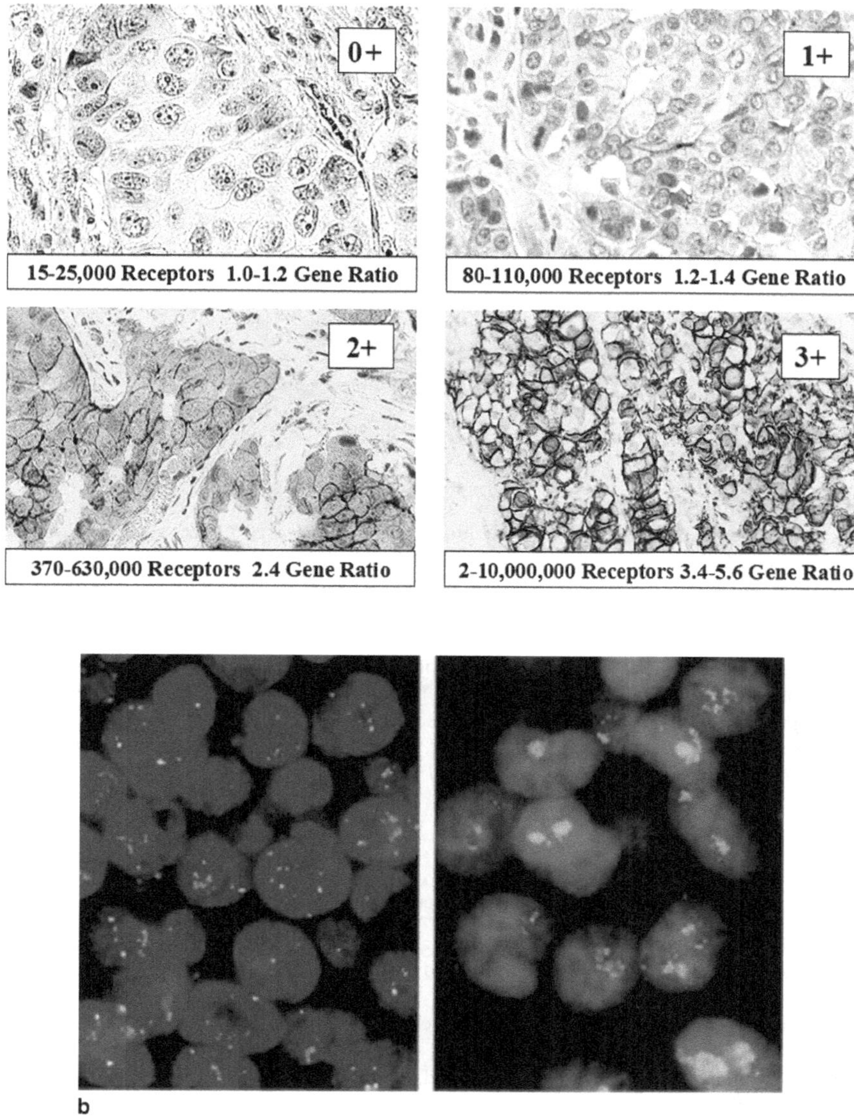

Fig. 14.1 HER-2/neu protein expression in infiltrating ductal breast cancer measured by immunohistochemistry using the Herceptest™ Slide Scoring System. **Upper Left:** 0+ (negative) staining for HER-2/neu protein. This level of staining is typically associated with 15,000–25,000 surface receptor molecules per cell and HER-2/*neu* gene copy to chromosome 17 copy ratios measured by FISH of 1.0 to 1.2. **Upper Right:** 1+ staining associated with 80,000–110,000 receptors and gene ratio of 1.2 to 1.4. **Lower Left:** 2+ staining with membranous distribution, but no total cell encirclement associated with 370,000–630,000 receptors and gene ratio of 1.4 to 2.4. **Lower Right:** 3+ staining with diffuse positive membranous distribution, total cell encirclement and "chicken wire" appearance associated with 2,000,000–10,000,000 receptors and gene ratio of 3.4 to 5.6. (peroxidase/antiperoxidase with Herceptest™ antibody X 200). [Receptor count and FISH gene ratio data provided by Dr. Kenneth Bloom, USLabs, Inc., Irvine, CA.]

(continued)

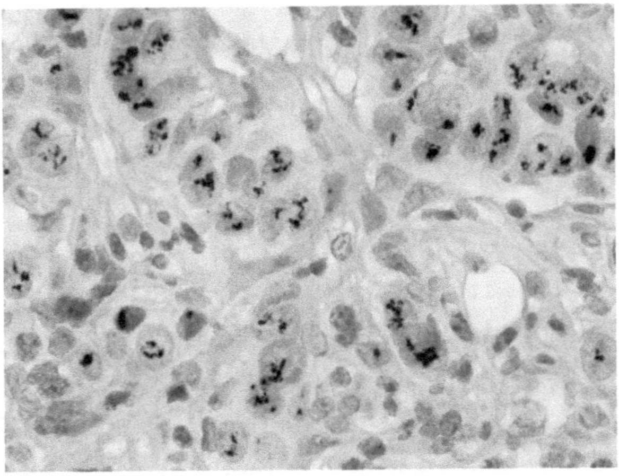

C

Fig. 14.1 (continued) **B**. HER-2/*neu* gene amplification in infiltrating ductal breast cancer detected by fluorescence in situ hybridization (FISH). **Left:** HER-2/*neu* gene amplification demonstrated by the Abbott-Vysis Pathvysion™ method showing significant increase in HER-2/*neu* gene signals (red) compared to chromosome 17 signals (green) with a HER-2/*neu* gene ratio of 3.9. **Right:** HER-2/*neu* gene amplification using the Ventana Inform™ method showing another breast cancer specimen with an absolute (raw) HER-2/*neu* gene copy number of 24. **C.** HER-2/*neu* gene amplification in infiltrating breast cancer detected by chromogenic in situ hybridization (CISH) using anti-HER-2/*neu* probe and IHC with diaminobenzidine chromagen (SpotLight™ HER-2/*neu* probe, Zymed Corp., South San Francisco, CA). *[Reprinted from Ross JS, Hortobagyi GH, eds., The molecular oncology of breast cancer. Sudbury, MA: Jones and Bartlett, Inc., with permission by the publisher]*

Table 14.1 Features of the ideal anti-cancer target

- □ Crucial to the malignant phenotype
- □ Not significantly expressed in vital organs and tissues
- □ A biologically-relevant molecular feature
- □ Reproducibly measurable in readily obtained clinical samples
- □ Correlated with clinical outcome
- □ When interrupted, interfered with, or inhibited, the result is a clinical response in a significant proportion of patients whose tumors express the target
- □ Responses in patients whose tumors do not express the target are minimal

[Reprinted from Ross JS, Hortobagyi GH, eds., The molecular oncology of breast cancer. Sudbury, MA: Jones and Bartlett, Inc., with permission by the publisher.]

the interruption, interference, or inhibition of which yields a clinical response in a significant proportion of patients whose tumors express the target, with minimal to absent responses in patients whose tumors do not express the target. For antibody therapeutics, additional important criteria include the use of cell surface targets that, when complexed with the therapeutic naked or conjugated antibody, internalize the antigen–antibody complex by reverse pinocytosis, thus facilitating tumor cell killing.

4 The First Diagnostic-Therapeutic Combination in Cancer Therapy: Hormonal Therapy for Breast Cancer

Targeted therapy for cancer began in the early 1970s with the introduction of the estrogen receptor (ER) biochemical assay to select patients with painful metastatic breast cancer for surgical ablation of estrogen-producing organs (ovaries, adrenals) (Figure 14.2) *(9)*. The ER assay was followed by a similar dextran-coated charcoal biochemical assay for the progesterone receptor (PR) and subsequently converted to an immunohistochemistry (IHC) platform, when the decreased size of primary tumors associated with self-examination and mammography-based screening programs prevented the use of the biochemical test *(10)*. The drug tamoxifen (Nolvadex®), which has both hormonal and nonhormonal mechanisms of action, has been the most widely prescribed antiestrogen for the treatment of metastatic breast cancer and chemoprevention of the disease in high risk women *(11, 12)*. Although ER and progesterone receptor testing is the front line for predicting tamoxifen response, additional biomarkers, including HER-2/neu (HER-2) and cathepsin D testing, have been used to further refine therapy selection *(13)*. The introductions of specific estrogen response modulators and aromatase inhibitors such as anastrozole (Arimidex®), letrozole (Femara®), and the combination chemotherapeutic, estramustine (Emcyt®)*(14–18)* have added new strategies for evaluating tumors for hormonal therapy.

Most recently, the Oncotype Dx® (Genomic Health, Redwood City, CA) multigene RT-PCR multiplex assay, using a 21-gene probe set and mRNA extracted from paraffin blocks of stored breast cancer tissues, was introduced as a new guide to the use of tamoxifen in ER positive node negative breast cancer patients *(19)*. The assay features 16 cancer-related genes and 5 reference genes that were selected based on a series of transcriptional profiling experiments. The cancer-related genes include markers of proliferation such as Ki-67; markers of apoptosis such as survivin; invasion associated protease genes such as MMP11 and cathepsin L2, ER, and HER2/*neu* gene family members; the glutathione S transferase genotype M1; CD68, a lysosomal monocyte/macrophage marker; and BAG1, a co-chaperone glucocorticoid receptor associated with bcl-2 and apoptosis. Using a cohort of 688 lymph node negative, ER+ tumors obtained from patients enrolled in the NSABP B-14 clinical trial treated with tamoxifen alone, the 21-gene assay produced three prognosis scores of low, intermediate, and high risk. The recurrence rates for these patients at ten years follow-up was 7% for the low risk, 14% for the intermediate risk, and 31% for the high risk groups. The difference in relapse rates between the

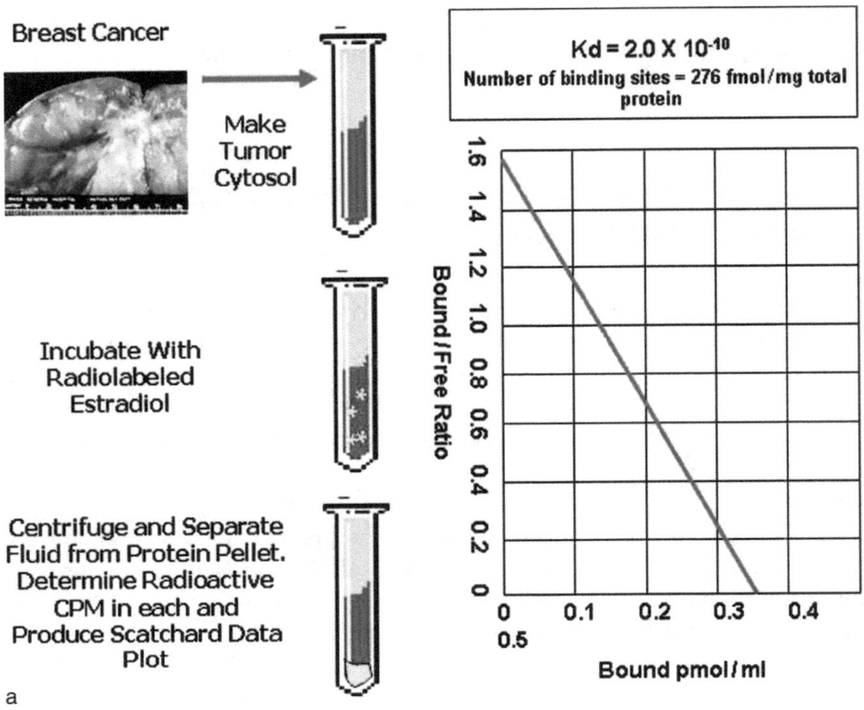

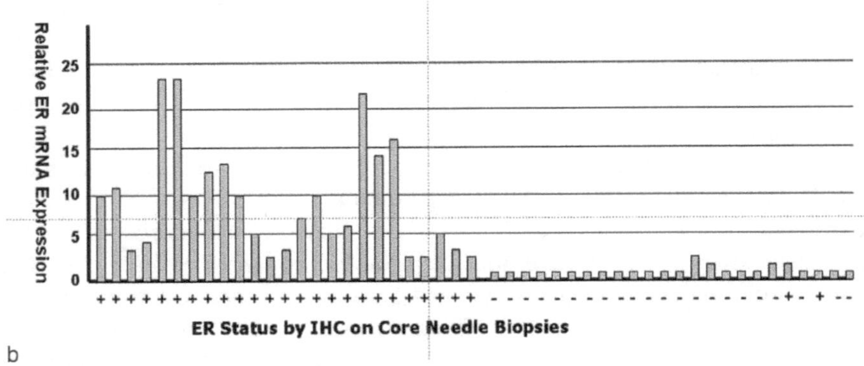

Fig. 14.2 ER status determination. **(A)** Comparison of ER messenger RNA expression detected by microarray profiling and corresponding ER protein expression measured by IHC. The concordance between ER levels determined by IHC and ER levels determined by gene expression profiling was about 95%. **(B)** Genes expressed in ER-positive cases. **(C)** Genes expressed in ER-negative cases. *[Reprinted from Ross JS, Hortobagyi GH, eds., The molecular oncology of breast cancer. 2004. Sudbury, MA: Jones and Bartlett, Inc., with permission by the publisher]*

low risk and high risk patients was highly significant ($p < 0.001$). On multivariate analysis this assay predicted adverse outcome independent of tumor size and also predicted overall survival *(19)*. Although not currently approved by the FDA, the interest in this new assay has been intense and it has become commercially available in a centralized format for new patients. Recent data presented at the 2005 ASCO Meeting showed that the Oncotype Dx® is also capable of performing as a stand-alone prognostic test based on the test results in an untreated patient population *(20)*. Detailed evaluation of the gene set in the Oncotype Dx® assay indicates that the mRNA levels of ER appear to be the most significant predictors in the node-negative ER- (IHC) positive population. Further studies are needed to validate the assay and learn its best uses and limitations, given the evolving approach to hormonal therapy with non-tamoxifen drugs, the wide use of cytotoxic agents in the adjuvant setting for node-negative patients, and the availability of both RT-PCR based and non-RT-PCR approaches to predicting breast cancer response to anti-estrogen and other anti-neo-plastic agents used for treatment of the disease *(21)*. In current practice, unlike breast cancer, the routine testing of tumor samples for androgen receptor status has not been incorporated into the selection of hormonal therapy for the disease.

5 Diagnostic-Therapeutic Combinations for Leukemia and Lymphoma

The introduction of immunophenotyping for leukemia and lymphoma was followed by the first applications of DNA-based assays, the polymerase chain reaction, and RNA-based molecular technologies in these diseases that complemented continuing advances in tumor cytogenetics *(22, 23)*. In addition to the imatinib (Gleevec®) targeted therapy for chronic myelogenous leukemia, other molecular targeted therapy in hematologic malignancies includes the use of all-*trans*-retinoic acid (ATRA) for the treatment of acute promyelocytic leukemia *(24)*; anti-CD20 antibody therapeutics targeting non-Hodgkin lymphomas, including rituximab (Rituxan®) *(25)*; and the emerging Flt-3 target for a subset of acute myelogenous leukemia patients (see below) *(26)*.

6 HER-2 Positive Breast Cancer and Trastuzumab (Herceptin®)

After the introduction of hormone receptor testing, some 30 years then elapsed before the next major targeted cancer chemotherapy program for a solid tumor was developed. In the mid 1980s, the discovery of the *HER-2* (c-*erb*B2) gene and protein and subsequent association with an adverse outcome in breast cancer provided clinicians with a new biomarker that could be used to guide adjuvant chemotherapy *(27)*. The development of trastuzumab (Herceptin®), a humanized monoclonal antibody designed to treat advanced metastatic breast cancer that had failed first- and second-line chemotherapy, caused a rapid wide adoption of HER-2 testing of the patients' primary tumors *(28)*; However, soon after its approval, widespread confusion concerning the most appropriate diagnostic test to determine HER-2 status in formalin-fixed paraffin-embedded breast cancer tissues substantially impacted trastuzumab use *(29–36)*. Since its launch in 1998, trastuzumab has become an important therapeutic option for patients with HER-2–positive breast cancer *(37–40)*.

In general, when specimens have been carefully fixed, processed, and embedded, there has been excellent correlation between *HER-2* gene copy status determined by FISH and HER-2 protein expression levels determined by IHC *(27)*. The main use of either method in current clinical practice is focused on the negative prediction of response to trastuzumab. Currently, both the American Society of Clinical Oncology and the College of American Pathologists consider HER-2 testing to be part of the standard workup and management of breast cancer *(41, 42)*. Recently, the chromogenic (nonfluorescent) in situ hybridization technique has been used to determine the *HER-2* gene amplification status with promising results (Figure 14.1) *(35, 36)*. Nonmorphologic approaches for determining HER-2 status have also been developed. The RT-PCR technique, which has been predominantly used to detect HER-2 mRNA in peripheral blood and bone marrow samples, has correlated more with gene amplification status than IHC levels of primary tumors, but has been less successful as a predictor of survival *(43, 44, 45)*. With the advent of laser capture microscopy and the acceptance of RT-PCR as a routine and reproducible laboratory technique, the use of RT-PCR for the determination of HER-2 status may increase in the future. The cDNA microarray-based method of detecting HER-2 mRNA expression levels has recently received interest as an alternative method for measuring HER-2/neu status in breast cancer *(46, 47)*. Finally, the serum HER-2/ELISA test measuring circulating HER-2 (p185neu) protein is an FDA-approved test that has seen increased clinical use as a method for monitoring the response to trastuzumab *(48)*. A summary of HER-2 testing methods in breast cancer is shown in Table 14.2.

7 Other Targeted Anticancer Therapies Using Antibodies

An unprecedented number and variety of targeted small molecule and antibody-based therapeutics are currently in early development and clinical trials for the treatment of cancer. Therapeutic antibodies have become a major strategy in clinical oncology, because of their ability to specifically bind to primary and metastatic cancer cells with high affinity, and to create antitumor effects by complement-mediated cytolysis and antibody-dependent cell-mediated cytotoxicity (naked antibodies), or by the focused delivery of radiation or cellular toxins (conjugated antibodies) *(48–53)*. Currently, there are eight anticancer therapeutic antibodies approved by the U.S. Food and Drug Administration (FDA) for sale in the United States (Table 14.3). Therapeutic monoclonal antibodies are typically of the IgG class, containing two heavy and two light chains. The heavy chains form a fused "Y" structure, with two light chains running in parallel to the open portion of the heavy chain. The tips of the heavy–light chain

Table 14.2 Methods of detection of HER-2/neu status in breast cancer

Method	Target	FDA-Approved	Slide-Based
IHC	Protein	Yes*	Yes
FISH	Gene	Yes*	Yes
CISH	Gene	No	Yes
Southern Blot	Gene	No	No
RT-PCR	mRNA	No	No
Microarray TP	mRNA	No	No
Tumor ELISA	Protein	No	No
Serum ELISA	Protein	Yes#	No

* For prognosis and prediction of response and eligibility to receive trastuzumab therapy
# For monitoring response of breast cancer to treatment
IHC = immunohistochemistry
FISH = fluorescence in situ hybridization
CISH = chromogenic in situ hybridization
RT-PCR = reverse transcriptase polymerase chain reaction
TP = transcriptional profiling
ELISA = enzyme-linked immunosorbent assay
[Table reprinted from Ross JS, Hortobagyi GH, eds., The molecular oncology of breast cancer. Sudbury, MA: Jones and Bartlett, Inc., with permission by the publisher.]

pairs form the antigen binding sites, with the primary antigen recognition regions known as the complementarity determining regions.

The early promise of mouse monoclonal antibodies for the treatment of human cancers was not realized because (1) unfocused target selection led to the identification of target antigens that were not critical for cancer cell survival and progression; (2) there was a low overall potency of naked mouse antibodies as anticancer drugs; (3) antibodies penetrated tumor cells poorly; (4) there was limited success in producing radioisotope and toxin conjugates; and (5) the development of human antimouse antibodies (HAMA) prevented the use of multiple dosing schedules *(54)*.

The next advance in antibody therapeutics began in the early 1980s when recombinant DNA technology was applied to antibody design to reduce the antigenicity of murine and other rodent-derived monoclonal antibodies. Chimeric antibodies were developed in which the constant domains of the human IgG molecule were combined with the murine variable regions by transgenic fusion of the immunoglobulin genes; the chimeric monoclonal antibodies were produced from engineered hybridomas and CHO cells *(55, 56)*. The use of chimeric antibodies significantly reduced the HAMA responses but did not completely eliminate them *(56, 57)*. Although several chimeric antibodies achieved regulatory approval, certain targets required humanized antibodies to achieve appropriate dosing. Partially humanized antibodies were then developed in which the six complementarity determining regions of the heavy and light chains and a limited number of structural amino acids of the murine monoclonal antibody were grafted by recombinant technology to the complementarity determining region depleted human IgG scaffold *(53)*. Although this process further reduced or eliminated the HAMA responses, in many cases significant further antibody design procedures were needed to reestablish the required specificity and affinity of the original murine antibody *(60, 61)*.

Table 14.3 Antibody therapeutics for cancer

Name	FDA Approval	Source *Partners*	Type	Target	Indication(s) (both approved and investigational)
Alemtuzumab *Campath®*	05/01	BTG *ILEX Oncology* *Schering AG*	Monoclonal antibody, humanized Anticancer, immunological Multiple sclerosis treatment Immunosuppressant	CD52	Cancer, leukemia, chronic lymphocytic Cancer, leukemia, chronic myelogenous Multiple sclerosis, chronic progressive Transplant rejection, general
Daclizumab *Zenapax®*	03/02	Protein Design Labs *Hoffmann-La Roche*	Monoclonal IgG_1 Chimeric Immunosuppressant Antipsoriasis Antidiabetic Ophthalmological Multiple sclerosis treatment		Transplant rejection, bone marrow Uveitis Multiple sclerosis, relapsing-remitting Multiple sclerosis, chronic progressive Cancer, leukemia, general Psoriasis Diabetes, Type I Asthma
Rituximab *Rituxan®*	11/97	IDEC *Genentech* *Hoffmann-La Roche* *Zenyaku Kogyo*	Monoclonal IgG_1 Chimeric Anticancer, immunological Antiarthritic, immunological Immunosuppressant	CD20	Colitis, ulcerative Cancer, lymphoma, non-Hodgkin's Cancer, lymphoma, B-cell Arthritis, rheumatoid Cancer, leukaemia, chronic lymphocytic Thrombocytopenic purpura
Trastuzumab *Herceptin®*	09/98	Genentech *Hoffmann-La Roche* *ImmunoGen*	Monoclonal IgG_1 Humanized Anticancer, immunological	p185neu	Cancer, breast Cancer, lung, non-small cell Cancer, pancreatic
Gemtuzumab *Mylotarg®*	05/00	Wyeth/AHP	Monoclonal IgG_4 Humanized	CD33 / coleacheamycin	Cancer, leukemia, AML (patients older than 60 years)
Ibritumomab *Zevalin®*	02/02	IDEC	Monoclonal IgG_1 Murine Anticancer	CD20 /(*90*)Yttrium	Cancer, lymphoma, low grade, follicular, transformed non-Hodgkin's (relapsed or refractory)

Tositomumab *Bexxar®*	06/03	Corixa	Anti-CD 20 Murine Monocolonal antibody with (131) I conjugation	CD20	Cancer, lymphoma, non-Hodgkin's
Cetuximab *Erbitux®*	02/04	Imclone Bristol Myers Squibb	Anti-EGFR monoclonal antibody	EGFR	Approved for third line treatment of metatstatic colorectal cancer that has failed primary chemotherapy. Requires positive PharmDx IHC immunostain.
Panitumumab *Vectibix®*	/06	Abgenix/Amgen	Anti-EGFR monoclonal antibody	EGFR	Approved for third line treatment of metatstatic colorectal cancer that has failed primary chemotherapy. Requires positive PharmDx IHC immunostain.
Bevacizumab *Avastin®*	02/04	Genentech	Anti-VEGF (ligand)	VEGF	Avastin is approved for use in combination with intravenous 5-Fluorouracil-based chemotherapy as a treatment for patients with first-line — or previously untreated — metastatic colorectal cancer.
Edrecolomab *PanorexTM*	01/95 (Europe Only, nut FDA-approved)	Glaxo-Smith-Kline	Monoclonal IgG_{2A} Murine Anticancer	Epithelial cell adhesion molecule (EpCAM)	Cancer, colorectal

[Adapted from Ross JS, Hortobagyi GH, eds., The molecular oncology of breast cancer. Sudbury, MA: Jones and Bartlett, Inc., with permission by the publisher.]

A second approach to reducing the immunogenicity of monoclonal antibodies has been to replace immunogenic epitopes in the murine variable domains with benign amino acid sequences, resulting in a deimmunized variable domain. The deimmunized variable domains are genetically linked to human IgG constant domains to yield a deimmunized antibody (Biovation, Aberdeen, Scotland). Additionally, primatized antibodies were subsequently developed that featured a chimeric antibody structure of human and monkey that, as a near exact copy of a human antibody, further reduced immunogenicity and enabled the capability for continuous repeat dosing and chronic therapy *(62)*. Finally, fully human antibodies have now been developed using murine sources and transgenic techniques *(62)*.

Using modern antibody design and deimmunization technologies, scientists and clinicians have attempted to improve the efficacy and reduce the toxicity of anticancer antibody therapeutics *(48,* 54, 63*–65)*. The bacteriophage antibody design system has facilitated the development of high affinity antibodies by increasing antigen binding rates and reducing corresponding detachment rates *(65)*. Increased antigen binding is also achieved in bivalent antibodies with multiple attachment sites, a feature known as avidity. Modern antibody design has endeavored to create small antibodies that can penetrate to cancerous sites but maintain their affinity and avidity. A variety of approaches has been used to increase antibody efficacy *(48)*. Clinical trials have recently combined anticancer antibodies with conventional cytotoxic drugs, yielding promising results *(48–53)*. The applications of radioisotope, small molecule cytotoxic drug, and protein toxin conjugation have resulted in promising results in clinical trials and achieved regulatory approval for several drugs now on the market (see below). Antibodies have also been designed to increase their enhancement of effector functions of antibody-dependent cellular cytotoxicity. Another cause of toxicity of conjugated antibodies has been the limitations of the conjugation technology, which can restrict the ratio of the number of toxin molecules per antibody molecule *(48, 49, 61)*. Methods designed to overcome the toxicity of conjugated antibodies include the use of antibody targeted liposomal small molecule drug conjugates and the use of antibody conjugates with drugs in nanoparticle formats to enhance bonding strength that enable controlled release of the cytotoxic agent. Another technique that uses site selective prodrug activation to reduce bystander tissue toxicity is the antibody directed enzyme prodrug therapy. An antibody bound enzyme is targeted to tumor cells. This allows for selective activation of a nontoxic prodrug to a cytotoxic agent at the tumor site for cancer therapy.

A variety of factors can reduce antibody efficacy *(54)*: (1) limited penetration of the antibody into a large solid tumor or into vital regions such as the brain; (2) reduced extravasations of antibodies into target sites due to decreased vascular permeability; (3) cross-reactivity and nonspecific binding of antibody to normal tissues, reducing the targeting effect; (4) heterogeneous tumor uptake, resulting in untreated zones; (5) increased metabolism of injected antibodies, reducing the therapeutic effects; and (6) HAMA and human antihuman antibodies forming rapidly and inactivating the therapeutic antibody.

Toxicity has been a major obstacle in the development of therapeutic antibodies for cancer.*(48–51)* Cross-reactivity with normal tissues can cause significant side effects for unconjugated (naked) antibodies, which can be enhanced when the antibodies are conjugated with toxins or radioisotopes. Immune mediated complications can include dyspnea from pulmonary toxicity, occasional central and peripheral nervous system complications, and decreased liver and renal function. On occasion, unexpected toxic complications can be seen, such as the cardiotoxicity associated with the HER-2 targeting antibody trastuzumab. Radioimmunotherapy with isotopic-conjugated antibodies can also cause bone marrow suppression (see below).

Unconjugated or naked antibodies include a variety of targeting molecules both on the market and in early and late clinical development. A variety of mechanisms has been cited to explain the therapeutic benefit of these drugs, including enhanced immune effector functions and direct inactivation of the targeted pathways as seen in the antibodies directed at surface receptors such as HER-1 (EGFR) and HER-2 *(2–5)*. Surface receptor targeting can reduce intracellular signaling, resulting in decreased cell growth and increased apoptosis *(62)*.

As seen in Table 14.3, of the ten anticancer antibodies on the market in the US, two are conjugated with a radioisotope Y*(90)*-ibritumomab tiuxetan (Zevalin®) and I*(131)* –tositomumab (Bexxar®), and one is conjugated with a complex natural product toxin gemtuzumab ozogamicin (Mylotarg®). Conjugation procedures have been designed to improve antibody therapy efficacy and have used a variety of methods to complex the isotope, toxin, or cytotoxic agent to the antibody *(48, 49)*. Cytotoxic small molecule drug conjugates have been widely tested, but enthusiasm for this approach has been limited by the relatively low potency of these compounds *(48)*. Fungal derived potent toxins have yielded greater success with the calicheamicin conjugated anti-CD33 antibody gemtuzumab ozogamicin, approved for the treatment of acute myelogenous leukemia, and a variety of antibodies conjugated with the fungal toxin maytansanoid (DM-1) in preclinical development and early clinical trials. The interest in radioimmunotherapy increased significantly in 2001 with the FDA approvals of the *(90)*Y-conjugated anti-CD20 antibody Y*(90)*-ibritumomab tiuxetan and the *(131)*I-conjugated anti-CD20 antibody I*(131)*-tositumomab. A variety of isotopes is under investigation in addition to *(90)*Y as potential conjugates for anticancer antibodies *(49)*. Radioimmunotherapy features the phenomenon of the bystander effect, in which if antigen expression is heterogeneous, extensive tumor cell killing can still take place, even on nonexpressing cells, but can also lead to significant toxicity when the neighboring cells are vital non-neoplastic tissues such as the bone marrow and liver.

7.1 Antibody Therapeutics for Hematologic Malignancies

The earliest and most successful clinical use of antibodies in oncology has been for the treatment of hematologic malignancies *(48–51, 62, 66–69)*. By taking advantage of improved recombinant technologies generating more specific and higher affinity monoclonal antibodies with reduced immunogenicity after humanization or deimmunization, and the emerging conjugation capabilities, antibody therapeutics have become a major weapon in the treatment of leukemias and lymphomas *(66–69)*.

7.1.1 Rituximab (Rituxan®)

Approved in 1997, rituximab (Rituxan®) is arguably the most commercially successful anticancer drug of any type since the introduction of taxanes. Rituximab sales exceeded $700 million in the United States in 2001 *(50)*. Targeting the CD20 surface receptor common to many B cell non-Hodgkin lymphoma subtypes, rituximab is a chimeric monoclonal IgG_1 antibody that induces apoptosis, antibody-dependent cell cytotoxicity, and complement-mediated cytotoxicity *(62)* and has achieved significantly improved disease-free survival rates compared with patients receiving cytotoxic agents alone *(70–73)*.

7.1.2 Y(90)-ibritumomab tiuxetan (Zevalin®)

Y*(90)*-ibritumomab tiuxetan (Zevalin®) consists of the murine version of the anti-CD20 chimeric monoclonal antibody, rituximab, which has been covalently linked to the metal chelator, MD-DTPA, permitting stable binding of *(111)* In when used for radionucleotide tumor imaging and *(90)*Y when used to produce enhanced targeted cytotoxicity *(74–77)*. In early 2002, Y*(90)*-ibritumomab tiuxetan became the first radioconjugated antibody therapeutic for cancer approved by the FDA. Since its FDA approval, numerous patients who have received Y*(90)*-ibritumomab tiuxetan after becoming refractory to a rituximab-based regimen have achieved significant responses *(75, 77)*.

7.1.3 Gemtuzumab ozogamicin (Mylotarg®)

The approval of gemtuzumab ozogamicin (Mylotarg®) by the FDA in 2000 marked the first introduction of a plant toxin conjugated antibody therapeutic *(78–82)*. Gemtuzumab ozogamicin is targeted against CD33, a surface marker expressed by 90% of myeloid leukemic blasts but absent from stem cells, armed with calicheamicin, a potent cytotoxic antibiotic that inhibits DNA synthesis and induces apoptosis *(78)*. The current indication for use of gemtuzumab ozogamicin is in acute myelogenous leukemia patients older than 60 years with the recommendation that before the initiation of therapy, the leukemic blast count be below 30,000/mL *(79–81)*.

7.1.4 Alemtuzumab (Campath®)

Alemtuzumab (Campath®), a humanized monoclonal antibody, was approved in mid-2001 for the treatment of B-cell chronic lymphocytic leukemia in patients who have been treated with alkylating agents and who have failed fludarabine therapy *(83, 84)*.

7.1.5 Daclizumab (Zenapax®)

Daclizumab (Zenapax®) is a chimeric monoclonal antibody that targets the interleukin-2 receptor. This antibody is primarily used to prevent and treat patients with organ transplant rejection, but has also been used in a wide variety of chronic inflammatory conditions, including psoriasis, multiple sclerosis, ulcerative colitis, asthma, type I diabetes mellitus, uveitis, and also in a variety of leukemias *(85, 86).*

7.1.6 I(*131*)-tositumomab (Bexxar®)

I*(131)*-tositumomab (Bexxar®) is a radiolabeled anti-CD20 murine monoclonal antibody approved in 2003 for the treatment of relapsed and refractory follicular/ low grade and transformed non-Hodgkin lymphoma *(87, 88).*

7.2 Antibody Therapeutics for Solid Tumors

Interest in the development of antibody therapeutics for solid tumors among many commercial organizations and universities has been significantly impacted by the technologic advances in antibody engineering and the approval and recent clinical and commercial success of trastuzumab, the only therapeutic antibody approved by the FDA for the treatment of solid tumors (edrecolomab is approved in Germany, but not in the United States).

7.2.1 Trastuzumab (Herceptin®)

Trastuzumab (Herceptin®) has been described above. During the six years since the FDA approval of trastuzumab, two additional antibodies have been approved for the treatment of solid tumors (cetuximab and bevacizumab). In addition, continuing progress has been made in this field, and there are a number of both late stage and early stage products in development which show substantial promise.

7.2.2 Cetuximab (Erbitux®) and Panitumumab (Vectibix®)

The epidermal growth factor receptor (EGFR), also known as HER-1, is the target of two FDA-approved small molecule drugs (see below) and one FDA-approved antibody. 89 Cetuximab (Erbitux®) is a chimeric monoclonal antibody that binds to the EGFR with high affinity, blocking growth factor binding, receptor activation, and subsequent signal transduction events, and leading to cell proliferation *(90).* Cetuximab enhanced the antitumor effects of chemotherapy and radiotherapy in preclinical models by inhibiting cell proliferation, angiogenesis, and metastasis, and by promoting apoptosis *(90)*. Cetuximab has been evaluated both alone and in combination with radiotherapy and various cytotoxic chemotherapeutic agents in a series of phase II/III studies that primarily treated patients with either head and neck or colorectal cancer *(90, 91)*. Breast cancer trials are also underway *(92)*. Although the FDA approval process for cetuximab was initially slowed because of concerns over clinical trial design and outcome data management, *(93)* the antibody was approved for use in the treatment of advanced metastatic colorectal cancer in February 2004. Similar to trastuzumab, the development of cetuximab also included an immunohistochemical test for determining EGFR overexpression to define patient eligibility to receive the antibody *(94)*. Thus, cetuximab has joined trastuzumab as an FDA-approved targeted therapy featuring an unconjugated antibody. However, there have been conflicting reports suggesting that the use of a pharmacodiagnostic test (EGFR immunostaining) is unnecessary for the selection of cetuximab in colorectal cancer therapy *(95)*. Recent clinical trials have found significant efficacy for cetuximab in the treatment of head and neck squamous cell cancers, often in combination with radiation treatment *(96)*. Joining cetuximab, and approved by the FDA in September 2006, panitumumab (Vectibix™) is also indicated for the treatment of patients with EGFR-expressing metastatic colorectal cancer who have disease progression, on or following fluoropyrimidine-, oxaliplatin-, and irinotecan-containing regimens *(97)*. Also, as with cetuximab, in order for patients to be eligible to receive panitumumab, their tumors must immunostain positively with the previously approved anti-EGFR IHC kit (PharmDx™, Dako Corp, Glosstrup, Denmark).

7.2.3 Bevacizumab (Avastin®)

Bevacizumab (rhuMAb-VEGF) is a humanized murine monoclonal antibody targeting the vascular endothelial growth factor ligand (VEGF) approved by the FDA in 2004 for the front line or first line treatment, in combination with chemotherapy, of metatstatic colorectal cancer. VEGF regulates both vascular proliferation and permeability and functions as an antiapoptotic factor for newly formed blood vessels *(98–100)*. In addition to its approved indication in colorectal cancer, bevacizumab has shown promising efficacy in combination with cytotoxic drugs for the treatment of non-small cell lung cancer *(101)*, renal cell carcinoma *(102)*, pancreatic cancer *(103)*, breast cancer *(104)*, and prostate cancer *(105)*. Unlike cetuximab, the development of bevacizumab has not included a diagnostic eligibility test. Neither direct measurement of VEGF expression in tumor, circulating VEGF levels in serum or urine, or assessment of tumor microvessel density have been incorporated into the clinical trials or linked to the response rates to the antibody. To date a number of theories have been proposed as to the actual mechanism of action of bevacizumab and the relative contributions of direct antiangiogenesis and other tumor vasculature stabilization and cytotoxic chemotherapy potentiation effects of the antibody *(107, 107)*. In summary, currently used without an integrated diagnostic eligibility test, bevacizumab cannot be considered a true targeted therapy, and further development of this agent for use in prostatic, breast, lung, renal, and other cancers may well be inhibited by the inability to individually select patients who will be more likely to benefit from its use, either alone or in combination with other traditional cytotoxic drugs, antibodies, and novel drugs.

7.2.4 Edrecolomab (Panorex®)

Edrecolomab is a murine IgG_{2A} monoclonal antibody that targets the human tumor-associated antigen Ep-CAM (17–1A). Edrecolomab has been approved in Europe (Germany) since 1995, but to date has not been approved by the FDA. In a study of 189 patients with resected stage III colorectal cancer, treatment with edrecolomab resulted in a 32% increase in overall survival compared with no treatment ($P<0.01$) *(108)*. Edrecolomab's antitumor effects are mediated through antibody-dependent cellular cytotoxicity, complement-mediated cytolysis, and the induction of an antiidiotypic network *(109)*. Edrecolomab is also currently being tested in large multicenter adjuvant phase III studies in stage II/III rectal cancer and stage II colon cancer. Edrecolomab was well tolerated when used as monotherapy, and added little to chemotherapy-related side effects when used in combination. Sequential treatment of patients with metastatic breast cancer with edrecolomab after adjuvant chemotherapy reduced levels of disseminated tumor cells in the bone marrow and eliminated Ep-CAM–positive micrometastases *(110)*.

7.2.5 huJ-591 (Anti-$PSMA_{EXT}$)

Prostate-specific membrane antigen (PSMA) is a membrane-bound glycoprotein restricted to normal prostatic epithelial cells, prostate cancer, and the endothelium of the neovasculature of a wide variety of nonprostatic carcinomas and other solid tumors (Fig. 14.4) *(111–113)*. PSMA expression per cell progressively increases in primary prostate cancer, metastatic hormone sensitive prostate cancer, and hormone refractory metastatic disease. PSMA expression is increased further in association with clinically advanced prostatic cancer, particularly in hormone refractory disease, and appears to be an ideal molecule for use in targeting prostatic cancer cells. Increasing expression levels of PSMA in resected primary prostate cancer is associated with increased rates of subsequent disease recurrence *(114)*. Humanized and fully human antibodies specific for the extracellular domain of PSMA have been developed. A phase I clinical trial of one these antibodies, huJ591 conjugated with *(90)*Y, has yielded promising results *(115)*. Programs using toxin conjugates with anti-PSMA antibodies have completed preclinical development *(116* and are being developed in early stage clinical trials for hormone-refractory advanced metastatic prostate cancer *(117)*. Finally, antibodies to PSMA have been used as diagnostic imaging agents (Fig. 14.3), including the commercially available Prostascint® *(118)*. PSMA is also expressed in the neovasculature of many nonprostate cancers *(119)*. In a recent study, near perfect correlation was seen between endothelial cell expression of PSMA in nonprostate cancers and the ability to visualize them in vivo with radioconjugates of the huJ591 antibody *(119)*.

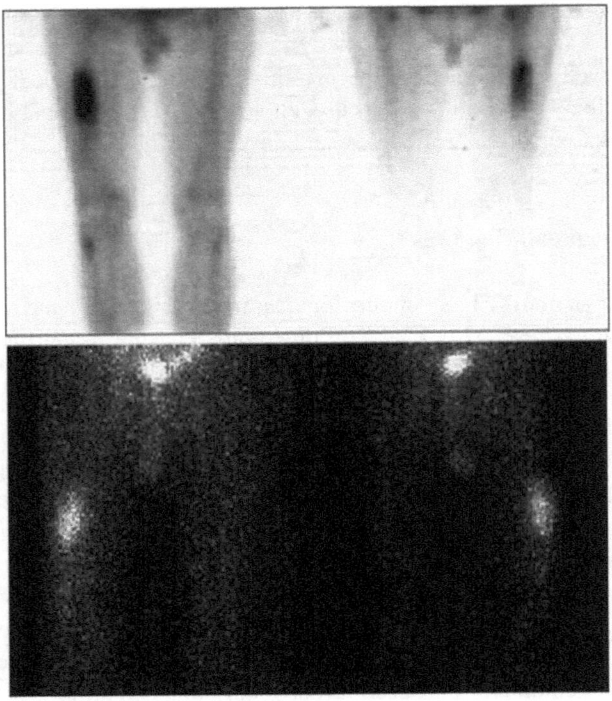

Fig. 14.3 PSMA expression in nonprostate cancer. **(Top)** Traditional bone scan demonstrating bilateral activity in the femur indirectly indicating the presence of metastatic renal cell carcinoma. **(Bottom)** (*111*)I-huJ591$_{\text{EXT}}$ diagnostic immunoscintiscan of the same patient showing direct localization of the anti-PSMA antibody conjugate to the sites of metastatic renal cell carcinoma that feature PSMA expression in the tumor neovasculature. *[Reprinted from Ross JS, Foster CS, eds., The molecular oncology of prostate cancer. 2006. Sudbury, MA: Jones and Bartlett, Inc., with permission by the publisher]*

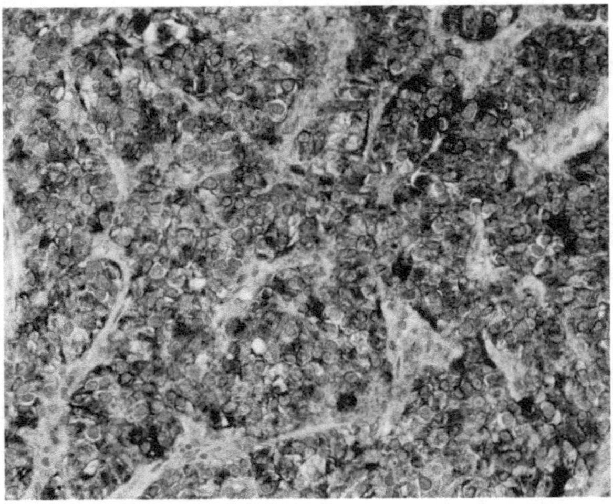

Fig. 14.4 Src kinase overexpression in breast cancer. The overexpression of Src kinase in a subset of breast cancer patients with an adverse prognosis associated with the "triple" (ER/PR/HER2) negative phenotype has led to the development of dasatinib as a potential antitumor agent for this disease

8 Selected Targeted Anticancer Therapies Using Small Molecules

Table 14.4 lists selected small molecule drugs designed to target specific genetic events and biologic pathways critical to cancer growth, invasion, and metastasis.

8.1 Targeted Small Molecule Drugs for Hematologic Malignancies

8.1.1 ATRA

Arguably the first truly targeted therapy after the development of hormonal therapy for breast cancer was the development of ATRA for the treatment of acute promyelocytic leukemia, a subset of acute nonlymphocytic leukemia featuring a disease-defining retinoic acid receptor activating t(15:17) reciprocal translocation *(120, 121)*. For these selected patients, direct targeting of the retinoic acid receptor with ATRA has resulted in very high response rates, delay in disease progression, and long-term cures for these patients *(118, 119)*.

8.1.2 Imatinib (Gleevec®)

The development of imatinib in 2001 for patients with chronic myelogenous leukemia ushered in a new excitement in both the scientific and the public communities for targeted anticancer therapy. Imatinib received fast-track approval by the FDA as an ATP-competitive selective inhibitor of *bcr-abl* and has unprecedented efficacy for the treatment of early stage chronic myelogenous leukemia, typically achieving durable complete hematologic and complete cytogenetic remissions, with minimal toxicity *(122–124)*. Imatinib is a true targeted therapy for leukemia, in that a test for the bcr/abl translocation must be performed before a patient will be considered as eligible to receive the drug. The prediction of resistance to imatinib in early phase CML has been the subject of numerous studies *(125, 126)*. It is the current goal to predict resistance emergence with gene mutation testing and employ novel tyrosine kinase inhibitors to attempt to overcome blast cells that have lost the ability to bind imatinib to the ATP binding pocket of the fusion gene *(125, 126)*.

Imatinib has also achieved regulatory approval for the treatment of relapsed and metastatic gastrointestinal stromal tumors (GISTs), which characteristically feature an activating point mutation in the c-*kit* receptor tyrosine kinase gene *(127)*. For GISTs, the response to imatinib treatment appears to be predictable based on the location of the c-*kit* mutation *(128)*. The use of imatinib in GIST is also an example of targeted therapy, as a measurement of c-*kit* expression usually performed by IHC is required to confirm the diagnosis and render the patient eligible for treatment. Interestingly, most commercially available antibodies for c-*kit* recognize the total c-*kit* and do not distinguish the activated or phosphorylated version, which is the actual target of imatinib. Currently, the high treatment failure rate is directly linked to the test used to characterize the patients. It is anticipated that either the use of specific antibodies designed to identify the activated c-*kit* gene or directed sequencing of the c-*kit* gene may be required before imatinib is prescribed for patients with recurrent or metastatic GIST. An alternative to c-kit mutation testing for the prediction of resistance to imatininb, functional imaging after initial dosing of the drugs, has been employed for patients with metastatic GIST *(129)*.

8.1.3 Dasatinib (Sprycel®)

This tyrosine kinase inhibitor targets the bcr/abl translocation and was approved in 2006 by the FDA for the treatment of imatinib-resistant chronic myelogenous leukemia *(130)*. Dasatinib is capable of blocking the tyrosine kinase signaling in patients who have developed mutations in the bcr/abl gene that have caused imatinib resistance *(130)*. Dasatinib is also an inhibitor of the Src kinase (Fig. 14.4) which has led to an interest in developing this agent for solid tumors such as the Src overexpressing subset of breast cancers featuring the "triple negative" (ER/PR/HER2 negative) phenotype *(131)*.

8.1.4 Flt-3 Targeted Therapy

In approximately 30% of cases of acute myelogenous leukemia and less frequently in other forms of leukemia, a *flt-3* gene mutation creates an internal tandem duplication that creates an abnormal FLT3 receptor that promotes the growth and survival of the leukemic cells *(132–134)*. Three small molecule compounds are in clinical trials for the treatment of acute myelogenous leukemia by targeting the flt-3 internal tandem duplication. These drugs are also examples of potential true targeted therapies, in that a test for detecting an internal tandem duplication that causes the *flt-3* gene activation will likely be required and incorporated into the FDA drug approval label, should these agents be successful in future clinical trials.

8.2 Targeted Small Molecule Drugs for Solid Tumors

8.2.1 Gefitinib (Iressa®)

Gefitinib was originally approved by the FDA in 2003 as a monotherapy for the treatment of patients with locally advanced or metastatic non–small cell lung cancer after failure of both platinum-based and docetaxel chemotherapies *(135, 136)*. Gefitinib is a small molecule drug that targets the EGFR. In contrast with the approval of

Table 14.4 Selected small molecule drugs designed to target specific genetic events and biologic pathways critical to cancer growth and progression

Target	Drug	Source	Clinical Development Status	Comment
PML-RAR- αin PML	ATRA	Promega	Approved	First true targeted therapy since the introduction of ER testing and hormonal therapy for breast cancer
Bcr/abl in CML	Imatinib	Novartis	Approved	Has emerged as standard of care for early stage CML
c-Kit in GIST PDGF-α	Imatinib Sunitumib	Novartis Pfizer	Approved Approved	Responses in relapsed/ metastatic GIST can be predicted by the location of the activating c-kit mutation
Flt-3 in AML	SU5416 PKC412 MLN-518	Pfizer Novartis Millennium	Early Stage Clinical Trials	Small molecule drugs that target the flt-3 internal tandem duplication seen in 30% of AML
EGFR in NSCLC	Gefitinib	Astra Zeneca	Approved/ withdrawn	No survival benefit. Returned to clinical trials.
EGFR in NSCLC and Pancreatic Cancer	Erlotinib	Genentech/ OSI	Approved	Survival benefit demonstrated. No diagnostic test currently used to select patients.
Anti-angiogenesis in Renal Cell Carcinoma	Sorafenib	Bayer	Approved	Raf kinase inhibitor also targets PDGFR and VEGFR.
Anti-angiogenesis in Myelodys-plastic Syndrome	Lenolidamide	Celgene	Approved	Also in clinical trials for the treatment of multiple myeloma.
Other Anti-angiogenesis	Thalidomide SU 5416 ZD6474 Endostatin Marimastat Others	Celgene Pfizer/Sugen Astra Zeneca Entremed British Biotech Others	Approved	Thalidomide is approved for treatment of leprosy and widely used to treat multiple myeloma. Other agents are in early and mid-stage clinical trials
Bcl-2	G3135	Genta	Failed Approval	Anti-sense oligonucleotide targets the anti-apoptotic gene, *bcl-2*
Proteasome in Multiple Myeloma	Bortezomib	Millennium	Approved	Proteasome inhibition effective in hematologic malignancies, but of uncertain potential for the treatment of solid tumors

[Adapted from Ross JS, Hortobagyi GH, eds., The molecular oncology of breast cancer. Sudbury, MA: Jones and Bartlett, Inc., with permission by the publisher.]

trastuzumab, this approval of gefitinib did not include an eligibility requirement reference to a specific tumor diagnostic test designed to select patients that were more likely to respond to the drug. Overexpression of EGFR typically identified by IHC is extremely common in both lung and breast cancers *(135–137)*, but in contrast with HER-2 overexpression, which is virtually limited to cases with gene amplification, multiple mechanisms of dysregulation of EGFR and associated activation of signaling pathways have been described for both of these tumors *(135–137)*. Thus, it has been difficult to develop this drug for expanded indications or combination therapies in the absence of a well-defined efficacy test. However, more recently, two independent groups reported their similar discovery of a specific activating mutation in the tyrosine kinase domain of the EGFR receptor that was associated with a high response to gefitinib in patients with non-small cell lung cancer *(138–139)*. Of interest have been the consistent observations that both a bronchioloalveolar histology and a persistent skin rash have been the best clinical signals of gefitinib response in lung cancer.140 In addition, although specific activating mutations in the EGFR gene have been reproduced in a number of studies *(141)*, some studies have failed to demonstrate this association, and other biomarkers including EGFR gene amplification have also been found to be predictive of tumor response *(142–143)*. Most recently, follow-on studies of gefitinib in lung cancer revealed that the increased response rates that led to the approval of the drug were not accompanied by a clinical survival advantage *(144)*. This has led to the current withdrawal of the drug while further research and clinical trials are performed. It is possible that gefitinib will reappear on the market for the treatment of lung cancer with an integrated diagnostic test designed to boost the response rates by limiting the treatment to tumors with specific histologic and molecular features.

8.2.2 Erlotinib (Tarceva®)

Erlotinib is another targeted small molecule inhibitor of EGFR that was approved by the FDA in 2005 for the treatment of non–small cell lung cancer and pancreatic cancer *(145,146)*. To date, as with gefitinib, the clinical trials and FDA approval for erlotinib have not included an assessment of the EGFR status or other diagnostic test for eligibility to receive the drug. In lung cancer the predictors of tumor response, including skin rash and brochioloalveolar histology, have also applied to erlotinib, as have the somewhat conflicting associations of both activating EGFR mutations and EGFR gene amplification as predictors of drug response *(141, 147)*. Clinical trials have demonstrated that erlotinib does add a survival benefit to the treatment of both lung and pancreatic cancers, and the drug remains on the market currently without an integrated diagnostic eligibility test.

8.2.3 BAY 43–9006 (Sorafenib®)

BAY 43–9006 is a RAF kinase inhibitor that also inhibits the VEGFR and PDGFR growth factor receptors. It is thus considered to be an antiangiogenesis drug. This oral agent was approved in late 2005 by the FDA for the treatment of metastatic renal cell carcinoma *(148)*. Currently, there are no diagnostic tests associated with the selection of this agent, and clinical trials for other types of cancer are ongoing.

8.2.4 Sunitinib (Sutent®)

Sunitinib is a small molecule receptor tyrosine kinase inhibitor approved by the FDA in 2006 for the treatment of gastrointestinal stromal tumor (GIST) and renal cell carcinoma (RCC). Sunitinib inhibits signaling through multiple receptor tyrosine kinases, including platelet-derived growth factor receptor, vascular endothelial growth factor receptor, and kit kinase *(149)*. Sunitinib is currently indicated for patients with GIST who have disease progression during prior treatment with imatinib or who did not tolerate imatinib. No diagnostic test is currently used to select patients for sunitinib therapy.

8.2.5 Other Small Molecule Antiangiogenesis Agents (SU5416, Thalidomide (Thalomid®), Lenalidamide (Revlimid®), Endostatin/Angiostatin, and Marimastat)

A variety of small molecule drugs are currently in clinical trials for the treatment of solid tumors that target the establishment and growth of tumor blood vessels *(150–153)*. Additional compounds that target matrix metalloproteases, such as the drug marimastat, are also considered to be angiogenesis inhibitors *(154–156)*. The antiangiogenesis drug lenalidomide (Revlimid®) was approved by the FDA in late 2005 for the treatment of myelodysplastic syndrome *(157)*. To date, none of these compounds has linked a diagnostic test such as tumor microvessel density or the expression of an angiogenesis promoting gene or protein in their clinical development plans.

8.2.6 G3139 (Genasense®)

Another strategy in anticancer therapy is the targeting of chemotherapy resistance by overcoming the antiapoptosis mechanisms of cancer cells. An example of this approach is the novel antisense oligonucleotide G3139, which targets the antiapoptotic gene *bcl-2 (158, 159)*. This agent has been the most widely tested antisense therapy and has been mostly focused on hematologic malignancies *(160)*.

8.2.7 Bortezomib (Velcade®)

Recently, drugs targeting the proteasome have been developed that are designed to impact downstream pathways regulating angiogenesis, tumor growth, adhesion, and resistance to apoptosis *(161, 162)*. One of these agents, bortezomib (PS-341), has recently been approved for the treatment of advanced refractory multiple myeloma *(163)*. Bortezomib has shown both preclinical activity in animal studies and biologic activity in early clinical trials involving patients with a variety of solid tumors, but to date, no trials using this agent alone or in combination with other drugs has progressed to Phase III. Although pharmacogenomic studies of bortezomib use in multiple myeloma have recently been published, to date no specific pattern of gene expression or other specific test has emerged that could be a guide to the selection of patients for treatment *(164)*.

9 Pharmacogenomics

Targeted therapy in oncology has been a major stimulus for the evolving field of pharmacogenomics. In its broadest definition, pharmacogenomics can encompass both germline and somatic (disease) gene and protein measurements used to predict the likelihood that a patient will respond to a specific single or multiagent chemotherapy regimen, and to predict the risk of toxic side effects *(165,166)*. In breast cancer, whole genome transcriptional profiling has been used as a technique for classification and prognosis *(167–170)*. Gene expression profiles can define cellular functions, biochemical pathways, cell proliferation activity, and regulatory mechanisms. The hierarchical clustering technique of data analysis from transcriptional profiling of clinical samples known to have responded or been resistant to a single agent or combination of anticancer drugs has recently been employed as a guide to anticancer drug therapy in cancers of the breast and other organs *(171)*. Using transcriptional profiling, the microarray technique has been able to generate 81% accuracy for predicting the presence or absence of pathologic complete response after preoperative chemotherapy with sequential weekly paclitaxel and 5-FU, doxorubicin, and cyclophosphamide (FAC) in breast cancer *(172)*. Interestingly, the highest rated single gene predictor in this study has also predicted paclitaxel response in an on-slide immunohistochemistry format *(173)*. These microarray-based gene expression profiling studies have been significantly limited by a number of factors, including 1) the difficulty in standardizing the specimen collection and storage procedures; 2) the differing microarray profiling technologies available commercially or in an investigator-managed laboratory; 3) the relatively small numbers of patients available for profiling compared with the thousands of genes under study, leading to a high false discovery rate; and 4) the wide variety of mathematic models, interpretive tools, and software used to evaluate the profiling results. Nonetheless, there remains great interest in both the scientific and the commercial communities in learning whether the high density genomic microarrays will ultimately be used as diagnostic assays themselves, or yield to more familiar technologies testing small subsets of the discovered markers on platforms already entrenched in the clinical laboratory *(174)*.

References

1. O'Dwyer ME, Druker BJ. Chronic myelogenous leukaemia—new therapeutic principles. J Intern Med 2001;250:3–9.
2. Mauro MJ, Druker BJ. STI571: targeting BCR-ABL as therapy for CML. Oncologist 2001;6:233–8.

3. Lemonick MD, Park A. New hope for cancer. Time 2001;157:62–69.
4. Brown E, Lewis PH, Nocera J. In search of the silver bullet. Fortune 2001;143:166–170.
5. Amos J, Patnaik M. Commercial molecular diagnostics in the U.S.: the Human Genome Project to the clinical laboratory. Hum Mutat 2002;19:324–333.
6. Bottles K. A revolution in genetics: changing medicine, changing lives. Physician Exec 2001;27:58–63.
7. Evans WE, McLeod HL. Pharmacogenomics—drug disposition, drug targets, and side effects. N Engl J Med 2003;348:538–549.
8. Weinshilboum R. Inheritance and drug response. N Engl J Med 2003;348:529–537.
9. Osborne CK. Steroid hormone receptors in breast cancer management. Breast Cancer Res Treat 1998;51:227–238.
10. Wilbur DC, Willis J, Mooney RA, et al. Estrogen and progesterone detection in archival formalin-fixed paraffin embedded tissue from breast carcinoma: a comparison of immunocytochemistry with dextran coated charcoal assay. Mod Pathol 1992;5:79–84.
11. Ciocca DR, Elledge R. Molecular markers for predicting response to tamoxifen in breast cancer patients. Endocrine 2000;13:1–10.
12. Jordan VC. Tamoxifen: a most unlikely pioneering medicine. Nat Rev Drug Discov 2003;2:205–213.
13. Locker GY. Hormonal therapy of breast cancer. Cancer Treat Rev 1998;24:221–240.
14. Ibrahim NK, Hortobagyi GN. The evolving role of specific estrogen receptor modulators (SERMs) Surg Oncol 1999;8:103–123.
15. Miller WR, Anderson TJ, Dixon JM. Anti-tumor effects of letrozole. Cancer Invest 2002;20:15–21.
16. Buzdar AU, Robertson JF, Eiermann W, et al. An overview of the pharmacology and pharmacokinetics of the newer generation aromatase inhibitors anastrozole, letrozole, and exemestane. Cancer 2002;95:2006–2016.
17. Jordan VC. Antiestrogens and selective estrogen receptor modulators as multifunctional medicines. 1. Receptor interactions. J Med Chem 2003;46:883–908.
18. Jordan VC. Antiestrogens and selective estrogen receptor modulators as multifunctional medicines. 2. Clinical considerations and new agents. J Med Chem 2003;46:1081–111.
19. Paik S, Shak S, Tang G, et al. A multigene assay to predict recurrence of tamoxifen-treated, node-negative breast cancer. N Engl J Med 2004;351:2817–26.
20. Paik S, Shak S, Tang G, et al. Expression of the 21 genes in the Recurrence Score assay and tamoxifen clinical benefit in the NSABP study B-14 of node negative, estrogen receptor positive breast cancer. Proc ASCO 2005;24:510.
21. Bast RC Jr, Hortobagyi GN. Individualized care for patients with cancer - a work in progress. N Engl J Med 2004;351:2865–7.
22. Rubnitz JE, Pui CH. Molecular diagnostics in the treatment of leukemia. Curr Opin Hematol 1999;6:229–5.
23. Gleissner B, Thiel E. Detection of immunoglobulin heavy chain gene rearrangements in hematologic malignancies. Expert Rev Mol Diagn 2001;1:191–200.
24. Grimwade D, Lo Coco F. Acute promyelocytic leukemia: a model for the role of molecular diagnosis and residual disease monitoring in directing treatment approach in acute myeloid leukemia. Leukemia 2002;16:1959–1973.
25. Collins-Burow B, Santos ES. Rituximab and its role as maintenance therapy in non-Hodgkin lymphoma. Expert Rev Anticancer Ther 2007;7:257–73.
26. Kiyoi H, Naoe T. FLT3 in human hematologic malignancies. Leuk Lymph 2002;43: 1541–1547.
27. Ross JS, Fletcher JA, Linette GP, et al. The Her-2/neu gene and protein in breast cancer 2003: biomarker and target of therapy. Oncologist 2003;8:307–325.
28. Slamon DJ, Leyland-Jones B, Shak S, et al. Use of chemotherapy plus a monoclonal antibody against HER2 for metastatic breast cancer that overexpresses HER2. N Engl J Med 2001;344:783–792.
29. Schnitt SJ, Jacobs TW. Current status of HER2 testing: caught between a rock and a hard place. Am J Clin Pathol 2001;116:806–810.

30. Hayes DF, Thor AD. c-erbB-2 in breast cancer: development of a clinically useful marker. Semin Oncol 2002;29:231–245.
31. Masood S, Bui MM. Prognostic and predictive value of HER2/neu oncogene in breast cancer. Microsc Res Tech 2002;59:102–108.
32. Paik S, Tan-chui E, Bryan J, et al. Successful quality assurance program for HER-2 testing in the NSAPB trial for Herceptin. Breast Cancer Res Treat 2002;76(suppl 1):S31.
33. Wang S, Saboorian MH, Frenkel EP, et al. Assessment of HER-2/neu status in breast cancer. Automated Cellular Imaging System (ACIS)-assisted quantitation of immunohistochemical assay achieves high accuracy in comparison with fluorescence in situ hybridization assay as the standard. Am J Clin Pathol 2001;116:495–503.
34. Wang S, Saboorian MH, Frenkel E, et al. Laboratory assessment of the status of Her-2/neu protein and oncogene in breast cancer specimens: comparison of immunohistochemistry assay with fluorescence in situ hybridization assays. J Clin Pathol 2000;53:374–381.
35. Tanner M, Gancberg D, Di Leo A, et al. Chromogenic in situ hybridization: a practical alternative for fluorescence in situ hybridization to detect HER–2/neu oncogene amplification in archival breast cancer samples. Am J Pathol 2000;157:1467–1472.
36. Zhao J, Wu R, Au A, et al. Determination of HER2 gene amplification by chromogenic in situ hybridization (CISH) in archival breast carcinoma. Mod Pathol 2002;15:657–665.
37. Hortobagyi GN. Overview of treatment results with trastuzumab (Herceptin) in metastatic breast cancer. Semin Oncol 2001;28:43–47.
38. McKeage K, Perry CM. Trastuzumab: a review of its use in the treatment of metastatic breast cancer overexpressing HER2. Drugs 2002;62:209–243.
39. Shawver LK, Slamon D, Ullrich A. Smart drugs: tyrosine kinase inhibitors in cancer therapy. Cancer Cell 2002;1:117–123.
40. Ligibel JA, Winer EP. Trastuzumab/chemotherapy combinations in metastatic breast cancer. Semin Oncol 2002;29:38–43.
41. Bast RC Jr, Ravdin P, Hayes DF et al. 2000 update of recommendations for the use of tumor markers in breast and colorectal cancer: clinical practice guidelines of the American Society of Clinical Oncology. J Clin Oncol 2001;19:1865–78.
42. Hammond ME, Fitzgibbons PL, Compton CC et al. College of American Pathologists Conference XXXV: solid tumor prognostic factors-which, how and so what? Summary document and recommendations for implementation. Cancer Committee and Conference Participants. Arch Pathol Lab Med 2000;124:958–65.
43. Pawlowski V, Revillion F, Hornez L et al. A real-time one-step reverse transcriptase-polymerase chain reaction method to quantify c-erbB-2 expression in human breast cancer. Cancer Detect Prev 2000;24:212–223.
44. Bieche I, Onody P, Laurendeau I et al. Real-time reverse transcription-PCR assay for future management of ERBB2-based clinical applications. Clin Chem 1999;45:1148–1156.
45. Tubbs RR, Pettay JD, Roche PC et al. Discrepancies in clinical laboratory testing of eligibility for trastuzumab therapy: apparent immunohistochemical false-positives do not get the message. J Clin Oncol 2001;19:2714–2721.
46. Dressman MA, Baras A, Malinowski R et al. Gene expression profiling detects gene amplification and differentiates tumor types in breast cancer. Cancer Res 2003;63:2194–9.
47. Pusztai L, Ayers M, Stec J et al. Gene expression profiles obtained from fine-needle aspirations of breast cancer reliably identify routine prognostic markers and reveal large-scale molecular differences between estrogen-negative and estrogen-positive tumors. Clin Cancer Res 2003;9:2406–15.
48. Fornier MN, Seidman AD, Schwartz MK et al. Serum HER2 extracellular domain in metastatic breast cancer patients treated with weekly trastuzumab and paclitaxel: association with HER2 status bimmunohistochemistry and fluorescence in situ hybridization and with response rate. Ann Oncol 2005;16:234–9.
48. Carter P. Improving the efficacy of antibody-based cancer therapies. Nat Rev Cancer 2001;1:118–129.

49. Goldenberg DM. Targeted therapy of cancer with radiolabeled antibodies. J Nucl Med 2002;43:693–713.
50. Reichert JM. Therapeutic monoclonal antibodies: trends in development and approval in the US. Curr Opin Mol Ther 2002;4:110–118.
51. Ross JS, Gray K, Gray GS et al. Anticancer antibodies. Am J Clin Pathol 2003;119:472–485.
52. Hemminki A. From molecular changes to customised therapy. Eur J Cancer 2002;38:333–338.
53. Milenic DE. Monoclonal antibody-based therapy strategies: providing options for the cancer patient. Curr Pharm Des 2002;8:1749–1764.
54. Reilly RM, Sandhu J, Alvarez-Diez TM, et al. Problems of delivery of monoclonal antibodies. Pharmaceutical and pharmacokinetic solutions. Clin Pharmacokinet 1995;28: 126–142.
55. Winter G, Harris WJ. Humanized antibodies. Immunol Today 1993;14:243–246.
56. Merluzzi S, Figini M, Colombatti A, et al. Humanized antibodies as potential drugs for therapeutic use. Adv Clin Path 2000;4:77–85.
57. Kuus-Reichel K, Grauer LS, Karavodin LM, et al. Will immunogenicity limit the use, efficacy, and future development of therapeutic monoclonal antibodies? Clin Diagn Lab Immunol 1994;1:365–372.
58. Pimm MV. Possible consequences of human antibody responses on the biodistribution of fragments of human, humanized or chimeric monoclonal antibodies: a note of caution. Life Sci 1994;55:PL45–PL49.
59. Jones PT, Dear PH, Foote J, et al. Replacing the complementarity-determining regions in a human antibody with those from a mouse. Nature 1986;321:522–525.
60. Isaacs JD. From bench to bedside: discovering rules for antibody design, and improving serotherapy with monoclonal antibodies. Rheumatology 2001;40:724–738.
61. Watkins NA, Ouwehand WH. Introduction to antibody engineering and phage display. Vox Sang 2000;78:72–79.
62. Reff ME, Hariharan K, Braslawsky G. Future of monoclonal antibodies in the treatment of hematologic malignancies. Cancer Control 2002;9:152–166.
63. Chester KA, Hawkins RE. Clinical issues in antibody design. Trends Biotechnol 1995;13:294–300.
64. Reff ME, Heard C. A review of modifications to recombinant antibodies: attempt to increase efficacy in oncology applications. Crit Rev Oncol Hematol 2001;40:25–35.
65. Nielsen UB, Marks JD. Internalizing antibodies and targeted cancer therapy: direct selection from phage display libraries. PSTT 2000;3:282–291.
66. Burke JM, Jurcic JG, Scheinberg DA. Radioimmunotherapy for acute leukemia. Cancer Control 2002;9:106–113.
67. Linenberger ML, Maloney DG, Bernstein ID. Antibody-directed therapies for hematological malignancies. Trends Mol Med 2002;8:69–76.
68. Stevenson GT, Anderson VA, Leong WS. Engineered antibody for treating lymphoma. Recent Results Cancer Res 2002;159:104–112.
69. Wiseman GA, Gordon LI, Multani PS, et al. Ibritumomab tiuxetan radioimmunotherapy for patients with relapsed or refractory non-Hodgkin lymphoma and mild thrombocytopenia: a phase II multicenter trial. Blood 2002;99:4336–4342.
70. Dillman RO. Monoclonal antibody therapy for lymphoma: an update. Cancer Pract 2001;9:71–80.
71. Grillo-Lopez AJ, Hedrick E, Rashford M, et al. Rituximab: ongoing and future clinical development. Semin Oncol 2002;29(1 suppl 2):105–112.
72. Coiffier B. Rituximab in the treatment of diffuse large B-cell lymphomas. Semin Oncol 2002;29(1 suppl 2):30–35.
73. Grillo-Lopez AJ. AntiCD20 mAbs: modifying therapeutic strategies and outcomes in the treatment of lymphoma patients. Expert Rev Anticancer Ther 2002;2:323–329.
74. Krasner C, Joyce RM. Zevalin: 90yttrium labeled anti-CD20 (ibritumomab tiuxetan), a new treatment for non-Hodgkin's lymphoma. Curr Pharm Biotechnol 2001;2:341–349.

75. Gordon LI, Witzig TE, Wiseman GA, et al. Yttrium 90 ibritumomab tiuxetan radioimmunotherapy for relapsed or refractory low-grade non-Hodgkin's lymphoma. Semin Oncol 2002;29(1 suppl 2):87–92.
76. Wagner HN Jr, Wiseman GA, Marcus CS, et al. Administration guidelines for radioimmunotherapy of non-Hodgkin's lymphoma with $^{(90)}$Y-labeled anti CD20 monoclonal antibody. J Nucl Med 2002;43:267–272.
77. Dillman RO. Radiolabeled anti-CD20 monoclonal antibodies for the treatment of B-cell lymphoma. J Clin Oncol 2002;20:3545–3557.
78. Stadtmauer EA. Trials with gemtuzumab ozogamicin (Mylotarg®) combined with chemotherapy regimens in acute myeloid leukemia. Clin Lymphoma 2002;2(suppl 1):S24–S28.
79. Nabhan C, Tallman MS. Early phase I/II trials with gemtuzumab ozogamicin (Mylotarg®) in acute myeloid leukemia. Clin Lymph 2002;2(suppl 1):S19–S23.
80. Sievers EL, Linenberger M. Mylotarg: antibody-targeted chemotherapy comes of age. Curr Opin Oncol 2001;13:522–527.
81. Bross PF, Beitz J, Chen G, et al. Approval summary: gemtuzumab ozogamicin in relapsed acute myeloid leukemia. Clin Cancer Res 2001;7:1490–1496.
82. Larson RA, Boogaerts M, Estey E, et al. Antibody-targeted chemotherapy of older patients with acute myeloid leukemia in first relapse using Mylotarg (gemtuzumab ozogamicin). Leukemia 2002;16:1627–1636.
83. Dumont FJ. CAMPATH (alemtuzumab) for the treatment of chronic lymphocytic leukemia and beyond. Expert Rev Anticancer Ther 2002;2:23–35.
84. Pangalis GA, Dimopoulou MN, Angelopoulou MK, et al. Campath-1H (anti-CD52) monoclonal antibody therapy in lymphoproliferative disorders. Med Oncol 2001;18:99–107.
85. Carswell CI, Plosker GL, Wagstaff AJ. Daclizumab: a review of its use in the management of organ transplantation. BioDrugs 2001;15:745–773.
86. Kreitman RJ, Chaudhary VK, Kozak RW, et al. Recombinant toxins containing the variable domains of the anti-Tac monoclonal antibody to the interleukin-2 receptor kill malignant cells from patients with chronic lymphocytic leukemia. Blood 1992;80:2344–2352.
87. Cheson BD. Bexxar (Corixa/GlaxoSmithKline). Curr Opin Investig Drugs 2002;3:165–170.
88. Zelenetz AD. A clinical and scientific overview of tositumomab and iodine I 131 tositumomab. Semin Oncol 2003;30(2 suppl 4):22–30.
89. Mendelsohn J, Baselga J. The EGF receptor family as targets for cancer therapy. Oncogene 2000;19:6550–6565.
90. Baselga J. The EGFR as a target for anticancer therapy—focus on cetuximab. Eur J Cancer 2001;37(suppl 4):S16–S22.
91. Herbst RS, Langer CJ. Epidermal growth factor receptors as a target for cancer treatment: the emerging role of IMC-C225 in the treatment of lung and head and neck cancers. Semin Oncol 2002;29(1 suppl 4):27–36.
92. Leonard DS, Hill AD, Kelly L, et al. Anti-human epidermal growth factor receptor 2 monoclonal antibody therapy for breast cancer. Br J Surg 2002;89:262–271.
93. Reynolds T. Biotech firm faces challenges from FDA, falling stock prices. J Natl Cancer Inst 2002;94:326–328.
94. Wong SF. Cetuximab: an epidermal growth factor receptor monoclonal antibody for the treatment of colorectal cancer. Clin Ther 2005;27:684–94.
95. Saltz L. Epidermal growth factor receptor-negative colorectal cancer: is there truly such an entity? Clin Colorectal Cancer 2005;5 Suppl 2:S98–100.
96. Harari PM, Huang S. Radiation combined with EGFR signal inhibitors: head and neck cancer focus. Semin Radiat Oncol 2006;16:38–44.
97. Saltz L, Easley C, Kirkpatrick P. Panitumumab. Nat Rev Drug Discov 2006;5:987–8.
98. Ferrara N. VEGF as a therapeutic target in cancer.Oncology 2005;69 Suppl 3:11–6.
99. Rosen LS. Clinical experience with angiogenesis signaling inhibitors: focus on vascular endothelial growth factor (VEGF) blockers. Cancer Control 2002;9(2 suppl):36–44.
100. Chen HX, Gore-Langton RE, Cheson BD. Clinical trials referral resource: current clinical trials of the anti-VEGF monoclonal antibody bevacizumab. Oncology 2000;15:1023–1026.

101. Wakelee H, Belani CP. Optimizing First-Line Treatment Options for Patients with Advanced NSCLC. Oncologist 2005;10 Suppl 3:1–10.
102. Stadler WM. Targeted agents for the treatment of advanced renal cell carcinoma. Cancer 2005;104:2323–33.
103. Bruckner HW, Hrehorovich VR, Sawhney HS. Bevacizumab as treatment for chemotherapy-resistant pancreatic cancer. Anticancer Res 2005;25:3637–9.
104. de Gramont A, Van Cutsem E. Investigating the potential of bevacizumab in other indications: metastatic renal cell, non-small cell lung, pancreatic and breast cancer. Oncology 2005;69 Suppl 3:46–56.
105. Berry W, Eisenberger M. Achieving treatment goals for hormone-refractory prostate cancer with chemotherapy. Oncologist 2005;10 Suppl 3:30–9.
106. Hurwitz H, Kabbinavar F. Bevacizumab combined with standard fluoropyrimidine-based chemotherapy regimens to treat colorectal cancer. Oncology 2005;69 Suppl 3:17–24.
107. Blagosklonny MV. How Avastin Potentiates Chemotherapeutic Drugs: Action and Reaction in Antiangiogenic Therapy. Cancer Biol Ther 2005;4:1307–10.
108. Schwartzberg LS. Clinical experience with edrecolomab: a monoclonal antibody therapy for colorectal carcinoma. Crit Rev Oncol Hematol 2001;40:17–24.
109. Haller DG. Update of clinical trials with edrecolomab: a monoclonal antibody therapy for colorectal cancer. Semin Oncol 2001;28(1 suppl 1):25–30.
110. Kirchner EM, Gerhards R, Voigtmann R. Sequential immunochemotherapy and edrecolomab in the adjuvant therapy of breast cancer: reduction of 17–1A-positive disseminated tumour cells. Ann Oncol 2002;13:1044–1048.
111. Israeli RS, Powell CT, Corr JG, et al. Expression of the prostate-specific membrane antigen. Cancer Res 1994;54:1807–1811.
112. Ross JS, Gray K, Webb IA, et al. Antibody based therapeutics: focus on prostate cancer. Cancer Metastasis Rev 2005;24:517–533.
113. Liu H, Moy P, Kim S, et al. Monoclonal antibodies to the extracellular domain of prostate-specific membrane antigen also react with tumor vascular endothelium. Cancer Res 1997;57:3629–3634.
114. Ross JS, Sheehan CE, Fisher HA, et al. Correlation of primary tumor prostate-specific membrane antigen expression with disease recurrence in prostate cancer. Clin Cancer Res 2003;9:6357–62.
115. Milowsky MI, Nanus DM, Kostakoglu L, et al. Phase I trial of yttrium-90–labeled anti–prostate-specific membrane antigen monoclonal antibody J591 for androgen-independent prostate cancer. J Clin Oncol 2004;22:2522–2531.
116. Fracasso G, Bellisola G, Cingarlini S, et al. Anti-tumor effects of toxins targeted to the prostate specific membrane antigen. Prostate 2002;53:9–23.
117. Galsky MD, Eisenberger M, Moore-Cooper S, et al. Phase 1/2 dose escalation trial of the prostate specific membrane antigen (PSMA)-targeted immunoconjugate, MLN2704, in patients with progressive metastatic androgen-independent prostate cancer. J Clin Oncol 2006;24(18S):4500.
118. Freeman LM, Krynyckyi BR, Li Y, et al. National prostascint study group. The role of (111)In capromab pendetide (Prosta-ScintR) immunoscintigraphy in the management of prostate cancer. Q J Nucl Med 2002;46:131–137.
119. Milowsky MI, Nanus DM, Kostakoglu L, Sheehan CE, Vallabhajosula S, Goldsmith SJ, Ross JS, Bander NH. Vascular targeted therapy with anti-prostate-specific membrane antigen monoclonal antibody J591 in advanced solid tumors. J Clin Oncol 2007;25:540–7.
120. Parmar S, Tallman MS. Acute promyelocytic leukaemia: a review. Expert Opin Pharmacother 2003;4:1379–1392.
121. Fang J, Chen SJ, Tong JH, et al. Treatment of acute promyelocytic leukemia with ATRA and As2O3: a model of molecular target-based cancer therapy. Cancer Biol Ther 2002;1:614–620.
122. Druker BJ. Imatinib alone and in combination for chronic myeloid leukemia. Semin Hematol 2003;40:50–58.

123. O'Brien SG, Guilhot F, Larson RA, et al. Imatinib compared with interferon and low-dose cytarabine for newly diagnosed chronic-phase chronic myeloid leukemia. N Engl J Med 2003;348:994–1004.
124. Goldman JM, Melo JV. Chronic myeloid leukemia—advances in biology and new approaches to treatment. N Engl J Med 2003;349:1451–1464.
125. O'hare T, Corbin AS, Druker BJ. Targeted CML therapy: controlling drug resistance, seeking cure. Curr Opin Genet Dev 2006;16:92–99.
126. Lange T, Park B, Willis SG, et al. BCR-ABL kinase domain mutations in chronic myeloid leukemia: not quite enough to cause resistance to imatinib therapy? Cell Cycle 2005;4:1761–6.
127. von Mehren M. Gastrointestinal stromal tumors: a paradigm for molecularly targeted therapy. Cancer Invest 2003;21:553–563.
128. Verweij J, van Oosterom A, Blay JY, et al. Imatinib mesylate (STI-571 Glivec, Gleevec) is an active agent for gastrointestinal stromal tumours, but does not yield responses in other soft-tissue sarcomas that are unselected for a molecular target. Results from an EORTC Soft Tissue and Bone Sarcoma Group phase II study. Eur J Cancer 2003;39:2006–2011.
129. Heinicke T, Wardelmann E, Sauerbruch T, et al. Very early detection of response to imatinib mesylate therapy of gastrointestinal stromal tumours using 18fluoro- deoxyglucose-positron emission tomography. Anticancer Res 2005;25:4591–4.
130. Chu SC, Tang JL, Li CC. Dasatinib in chronic myelogenous leukemia. N Engl J Med 2006;355: 1062–3.
131. Gilliland DG, Griffin JD. The roles of FLT3 in hematopoiesis and leukemia. Blood 2002;100:1532–1542.
132. Sawyers CL. Finding the next Gleevec: FLT3 targeted kinase inhibitor therapy for acute myeloid leukemia. Cancer Cell 2002;1:413–415.
133. Kelly LM, Yu JC, Boulton CL, et al. CT53518, a novel selective FLT3 antagonist for the treatment of acute myelogenous leukemia (AML). Cancer Cell 2002;1:421–432.
134. Advani AS. FLT3 and acute myelogenous leukemia: biology, clinical significance and therapeutic applications. Curr Pharm Des 2005;11:3449–57.
135. Schiller JH. New directions for ZD1839 in the treatment of solid tumors. Semin Oncol 2003;30(1 suppl 1):49–55.
136. Ranson M. ZD1839 (Iressa): for more than just non-small cell lung cancer. Oncologist 2002;7(suppl 4):16–24.
137. Campiglio M, Locatelli A, Olgiati C, et al. Inhibition of proliferation and induction of apoptosis in breast cancer cells by the epidermal growth factor receptor (EGFR) tyrosine kinase inhibitor ZD1839 ("Iressa") is independent of EGFR expression level. J Cell Physiol 2004;198:259–268.
138. Paez JG, Janne PA, Lee JC, et al. EGFR mutations in lung cancer: correlation with clinical response to gefitinib therapy. Science 2004;304:1497–500.
139. Lynch TJ, Bell DW, Sordella R, et al. Activating mutations in the epidermal growth factor receptor underlying responsiveness of non-small-cell lung cancer to gefitinib. N Engl J Med 2004;350:2129–2139.
140. Dudek AZ, Kmak KL, Koopmeiners J, et al. Skin rash and bronchoalveolar histology correlates with clinical benefit in patients treated with gefitinib as a therapy for previously treated advanced or metastatic non-small cell lung cancer. Lung Cancer 2006;51:89–96.
141. Chan SK, Gullick WJ, Hill ME. Mutations of the epidermal growth factor receptor in non-small cell lung cancer—search and destroy. Eur J Cancer 2006;42:17–23.
142. Carbone DP. Biomarkers of response to gefitinib in non-small-cell lung cancer. Nat Clin Pract Oncol 2004;1:66–7.
143. Kobayashi S, Boggon TJ, Dayaram T, et al. EGFR mutation and resistance of non-small-cell lung cancer to gefitinib. N Engl J Med 2005;352:786–92.
144. Twombly R. Failing survival advantage in crucial trial, future of Iressa is in jeopardy. J Natl Cancer Inst 2005;97:249–50.
145. Smith J. Erlotinib: small-molecule targeted therapy in the treatment of non-small-cell lung cancer. Clin Ther 2005;27:1513–34.

146. Moore MJ. Brief communication: a new combination in the treatment of advanced pancreatic cancer. Semin Oncol 2005;32:5–6.
147. Silvestri GA, Rivera MP. Targeted therapy for the treatment of advanced non-small cell lung cancer: a review of the epidermal growth factor receptor antagonists. Chest 2005; 128:3975–84.
148. Staehler M, Rohrmann K, Haseke N, et al. Targeted agents for the treatment of advanced renal cell carcinoma. Curr Drug Targets 2005;6:835–46.
149. Chow LQ, Eckhardt SG. Sunitinib: from rational design to clinical efficacy. J Clin Oncol 2007;25:884–96.
150. Khalil MY, Grandis JR, Shin DM. Targeting epidermal growth factor receptor: novel therapeutics in the management of cancer. Expert Rev Anticancer Ther 2003;3:367–380.
151. Zogakis TG, Libutti SK. General aspects of anti-angiogenesis and cancer therapy. Expert Opin Biol Ther 2001;1:253–275.
152. Thomas DA, Kantarjian HM. Current role of thalidomide in cancer treatment. Curr Opin Oncol 2000;12:564–573.
153. Mendel DB, Laird AD, Smolich BD, et al. Development of SU5416, a selective small molecule inhibitor of VEGF receptor tyrosine kinase activity, as an anti-angiogenesis agent. Anticancer Drug Des 2000;15:29–41.
154. Dell'Eva R, Pfeffer U, Indraccolo S, et al. Inhibition of tumor angiogenesis by angiostatin: from recombinant protein to gene therapy. Endothelium 2002;9:3–10.
155. Brown PD. Ongoing trials with matrix metalloproteinase inhibitors. Expert Opin Investig Drugs 2000;9:2167–2177.
156. Miller KD, Gradishar W, Schuchter L, et al. A randomized phase II pilot trial of adjuvant marimastat in patients with early-stage breast cancer. Ann Oncol 2002;13:1220–1224.
157. List AF. Emerging data on IMiDs in the treatment of myelodysplastic syndromes (MDS). Semin Oncol 2005;32:S31–5.
158. Tolcher AW. Regulators of apoptosis as anticancer targets. Hematol Oncol Clin North Am 2002;16:1255–1267.
159. Tamm I, Dorken B, Hartmann G. Antisense therapy in oncology: new hope for an old idea? Lancet 2001;358:489–497.
160. Stein CA, Benimetskaya L, Mani S. Antisense strategies for oncogene inactivation. Semin Oncol 2005;32:563–72.
161. Adams J. Development of the proteasome inhibitor PS-341. Oncologist 2002;7:9–16.
162. Elliott PJ, Ross JS. The proteasome: a new target for novel drug therapies. Am J Clin Pathol 2001;116:637–646.
163. Richardson PG, Barlogie B, Berenson J, et al. A phase 2 study of bortezomib in relapsed, refractory myeloma. N Engl J Med 2003;348:2609–2617.
164. Mulligan G, Mitsiades C, Bryant B, et al. Gene expression profiling and correlation with outcome in clinical trials of the proteasome inhibitor bortezomib. Blood 2007;109:3177–88.
165. Weinstein JN. Pharmacogenomics—teaching old drugs new tricks. N Engl J Med 2000;343:1408–1409.
166. Ross JS, Schenkein DP, Kashala O, et al. Pharmacogenomics. Adv Anat Pathol 2004;11:211–20.
167. Sorlie T, Perou CM, Tibshirani R, et al. Gene expression patterns of breast ccarcinomas distinguish tumor subclasses with clinical implications. Proc Natl Acad Sci USA 2001;98: 10869–74.
168. Bertucci F, Houlgatte R, Benziane A, et al. Gene expression profiling of primary breast carcinomas using arrays of candidate genes. Hum Mol Genet 2000;9:2981–91.
169. van 't Veer LJ, Dai H, van de Vijver MJ, et al. Gene expression profiling predicts clinical outcome of breast cancer. Nature 2002;415:530–6.
170. van de Vijver MJ, He YD, van't Veer LJ, et al. A gene-expression signature as a predictor of survival in breast cancer. N Engl J Med 2002;347:1999–2009.
171. Ntzani EE, Ioannidis JP. Predictive ability of DNA microarrays for cancer outcomes and correlates: an empirical assessment. Lancet 2003;362:1439–44.

172. Ayers M, Symmans WF, Stec J, et al. Gene expression profiles predict complete pathologic response to neoadjuvant paclitaxel and fluorouracil, doxorubicin, and cyclophosphamide chemotherapy in breast cancer. J Clin Oncol 2004;22:2284–93.
173. Rouzier R, Rajan R, Wagner P, et al. Microtubule-associated protein tau: a marker of paclitaxel sensitivity in breast cancer. Proc Natl Acad Sci U S A 2005;102:8315–20.
174. Ross JS. Genomic microarrays in cancer molecular diagnostics: just biomarker discovery tools or future bedside clinical assays? Expert Rev Mol Diagn 2005;5:837–8.

Chapter 15
Pharmacogenomics Applications in Epilepsy

Chantal Depondt

Contents

Abstract Epilepsy is one of the commonest neurological disorders. Although multiple antiepileptic drugs (AEDs) are available, treatment in individual patients is often problematic due to the unpredictability of efficacy, adverse drug reactions, and optimal dosage. Moreover, up to one third of patients develop drug refractory epilepsy despite optimal treatment.

Insights into the pathogenesis of epilepsy and the mechanism of action of AEDs have improved our understanding of the genetic determinants of AED response. Although there are numerous good candidate genes for epilepsy pharmacogenetics, only a limited number of genetic association studies have been published to date, and none have resulted in clinical applications so far.

Thanks to recent advances in genetics and decreasing genotyping costs, large-scale pharmacogenetic studies are now possible. Although clinical application of research findings is likely to take time, it is hoped that ultimately, epilepsy pharmacogenetics will lead to a more efficacious and less harmful treatment for patients with epilepsy, and to the development of new and more effective AEDs.

Chantal Depondt
Service de Neurologie, Université Libre de Bruxelles, Belgium
cdepondt@ulb.ac.be

N. Cohen (ed.) *Pharmacogenomics and Personalized Medicine*,

Glossary

Aplastic anaemia: a form of anaemia caused by suppression of blood cell production in the bone marrow.

Epilepsy: a neurological condition characterized by recurrent, unprovoked (i.e., without an obvious, immediate preceding cause such as a metabolic insult, an acute stroke, or trauma, etc.) epileptic seizures.

Epileptic seizure: the manifestation of an abnormal and excessive synchronized discharge of a set of cerebral neurons.

Epilepsy syndrome: an epileptic disorder characterized by a cluster of signs and symptoms customarily occurring together.

Epoxide: a cyclic ether with only three ring atoms.

(Haplotype) tagging SNP: a SNP that represents other common variants in the same genetic region because of linkage disequilibrium, and distinguishes haplotypes from one another.

Idiosyncratic drug reaction: a rare type of adverse drug reaction that is unpredictable based on the known pharmacological properties of the drug, and shows no simple dose-response relationship.

Linkage disequilibrium (LD): the co-occurrence of alleles on the same haplotype more often than expected by chance.

Stevens-Johnson syndrome: a severe type of allergic rash that is often drug-induced.

Keywords Epilepsy, antiepileptic drugs, drug response, adverse drug reaction, refractory, pharmacogenetics, gene, association

1 Introduction

Epilepsy is a chronic disorder, characterized by recurrent, unprovoked epileptic seizures. It is the commonest chronic neurological disorder after headache, with a prevalence of 5–10 per 1000 persons and an incidence of 50–120 per 100.000 per year *(1)*. An estimated 50 million people are affected worldwide.

Epilepsy and epileptic seizures are symptoms of abnormal brain function. They can be caused by a very wide range of different aetiologies, ranging from purely genetic factors (the so-called idiopathic epilepsies) to identifiable brain disorders such as structural brain abnormalities (e.g., stroke, posttraumatic changes, etc.) or metabolic disorders (the so-called symptomatic epilepsies). In many cases however, no cause can be identified (the so-called cryptogenic epilepsies). Overall, the different epileptic syndromes are caused by differing degrees of interaction between genetic and environmental factors. This is partially reflected in the International League Against Epilepsy (ILAE) classifications of epileptic seizures, epilepsies, and epileptic syndromes *(2, 3)*.

The exact pathophysiology of epilepsy remains unknown, but hyperexcitability and altered synaptic transmission of brain neurons are known to be cardinal features in epileptogenesis. In recent years, mutations have been identified in a number of genes encoding voltage-gated and ligand-gated neuronal ion channels in some rare forms of human monogenic epilepsy *(4, 5)*. These findings have contributed to a greater understanding of epileptogenesis, at least in some types of epilepsy. The genetic factors contributing to common, sporadic forms of epilepsy remain largely unknown so far. Epilepsy susceptibility candidate genes are numerous, and include mainly genes encoding brain-expressed ion channels and neurotransmitter receptors (see Table 15.1).

Antiepileptic drugs (AEDs) form the mainstay of the treatment of epilepsy. Although for many years only a handful of AEDs were available, a large number of new AEDs have been developed over the last 15–20 years, such that there are currently over 15 different AEDs available (see Table 15.2), with more in the pipeline. Most available AEDs have been discovered by chance or through screening in animal models of epilepsy, rather than being designed based on specific mechanisms of action.

Although a substantial proportion of patients can be rendered seizure free with the available AEDs, a number of important problems are inherent to current AED treatment. The optimal AED and its efficacy in terms of seizure response and adverse drug reactions (ADR) are generally unpredictable in an individual patient. Nowadays, clinicians wanting to start a patient on AED treatment take into account factors such as epilepsy type, concomitant disease, and comedication when choosing between available AEDs. Other factors influencing their choice are restrictions by local regulatory instances, such as reimbursement of newer AEDs. Guided by these variables, they will choose the AED which they think is most suited for the patient, i.e., the AED with the highest chance of rendering the patient seizure free while causing the least possible ADRs. ADRs are common with AED treatment, and may be classified as dose-related, idiosyncratic, long-term, or teratogenic. Moreover, it is currently impossible to predict the optimum dose of an AED for individual patients that best balances seizure control against ADRs. The optimal dose is determined in the same empirical way, judging by seizure frequency and the occurrence of ADRs. In about 50% of patients treated this way, the first AED will be effective *(6)*. In the remaining cases, the clinician will either replace the AED or add a second AED, of which the choice will be determined along the same lines, until a drug or combination of drugs is found on which the patient has maximal seizure control with minimal ADRs. However, only a small proportion of patients will be rendered seizure free on subsequent AED trials and up to one third of all patients with epilepsy are drug-refractory despite optimal AED treatment *(7)*. A variety of definitions have been used for refractory epilepsy. Broadly speaking, refractory epilepsy can be defined as the continued occurrence of seizures despite the use of several AEDs, even as polytherapy at maximal tolerated doses. In practical terms, epilepsy is usually called refractory if seizures do not respond to at least three different AEDs that are appropriate for the specific type of epilepsy at the maximum tolerated doses *(8)*. Although a number of clinical variables may predict to some

Table 15.1 Major epilepsy candidate genes

Gene category	Major subtypes	Main genes and gene families
Ion channel and neurotransmitter-related genes		
1. Sodium channel genes	Voltage-gated	SCNA, SCNB
	Non voltage-gated	ACCN
2. Potassium channel genes	Voltage-gated	KCNA,KCNAB, KCNB, KCNC, KCND, KCNG, KCNS
	Voltage-gated, KQT-like subfamily	KCNE, KCNQ
	Eag-like family	KCNH
	Hyperpolarization-activated cyclic nucleotide-gated	HCN
	Calcium-activated	KCNM, KCNN
	Inwardly rectifying	KCNJ
	Weakly inwardly rectifying	KCNK
3. Calcium channels	Voltage-gated	CACNL1A, CACNA2D, CACNLB, CACNLG
	Ligand-gated	RYR, ITPR
4. Chloride channels	Voltage-gated	CLCN
5. GABA-related genes	$GABA_A$ receptors	GABRA, GABRB, GABRD, GABRE, GABRG, GABRQ
	$GABA_B$ receptors	GABBR
	GABA transporters	SLC6A
	GABA anabolism	GAD, ALPL
	GABA catabolism	ABAT, ALDH5A1
6. Glycine-receptor genes		GLRA, GLRB
7. Glutamate-related genes	Ionotropic glutamate receptors	GRIN, GRIA, GRIK
	Metabotropic glutamate receptors	GRM
	Glutamate transporters	SLC1
	Glutamate anabolism	GLS
	Glutamate catabolism	GLUD, GLUL, GSS, PYCS
8. Acetylcholine-related genes	Nicotinic acetylcholine receptors	CHRNA, CHRNB
	Muscarinic acetylcholine receptors	CHRM
	Acetylcholine transporters	SLC18A3
	Acetylcholine anabolism	CHAT
	Acetylcholine catabolism	ACHE
Epilepsy-associated repeat (EAR)-containing genes		LGI, VLGR1/MASS1
Ion pumps and transporters		ATP1, SLC
Ion-channel regulators and associated proteins		BDNF, genes encoding phosphatases / kinases…
Other neurotransmitter-related genes		Adenosine, serotonine, dopamine, opioid, NPY receptor genes
Genes encoding synaptic proteins		SYN, SNAP, SNARE, VAMP, STX, SV2, SYT
Genes involved in apoptosis		CASP, AKT, BCL, TSC
Genes encoding gap-junction proteins		GJA, GJB
Genes involved in brain development		OTX, EMX, PAX, ARX, SOX
Immune system genes		IL, IL receptor genes, HLA
Homologues of mouse epilepsy genes, (e.g. Jh8, Pcmt1, Pmp22…)		

Table 15.2 Major AEDs and their presumed transporter proteins, metabolizing enzymes and main targets

AED	Transporter	Metabolism	Main target
Carbamazepine	PGP ?, MRP2 ?	Epoxidation (CYP3A4 > CYP1A2, CYP2C8), hydrolysis (mEH); glucuronidation	VG Na^+ channels
Clobazam	?	Oxidation (CYP3A4); conjugation	$GABA_A$ α-subunit
Clonazepam	?	Acetylation; reduction and nitration	$GABA_A$ α-subunit
Ethosuximide	?	Oxidation (CYP3A4 > CYP2B, CYP2C9, CYP2E1); conjugation	T-type Ca^{2+} channel
Felbamate	PGP	–60% hydroxylation (CYP3A4, CYP2E1 > CYP2C19); conjugation –40% unchanged renal excretion	NMDA receptors
Gabapentin	PGP, LNAA	>95% unchanged renal excretion	GABA synthesis and metabolism ?
Lamotrigine	PGP	Glucuronidation (UGT1A4)	VG Na^+ channels
Levetiracetam	?	Hydrolysis in blood and other tissues + unchanged renal excretion	SV2A
Oxcarbazepine	PGP, MRP	Hydroxylation (limited); glucuronidation	VG Na^+ channels
Pregabalin	?	98% unchanged renal excretion	VG Ca^{2+} channel α2δ-subunit
Phenobarbitone	PGP	–8-34% hydroxylation (CYP2C9, CYP2C19 > CYP2E1); glucuronidation -N-glucosidation-epoxidation, hydrolysis (mEH)	$GABA_A$ receptor
Phenytoin	PGP ?, MRP2 ?, RLIP76 ?	Hydroxylation (~90% CYP2C9, ~10% CYP2C19), hydrolyse (mEH), or GSH and GST; glucuronidation	VG Na^+ channels
Tiagabine	?	Oxidation (>90% CYP3A4); glucuronidation	GAT-1
Topiramate	PGP	–80% unchanged renal excretion –20% hydroxylation (CYP2C19) and glucuronidation	VG Na^+ channels
Valproic acid	MRP ?	-β-oxidation; glucuronidation - CYP2A6, CYP2C9, CYP2C19	GABA synthesis and metabolism ?
Vigabatrin	SLC36A1	>95% unchanged renal excretion	GABAT
Zonisamide	?	Acetylation (CYP3A4), isoxazole ring cleavage; glucuronidation	VG Na^+ channels

Adapted from (18), (63–73)

For DMEs, specific (iso)enzymes are mentioned if known.

LNAA = large neutral amino acid transporter; GSH = glutathion; GST = glutathione S-transferase; VG = voltage gated; SV2A = synaptic vesicle protein 2A; GAT-1 = GABA transporter 1; GABAT = GABA transaminase.

degree which patients are likely to become refractory, it remains currently impossible to predict treatment resistance at an early stage in many of these patients. Although selected subgroups of these refractory patients may become seizure free with surgery or other specialized treatments, many of them will have ongoing seizures. It is obvious that this treatment strategy of trial and error is entailing a significant cost, in terms of the actual cost related to multiple AED trials and the medical costs related to ongoing seizures and ADRs, as well as in terms of precious time lost in titrating one AED after the other and awaiting its effect, and the human cost related to patient morbidity and mortality. Identifying the factors that contribute to drug response and resistance is therefore a major challenge, with a potentially very significant impact on clinical practice.

How can pharmacogenetics improve AED therapy? AED efficacy, toxicity, and resistance are all multifactorially determined, i.e., influenced by interactions of multiple genetic, environmental, disease-related, and drug-related factors. If it were possible to identify factors that predict AED response in terms of efficacy and/or ADRs, then the current practice of trial and error in the treatment of epilepsy could evolve towards a more targeted, more efficacious, and less harmful treatment; and patients likely to be refractory could be referred for surgery earlier on during the course of their disease. Moreover, identification of genetic factors that predict AED responses could lead to the development of new, more efficacious AEDs, and could have important implications for the conduct of new AED trials.

2 Candidate Genes in Epilepsy Pharmacogenetics

Although whole genome screening is becoming increasingly feasible, until now the usual strategy to identify possible genetic determinants of AED response has been to start from biology, and to draw up a focused list of genes with the potential to influence drug response, based on this knowledge. The major classes of candidate genes for epilepsy pharmacogenetics are those affecting pharmacokinetics and those affecting pharmacodynamics.

Pharmacokinetics consists of drug absorption, distribution, and elimination. AED absorption is dependent both on the properties of the drug (e.g., formulation, lipid solubility) and on the biological properties of the person, which are both exogenic (e.g., intake of food or concurrent medication) and endogenic. AEDs are distributed throughout the body partly by passive, concentration-driven transfer and partly through active transport mechanisms. Again, this process is influenced by drug-dependent (e.g., lipid solubility) and patient-dependent (e.g., altered protein binding) factors. AED elimination from the body is usually through metabolism or biotransformation in the liver, followed by excretion in the kidney. Many of the newer AEDs are eliminated through the kidneys without liver biotransformation. Most biotransformation happens by hepatocyte microsomal enzymes in two phases. Phase I is usually a process of oxidation, reduction, or hydroxylation, mostly carried out by enzymes of the CYP450 family. In phase II, the resulting metabolite is conjugated, usually by glucuronidation. The resulting conjugate is then excreted.

Pharmacodynamics is the interaction of a drug with its target(s) at the cellular level, e.g., binding to a receptor or inhibition of an enzyme. Except for levetiracetam, which acts on synaptic vesicle protein SV2A *(9)*, all currently licensed AEDs of which the mechanism of action is known act through one or several of the following three mechanisms: modulation of voltage-dependent ion channels (Na^+, Ca^{2+}, K^+), enhancement of GABA-mediated inhibitory neurotransmission, and attenuation of excitatory (particularly glutamate-mediated) transmission *(10)*. The mechanism of action of some AEDs is not fully understood.

Based on what is currently known about the disposition and mechanism of action of AEDs, it emerges that there are three main gene categories of interest: 1) genes encoding drug transporters of which AEDs are known substrates; 2) genes encoding drug metabolizing enzymes (DMEs) involved in the breakdown of AEDs; and 3) genes encoding AED targets.

1) Genes Encoding Drug Transporters:

Functional polymorphisms in genes encoding drug transporters of which AEDs are known substrates can be expected to alter AED uptake, distribution, or efflux, and thus result in interindividual differences in AED concentration, effectiveness, and/or occurrence of ADRs. Most drug transporters show a broad substrate specifity, and several AEDs are thought to be transported by more than one transporter protein. Thus, one may expect that a functional polymorphism in one of the encoding genes would affect the kinetics of several AEDs, which is in agreement with the clinical observation that patients with refractory epilepsy are usually resistant to a broad range of AEDs with different mechanisms of action *(8)*. The substrate specificity of drug transporters with regards to AEDs is a matter of debate. Table 15.2 summarizes the currently available data.

The most studied drug transporters with regards to AED transport are those belonging to the superfamily of ATP-binding cassette (ABC) proteins. The two principal families within the ABC superfamily are the multidrug-resistance proteins (MDR or ABCB) and the multidrug-resistance associated proteins (MRP or ABCC). They act as active efflux pumps, transferring substances from the inside of cells to the outside *(11, 12)*. They may pump AEDs back from the brain into blood, and perhaps from blood into the gut, thus lowering the concentration of AEDs and contributing to AED resistance. Several studies have demonstrated overexpression of multidrug transporter proteins in the brain tissue of patients with drug resistant epilepsy of different origins *(13)–(16)*. However, a definite proof of a causal relationship between this overexpression and resistance to AEDs in humans is currently lacking.

2) Genes Encoding Drug Metabolizing Enzymes:

The metabolic pathways and specific metabolizing enzymes for most AEDs are known, and functional variants in the encoding genes are again expected to result in interindividual differences in concentration, effectiveness, and/or occurrence of ADRs. It is unlikely that these functional variants would also contribute significantly to true drug resistance, as their effects are expected to be reflected in drug plasma levels, which can be readily monitored for most AEDs.

The main candidate genes in this category are those encoding the different enzymes of the cytochrome P450 (CYP450) superfamily. Each individual enzyme may have several different substrates and can effect several types of biotransformation, and each biotransformation can be catalyzed by more than one enzyme. There are four main enzyme families (CYP1–4), encoded by at least 25 different genes *(17, 18)*. involved in the metabolism of drugs. At least eight isoenzymes are known to be involved in the metabolism of AEDs (see Table 15.2). The functional polymorphisms underlying alleles with variable metabolization rates are known for several of these genes *(19)*.

Much less is known about the phase II enzymes, which are responsible for conjugation and detoxication of reactive metabolites, in relation to AEDs. The most important enzyme family in this category is that of the UGTs (UDP-glucuronosyltransferases), which conjugate their substrates through the addition of a glycosyl group or glucuronidation. The UGT family comprises two major subfamilies, UGT1 and UGT2 *(20, 21)*. The UGT isoenzymes have few specific substrates and show wide degrees of overlapping substrate specificity. Other phase II enzymes with a role in AED metabolism include the N-acetyltransferases (NAT1 and NAT2) and glutathione S-transferase (GST).

3) Genes Encoding AED Targets:

The genetic determinants of pharmacodynamics have only recently become the focus of attention. Altered pharmacosensitivity of drug targets due to polymorphisms in the encoding genes may explain some of the interindividual variation in AED response. In contrast to polymorphisms affecting genes encoding drug metabolizing enzymes, genetic variation in target encoding genes will not be reflected by differences in AED levels or dose requirements.

As most AEDs are known to act through binding to brain ion channels and neurotransmitter receptors, the most obvious candidates in this category are genes encoding sodium channels, potassium channels, calcium channels, GABA and glutamate receptors. Other AED targets include GABA transporters (tiagabine) and GABA transaminase (vigabatrin). Levetiracetam was recently shown to act through binding to synaptic vesicle protein 2A (SV2A), suggesting a novel mechanism of action for AEDs *(9)*. Besides the genes encoding the actual AED target, this category also includes effector genes downstream in the pathway of AED action and target.

4) Others:

A number of other potentially interesting gene categories exist besides these three major classes of candidate genes. One includes genes relating specifically to idiosyncratic drug reactions. Idiosyncratic drug reactions are relatively rare with AED treatment, but they are important because they pose a potentially life-threatening risk for the patient. The best known examples are the hypersensitivity syndrome induced by aromatic AEDs (phenytoin, phenobarbital, carbamazepine) and lamotrigine *(22)*, and felbamate-induced aplastic anaemia *(23)*. Although the physiological basis of idiosyncratic drug reactions is not entirely elucidated yet, it is thought that they are immune-mediated, probably involving the formation of reactive metabolites *(24)*. It is likely that genetic factors play a role in an individual's predisposition to develop an idiosyncratic drug reaction. Candidate genes are those encoding the enzymes involved in the generation of toxic metabolites (mainly CYP450 isoenzymes), genes encoding enzymes involved in the detoxification of reactive metabolites (for instance, microsomal epoxide hydrolase or mEH), and genes encoding components of the immune system.

Another interesting but so far less explored group of candidate genes consists of genetic factors relating to the molecular pathology of epilepsy itself. It is well known that patients' responses to drug treatment may differ according to the underlying molecular disease pathogenesis. In epilepsy, the type and aetiology of the epilepsy are important determinants in response to treatment, with idiopathic (i.e., genetically determined) epilepsies showing a higher response rate than symptomatic and cryptogenic epilepsies (i.e., those with a defined or presumed underlying cerebral abnormality) *(6)*. Therefore, it would not be surprising if genes harbouring mutations causing epilepsy, susceptibility genes for common epilepsies, or genes affecting the inherent severity of the disease would also influence responses to AEDs. As AEDs act on those mechanisms thought to be involved in the generation of seizures/epilepsy, this class of candidate genes will obviously overlap with those genes encoding drug targets.

Finally, it is worth mentioning that besides genetic polymorphisms resulting in a direct alteration of the encoded protein, genetic variants may also exert their functional effects indirectly, such as through transcriptional effects, differential splicing, or posttranslational influences. Therefore, candidate genes also include genes encoding for instance transcription factors, regulators, kinases, phosphatases, etc.

Table 15.3 gives a schematic overview of potential candidate genes in epilepsy pharmacogenetics.

3 Reported Pharmacogenetic Associations in Epilepsy

This section reviews current knowledge in epilepsy pharmacogenetics for each of the above classes of candidate genes. Although other approaches such as mRNA expression profiling and proteomics are likely to contribute in the future, most currently available data come from genetic association studies. Table 15.4 summarizes the pharmacogenetic associations reported to date.

Table 15.3 Epilepsy pharmacogenetics candidate genes

Gene category	Major gene families
AED transporter genes	MDR, MRP
Drug metabolizing enzyme genes	CYP450, UGT, NAT, GST
AED target genes	Sodium, potassium, calcium channels; GABA & glutamate receptors; GABA transporters; GABA transaminase; SV2A
Immune response genes	CYP450, mEH, HLA, TNF
Epilepsy genes	Ion channels, neurotransmitter receptors
Genes with indirect influence	Transcription factors, regulators, kinases, phosphatases…

Table 15.4 Reported pharmacogenetic associations in epilepsy

Gene category	Gene	Phenotype	Main references
Transporter	MDR1	Drug refractory epilepsy	*(26–34)*[a]
Drug metabolizing enzyme	CYP2C9	Phenytoin toxicity	*(35, 37, 38)*
		Phenytoin dose	*(35, 37–39)*
AED target	SCN1A	Phenytoin and carbamazepine dose	*(35)*
		Phenytoin levels	*(47)*
Immune response	TNFα	carbamazepine hypersensitivity	*(48)*
	HLA-B (*1502 allele)	Stevens-Johnson syndrome on carbamazepine	*(49, 50)*

[a]not exact replications

1) Genes Encoding Drug Transporters:

The single nucleotide polymorphism (SNP) C3435T in exon 26 of the MDR1 (also called P-glycoprotein [PGP] or ABCB1) gene is significantly correlated with expression levels and function of MDR1 in Caucasians *(25)*. This SNP has been the subject of several genetic association studies in patients with refractory epilepsy. One group initially reported an association of the C3435T polymorphism with multidrug resistance in patients with different types of epilepsy *(26)*. This is the only genetic polymorphism that has been associated with multidrug resistance in epilepsy to date. Several groups have attempted to confirm this association since *(27–34)*. Although three were reported as positive, none of them could exactly replicate the initial association. The contradictory results can probably be explained in part by methodological problems, such as small sample sizes and the use of different populations and phenotype definitions between studies. Another study failed to find any significant correlation between the MDR1 C3435T polymorphism and dosage of the AEDs phenytoin or carbamazepine *(35)*. In conclusion, the role of genetic variation in MDR1 in epilepsy remains uncertain at present.

2) Genes Encoding Drug Metabolizing Enzymes:

Several studies have addressed the relation of genetic variants in genes encoding drug metabolizing enzymes to AED response, mostly with regards to drug toxicity.

The most studied in this category is CYP2C9, which accounts for up to 90% of the metabolism of phenytoin *(36)*. The encoding gene has at least 12 different alleles (CYP2C9*1–CYP2C9*12) *(101)*. Low activity alleles are associated with decreased phenytoin clearance and thus higher plasma levels and increased toxicity *(37)*, *(38)*. A small study identified an association between the low activity alleles CYP2C9*2 and CYP2C9*3 and a lower dose requirement of phenytoin *(39)*. A larger study identified a significant correlation between the CYP2C9*3 but not the CYP2C9*2 allele and the maximum dose of phenytoin that patients took, with patients carrying the *3 allele taking lower doses *(35)*. There were no significant associations between *2 or *3 alleles and the presence of phenytoin ADRs in this study.

The genes encoding the different CYP3A isoforms are clustered on chromosome 7q, with CYP3A4 being the most important isoform with respect to AED metabolism (see Table 15.2). Although several polymorphisms in CYP3A4 are known, current evidence suggests that genetic variation in CYP3A4 is not a major factor in interindividual variability in drug clearance *(40)*.

The gene encoding mEH, which is responsible for detoxification of epoxide intermediates, is a candidate for variation in response to carbamazepine, phenobarbitone, and phenytoin. An early study proposed a correlation between a genetic defect in arene oxide detoxification and major birth defects induced by phenytoin *(41)*. However, two small studies found no correlation between mutations in the mEH encoding gene and AED toxicity *(42, 43)*.

No genetic association studies of genes encoding phase II metabolism enzymes have been reported in epilepsy so far.

3) Genes Encoding AED Targets:

One study compared sensitivity to the AEDs valproate and carbamazepine of wild-type nicotinic acetylcholine receptors (nAchR) versus those with mutations in the CHRNA4 gene causing the monogenic epilepsy syndrome autosomal dominant nocturnal frontal lobe epilepsy (ADNFLE) in Xenopus oocytes *(44)*. The results showed that carbamazepine acts as a noncompetitive inhibitor of acetylcholine currents, and that this effect was greater in mutant $\alpha4\beta2$ nAchR compared to wild-type receptors. A similar study demonstrated that neuronal sodium channels expressing a mutant auxiliary $\beta1$-subunit, encoded by the SCN1B gene and responsible for the monogenic epilepsy syndrome GEFS+ (generalized epilepsy with febrile seizures plus), display a reduced sensitivity to phenytoin *(45)*. These results suggest that mutations in genes encoding AED targets can affect drug response. As a consequence, common polymorphisms in these genes may also contribute to individual variations in AED response.

A study assessing the correlation of four tagging SNPs in the SCN1A gene, encoding the α-subunit of the neuronal voltage-gated sodium channel, with AED response did not show any statistically significant associations *(46)*. In a different study, the same variants were related to clinical dosing of phenytoin and carbamazepine *(35)*. One SNP (rs3812718) was found to be highly associated with the maximum dose of both AEDs ($p = 0.0014$ and $p = 0.0045$, respectively). This polymorphism is predicted to disrupt the consensus sequence of the 5' splice donor site of a highly conserved alternative exon ("exon 5N"), and significantly affects the proportions of the alternative transcripts in brains of individuals with a history of refractory epilepsy. A followup study assessed the correlation of this SCN1A variant with serum levels of phenytoin in a different patient cohort, and showed that the polymorphism was also significantly associated with phenytoin serum levels at a maintenance dose ($p = 0.03$) *(47)*. These results provide the first evidence of a drug target polymorphism associated with the clinical use of AEDs.

The role of common genetic variation in five other sodium channel genes (SCN2A, SCN3A, SCN8A, SCN1B, and SCN2B) in AED response was also examined using a haplotype tagging approach *(46)*. None of the results reached statistical significance after correction for multiple testing. Therefore, it seems unlikely that common variation in these genes plays a significant role in AED response.

4) Others:

Two associations of immune response gene variants with severe ADRs in patients on AEDs have been reported. The first is an association between the TNF2 allele of the tumour necrosis factor α (TNFα) gene, resulting in elevated expression of TNFα, and carbamazepine hypersensitivity *(48)*. The TNFα gene is in linkage disequilibrium (LD) with the HLA-DR3 and α-DQ2 genes, and the TNF-DR3-DQ2 haplotype was also shown to be associated with severe drug toxicity. The second is an exceptionally strong association of the HLA-B*1502 allele in Chinese patients who developed Stevens-Johnson syndrome on carbamazepine therapy, with 100% of the patients carrying the allele, versus 3% of those on carbamazepine without Stevens-Johnson syndrome, and 8.6% of controls *(49)*. The strength of the association in this population is such that it might lead to development of a predictive test. A small study in Caucasian patients with Stevens-Johnson syndrome on carbamazepine found that only 33% of the patients carried the HLA-B*1502 allele *(50)*. However, all patients carrying the allele appeared to have Asian ancestry, suggesting that the HLA-B*1502 allele is a population-specific marker for Stevens-Johnson syndrome.

4 Potential Implications

The main implications of epilepsy pharmacogenetics are twofold: improvement of clinical treatment of epilepsy, and development of new AEDs.

1) Improving Clinical Treatment of Epilepsy:

The ultimate goal of pharmacogenetics is to replace the current treatment practice of trial and error with a more rationalized and perhaps even personalized treatment. The idea of such treatment is to tailor drug therapy to an individual patient's genetic constitution. For instance, clinicians could avail themselves of a set of genotyping tests—including a few polymorphisms each in one or more genes encoding drug transporters, drug metabolizing enzymes, AED targets, and immune-related factors—to assist their choice of AED. The outcome of these tests could then be converted into an individualized ranking order of AEDs. Additionally, the results could help predict which dose should be aimed to control seizures without causing ADRs, and perhaps how quickly the dose can be increased. Moreover, if genetic testing could help predict which patients are more likely to be AED refractory, the delay prior to surgical or other second-line treatment could be shortened. In the end, all these factors should significantly improve the quality of life for epilepsy patients. However, it must be noted that experience from pharmacogenetics in other disease domains has demonstrated that translating laboratory findings to clinical practice is often a long and slow process. Therefore, it is likely that it will take several years at least before personalized treatment in epilepsy becomes a reality.

2) AED Development:

Pharmacogenetics may contribute to AED development in two ways: through identification of new drug targets, and as a tool during clinical trials of new AEDs.

Despite the advent of around 10 new AEDs in recent years, up to one third of patients with epilepsy remain drug-refractory *(7)*. This illustrates the need for novel AEDs with mechanisms of action that are different from those of the currently available AEDs, i.e., modulation of ion channels, or central nervous system neurotransmission. It is hoped that pharmacogenetics will contribute to a better understanding of the molecular mechanisms underlying AED action and drug resistance, which may lead to the development of new, more efficient drugs. For example, elucidation of the role of multidrug-resistance proteins in cancer has led to clinical trials with MDR inhibitors *(51)*. Similarly, co-administration of MDR inhibitors with AEDs could be a novel therapeutic approach in epilepsy *(52, 53)*. Identification of drug-target polymorphisms associated with AED response could guide drug designers to develop AEDs that are more efficacious and/or produce fewer ADRs. For example, some drug designers are trying to create compounds that will bind to a target regardless of mutations.

More recently, pharmacogenetics is also becoming a tool during trials of new drugs *(54–56)*. Several of the larger pharmaceutical companies are now systematically collecting DNA from patients participating in phase II clinical trials. The purpose is to identify a) genetic variants that predict response to the drug ("efficacy pharmacogenetics") and b) genetic variants associated with toxicity ("safety pharmacogenetics"). Those variants are then typed prospectively both during later-stage trials and as a part of postmarketing surveillance. Drug trials may thus become faster and more targeted, and clinical drug use more efficient and safer. Moreover, drugs that are efficacious but cause severe toxicity in a relatively small subset of people, and thus would not normally obtain approval, could be rescued. An example in the field of epilepsy is felbamate, an efficacious drug that had to be withdrawn because of rare occurrences of potentially fatal aplastic anaemia and hepatic failure. If a (set of) genetic polymorphism(s) could be identified that would reliably predict the risk for these serious ADRs, then such drugs could be used safely in selected patients.

5 Conclusion and Future Directions

The pharmacogenetics of epilepsy is a promising but relatively unexplored field. There is ample evidence that response to AEDs is influenced by genetic factors, but only a handful of the numerous candidate genes for epilepsy pharmacogenetics have been studied to date. The most intensively studied gene is MDR1, but the results of association studies in refractory epilepsy are contradictory. The association between CYP2C9 polymorphisms and dosing requirements for phenytoin has been confirmed by several groups. However, the clinical usefulness of a CYP2C9 genotyping test seems limited, because the allele is only one of multiple factors influencing phenytoin dosage, and because serum phenytoin levels can be routinely measured, although genotyping offers the advantage of prospective application. The association of SCN1A with the dosages of phenytoin and carbamazepine, and the associations of TNFα and HLA-B with idiosyncratic ADRs on carbamazepine, are awaiting replication in independent cohorts. Numerous other good candidate genes remain to be studied.

With improved insights in the pathogenesis of epilepsy and the mechanism of action of AEDs on the one hand, and major advances in the field of genetics on the other hand, the scope of pharmacogenetic studies in epilepsy is changing rapidly. Thanks to major international efforts such as the Human Genome Project *(55, 102)* and the HapMap project *(58, 103)*, the availability of large numbers of SNP markers, the ever decreasing costs of high-throughput genotyping, and improved statistical tools, it has now become possible to study all common variation in an entire pathway, or even in the entire genome *(59)*. Such large-scale projects will also allow researchers to look at interactions between different variants in the same gene or variants in different genes *(60)*. Because drug response is a complex trait, influenced by multiple genetic and environmental factors, the effect size of any single genetic variant is likely to be small. Therefore, looking at interactions between multiple variants—and possibly exogenic factors—is likely to be more fruitful than looking at single variants.

Moreover, it is likely that other strategies besides association studies will soon contribute to the field of epilepsy pharmacogenetics. For example, microarrays can be used to compare mRNA expression profiles between drug-responsive and drug-refractory patients, or between patients with and without ADRs. Aberrantly expressed genes could provide insight into the pathophysiology of drug resistance or the development of ADRs, and the encoded proteins are plausible targets for new drugs. A small number of studies in human tissue have already hinted at some interesting gene categories, involved in apoptosis *(61)*, gene transcription control, and calcium homeostasis *(62)*. Proteomics, although currently unexplored in drug response in epilepsy, could lead to the identification of particular protein profiles, which might be useful for predicting drug response or ADRs. A potential obstacle to both mRNA expression studies and proteomics is the availability of human brain tissue, particularly from patients with drug-sensitive epilepsy. Brain specimens from drug refractory patients can be obtained relatively easily from surgical resections that are performed to treat some refractory epilepsies. Other potential problems are the interpretation of the large amount of data and the confirmation of functional relevance. Whatever strategy is applied, future studies should ideally be conducted in large sample sizes of rigorously phenotyped patients. Results should be corrected for multiple testing, and independent replication should always be aimed for. Also, although retrospective studies are valuable, prospective studies are superior in assessing potential clinical relevance; i.e., ideally, patients should be characterized on the basis of their DNA-, RNA-, or protein signatures before or at the time they start a specific drug, and then have their response studied over time and correlated to those signatures. It is clear that such large-scale projects will require collaboration between multiple centres, as well as between clinicians and geneticists. The next step will then be to translate relevant research findings into useful clinical applications. The ultimate goal of epilepsy pharmacogenetics is to pave the way for an improved, more efficacious and less harmful therapy for patients, and to lead to the development of novel AEDs, targetting particularly the ~33% of the epileptic population with drug-refractory epilepsy.

References

1. Shorvon S. Handbook of epilepsy treatment: Blackwell Science, 2000.
2. Commission on Classification and Terminology of the International League Against Epilepsy. Proposal for revised clinical and electroencephalographic classification of epileptic seizures. Epilepsia 1981;22:489–501.
3. Commission of Classfication and Terminology of the International League Against Epilepsy. Proposal for revised classification of epilepsies and epileptic syndromes. Epilepsia 1989;30(4):389–99.
4. Scheffer IE, Berkovic SF. The genetics of human epilepsy. Trends Pharmacol Sci 2003;24(8):428–33.
5. Suzuki T, Delgado-Escueta AV, Aguan K, et al. Mutations in EFHC1 cause juvenile myoclonic epilepsy. Nat Genet 2004;36(8):842–9.
6. Kwan P, Brodie MJ. Early identification of refractory epilepsy. N Engl J Med 2000; 342(5):314–9.
7. Devinsky O. Patients with refractory seizures. N Engl J Med 1999;340(20):1565–70.
8. Sisodiya SM. Mechanisms of antiepileptic drug resistance. Curr Opin Neurol 2003;16(2):197–201.
9. Lynch BA, Lambeng N, Nocka K, et al. The synaptic vesicle protein SV2A is the binding site for the antiepileptic drug levetiracetam. Proc Natl Acad Sci U S A 2004;101(26):9861–6.
10. Meldrum BS. Update on the mechanism of action of antiepileptic drugs. Epilepsia 1996;37 Suppl 6:S4–11.
11. Schinkel AH. Pharmacological insights from P-glycoprotein knockout mice. Int J Clin Pharmacol Ther 1998;36(1):9–13.
12. Seetharaman S, Barrand MA, Maskell L, Scheper RJ. Multidrug resistance-related transport proteins in isolated human brain microvessels and in cells cultured from these isolates. J Neurochem 1998;70(3):1151–9.
13. Dombrowski SM, Desai SY, Marroni M, et al. Overexpression of multiple drug resistance genes in endothelial cells from patients with refractory epilepsy. Epilepsia 2001;42(12):1501–6.
14. Sisodiya SM, Lin WR, Harding BN, Squier MV, Thom M. Drug resistance in epilepsy: expression of drug resistance proteins in common causes of refractory epilepsy. Brain 2002;125(Pt 1):22–31.
15. Sisodiya SM, Martinian L, Scheffer GL, et al. Major vault protein, a marker of drug resistance, is upregulated in refractory epilepsy. Epilepsia 2003;44(11):1388–96.
16. Tishler DM, Weinberg KI, Hinton DR, Barbaro N, Annett GM, Raffel C. MDR1 gene expression in brain of patients with medically intractable epilepsy. Epilepsia 1995;36(1):1–6.
17. Park BK, Pirmohamed M, Kitteringham NR. The role of cytochrome P450 enzymes in hepatic and extrahepatic human drug toxicity. Pharmacol Ther 1995;68(3):385–424.
18. Patsalos PN, Froscher W, Pisani F, van Rijn CM. The importance of drug interactions in epilepsy therapy. Epilepsia 2002;43(4):365–85.
19. Daly AK. Pharmacogenetics of the major polymorphic metabolizing enzymes. Fundam Clin Pharmacol 2003;17(1):27–41.
20. Burchell B, Brierley CH, Rance D. Specificity of human UDP-glucuronosyltransferases and xenobiotic glucuronidation. Life Sci 1995;57(20):1819–31.
21. King CD, Rios GR, Green MD, Tephly TR. UDP-glucuronosyltransferases. Curr Drug Metab 2000;1(2):143–61.

22. Knowles SR, Shapiro LE, Shear NH. Anticonvulsant hypersensitivity syndrome: incidence, prevention and management. Drug Saf 1999;21(6):489–501.
23. Dieckhaus CM, Thompson CD, Roller SG, Macdonald TL. Mechanisms of idiosyncratic drug reactions: the case of felbamate. Chem Biol Interact 2002;142(1–2):99–117.
24. Uetrecht J. Screening for the potential of a drug candidate to cause idiosyncratic drug reactions. Drug Discov Today 2003;8(18):832–7.
25. Hoffmeyer S, Burk O, von Richter O, et al. Functional polymorphisms of the human multidrug-resistance gene: multiple sequence variations and correlation of one allele with P-glycoprotein expression and activity in vivo. Proc Natl Acad Sci U S A 2000; 97(7):3473–8.
26. Siddiqui A, Kerb R, Weale ME, et al. Association of multidrug resistance in epilepsy with a polymorphism in the drug-transporter gene ABCB1. N Engl J Med 2003;348(15):1442–8.
27. Hung CC, Tai JJ, Lin CJ, Lee MJ, Liou HH. Complex haplotypic effects of the ABCB1 gene on epilepsy treatment response. Pharmacogenomics 2005;6(4):411–7.
28. Kim DW, Kim M, Lee SK, Kang R, Lee SY. Lack of association between C3435T nucleotide MDR1 genetic polymorphism and multidrug-resistant epilepsy. Seizure 2006;15(5):344–7.
29. Kim YO, Kim MK, Woo YJ, et al. Single nucleotide polymorphisms in the multidrug resistance 1 gene in Korean epileptics. Seizure 2006;15(1):67–72.
30. Leschziner G, Jorgensen AL, Andrew T, et al. Clinical factors and ABCB1 polymorphisms in prediction of antiepileptic drug response: a prospective cohort study. Lancet Neurol 2006;5(8):668–76.
31. Seo T, Ishitsu T, Ueda N, et al. ABCB1 polymorphisms influence the response to antiepileptic drugs in Japanese epilepsy patients. Pharmacogenomics 2006;7(4):551–61.
32. Sills GJ, Mohanraj R, Butler E, et al. Lack of association between the C3435T polymorphism in the human multidrug resistance (MDR1) gene and response to antiepileptic drug treatment. Epilepsia 2005;46(5):643–7.
33. Tan NC, Heron SE, Scheffer IE, et al. Failure to confirm association of a polymorphism in ABCB1 with multidrug-resistant epilepsy. Neurology 2004;63(6):1090–2.
34. Zimprich F, Sunder-Plassmann R, Stogmann E, et al. Association of an ABCB1 gene haplotype with pharmacoresistance in temporal lobe epilepsy. Neurology 2004;63(6):1087–9.
35. Tate SK, Depondt C, Sisodiya SM, et al. Genetic predictors of the maximum doses patients receive during clinical use of the anti-epileptic drugs carbamazepine and phenytoin. Proc Natl Acad Sci U S A 2005;102(15):5507–12.
36. Kupfer A, Preisig R. Pharmacogenetics of mephenytoin: a new drug hydroxylation polymorphism in man. Eur J Clin Pharmacol 1984;26(6):753–9.
37. Brandolese R, Scordo MG, Spina E, Gusella M, Padrini R. Severe phenytoin intoxication in a subject homozygous for CYP2C9*3. Clin Pharmacol Ther 2001;70(4):391–4.
38. Ninomiya H, Mamiya K, Matsuo S, Ieiri I, Higuchi S, Tashiro N. Genetic polymorphism of the CYP2C subfamily and excessive serum phenytoin concentration with central nervous system intoxication. Ther Drug Monit 2000;22(2):230–2.
39. van der Weide J, Steijns LS, van Weelden MJ, de Haan K. The effect of genetic polymorphism of cytochrome P450 CYP2C9 on phenytoin dose requirement. Pharmacogenetics 2001;11(4):287–91.
40. Lamba JK, Lin YS, Thummel K, et al. Common allelic variants of cytochrome P4503A4 and their prevalence in different populations. Pharmacogenetics 2002;12(2):121–32.
41. Strickler SM, Dansky LV, Miller MA, Seni MH, Andermann E, Spielberg SP. Genetic predisposition to phenytoin-induced birth defects. Lancet 1985;2(8458):746–9.
42. Gaedigk A, Spielberg SP, Grant DM. Characterization of the microsomal epoxide hydrolase gene in patients with anticonvulsant adverse drug reactions. Pharmacogenetics 1994;4(3):142–53.
43. Green VJ, Pirmohamed M, Kitteringham NR, et al. Genetic analysis of microsomal epoxide hydrolase in patients with carbamazepine hypersensitivity. Biochem Pharmacol 1995;50(9):1353–9.
44. Picard F, Bertrand S, Steinlein OK, Bertrand D. Mutated nicotinic receptors responsible for autosomal dominant nocturnal frontal lobe epilepsy are more sensitive to carbamazepine. Epilepsia 1999;40(9):1198–209.

45. Lucas PT, Meadows LS, Nicholls J, Ragsdale DS. An epilepsy mutation in the beta1 subunit of the voltage-gated sodium channel results in reduced channel sensitivity to phenytoin. Epilepsy Res 2005;64(3):77–84.
46. Depondt C. Susceptibility genes in epilepsy and antiepileptic drug responsiveness.. University College, London, 2005.
47. Tate SK, Singh R, Hung CC, et al. A common polymorphism in the SCN1A gene associates with phenytoin serum levels at maintenance dose. Pharmacogenet Genomics 2006;16(10): 721–6.
48. Pirmohamed M, Lin K, Chadwick D, Park BK. TNFalpha promoter region gene polymorphisms in carbamazepine-hypersensitive patients. Neurology 2001;56(7):890–6.
49. Chung WH, Hung SI, Hong HS, et al. Medical genetics: a marker for Stevens-Johnson syndrome. Nature 2004;428(6982):486.
50. Lonjou C, Thomas L, Borot N, et al. A marker for Stevens-Johnson syndrome: ethnicity matters. Pharmacogenomics J 2006;6(4):265–8.
51. Avendano C, Menendez JC. Inhibitors of multidrug resistance to antitumor agents (MDR). Curr Med Chem 2002;9(2):159–93.
52. Newman MJ, Dixon R, Toyonaga B. OC144–093, a novel P glycoprotein inhibitor for the enhancement of anti-epileptic therapy. Novartis Found Symp 2002;243:213–26; discussion 26–30, 31–5.
53. Summers MA, Moore JL, McAuley JW. Use of verapamil as a potential P-glycoprotein inhibitor in a patient with refractory epilepsy. Ann Pharmacother 2004;38(10):1631–4.
54. Evans WE, Relling MV. Moving towards individualized medicine with pharmacogenomics. Nature 2004;429(6990):464–8.
55. Roses AD. Genome-based pharmacogenetics and the pharmaceutical industry. Nat Rev Drug Discov 2002;1(7):541–9.
56. Roses AD. Pharmacogenetics and drug development: the path to safer and more effective drugs. Nat Rev Genet 2004;5(9):645–56.
57. Watson JD. The human genome project: past, present, and future. Science 1990;248(4951):44–9.
58. The International HapMap Project. Nature 2003;426(6968):789–96.
59. Wang WY, Barratt BJ, Clayton DG, Todd JA. Genome-wide association studies: theoretical and practical concerns. Nat Rev Genet 2005;6(2):109–18.
60. Marchini J, Donnelly P, Cardon LR. Genome-wide strategies for detecting multiple loci that influence complex diseases. Nat Genet 2005;37(4):413–7.
61. Kim SK, Wang KC, Hong SJ, et al. Gene expression profile analyses of cortical dysplasia by cDNA arrays. Epilepsy Res 2003;56(2–3):175–83.
62. Becker AJ, Chen J, Paus S, et al. Transcriptional profiling in human epilepsy: expression array and single cell real-time qRT-PCR analysis reveal distinct cellular gene regulation. Neuroreport 2002;13(10):1327–33.
63. Abbot EL, Grenade DS, Kennedy DJ, Gatfield KM, Thwaites DT. Vigabatrin transport across the human intestinal epithelial (Caco-2) brush-border membrane is via the H+ -coupled amino-acid transporter hPAT1. Br J Pharmacol 2006;147(3):298–306.
64. Awasthi S, Hallene KL, Fazio V, et al. RLIP76, a non-ABC transporter, and drug resistance in epilepsy. BMC Neurosci 2005;6:61.
65. Baltes S, Fedrowitz M, Tortos CL, Potschka H, Loscher W. Valproic acid is not a substrate for P-glycoprotein or multidrug resistance proteins 1 and 2 in a number of in vitro and in vivo transport assays. J Pharmacol Exp Ther 2007;320(1):331–43.
66. Baltes S, Gastens AM, Fedrowitz M, Potschka H, Kaever V, Loscher W. Differences in the transport of the antiepileptic drugs phenytoin, levetiracetam and carbamazepine by human and mouse P-glycoprotein. Neuropharmacology 2007;52(2):333–46.
67. Clinckers R, Smolders I, Meurs A, Ebinger G, Michotte Y. Quantitative in vivo microdialysis study on the influence of multidrug transporters on the blood-brain barrier passage of oxcarbazepine: concomitant use of hippocampal monoamines as pharmacodynamic markers for the anticonvulsant activity. J Pharmacol Exp Ther 2005;314(2):725–31.

68. Crowe A, Teoh YK. Limited P-glycoprotein mediated efflux for anti-epileptic drugs. J Drug Target 2006;14(5):291–300.
69. Jezyk N, Li C, Stewart BH, Wu X, Bockbrader HN, Fleisher D. Transport of pregabalin in rat intestine and Caco-2 monolayers. Pharm Res 1999;16(4):519–26.
70. Loscher W, Potschka H. Role of multidrug transporters in pharmacoresistance to antiepileptic drugs. J Pharmacol Exp Ther 2002;301(1):7–14.
71. Shorvon SD. The treatment of epilepsy: Blackwell Publishing; 2004.
72. Maines LW, Antonetti DA, Wolpert EB, Smith CD. Evaluation of the role of P-glycoprotein in the uptake of paroxetine, clozapine, phenytoin and carbamazapine by bovine retinal endothelial cells. Neuropharmacology 2005;49(5):610–7.
73. Owen A, Pirmohamed M, Tettey JN, Morgan P, Chadwick D, Park BK. Carbamazepine is not a substrate for P-glycoprotein. Br J Clin Pharmacol 2001;51(4):345–9.

Website References

101. http://www.imm.ki.se/CYPalleles/.
102. www.ornl.gov/techresources/Human_Genome/home.shtml.
103. www.hapmap.org.

Chapter 16
Pharmacogenomics in Alzheimer's Disease

Ramón Cacabelos

Contents

Abstract Structural genomics studies demonstrate that more than 200 genes might be involved in Alzheimer's disease (AD), regulating dysfunctional genetic networks that lead to premature neuronal death. Functional genomics studies in AD reveal that age of onset, brain atrophy, cerebrovascular hemodynamics, brain bioelectrical activity, cognitive decline, apoptosis, immune function, lipid metabolism dyshomeostasis, and amyloid deposition are associated with AD-related genes. Pharmacological treatment in AD accounts for 10–20% of direct costs, and less than 20% of AD patients are moderate responders to conventional drugs (donepezil, rivastigmine, galantamine, memantine) with doubtful cost-effectiveness. Both AD pathogenesis and drug metabolism are genetically regulated complex traits in which hundreds of genes cooperatively participate. Pioneering pharmacogenomics studies demonstrate that the therapeutic response in AD is genotype-specific, with APOE-4/4 carriers as the worst responders to conventional treatments. About 10–20% of Caucasians are carriers of defective CYP2D6 polymorphic variants that alter the metabolism and effects of AD drugs, as well as many psychotropic agents currently administered to patients with dementia. There is a moderate accumulation

---

Ramón Cacabelos
EuroEspes Biomedical Research Center, Institute for CNS Disorders 15166-Bergondo, Coruña; EuroEspes Chair of Biotechnology and Genomics, Camilo José Cela University, Madrid, Spain
rcacabelos@euroespes.com

N. Cohen (ed.) *Pharmacogenomics and Personalized Medicine*,

of AD-related genetic variants of risk in CYP2D6 poor metabolizers and ultrarapid metabolizers, who are the worst responders to conventional drugs. The association of the APOE-4 allele with specific genetic variants of other genes (e.g., CYP2D6, ACE) negatively modulate the therapeutic response to multifactorial treatments affecting cognition, mood, and behaviour. Pharmacogenetic factors may account for 60–90% of drug variability in drug disposition and pharmacodynamics. The incorporation of pharmacogenetic protocols to AD research and clinical practice can foster therapeutics optimization by helping to develop cost-effective pharmaceuticals and improving drug efficacy and safety.

Keywords Alzheimer's disease, genetics, genomics, APOE, ACE, CYP2D6, cholinesterase inhibitors, combination therapy, pharmacogenetics, pharmacogenomics, cognition, anxiety

Glossary

ACE: Angiotensin I-converting enzyme. Polymorphic variants of the ACE gene (17q23)(insertion/deletion variants in intron 16, ACE-I/D) are associated with risk for Alzheimer's disease, vascular dementia, hypertension, atherosclerosis, stroke, and cardiovascular disorders.

Alzheimer's Disease: Major form of dementia characterized by memory disorders, aphasia, apraxia, agnosia, behavioral disturbances, and progressive functional decline.

Aβ (ABP): Amyloid beta protein. Pathogenic fragment of APP which accumulates in senile plaques.

ADRs: Adverse drug reactions.

Animon Complex®: Nutraceutical compound with quenopodium quinoa, iron, folic acid, and vitamin B12.

APOE: Apolipoprotein E. The APOE gene (19q13.2) exhibits 3 major alleles (ε2, ε3, ε4) and 6 genotypes (APOE-2/2, <1%; APOE-3/3, 1–3%; APOE-2/2, <1%; APOE-3/3, 40–60%; APOE-3/4, 20–30%; APOE-4/4, 1–10%) in the population. The inheritance of the APOE-4 allele is a major risk factor for Alzheimer's disease. The APOE-2 allele may be protective.

APP: Amyloid Precursor Protein (21q21). Mutations in this gene are causative of Alzheimer's disease. Alterations in APP posttranslational processing are responsible for conformational changes leading to amyloid deposition in brain tissue (senile plaques) and vessels (amyloid angiopathy).

CDP-Choline: Citidine diphosphocholine. An endogenous nucleotide and choline donor currently used as a cognition enhancer and neuroprotectant.

Cholinesterase Inhibitors: Drugs currently given to patients with Alzheimer's disease, characterized by their capacity to enhance cholinergic neurotransmission. Main cholinesterase inhibitors in the international market (1991–2007) include the following: tacrine, donepezil, rivastigmine, galantamine.

CNS: Central Nervous System.

CYPs: Enzymes of the cytochrome P450 family associated with phase-I drug metabolism, integrated by more than 200 members.

(continued)

Glossary (continued)

CYP2D6: Cytochrome P450, family 2, subfamily D, polypeptide 6. Microsomal monooxygenase associated with debrisoquin and spartein metabolism. Products of the CYP2D6 gene (22q13.1) are associated with the metabolism of multiple types of drugs, including cholinesterase inhibitors (tacrine, donepezil, galantamine), antidepressants, neuroleptics, opioids, some β-blockers, class I antiarrhythmics, analgesics, and many other drug categories, acting as substrates, inhibitors, or inducers with which cholinesterase inhibitors may potentially interact, leading to ADRs. Approximately 30–40% of CNS drugs are processed via CYP2D6 enzymes.

Donepezil: Cholinesterase inhibitor currently used in Alzheimer's disease.

EMs: Extensive metabolizers. Subjects with a normal CYP-related metabolism of drugs.

E-SAR-94010: Marine lipoprotein with antiatherosclerotic and lipid-lowering activities.

Genetic Variation: Differences in the genetic profile between two or more populations. The spectrum of variation can be represented by allelic differences and/or genomic changes including SNPs, binary insertion/deletion events of short sequences, short tandem repeats, deletions, dulications, inversions, retroelements insertions, large tandem repeats, and chromosomal variation.

Genotype-Phenotype Correlations: Assigment of defined phenotypic features to a specific genotype (either monogenic or polygenic profiles).

HRS-A: Hamilton Rating Scale for Anxiety.

Liver Transaminases: GOT: glutamic-oxalacetic transaminase; GGT: Gamma-glutamyl transpeptidase; GPT: Glutamic-piruvic transaminase.

MAPT: Microtubule associated protein tau. Mutations in the MAPT gene (17q21.1) cause tauopathies with accumulation of intracellular neurofibrillary tangles in neurons. Examples of tauopathies include Alzheimer disease, corticobasal degeneration, dementia pugilistica, dementia with tangles only, dementia with tangles and calcification, Down syndrome, frontotemporal dementias, and Parkinsonism linked to chromosome 17 mutations, myotonic dystrophy, Niemann-Pick disease type C, Parkinsonism-dementia complex of Guam, Pick's disease, postencephalitic Parkinsonism, prion diseases with tangles, progressive supranuclear palsy, and subacute sclerosing panencephalitis.

MMSE: Mini-Mental State Examination. Psychometric scale for cognition assessment in Alzheimer's disease and other dementias.

NFT: Neurofibrillary tangles. Intracellular aggregates of paired helical filaments formed by hyperphosphorylation of the tau protein present in Alzheimer's disease neurons.

Nicergoline: A vasoactive substance currently used in cerebrovascular disorders.

NMDA Antagonists: Drugs with action on glutamatergic NMDA receptors (e.g., Memantine, for the treatment fo Alzheimer's disease).

Piracetam: A nootropic substance with neuroprotective activity.

PMs: Poor metabolizers. Patients with deficient CYP enzymes (cytochrome P450).

Presenilins (PSs): Proteins which are altered in Alzheimer's disease. Mutations in the PS1 (14q24.3) and PS2 (1q31-q42) genes are potentially causative of Alzheimer's disease.

Secretase Inhibitors: Drugs under development for the treatment of Alzheimer's disease, characterized by their potential capacity to inhibit β- and γ-secretases precluding amyloid formation and deposition.

UMs: Ultrarapid metabolizers. Subjects with a CYP gene duplication (or multiplication) and consequent ultrarapid clearance of drugs.

1 Introduction

Senile dementia is becoming a major health problem in developed countries, and the primary cause of disability in the elderly. Alzheimer's disease (AD) is the most frequent form of dementia (50–70%), followed by vascular dementia (30–40%), and mixed dementia (15–20%). These prevalent forms of age-related neurodegeneration affect more than 25 million people at present, and probably more than 75 million people will be at risk in the next 20–25 years worldwide. The prevalence of dementia increases exponentially from approximately 1% at 60–65 years of age to more than 30–35% in people older than 80 years. It is very likely that in those patients older than 75–80 most cases of dementia are mixed in nature (degenerative + vascular), whereas pure AD cases are very rare after 80 years of age. The average annual cost per person with dementia ranges from US$15,000 to US$50,000, depending upon disease stage and country, with a lifetime cost per patient of more than US$175,000. In some countries, approximately 80% of the global costs of dementia (direct + indirect costs) are assumed by the patients and/or their families. About 10–20% of the costs in dementia are attributed to pharmacological treatment, including antidementia drugs, psychotropics, and other drugs currently prescribed for the elderly. In addition, during the past 20 years more than 300 drugs have been partially or totally developed for AD, with subsequent costs for the pharmaceutical industry, and only five drugs with moderate-to-poor efficacy and questionable cost-effectiveness have been approved in developed countries *(1–3)*.

With the advent of recent knowledge on the human genome and the identification and characterization of Alzheimer's disease (AD)-related genes *(4)*, as well as novel data regarding CYP family genes and other genes whose enzymatic products are responsible for drug metabolism in the liver (e.g., NATs, ABCBs/MDRs, TPMT), it has been convincingly postulated that the incorporation of pharmacogenetic and pharmacogenomic procedures (Fig. 16.1) in drug development might bring about substantial benefits in terms of therapeutics optimization in dementia, assuming that genetic factors are determinant for both premature neuronal death in AD and drug metabolism *(4–14)*.

The natural course of technical events to achieve efficient goals in pharmacogenetics and pharmacogenomics include the following steps: (a) genetic testing of mutant genes and/or polymorphic variants of risk; (b) genomic screening, and understanding of transcriptomic, proteomic, and metabolomic networks; (c) functional genomics studies and genotype-phenotype correlation analysis; and (d) pharmacogenetics and pharmacogenomics developments, addressing drug safety and efficacy, respectively *(5–12)*.

The application of these procedures to dementia is a very difficult task, since dementia is a complex disorder in which more than 200 genes might be involved *(4, 15)* (Table 16.1). In addition, it is very unlikely that a single drug would be able to reverse the multifactorial mechanisms associated with premature neuronal death in most dementing processes with a complex phenotype represented by memory decline, behavioural changes, and progressive functional deterioration. This clinical picture usually requires the utilization of different drugs administered simultaneously, including memory enhancers such as the conventional antidementia drugs (tacrine,

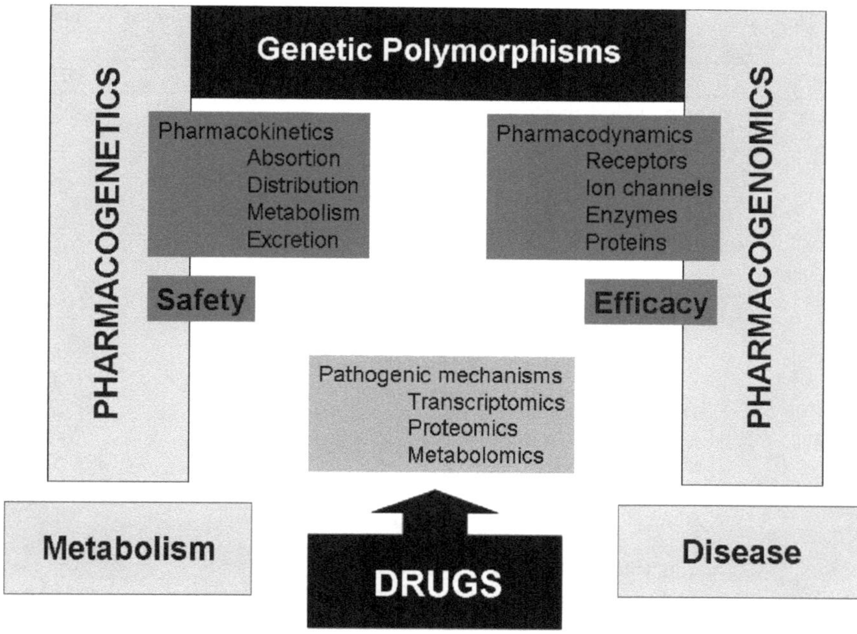

Fig. 16.1 Efficacy and safety issues associated with pharmacogenetics and pharmacogenomics (Adapted from [12])

donepezil, rivastigmine, galantamine, memantine) approved by the FDA; psychotropics (antidepressants, neuroleptics, anxiolytics); anticonvulsants; antiparkinsonians; and also other types of drugs of current use in the elderly due to the presence of concomitant ailments (i.e., hypertension, cardiovascular disorders, diabetes, hypercholesterolemia, etc). In fact, the average number of drugs taken by patients with dementia ranges from 6 to more than 10 per day depending upon their physical and mental conditions. Nursing home residents receive, on average, 7–8 medications each month, and more than 30% of residents have monthly drug regimes of 9 or more medications, including (in descending order) analgesics, antipyretics, gastrointestinal agents, electrolytic and caloric preparations, central nervous system (CNS) agents, antiinfective agents, and cardiovascular agents *(16)*. Polypharmacy, drug-drug interactions, adverse reactions, and noncompliance are substantial therapeutic problems in the pharmacological management of elderly patients *(17)*, adding further complications and costs to the patients and their caregivers. In 2000–2001, 23.0–36.5% of elderly individuals received at least one of 33 potentially inappropriate medications in 10 health maintenance organizations (HMOs) of the USA (N = 157,517) *(18)*. Although drug effect is a complex phenotype that depends on many factors, it is estimated that genetics accounts for 20–95% of variability in drug disposition and pharmacodynamics *(19)*. Under these circumstances, therapeutics optimization is a major goal in the elderly population, and novel pharmacogenetic and pharmacogenomic procedures may help in this endeavour *(10–12)*.

Table 16.1 Selected human genes investigated as potential candidate genes associated with dementia and age-related neurodegenerative disorders

Locus	Symbol	Title/Gene	MIM
1p21.3-p13.1	SORT1	Sortilin	602458
1p31	BBP	Beta-amyloid binding protein precursor	
1p32	ZFYVE9 SARA MADHIP	Zinc finger, FYVE domain containing 9 SMAD anchor for receptor activation MADH-interacting protein	
1p34	LRP8 APOER2	Low-density lipoprotein receptor-related protein 8	602600
1p36	AD7CNTP	Alzheimer disease neuronal thread protein (ADNTP)	607413
1p36.3	MTHFR	Methylenetetrahydrofolate reductase	236253 104300
1q21	S100A	S100 Calcium-binding protein A1	176940
1q21-q23	APCS	Serum amyloid P component	104770
1q23	NCSTN APH2	Nicastrin	605254
1q25	SOAT1 STAT ACAT	Acyl-CoA:Cholesterol acyltransferase Sterol O-acyltransferase 1	102642
1q31-q42	AD4 PSEN2 STM2	Presenilin-2	600759 104300
Chr. 1	APH1A	C. elegans anterior pharynx defective homolog	607629
2p14-p13	RTN4 NOGO	Neurite outgrowth inhibitor (reticulon 4)	604475
2p25	ADAM17 TACE	A desintegrin and metalloproteinase domain 17 Tumor necrosis factor-alpha converting enzyme	603639
2q14	IL1A	Interleukin-1-Alpha	147760
2q21.1	CSEN DREAM KCNIP3	Calsenilin	604662
2q21.2	LRP1B	Low density lipoprotein receptor-related protein 1B	608766
3q26.1-q26.2	BCHE	Butyrylcholinesterase	177400
3q32.3-q34	CREB1	cAMP response element-binding protein	123810
Chr. 4	APBB2 FE65L1	Amyloid beta-A4 precursor protein-binding, family B, member 2	602710
5q15-q21	CAST	Calpastatin	114090
5q31	APBB3 FE65L2	Amyloid beta A4 precursor protein-binding, family B, member 3	602711
5q35.3	DBN1	Drebrin E	12660
6p21.3	AGER RAGE	Advance glycosylation end product-specific receptor	600214
6p21.3	TNFA	Tumor necrosis factor-α Cachectin	191160
7p21	IL-6 IFNB2	Interleukin-6 Beta-2 interferon	147620
7q36	NOS3	Nitric Oxide Synthase-3	163729
8p22	CTSB CPSB	Cathepsin B Amyloid precursor protein secretase	116810

(continued)

Table 16.1 (continued)

Locus	Symbol	Title/Gene	MIM
9q13	APBA1 X11 MINT1 LIN10	Amyloid beta-A4 precursor protein-binding, family A, member 1	602414
10p13	AD7	Alzheimer disease-7	606187
10q23-q25	IDE	Insulin-degrading enzyme	146680
10q24	AD6	Alzheimer disease-6	605526 104300
10q24	PLAU URK	Plasminogen activator, urokinase	191840
11p15	APBB1 F65	Amyloid beta-A4 precursor protein-binding, family B, member 1	602709
11p15.1	SAA1	Serum amyloid A1	104750
11q23.2-q24.2	SORL1	Sortilin-related receptor 1	602005
11q23.3	BACE1	Beta-site amyloid beta A4 precursor protein-cleaving enzyme	604252
	BACE	Beta-secretase Memapsin-2	
11q24	APLP2	Amyloid beta-A4 precursor-like protein 2	104776
12p11.23-q13.12	AD5	Familial AD-5	602096
12p12.3-p12.1	IAPP	Islet amyloid polypeptide	147940
	IAP	Amylin	
	DAP	Diabetes-associated peptide	
12p13.3-p12.3	A2M	Alpha-2-Macroglobulin	103950
12q13.1-q13.3	LRP1	Low density lipoprotein-related protein-1	107770
	A2MR	Alpha-2-macroglobulin receptor	
14q24.3	FOS	FBJ murine osteosarcoma viral (v-fos) oncogene homolog Oncogene Fos	164810
14q24.3	AD3 PSEN1	Presenilin-1	104311
14q32.1	SERPINA3 AACT ACT	Alpha-1-antichymotrypsin	107280
14q32.1	CYP46	Cytochrome P450	604087
	CYP46A1	Family 46, Subfamily A Polypeptide 1 Cholesterol 24-hydrolase	
Chr. 15	APH1B	Homolog of C. elegans anterior pharynx defective 1B	607630
15q11-q12	APBA2	Amyloid beta-A4 precursor protein-binding, family A, member 2	602712
	X11L		
16q22	APPBP1	Amyloid beta precursor protein-binding protein 1	603385
17q11.2	BLMH BMH	Bleomycin hydrolase	602403
17q21	STH	Saitohin	607067
17q21.1	MAPT	Macrotubule-associated protein tau	157140
	MTBT1		600274

(continued)

Table 16.1 (continued)

Locus	Symbol	Title/Gene	MIM
	DDPAC		168610
	MST		172700
17q21-q22	GPSC	Familial progressive subcortical gliosis	221820
17q22-q23	APPBP2	Amyloid beta precursor protein-binding protein 2	605324
	PAT1		
17q23	ACE	Angiotensin I converting enzyme	106180
	ACE1	Dipeptidyl carboxipeptidase-1	104300
	DCP1		
17q23.1	MPO	Myeloperoxidase	254600
17q24	FALZ	Fetal Alzheimer antigen	601819
	FAC1		
18q11.2-q12.2	TTR	Transthyretin	176300
	PALB	Prealbumin	
19p13.2	NOTCH3	Drosophila Notch 3 homolog	600276
	CADASIL		
	CASIL		
19p13.2	AD8	Alzheimer disease 9	608907
19p13.3-p13.2	ICAM	Intercellular adhesion molecule 1	147840
	CD54		
	BB2		
19p13.3	APBA3	Amyloid beta-A4 precursor protein binding, family A, member 3	604262
	X11L2		
19q13.12	PEN2	Presenilin enhancer 2	607632
19q13.2	APOE	Apolipoprotein E	107741
19q13.2	APOC1	Apolipoprotein C-I	107710
19cen-q13.2	AD2	Alzheimer disease-2	104310
19cen-q13.2	APLP1	Amyloid beta-A4 precursor-like protein 1	104775
19q31-qter	APPL1	Amyloid beta-A4 precursor protein-like 1	104740
20p	AD8	Alzheimer disease-8	607116 104300
20p11.2	CST3	Cystatin 3	604312
20p11.2	CST3	Cystatin C	604312
21q21	AD1	Amyloid beta (A4) precursor protein	104760
	APP	Amyloid of aging and Alzheimer disease	
	AAA	Cerebrovascular amyloid peptide	
	CVAP	Protease nexin II	
21q22.3	BACE2	Beta-site amyloid beta A4 precursor protein-cleaving enzyme 2	605668
	ALP56	Down syndrome-region aspartic protease	
	DRAP		
22q11	RTN4R, NOGOR	NOGO receptor (reticulon 4 receptor)	605566
	HN	Humanin	606120

Adapted from (4, 12)

2 Pathogenetics of Alzheimer's disease

A few years after the pioneering studies of Alois Alzheimer (1864–1915) with August D, Johann F, and other patients, reported between 1907 and 1911, it soon became clear that AD was a clinical entity that accumulated in some families, suggesting that an important genetic component might be influencing the pathogenesis of this neurodegenerative disorder. Familial predisposition to dementia has been documented in the second patient of Alzheimer's, who died in October 1910 at age 57 years, representing the index case of a family with a clear predisposition to presenile dementia. Our present knowledge of AD genetics derives from population studies, family studies, twin studies, adoption studies, and molecular biology studies carried out during the past 50 years *(4)*. After the pioneering work of Schotky, Lowenberg, Waggoner, and MacManemey in the 1930s, Sjögren in the 1950s, and Heston and associates in the 1960s and 1970s, complex segregation analysis in the early 1990s led to the conclusion that AD is determined, in part, by a major autosomal dominant allele with an additional multifactorial component. Autosomal recessive forms of AD cannot be ruled out in specific populations. Epidemiological studies also suggested that most cases of AD (>80%) are familial. Advances in molecular genetics during the past two decades allowed the identification of several genetic loci associated with AD (Table 16.1) and the genetic classification of AD (AD1 to ADn) as depicted in the OMIM database *(4, 20)*.

The genetic defects identified in AD during the past 25 years can be classified into three main categories: (a) Mendelian or mutational defects in genes are directly linked to AD, including (i) 32 mutations in the amyloid beta (Aβ)(ABP) precursor protein (APP) gene (21q21), (ii) 165 mutations in the presenilin 1 (PS1) gene (14q24.3), and (iii) 12 mutations in the presenilin 2 (PS2) gene (1q31-q42) *(4, 20, 21)* (Table 16.1). (b) Multiple polymorphic variants of risk characterized in more than 200 different genes distributed across the human genome can increase neuronal vulnerability to premature death *(4)* (Table 16.1). Among these genes of susceptibility, the apolipoprotein E (APOE) gene (19q13.2) is the most prevalent as a risk factor for AD, especially in those subjects harbouring the APOE-4 allele; whereas carriers of the APOE-2 allele might be protective against dementia *(4, 12)*. APOE-related pathogenic mechanisms are also associated with brain aging and with the neuropathological hallmarks of AD *(4–12, 22, 23)*. (c) Diverse mutations located in mitochondrial DNA (mtDNA) through heteroplasmic transmission can influence aging and oxidative stress conditions, conferring phenotypic heterogeneity *(4, 24)*. It is also likely that defective functions of genes associated with longevity may influence premature neuronal survival, since neurons are potential pacemakers, defining life span in mammals *(4)*. All these genetic factors may interact in still unknown genetic networks leading to a cascade of pathogenic events characterized by abnormal protein processing and misfolding, with subsequent accumulation of abnormal proteins (conformational changes), ubiquitin-proteasome system dysfunction, excitotoxic reactions, oxidative and nitrosative stress, mitochondrial injury, synaptic failure, altered metal homeostasis, dysfunction of axonal and dendritic transport, and chaperone misoperation *(4, 12)* (Fig. 16.2). These pathogenic events may exert an additive effect, converging in final pathways leading to premature neuronal death. Some of these mechanisms are common to several neurodegenerative disorders which differ depending upon the gene(s) affected and the involvement of specific genetic networks, together with cerebrovascular factors, epigenetic factors (DNA methylation), and environmental conditions (nutrition, toxicity, social factors, etc.) *(4, 11, 12, 25–27)*. The higher the number of genes involved in AD pathogenesis, the earlier the onset of the disease, the faster its clinical course, and the poorer its therapeutic outcome *(5–8, 10–12)*.

Association studies of diverse genes in different populations show contradictory results of difficult validation. Although the amyloid hypothesis is recognized as the *primum movens* of AD pathogenesis *(15, 28)*, mutational genetics associated with APP and PSs genes alone (<10% of AD cases) does not explain in full the neuropathological findings present in AD, represented by amyloid deposition in senile plaques and vessels (amyloid angiopathy), neurofibrillary tangle (NFT) formation due to hyperphosphorylation of tau protein, synaptic and dendritic desarborization, and neuronal loss, accompanied by neuroinflammatory reactions, oxidative stress and free radical formation probably associated with mitochondrial dysfunction, excitotoxic reactions, alterations in cholesterol metabolism and lipid rafts, deficiencies in neurotransmitter and neurotrophic factor function, defective activity of the ubiquitin-proteasome and chaperone systems, and cerebrovascular dysregulation *(4)*. All these neurochemical events are potential targets for treatment *(10–12)* (Fig. 16.2).

2.1 Genetic Variation

Approximately 5% of the human genome is structurally variant in the normal population, involving more than 800 genes *(29)*. The spectrum of variation in the human genome includes: (a) single changes (single nucleotide polymorphisms (SNPs), point mutations)(1 bp), (b) small insertions/deletions (binary insertion/deletion events of short sequences)(1–50 bp), (c) short tandem repeats (microsatellites)(1–500 bp), (d) fine-scale structural variation (deletions, duplications, tandem repeats, inversions)(50 bp–5 kb), (e) retroelements insertions (SINEs, LINEs, LTRs, ERVs)(300 bp–10 kb), (f) intermediate-scale structural variations (deletions, duplications, tandem repeats, inversions)(5 kb–50 kb), (g) large-scale structural variation (deletions, duplications, large tandem repeats)(50 kb–5 Mb), and (h) chromosomal variations (euchromatic variations, cytogenetic deletions, duplications, translocations, inversions, and aneuplidy)(>5 Mb) *(29)*. Segmental duplications of low copy repeats are blocks of DNA ranging from 1–400 kb in length that occur at multiple sites within the genome and typically share a high level (>95%) of sequence identity. Segmental duplications frequently mediate polymorphic rearrangements of intervening sequences via nonallelic homologous recombination (NAHR) with major implications for human disease. SNPs and insertion (I)/deletion (D) events are the most frequent types of structural variation. I/D polymorphisms of several genes with functions in enzymatic pathways or in drug metabolizing

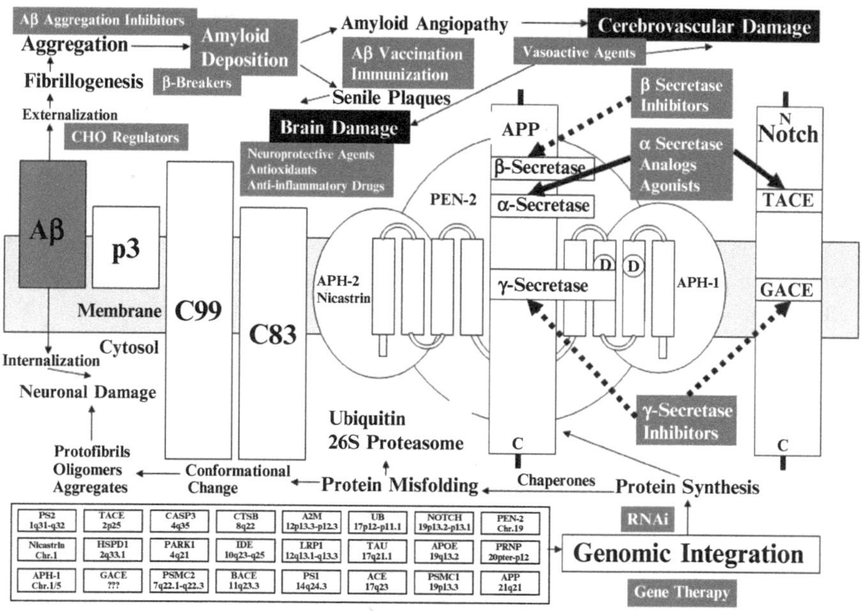

Fig. 16.2 Brain amyloidogenesis and potential therapeutic interventions in Alzheimer's disease (Adapted from [11])

enzymes (e.g., CYP2D6) may drastically influence a variety of common phenotypes with pathogenic and/or pharmacogenetic relevance. The differential expression of common variants is a major source of genetic variation with important repercussions in human diversity and disease heterogeneity. Prior to the completion of the Human Genome Project and the emergence of dense genetic maps, scientists used linkage studies and positional cloning to identify DNA mutations in rare diseases, but in the past two decades association study designs became more powerful compared with linkage study designs in identifying susceptibility loci and SNP variation. Currently, more than 10 million DNA sequence variations have been uncovered in the human genome *(30)*.

It has been observed that the genetic variation rate (GVR) is higher in AD patients than in the general population *(4, 5, 12, 31)*. The variability of bigenic, trigenic, tetragenic, and polygenic genotypes of AD-related genes is currently higher in AD than in controls, with an absolute genetic variation (AGV) of 40–60% and a relative genetic variation (RGV) of 0.85–1.89%, depending on the number of genes included in the haplotype-like cluster. Approximately, 40% of AD cases exhibit a GVR higher than 1%, as compared to controls, when a trigenic cluster integrated by combinations of APOE+PS1+PS2 polymorphic variants is examined. Increased GVR in AD might indicate that the over-representation of a series of genes involved in brain maturation and in the maintenance of higher activities of the CNS has surpassed a natural selection threshold (excessive genome complexity, genomic overdiversification), constituting a Darwinian disadvantage that shortens life span in humans *(4, 31)*.

AD is a perfect paradigm to potentially explain how the stochastic process of aging interacts with genetic factors leading to reduce neuronal survival and consequently human longevity, since neurons are major sensors of longevity, and longevity depends on genome stability, metabolic factors, and environmental factors. In this regard, increased genetic variation in AD might represent an evolutionary disadvantage capable of reducing human longevity due to the induction of premature neuronal death *(4, 12, 31)*. At the base of this deleterious mechanism, epigenetic factors and chaperone dysfunction-related protein misfolding might be present. The accumulation of misfolded proteins, with loss-of-function and/or toxic gain-of-function, can have cellular consequences such as stress response, proteasome inhibition, chaperone sequestration, transcription/cell cycle factor sequestration, fibril pore formation, calcium overload, oxidative stress, glutamate overload, mitochondrial dysfunction, and cell death *(32)*, all present in AD brains *(4)*.

2.2 Genotype-Phenotype Correlations

Functional genomics studies have demonstrated the influence of many genes on AD pathogenesis and phenotype expression (Table 16.1). Mutations in the APP, PS1, PS2, and MAPT genes give rise to well-characterized differential neuropathological and clinical phenotypes of dementia *(4)*. The analysis of genotype-phenotype correlations has also revealed that the presence of the APOE-4 allele in AD, in conjunction with other genes, influences disease onset, brain atrophy, cerebrovascular perfusion, blood pressure, β-amyloid deposition, ApoE secretion, lipid metabolism, brain bioelectrical activity, cognition, apoptosis, and treatment outcome *(4–8, 10–12, 22, 23, 33, 34)*. The characterization of phenotypic profiles according to age, cognitive performance (MMSE and ADAS-Cog score), serum ApoE levels, serum lipid levels including cholesterol (CHO), HDL-CHO, LDL-CHO, VLDL-CHO, and triglyceride (TG) levels, as well as serum nitric oxide (NO), β-amyloid, and histamine levels *(12, 35, 36)*, reveals sex-related differences in 25% of the biological parameters, and almost no differences (0.24%) when patients are classified as APOE-4(–) and APOE-4(+) carriers, probably indicating that gender-related factors may influence these parametric variables more powerfully than the presence or absence of the APOE-4 allele; in contrast, when patients are classified according to their APOE genotype, dramatic differences emerge among them (>45%), with a clear biological disadvantage in APOE-4/4 carriers who exhibit (i) earlier age of onset, (ii) low ApoE levels, (iii) high CHO and LDL-CHO levels, and (iv) low NO, β-amyloid, and histamine levels in blood *(4, 5, 11, 12, 34–36)*. These phenotypic differences are less pronounced when AD patients are classified according to their PS1 (15.6%) or ACE genotypes (23.52%), reflecting a weak impact of PS1- and ACE-related genotypes on the phenotypic expression of biological markers in AD. PS1-related genotypes appear to influence age of onset, blood histamine levels, and cerebrovascular hemodynamics, as reflected by significant changes in systolic (Sv), diastolic (Dv), and mean velocities (Mv) in the left middle cerebral arteries (MCA) (12). ACE-related phenotypes seem to be more influential than PS1 genotypes in defining biological phenotypes, such as age of onset, cognitive performance, HDL-CHO levels, serum Ace and NO levels, and brain blood flow Mv in MCA. However, when APOE and PS1 genotypes are integrated in bigenic clusters and the resulting bigenic genotypes are differentiated according to their corresponding phenotypes, an almost logarithmic increased expression of differential phenotypes is observed (61.46% variation), indicating the existence of a synergistic effect of the bigenic (APOE+PS1) cluster on the expression of biological markers, apparently unrelated to APP/PS1 mutations *(12, 35, 36)*. These examples illustrate the potential additive effects of AD-related genes on the phenotypic expression of biological markers. Furthermore, the analysis of genotype-phenotype correlations with a monogenic or bigenic approach documents a modest genotype-related variation in serum amyloid-β (ABP) levels, suggesting that peripheral levels of ABP are of relative value as predictors of disease stage or as markers of disease progression and/or treatment-related disease-modifying effects *(12, 35, 36)*. The peripheral levels of ABP in serum exhibit an APOE-dependent pattern according to which both APOE-4(+) and APOE-2(+) carriers tend to show higher ABP levels than APOE-4(–) or APOE-3 carriers *(12, 22, 35, 36)*. This trend is even clearer when APOE, PS1, and PS2 genotypes are integrated in bigenic or trigenic clusters, where the 3322, 3212, and 4412 genotypes show the highest ABP levels as compared with other genotypes *(12, 22, 35, 36)*. The incorporation of genotype assessment to biochemical studies (e.g., phenotype expression profile) in AD would avoid inconsistencies and unnecessary controversies such as those reflected in recent papers concerning variability in ABP levels in AD *(37)*. Likewise, in drug clinical trials with β-breakers or amyloid scavengers, as well as in cases of vaccination against ABP deposits or treatment with β-secretase inhibitors, at least APOE genotyping should be included to discriminate specific genotype-related responses.

In contrast to the inconsistent variability in ABP levels, genotype-related serum histamine changes exhibit an outstanding variation that can be modified by therapeutic intervention *(38, 39)*. APOE-related serum histamine levels exhibit an opposite pattern to that observed in ABP levels. The lowest concentration of serum histamine is systematically present in APOE-2(+) and APOE-4(+) carriers, and the highest levels of histamine are seen in APOE-3(+) carriers. Central and peripheral histaminergic mechanisms may regulate cerebrovascular function in AD, which is significantly altered in APOE-4/4 carriers *(4, 12, 38, 39)*. These observations can lead to the conclusion that the simple quantification of biochemical markers in fluids or tissues of AD patients with the aim of identifying pathogenic mechanisms and/or monitoring therapeutic effects, when they are not accompanied by differential genotyping for sample homogenization, are of very poor value.

It has been demonstrated that brain activity slowing correlates with progressive GDS staging in dementia *(4, 11, 12)*. In the general population subjects harbouring the APOE-4/4 genotype exhibit a premature slowing in brain mapping activity represented by increased slow delta and theta activities as compared with other APOE genotypes *(4, 11, 12)*. In patients with AD, slow activity predominates in APOE-4 carriers with similar GDS stage *(4, 5, 11, 12)*. Similarly, when brain metabolism and neuronal oxygen consumption (oxy-, deoxy-, and total hemoglobin variation)

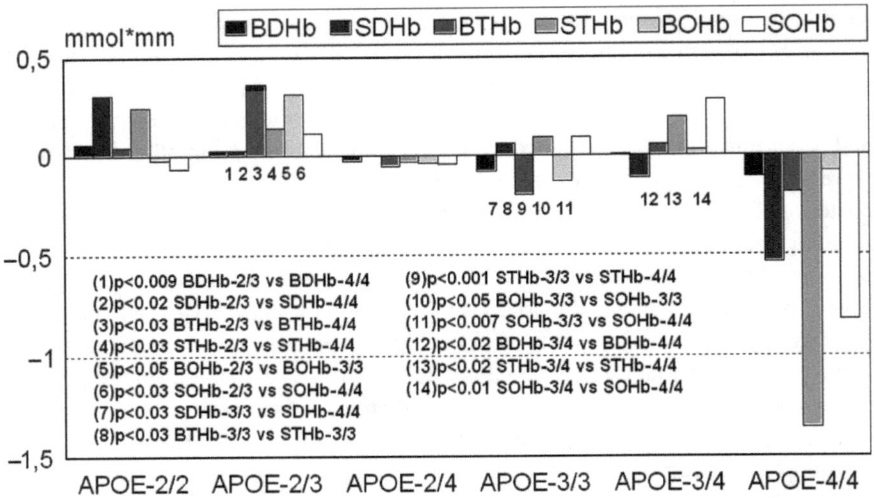

Fig. 16.3 APOE-related variation in the concentration of deoxy (DHb)-, total (THb)-, and oxy-hemoglobin (OHb) in the occipital cortex of patients with dementia in basal conditions and after visual stimulation as assessed by brain optical topography (Source: R. Cacabelos and I. Tellado, EuroEspes Biomedical Research Center, Optical Topography System, Hitachi Medical Corporation)

are assessed by optical topography, again an APOE-dependent topographic pattern is observed (Fig. 16.3). With this new technology it is possible to quantify online brain activation and cortical hemoglobin (Hb) variation after somatosensory stimulation (visual, auditory, mental tasks) in freely moving patients. Under this experimental paradigm, APOE-4/4 carriers are the worst responders to different sensory stimuli (Fig. 16.3).

All these examples of genotype-phenotype correlations, as a gross approach to functional genomics, illustrate the importance of genotype-related differences in AD and their impact on phenotype expression *(4, 5, 11, 12, 35, 36)*. Most biological parameters, potentially modifiable by monogenic genotypes and/or polygenic cluster profiles, can be used in clinical trials for monitoring efficacy outcomes. These parametric variables also show a genotype-dependent profile in different types of dementia. For instance, striking differences have been found between AD and vascular dementia in structural and functional genomics studies *(4, 5, 11, 12, 22, 35, 36)*.

3 Alzheimer's Disease Therapeutics

Drugs approved by the FDA and other regulatory authorities in Europe and Japan include the cholinesterase inhibitors (ChEIs) tacrine, donepezil, rivastigmine, and galantamine, and the NMDA receptor partial antagonist memantine *(11, 12)*. Some studies assessing the cost-effectiveness of ChEIs suggest that ChEI therapy provides benefit at every stage of disease, with better outcomes resulting from persistent, uninterrupted treatment; whereas other studies indicate that ChEIs are not cost-effective, with benefits below minimally relevant thresholds or cost-neutral *(3)*. Methological limitations in some studies reduce the confidence of independent evaluators in the validity of the conclusions drawn in published reports *(40)*. Although the therapeutic value and cost-effectiveness of current antidementia treatment is very questionable *(3)*, these drugs are of common use in AD *(10–12)* and still require further evaluation from a pharmacogenetic/pharmacogenomic perspective in order to avoid side effects and unnecessary costs *(12)*.

3.1 Potential Therapeutic Strategies

Modern therapeutic strategies in AD are addressed to interfere with the main pathogenic mechanisms potentially involved in AD. Major pathogenic events (drug targets) and their respective therapeutic alternatives (Figs. 16.2 & 16.4) include the following: (a) genetic defects: gene therapy and RNAi; (b) β-amyloid deposition: β-secretase inhibitors, γ-secretase inhibitors, α-secretase activators, Aβ-fibrillation

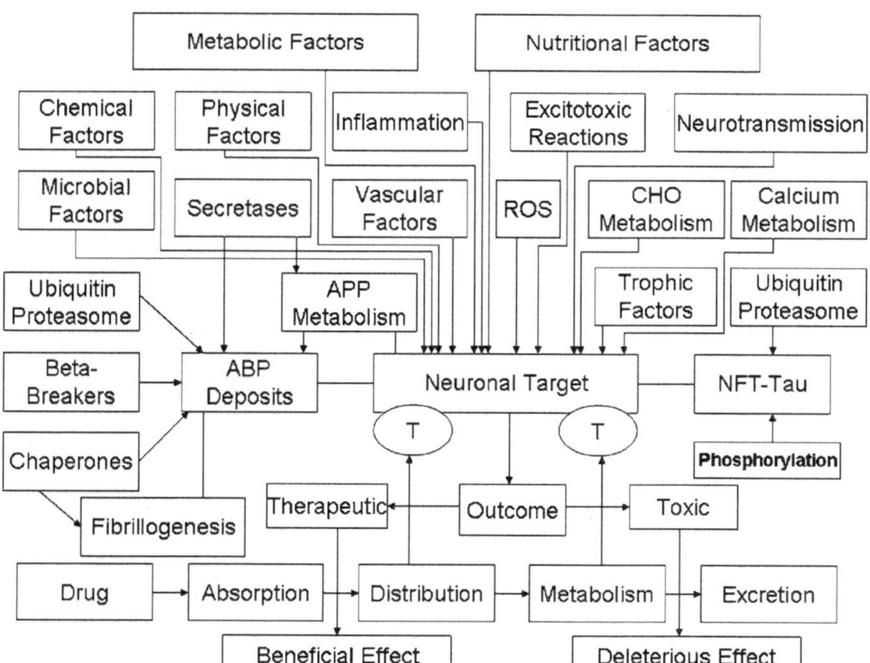

Fig. 16.4 Pathogenic factors acting on neuronal targets in Alzheimer's disease and potential pharmacological strategies (Adapted from *[68]*)

and aggregation inhibitors, amyloid immunotherapy (active and passive vaccination), copper chelating agents, solubilizers of Aβ aggregates, APP production inhibitors, and Aβ selective regulators (reticulons, chaperones); (c) tau-related pathology: phosphatase activators, GSK-3 inhibitors, Cdk5 inhibitors, p38 inhibitors, JNK inhibitors; (d) apoptosis: caspase inhibitors; (e) neurotransmitter deficits: acetylcholine enhancers (acetylcholine-release stimulants, acetylcholine reuptake inhibitors, cholinesterase inhibitors, choline-acetyl-transferase stimulants, muscarinic antagonists, nicotinic agonists), GABA modulators (inverse GABA-receptor agonists), glutamate modulators (NMDA antagonists, ampakines), dopamine reuptake inhibitors, adrenoreceptor modulators, histamine H3 antagonists, and serotonin modulators (5HT3 and 5HT1A receptor agonists, 5HT6 receptor antagonists, serotonin stimulants); (f) neurotrophic deficits: neurotrophic factors, growth factors, synthetic neuropeptides, and natural compounds with neurotrophic activity; (g) neuronal loss: neuronal stem cells, growth factors, neurite outgrowth activators, NOGO inhibitors, MOP inhibitors, GSK3 inhibitors, JNK inhibitors, and p38 inhibitors; (h) neuroinflammation: COX1 and COX2 inhibitors, complement activation inhibitors, p38 inhibitors, eNOS inhibitors, PPARα agonists, PPARγ agonists, novel NSAIDs, and cytokine inhibitors; (i) oxidative stress: antioxidants, caspase inhibitors, and antioxidating enzyme enhancers; (j) calcium dysmetabolism: calcium channel blockers; (k) neuronal hypometabolism: PPARγ agonists, and GSK3 inhibitors; (l) lipid metabolism dysfunction: HMG-CoA reductase inhibitors, PPARγ agonists, and novel biomarine lipoproteins; (m) cerebrovascular dysfunction: vasoactive substances, NO inhibitors, HIF inhibitors, dandrolene-related agents, novel lipoproteins with antiatherosclerotic activity, and liver X receptor agonists; (n) neuronal dysfunction associated with nutritional deficits: brain metabolism enhancers, nutrigenomic agents, and nutraceuticals; and (o) a miscellany of pathogenic mechanisms potentially manageable with diverse classes of chemicals or biopharmaceuticals *(1, 2, 10–12)*.

4 Pharmacogenetic Strategies in Alzheimer's Disease

4.1 General Concepts

Pharmacogenetics/pharmacogenomics is a novel science that refers to the genomic conditions by which different genes determine the behavior and sensitivity of drugs on a specific organism or genotype. Pharmacogenomics relates to the application of genomic technologies, such as genotyping, gene sequencing, gene expression, genetic epidemiology, transcriptomics, proteomics, metabolomics, and bioinformatics, to drugs in clinical development and on the market, applying the large-scale systematic approaches of genomics to speed the discovery of drug response markers, whether they act at the level of drug target, drug metabolism, or disease pathways *(12–14, 19, 41, 42)*. The potential implications of pharmacogenomics in clinical trials and molecular therapeutics is that a particular disease could be treated according to genomic and biological markers, selecting medications and diseases that are optimized for individual patients or clusters of patients with a similar genomic profile *(19, 41)*. For many medications, interindividual differences are mainly due to SNPs in genes encoding drug metabolizing enzymes, drug transporters, and/or drug targets (e.g., genome-related defective enzymes, receptors, and proteins that alter metabolic pathways leading to disease phenotype expression) *(19)*.

The therapeutic lessons obtained from pharmacogenetics in the past, as pointed out by Meyer *(43)*, can be the following: (i) all drug effects vary from person to person and all drug effects are influenced by genes; (ii) most drug responses are multifactorial; (iii) genetic polymorphisms of single genes, including mutations in coding sequences, gene duplications, gene deletions, and regulatory mutations affect numerous drug-metabolizing enzymes, including several cytochrome-P450 enzymes (CYP-related genes), N-acetyltransferases (NAT genes), thiopurine-methyltransferase (TPMT), and UDP-glucuronosyltransferases (UDP-GT); (iii) individuals that possess these polymorphisms are at risk of experiencing documented adverse reactions or inefficacy of drugs at usual doses; (iv) genetic polymorphisms of drug targets and drug transporters are increasingly recognized (receptors, ion channels, growth factors) as causing variation in drug responses; (v) several targets respond to treatment only in subgroups of patients who carry sensitizing mutations of these targets; (vi) the frequency of variation of drug effects, whether multifactorial or genetic, varies considerably in ethnically defined populations; and (vii) application of response-predictive genetic profiles on clinical outcomes has so far been done mostly in academic centers and has not yet reached clinical practice *(43)*.

The heterogeneity of AD, and how apparently identical phenotypes assessed with international clinical criteria (NINCDS-ADRDA, DSM-IV, ICD-10) do not always respond to the same drugs, have been very well known for many years *(10–12)*. This may be due to different factors, including pharmacokinetic and pharmacodynamic properties of drugs, nutrition, liver function, concomitant medications, and individual genetic factors. In fact, the therapeutic response of AD patients to conventional cholinesterase inhibitors is partially effective in only 10–20% of the cases, with side effects, intolerance, and noncompliance in more than 60% of the patients due to different reasons (e.g., efficacy, safety) (1–3). Therefore, the individualization of therapy or pharmacological tailorization in AD and other CNS disorders is just another step forward towards the longstanding goal of molecular pharmacology *(19, 44–46)*, taking advantage of the information and procedures provided by the sequencing of the entire human genome *(47)*.

4.2 Pharmacogenetics of Drug Metabolism

Although drug effect is a complex phenotype that depends on many factors, it is estimated that genetics accounts for 20–95% of variability in drug disposition and pharmacodynamics *(19)*. Cholinesterase inhibitors in current use with AD, such as donepezil and galantamine (and tacrine, as well), are metabolized via CYP-related enzymes. These drugs can interact with many other drugs which are substrates, inhibitors, or inducers of the cytochrome P-450 system; this interaction eliciting liver toxicity and other adverse drug reactions (ADRs) *(10–12)*.

AD patients are currently treated with cholinesterase inhibitors, neuroprotective drugs, antidepressants, anxyolitics, antiparkinsonian drugs, anticonvulsants, and neuroleptics at a given time of the clinical disease course to palliate memory dysfunction, behavioral changes, sleep disorders, agitation, depression, parkinsonism, myoclonus, and seizures or psychotic symptoms *(1, 12, 48)*. Many of these substances are metabolized by enzymes known to be genetically variable, including: (a) esterases: butyrylcholinesterase, paraoxonase/arylesterase; (b) transferases: N-acetyltransferase, sulfotransferase, thiol methyltransferase, thiopurine methyltransferase, catechol-O-methyltransferase, glutathione-S-transferases, UDP-glucuronosyltransferases, glucosyltransferase, histamine methyltransferase; (c) Reductases: NADPH:quinine oxidoreductase, glucose-6-phosphate dehydrogenase; (d) oxidases: alcohol dehydrogenase, aldehydehydrogenase, monoamine oxidase B, catalase, superoxide dismutase, trimethylamine N-oxidase, dihydropyrimidine dehydrogenase; and (e) cytochrome P450 enzymes, such as CYP1A1, CYP2A6, CYP2C8, CYP2C9, CYP2C19, CYP2D6, CYP2E1, CYP3A5 (Table 16.2) and many others *(12)*. Polymorphic variants in these genes can induce alterations in drug metabolism modifying the efficacy and safety of the prescribed drugs.

Drug metabolism includes phase I reactions (i.e., oxidation, reduction, hydrolysis) and phase II conjugation reactions (i.e., acetylation, glucuronidation, sulfation, methylation) *(45)*. The principal enzymes with polymorphic variants involved in phase I reactions are the following: CYP3A4/5/7, CYP2E1, CYP2D6, CYP2C19, CYP2C9, CYP2C8, CYP2B6, CYP2A6, CYP1B1, CYP1A1/2, epoxide hydrolase, esterases, NQO1 (NADPH-quinone oxidoreductase), DPD (dihydropyrimidine dehydrogenase), ADH (alcohol dehydrogenase), and ALDH (aldehyde dehydrogenase). Major enzymes involved in phase II reactions include the following: UGTs (uridine 5′-triphosphate glucuronosyl transferases), TPMT (thiopurine methyltransferase), COMT (catechol-O-methyltransferase), HMT (histamine methyl-transferase), STs (sulfotransferases), GST-A (glutathion S-transferase A), GST-P, GST-T, GST-M, NAT2 (N-acetyl transferase), NAT1, and others *(49)*.

4.3 The CYP Gene Family

The typical paradigm for the pharmacogenetics of phase I drug metabolism is represented by the cytochrome P450 enzymes, a superfamily of microsomal drug-metabolizing enzymes. P450 enzymes comprise a superfamily of heme-thiolate proteins widely distributed in bacteria, fungi, plants, and animals. The P450 enzymes are encoded in genes of the CYP superfamily (Table 16.2) and act as terminal oxidases in multicomponent electron transfer chains, which are called P450-containing monooxygenase systems. Some of the enzymatic products of the

Table 16.2 CYP genes encoding cytochrome P450-related enzymes involved in human pharmacogenetic activities

Gene	Locus	Name	Alternate Names	Related Drugs	Related Diseases	OMIM Phenotype	Alternate Symbols
CYP1A2	15q22-qter	Cytochrome P450, subfamily (aromatic compound-inducible), polypeptide 2	P450 form 4; aryl hydrocarbon hydroxylase; cytochrome P450, subfamily 1 (aromatic compound-inducible), polypeptide 2; dioxin-inducible P3-450; flavoprotein-linked monooxygenase; microsomal monooxygenase; xenobiotic monooxygenase	Amiodarone, caffeine, citalopram, clozapine, cyclobenzaprine, dexamethasone, Echinacea, estradiol, etoposide, fluvoxamine, haloperidol, imipramine, interferon alpha, lidocaine, mibefradil, midazolam, modafinil, naproxen, ondansetron, propranolol, ribavirin, riluzole, ropivacaine, tacrine, teniposide, theophylline, thiotepa, ticlopidine, verapamil, zolmitriptan, zoxazolamine	Chronic hepatitis C, Schizophrenia, psychosis		CP12; P3-450; P450(PA)
CYP1B1	2p21	Cytochrome P450, subfamily 1 (dioxin-inducible), polypeptide 1 (glaucoma 3, primary infantile)	Aryl hydrocarbon hydroxylase; cytochrome P450, subfamily 1 (dioxin-inducible), polypeptide 1 (glaucoma 3, primary infantile); flavoprotein-linked monooxygenase; microsomal monooxygenase; xenobiotic monooxygenase	Estrogens	Breast neoplasms	Primary congenital glaucoma 3A; early-onset digenic glaucoma; Peters anomaly	CP1B; GLC3A

(continued)

Table 16.2 (continued)

Gene	Locus	Name	Alternate Names	Related Drugs	Related Diseases	OMIM Phenotype	Alternate Symbols
CYP2A6	19q13.2	Cytochrome P450, family 2, subfamily A, polypeptide 6	Coumarin 7-hydroxylase; cytochrome P450, subfamily IIA (Phenobarbital-inducible), polypeptide 3; cytochrome P450, subfamily IIA (Phenobarbital-inducible), polypeptide 6; flavoprotein-linked monooxygenase; xenobiotic monooxygenase	5-Fluorouracil, dexamethasone, etoposide, fadrozole, fluorouracil, midazolam, nicotine, rifampin, teniposide	Neoplasms	Coumarin resistance, protection from nicotine addiction	CPA6; CYP2A3
CYP2B6	19q13.2	Cytochrome P450, family 2, subfamily B, polypeptide 6	Cytochrome P450, subfamily IIB (Phenobarbital-inducible), polypeptide 6	Aflatoxin B1, bupropion, cyclophosphamide, dexamethasone, etoposide, ifosfamide, midazolam, phenobarbital, propofol, rifampin, teniposide, thiotepa, vitamin D, xenobiotics	Nicotine addiction		CPB6; CYPIIB6; P450
CYP2C19	10q24.1-q24.3	Cytochrome P450, family 2, subfamily C, polypeptide 19	Cytochrome P450, subfamily IIC (mephenytoin 4-hydroxylase), polypeptide 19; flavoprotein-linked monooxygenase; mephenytoin 4,-hydroxylase; microsomal monooxygenase; xenobiotic monooxygenase	Amitriptyline, carisoprodol, citalopram, cyclophosphamide, diazepam, fluoxetine, fluvoxamine, glucorticoids, hexobarbital, lansoprazole, mephenytoin, modafinil, nelfinavir, nilutamide, omeprazole, pantoprazole, proguanil, rifampin, thiotepa, ticlopidine	Lupus nephritis, gastroesophageal reflux disease, peptic ulcer disease, visual disorders	Mephenytoin poor metabolizer	CPCJ; CYP2C; P450C2C; P450IIC19

CYP2C9	10q24	Cytochrome P450, family 2, subfamily C, polypeptide 9	Cytochrome P450, subfamily IIC (mephenytoin 4-hydroxylase), polypeptide 10; cytochrome P450, subfamily IIC (mephenytoin 4-hydroxylase), polypeptide 9; flavoprotein-linked monooxygenase; mephenytoin 4-hydroxylase; microsomal monooxygenase; xenobiotic monooxygenase	Acenocoumarol, amiodarone, celecoxib, coumadin, dexamethasone, diclofenac, etoposide, fluconazole, fluoxetine, fluvastatin, fluvoxamine, glimepiride, glipizide, glyburide, ibuprofen, irbesartan, isoniazid, losartan, midazolam, phenylbutazone, phenytoin, rifampin, teniposide, tenoxicam, thiotepa, tolbutamide, torsemide, vitamin D, warfarin	Arthritis, blood coagulation disorders, diabetes mellitus, epilepsy, hypertension, thrombolytic disease	Tolbutamide poor metabolizer, warfarin sensitivity	CPC9; CYP2C10; P450 MP-4; P450 PB-1; P450IIC9
CYP2D6	22q13.1	Cytochrome P450, family 2, subfamily D, polypeptide 6	Cytochrome P450, subfamily IID (debrisoquin, sparteine), polypeptide 6; cytochrome P450, subfamily IID (debrisoquine, sparteine)-like 1; debrisoquine 4-hydroxylase; flavoprotein-linked monooxygenase; microsomal monooxygenase; xenobiotic monooxygenase	Amitriptyline, caffeine, cimetidine, citalopram, clomipramine, clozapine, cocaine, codeine, debrisoquine, desipramine, dextromethorphan, diltiazem, flecainide, fluoxetine, fluvoxamine, haloperidol, imipramine, interferon alpha, metoprolol, mexiletine, morphine, paroxetine, perhexiline, perphenazine, propafenone, propranolol, ribavirin, risperidone, ritonavir, sparteine, tamoxifen, thioridazine, thiotepa, timolol, tramadol, venlafaxine, xenobiotics, yohimbine, zuclopenthixol	Breast neoplasms, cystic fibrosis, depression, chronic hepatitis C, lung neoplasms, neoplasms, codeine dependence pain, schizophrenia, codeine dependence, psychosis	Susceptibility to parkinsonism, debrisoquine sensitivity	CPD6; CYP2D; CYP2D6; CYP2DL1; P450-DB1; P450C2D

(continued)

Table 16.2 (continued)

Gene	Locus	Name	Alternate Names	Related Drugs	Related Diseases	OMIM Phenotype	Alternate Symbols
CYP2E1	10q24.3-qter	Cytochrome P450, subfamily IIE (ethanol-inducible)	Cytochrome P450, subfamily IIE (ethanol-inducible); cytochrome P450, subfamily IIE (ethanol-inducible), polypeptide 1; flavoprotein-linked monooxygenase; microsomal monooxygenase; xenobiotic monooxygenase	Dexamethasone, ethanol, etoposide, midazolam, nicotine, teniposide, thiotepa, xenobiotics	Alcoholic liver disease, lung neoplasms, nicotine dependency		CPE1; CYP2E; CYP2E1; P450-J; P450C2E
CYP3A	7q21.3-q22.1	Cytochrome P450, family 3, subfamily A	Cytochrome P450, subfamily IIIA (nifedipine oxidase)	Dexamethasone, docetaxel, erythromycin, midazolam, rifampin, tamoxifen, thiotepa, xenobiotics	Arrhythmia, lung neoplasms		CYP3
CYP3A4	7q21.1	Cytochrome P450, family 3, subfamily A, polypeptide 4	P450-III, steroid inducible; cytochrome P450, subfamily IIIA (nifedipine oxidase), polypeptide 3; cytochrome P450, subfamily IIIA (nifedipine oxidase), polypeptide 4; glucocorticoid-inducible P450; nifedipine oxidase	Alprazolam, anthracycline, cisapride, citalopram, dexamethasone, docetaxel, epipodophyllotoxin, etoposide, glucocorticoids, interferon alpha, irinotecan, losartan, midazolam, nifedipine, omeprazole, ribavirin, rifampin, tamoxifen, teniposide, testosterone, topotecan, vitamin D, xenobiotics	Breast neoplasms, chronic hepatitis C, leukaemia, L1 acute lymphocytic leukaemia, myeloid leukaemia, neoplasms, prostatic neoplasms, helycobarcter pylori gastric ulcers		CP33; CP34; CYP3A; CYP3A3; CYP3A4; HLP; NF-25; P450C3; P450PCN1

CYP3A5	7q21.1	Cytochrome P450, family 3, subfamily A, polypeptide 5	Aryl hydrocarbon hydrolase; cytochrome P450, subfamily IIIA (nifedipine oxidase), polypeptide 5; flavoprotein-linked monooxygenase; microsomal monooxygenase; nifedipine oxidase; xenobiotic monooxygenase	Aflatoxin B1, antrhacycline, cisapride, cyclosporine, dexamethasone, etoposide, glucocorticoids, irinotecan, midazolam, simvastatin, tacrolimus, teniposide, vitamin C, warfarin, xenobiotics	Blood coagulation disorders, L1 acute lymphocytic leukaemia, myeloid leukaemia		CYP35; CYP3A5; P450PCN3; PCN3
CYP3A7	7q21-q22.1	Cytochrome P450, family 3, subfamily A, polypeptide 7	Aryl hydrocarbon hydrolase; cytochrome P450, subfamily IIIA, polypeptide 7; flavoprotein-linked monooxygenase; microsomal monooxygenase; xenobiotic monooxygenase	Cisapride, midazolam, vitamin D, xenobiotics			CP37; P450-HFLA
CYP4B1	1p34-p12	Cytochrome P450, subfamily IVB, polypeptide 1	Cytochrome P450, subfamily IVB, member 1; cytochrome P450, subfamily IVB, polypeptide 1; microsomal monooxygenase	Xenobiotics			P-450HP
CYP11B2	8q21-q22	Cytochrome P450, family 11, subfamily B, polypeptide 2	Steroid 11-beta/18-hydrolase; aldosterone synthase; cytochrome P450, subfamily XIB (steroid 11-beta-hydrolase), polypeptide 2; steroid 11-beta-monooxygenase; steroid 11-beta/18-hydrolase	Candesartan		Aldosterone to renin ratio raised, congenital hypoaldosteronism due to CMO I deficit, congenital hypoaldosteronism due to CMO II deficit, low renin hypertension	ALDOS; CPN2; CYP11B; CYP11BL; P-450C-18; P450aldo

Adapted from (12)

CYP gene superfamily can share substrates, inhibitors, and inducers, whereas others are quite specific for their substrates and interacting drugs *(5, 11, 12, 43)*. There are more than 200 P450 genes identified in different species, with more than 1,000 variants among CYP450 genes *(50)*. These species-specific differences are important when performing comparative pharmacogenetic studies and/or pharmacological experiments in animal models *(51)*.

The microsomal, membrane-associated P450 isoforms CYP3A4, CYP2D6, CYP2C9, CYP2C19, CYP2E1, and CYP1A2 are responsible for the oxidative metabolism of more than 90% of marketed drugs; and CYP3A4 metabolizes more drug molecules than all other isoforms together. Most of these polymorphisms exhibit geographic and ethnic differences *(52–57)*. These differences influence drug metabolism in ethnic groups in which drug dosage should be adjusted according to their enzymatic capacity, differentiating normal or extensive metabolizers (EMs), poor metabolizers (PMs), and ultrarapid metabolizers (UMs). Most drugs act as substrates, inhibitors, or inducers of CYP enzymes. Enzyme induction enables some xenobiotics to accelerate their own biotransformation (auto-induction) or the biotransformation and elimination of other drugs *(11, 12)*. A number of P450 enzymes in human liver are inducible. Induction of the majority of P450 enzymes occurs by increase in the rate of gene transcription and involves ligand-activated transcription factors, aryl hydrocarbon receptor, constitutive androstane receptor (CAR), and pregnane X receptor (PXR) *(56, 58)*. In general, binding of the appropriate ligand to the receptor initiates the induction process that cascades through a dimerization of the receptors, their translocation to the nucleus and binding to specific regions in the promoters of CYPs *(58–60)*. CYPs are also expressed in the CNS, and a complete characterization of constitutive and induced CYPs in brain is essential for understanding the role of these enzymes in neurobiological functions and in age-related and xenobiotic-induced neurotoxicity *(61)*.

The most important enzymes of the P450 cytochrome family in drug metabolism in decreasing order are CYP3A4, CYP2D6, CYP2C9, CYP2C19, and CYP2A6 *(12, 49, 50, 57, 62, 63)*. The predominant allelic variants in the CYP2A6 gene are CYP2A6*2 (Leu160His) and CYP2A6del. The CYP2A6*2 mutation inactivates the enzyme and is present in 1–3% of Caucasians. The CYP2A6del mutation results in no enzyme activity and is present in 1% of Caucasians and 15% of Asians *(11, 12, 49)*. The most frequent mutations in the CYP2C9 gene are CYP2C9*2 (Arg144Cys), with reduced affinity for P450 in 8–13% of Caucasians, and CYP2C9*3 (Ile359Leu), with alterations in the specificity for the substrate in 6–9% of Caucasians and 2–3% of Asians *(11, 12, 49)*. The most prevalent polymorphic variants in the CYP2C19 gene are CYP2C19*2, with an aberrant splicing site resulting in enzyme inactivation in 13% of Caucasians, 23–32% of Asians, 13% of Africans, and 14–15% of Ethiopians and Saudi Arabians, and CYP2C19*3, a premature stop codon resulting in an inactive enzyme present in 6–10% of Asians, and almost absent in Caucasians *(11, 12, 49)*. The most important mutations in the CYP2D6 gene are the following: CYP2D6*2xN, CYP2D6*4, CYP2D6*5, CYP2D6*10, and CYP2D6*17 *(10–12, 57, 64)*. The CYP2D6*2xN mutation gives rise to a gene duplication or multiplication resulting in increased enzyme activity which appears in 1–5% of the Caucasian population, 0–2% of Asians, 2% of Africans, and 10–16% of Ethiopians. The defective splicing caused by the CYP2D6*4 mutation inactivates the enzyme and is present in 12–21% of Caucasians. The deletion in CYP2D6*5 abolishes enzyme activity and shows a frequency of 2–7% in Caucasians, 1% in Asians, 2% in Africans, and 1–3% in Ethiopians. The polymorphism CYP2D6*10 causes Pro34Ser and Ser486Thr mutations with unstable enzyme activity in 1–2% of Caucasians, 6% of Asians, 4% of Africans, and 1–3% of Ethiopians. The CYP2D6*17 variant causes Thr107Ile and Arg296Cys substitutions which produce a reduced affinity for substrates in 51% of Asians, 6% of Africans, and 3–9% of Ehtiopians, and is practically absent in Caucasians *(10–12, 49, 57, 64)*.

4.3.1 CYP2D6 Genotypes in Alzheimer's Disease

The CYP2D6 enzyme, encoded by a gene that maps on 22q13.1–13.2, catalyses the oxidative metabolism of more than 100 clinically important and commonly prescribed drugs such as cholinesterase inhibitors (tacrine, donepezil, galantamine), antidepressants, neuroleptics, opioids, some β-blockers, class I antiarrhythmics, analgesics, and many other drug categories, acting as substrates, inhibitors, or inducers with which cholinesterase inhibitors may potentially interact, this leading to the outcome of ADRs *(10–12, 65)*. The CYP2D6 locus is highly polymorphic, with more than 100 different CYP2D6 alleles identified in the general population, showing deficient (poor metabolizers, PM), normal (extensive metabolizers, EM) or increased enzymatic activity (ultrarapid metabolizers, UM) *(63)*. Most individuals (>80%) are EMs; however, remarkable interethnic differences exist in the frequency of the PM and UM phenotypes among different societies all over the world *(5, 10–12, 53, 55–57, 64)*. On the average, approximately 6.28% of the world population belongs to the PM category. Europeans (7.86%), Polynesians (7.27%), and Africans (6.73%) exhibit the highest rate of PMs, whereas Orientals (0.94%) show the lowest rate. The frequency of PMs among Middle Eastern populations, Asians, and Americans is in the range of 2–3% *(10–12, 57)*. CYP2D6 gene duplications are relatively infrequent among Northern Europeans, but in East Africa the frequency of alleles with duplication of CYP2D6 is as high as 29% *(19)*.

The most frequent CYP2D6 alleles in the European population are the following: CYP2D6*1 (wild-type)(normal), CYP2D6*2 (2850C>T)(normal), CYP2D6 *3 (2549A>del)(inactive), CYP2D6*4 (1846G>A)(inactive), CYP2D6*5 (gene deletion)(inactive), CYP2D6*6 (1707T>del)(inactive), CYP2D6*7 (2935A>C) (inactive), CYP2D6*8 (1758G>T)(inactive), CYP2D6*9 (2613–2615 delAGA) (partially active), CYP2D6*10 (100C>T)(partially active), CYP2D6* 11 (883G>C)(inactive), CYP2D6*12 (124G>A)(inactive), CYP2D6*17 (1023C>T) (partially active), and CYP2D6 gene duplications (with increased or decreased enzymatic activity depending upon the alleles involved) *(10–12, 66–68)*.

In the Spanish population, where the mixture of ancestral cultures has occurred for centuries, the distribution of the CYP2D6 genotypes differentiates four major categories of CYP2D6-related metabolyzer types: (i) extensive metabolizers (EM)(*1/*1, *1/*10); (ii) intermediate metabolizers (IM)(*1/*3, *1/*4, *1/*5, *1/*6, *1/*7, *10/*10, *4/*10, *6/*10, *7/*10); (iii) poor metabolizers (PM)(*4/*4,

*5/*5); and (iv) ultrarapid metabolizers (UM)(*1xN/*1, *1xN/*4, Dupl). In this sample we have found 51.61% EMs, 32.26% IMs, 9.03% PMs, and 7.10% UMs *(68)* (Fig. 16.5). The distribution of all major genotypes is the following: *1/*1, 47.10%; *1/*10, 4.52%; *1/*3, 1.95%; *1/*4, 17.42%; *1/*5, 3.87%; *1/*6, 2.58%; *1/*7, 0.65%; *10/*10, 1.30%; *4/*10, 3.23%; *6/*10, 0.65%; *7/*10, 0.65%; *4/*4, 8.37%; *5/*5, 0.65%; *1xN/*1, 4.52%; *1xN/*4, 1.95%; and Dupl, 0.65% *(68)* (Fig. 16.5). These results are similar to others in the Caucasian population previously reported by Sachse et al. *(64)*, Bernal et al. *(67)*, Cacabelos *(10–12, 68)*, Bernard et al. *(69)*, and others *(54–57, 70–72)*.

When comparing AD cases with controls, we observed that EMs are more prevalent in AD (*1/*1, 49.42%; *1/*10, 8.04%)(total AD-EMs: 57.47%) than in controls (*1/*1, 44.12%; *1/*10, 0%)(total C-EMs: 44.12%). In contrast, IMs are more frequent in controls (41.18%) than in AD (25.29%), especially the *1/*4 (C: 23.53%; AD: 12.64%) and *4/*10 genotypes (C: 5.88%; AD: 1.15%). The frequency of PMs was similar in AD (9.20%) and controls (8.82%), and UMs were more frequent among AD cases (8.04%) than in controls (5.88%) *(68)*.

Although initial studies postulated the involvement of the CYP2D6B mutant allele in Lewy body formation in both Parkinson's disease and the Lewy body variant of AD, as well as in the synaptic pathology of pure AD without Lewy bodies *(73)*, subsequent studies in different ethnic groups did not find an association between AD and CYP2D6 variants *(72, 74–79)*. Notwithstanding, the genetic variation between AD and controls associated with CYP2D6 genotypes is 13.35% in EMs, 15.89% in IMs, 0.38% in PMs, and 2.16% in UMs, with an absolute genetic variation of 31.78% between both groups, suggesting that this genetic difference might influence AD pathogenesis and therapeutics *(68)*.

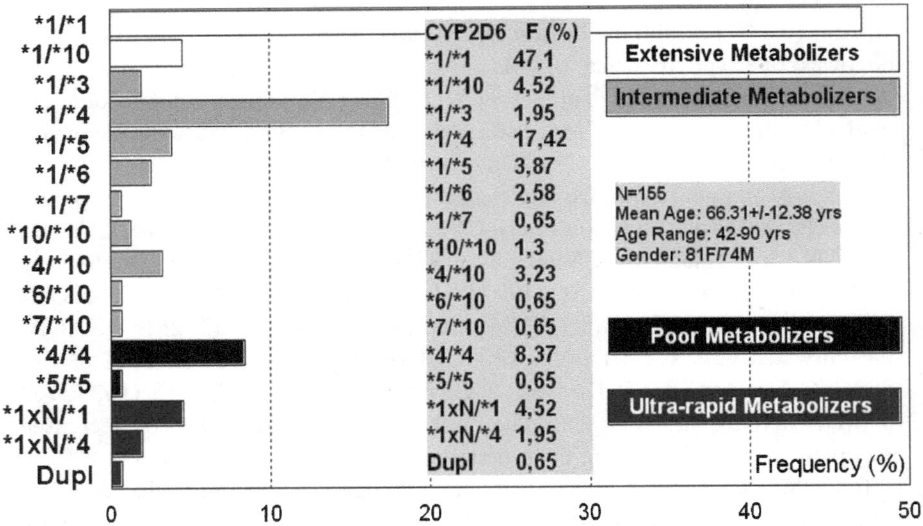

Fig. 16.5 Frequencies of major CYP2D5 genotypes in the Spanish population (Adapted from [64])

4.3.1.1 Association of CYP2D6 Variants with Alzheimer's Disease-Related Genes

We have also investigated the association of CYP2D6 genotypes with AD-related genes, such as APP, MAPT, APOE, PS1, PS2, A2M, ACE, AGT, FOS, and PRNP variants *(68)* (Table 16.3). No APP or MAPT mutations have been found in AD cases. Homozygous APOE-2/2 (12.56%) and APOE-4/4 (12.50%) accumulate in UMs, and APOE-4/4 cases were also more frequent in PMs (6.66%) than in EMs (3.95%) or IMs (0%). PS1–1/1 genotypes were more frequent in EMs (45%), whereas PS-1/2 genotypes were overrepresented in IMs (63.16%) and UMs (60%). The presence of the PS1–2/2 genotype was especially high in PMs (38.46%) and UMs (20%). A mutation in the PS2 gene exon 5 (PS2E5+) was markedly present in UMs (66.67%). About 100% of UMs were A2M-V100I-A/A, and the A2M-V100I-G/G genotype was absent in PMs and UMs. The A2M-I/I genotype was absent in UMs, and 100% of UMs were A2M-I/D and ACE-D/D. Homozygous mutations in the FOS gene (B/B) were only present in UMs as well. AGT-T235T cases were absent in PMs, and the AGT-M174M genotype appeared in 100% of PMs. Likewise, the PRNP-M129M variant was present in 100% of PMs and UMs *(68)* (Table 16.3). These association studies clearly show that in PMs and UMs there is an accumulation of AD-related polymorphic variants of risk which might be responsible for the defective therapeutic responses currently seen in these AD clusters *(68)*. Furthermore, CYP2D6-related AD PMs exhibit a poorer cerebrovascular function, which might affect drug penetration in the brain, with consequent therapeutic implications *(68)*.

4.3.1.2. Influence of CYP2D6 Genotypes on Liver Transaminase Activity

Some conventional antidementia drugs (tacrine, donepezil, galantamine) are metabolized via CYP-related enzymes, especially CYP2D6, CYP3A4, and CYP1A2, and polymorphic variants of the CYP2D6 gene can affect the liver metabolism, safety, and efficacy of some cholinesterase inhibitors *(10–12, 68, 80, 81)*. In order to elucidate whether or not CYP2D6-related variants may influence transaminase activity, we have studied the association of GOT, GPT, and GGT activity with the most prevalent CYP2D6 genotypes in AD (Table 16.4). Globally, UMs and PMs tend to show the highest GOT activity and IMs the lowest. Significant differences appear among different IM-related genotypes. The *10/*10 genotype exhibited the lowest GOT activity with marked differences as compared to UMs ($p < 0.05$ vs *1xN/*1; $p < 0.05$ vs *1xN/*4) *(68)*. GPT activity was significantly higher in PMs (*4/*4) than in EMs (*1/*10, $p < 0.05$) or IMs (*1/*4, *1/*5, $p < 0.05$). The lowest GPT activity was found in EMs and IMs *(68)*. Striking differences have been found in GGT activity between PMs (*4/*4), which showed the highest levels, and EMs (*1/*1, $p < 0.05$; *1/*10, $p < 0.05$), IMs (*1/*5, $p < 0.05$), or UMs (*1xN/*1, $p < 0.01$))(Table 16.4). Interestingly enough, the *10/*10 genotype, with the lowest values of GOT and GPT, exhibited the second highest levels of GGT after *4/*4, probably indicating that CYP2D6-related enzymes differentially regulate drug metabolism and transaminase activity in the liver. These results also clearly demonstrate the direct effect of CYP2D6 variants on transaminase activity *(68)* (Table 16.4).

Table 16.3 Distribution of AD-related genotypes associated with different CYP2D6 metabolizer types in Alzheimer disease

Gene	Polymorphic Variant	Extensive Metabolizers	Intermediate Metabolizers	Poor Metabolizers	Ultrarapid Metabolizers
APOE	2/2	0.00%	0.00%	0.00%	12.56%
	2/3	5.26%	8.51%	20.00%	0.00%
	2/4	0.00%	0.00%	0.00%	0.00%
	3/3	61.84%	63.83%	46.67%	50.00%
	3/4	28.95%	27.66%	26.67%	25.00%
	4/4	3.95%	0.00%	6.66%	12.50%
PS1	1/1	45%	23.68%	15.39%	20.00%
	1/2	46.67%	63.16%	46.15%	60.00%
	2/2	8.33%	13.16%	38.46%	20.00%
PS2	E5(-)	66.67%	79.49%	66.67%	33.33%
	E5(+)	33.33%	20.51%	33.33%	66.67%
A2Mins/del	II	65.72%	70.00%	87.50%	0.00%
	ID	34.28%	23.33%	12.50%	100.00%
	DD	0.00%	6.67%	0.00%	0.00%
A2Mpol	AA	44.45%	32.26%	37.50%	100.00%
A2M-V100I	AG	50.00%	51.62%	62.50%	0.00%
	GG	5.55%	16.12%	0.00%	0.00%
ACE	II	23.53%	3.57%	16.67%	0.00%
	ID	29.41%	50.00%	50.00%	0.00%
	DD	47.06%	46.43%	33.33%	100.0%
AGT-M235T	MM	0.00%	12.50%	20.00%	16.67%
	MT	84.21%	41.67%	80.00%	50.00%
	TT	15.79%	45.83%	0.00%	33.33%
AGT-T174M	MM	0.00%	0.00%	0.00%	25.00%
	TM	15.79%	20.00%	0.00%	25.00%
	TT	84.21%	80.00%	100.00%	50.00%
cFOS	B/B	2.18%	0.00%	0.00%	0.00%
	A/B	23.91%	33.33%	28.57%	25.00%
	A/A	73.91%	66.67%	71.43%	75.00%
PRNP-M129V	MM	52.94%	30.00%	100.00%	100.00%
	MV	41.18%	60.00%	0.00%	0.00%
	VV	5.88%	10.00%	0.00%	0.00%

Adapted from *(68)*

4.4 CYP2D6-Related Therapeutic Response to a Multifactorial Treatment

No clinical trials have been performed to date to elucidate the influence of CYP2D6 variants on the therapeutic outcome in AD in response to cholinesterase inhibitors or other antidementia drugs. To overcome this lack of pharmacogenetic information, we have performed the first prospective study in AD patients who received a combination therapy (CPND protocol) with (a) an endogenous nucleotide and choline donor, CDP-choline (500 mg/day), (b) a nootropic substance, piracetam (1600 mg/day), (c) a vasoactive compound, 1,6 dimethyl 8β-(5-bromonicotinoyl-oxymethyl)-10α-methoxyergoline (nicergoline)(5 mg/day), and (d) a cholinesterase inhibitor,

Table 16.4 CYP2D6-related liver transaminase activity in Alzheimer's disease

Phenotype	CYP2D6	GOT (IU/L)	GPT (IU/L)	GGT (IU/L)
Extensive	*1/*1	23.49 ± 8.70[1]	23.77 ± 16.04	31.16 ± 31.26[14-16]
Metabolizers	*1/*10	17.57 ± 6.29[2]	16.28 ± 7.40[11]	18.14 ± 6.79[17]
Intermediate	*1/*3	22.33 ± 1.52[3,4]	24.66 ± 10.59	22.00 ± 8.71
Metabolizers	*1/*4	21.76 ± 3.57[5,6]	21.88 ± 8.40	32.23 ± 25.53
	*1/*5	18.33 ± 2.33[7,8]	16.16 ± 5.60[12,13]	18.50 ± 6.47[18,19]
	*1/*6	23.00 ± 4.83	23.25 ± 5.31	33.50 ± 26.41
	*10/*10	16.00 ± 1.41[9,10]	16.50 ± 3.53	39.00 ± 11.31[20]
	*4/*10	20.00 ± 3.87	20.60 ± 4.03	34.20 ± 16.20
Poor Metabolizers	*4/*4	21.78 ± 6.48	17.64 ± 15.05	59.71 ± 113.58[21]
Ultra-rapid Metabolizers	*1xN/*1	20.50 ± 3.01	18.00 ± 5.32	21.50 ± 9.22
	*1xN/*4	23.33 ± 4.04	23.00 ± 5.01	25.66 ± 6.02

Values: mean ± SD.

GGT: Gamma-Glutamyl Transpeptidase; GOT: Glutamic-Oxalacetic Transaminase; GGT: Glutamic-Pyruvic Transaminase.(1) p<0.05 vs *1/*10; (2) p<0.05 vs *1/*4; (3) p<0.03 vs *1/*5; (4) p<0.001 vs *1/*10; (5) p<0.03 vs *1/*5; (6) p<0.03 vs *10/*10;(7) p<0.05 vs *1/*6; (8) p<0.04 vs *1xN/*4; (9) p<0.05 vs *1xN/*1; (10) p<0.05 vs *1xN/*4; (11) p<0.05 vs *4/*4;(12) p<0.05 vs *1/*6; (13) p<0.05 vs *4/*4; (14) p<0.05 vs *4/*4; (15) p<0.01 vs *10/*10; (16) p<0.01 vs *4/*10; (17) p<0.05 vs *4/*4; (18) p<0.01 vs *10/*10; (19) p<0.05 vs *4/*10; (20) p<0.05 vs *1xN/*1; (21) p<0.05 vs *1xN/*1. (Adapted from [68])

donepezil (5 mg/day), for one year. With this multifactorial therapeutic intervention, EMs improved their cognitive function (MMSE score) from 21.58±9.02 at baseline to 23.78 ± 5.81 after 1-year treatment (r=+0.82; a Coef.=+20.68; b Coef.: +0.4). IMs also improved from 21.40 ± 6.28 to 22.50±5.07 (r=+0.96; a Coef. =+21.2; b Coef. =+0.25), whereas PMs and UMs deteriorate from 20.74±6.72 to 18.07±5.52 (r=−0.97; a Coef.=+21.63; b Coef.=−0.59), and from 22.65±6.76 to 21.28±7.75 (r=−0.92; a Coef.=+23.35; b Coef.=−0.36), respectively. According to these results, PMs and UMs were the worst responders, showing a progressive cognitive decline with no therapeutic effect; and EMs and IMs were the best responders, with a clear improvement in cognition after one year of treatment (Fig. 16.6). Among EMs, AD patients harbouring the *1/*10 genotype (r=+0.97; a Coef.=+19.27; b Coef.=+0.55) responded better than patients with the *1/*1 genotype (r=+0.44; a Coef.=+22.10; b Coef.=+0.25). The best responders among IMs were the *1/*3 (r=+0.98; a Coef.=+20.65; b Coef.=1.18), *1/*6 (r=0.93; a Coef.=+22.17; b Coef.=+0.44) and *1/*5 genotypes (r=+0.70; a Coef.=+19.96; b Coef.=+0.25), whereas the *1/*4, *10/*10, and *4/*10 genotypes were poor responders (Fig. 16.6). Among PMs and UMs, the poorest responders were carriers of the *4/*4 (r=−0.98; a Coef.=+19.72; b Coef.=−0.91) and *1xN/*1 genotypes (r=−0.97; a Coef.=+24.55; b Coef.=−0.98), respectively *(68)* (Fig. 16.6).

From all these data we can conclude the following: (i) The most frequent CYP2D6 variants in the Spanish population are the *1/*1 (47.10%), *1/*4 (17.42%), *4/*4 (8.37%), *1/*10 (4.52%), and *1xN/*1 (4.52%), accounting for more than 80% of the population; (ii) the frequency of EMs, IMs, PMs, and UMs is about 51.61%, 32.26%, 9.03%, and 7.10%, respectively; (iii) EMs are more prevalent in AD

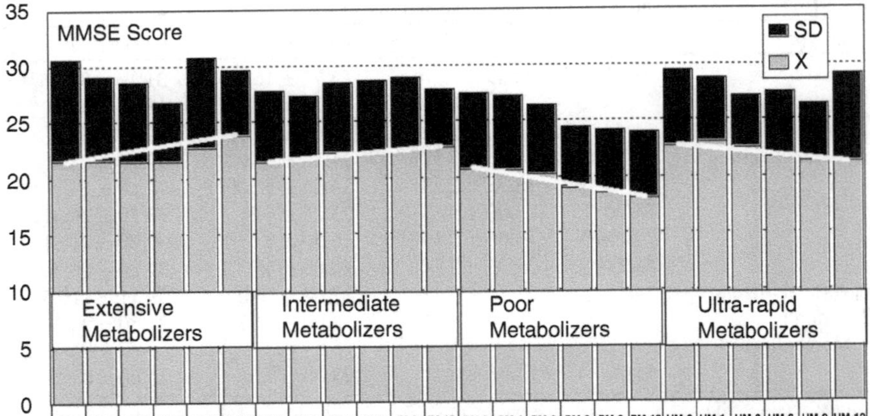

	EM-0	EM-1	EM-3	EM-6	EM-9	EM-12	IM-0	IM-1	IM-3	IM-6	IM-9	IM-12
SD	9,02	7,46	6,99	5,17	8,09	5,81	6,28	5,58	6,2	6,48	6,39	5,07
X	21,58	21,57	21,53	21,54	22,66	23,78	21,4	21,67	22,2	22,1	22,5	22,71

	PM-0	PM-1	PM-3	PM-6	PM-9	PM-12	UM-0	UM-1	UM-3	UM-6	UM-9	UM-12
SD	6,72	6,52	6,11	5,39	5,52	5,86	6,76	5,67	4,62	5,68	4,99	7,75
X	20,74	20,65	20,24	19,04	18,57	18,07	22,65	23,02	22,49	21,73	21,34	21,28

Fig. 16.6 CYP2D6-related therapeutic response to a multifactorial treatment in Alzheimer's disease (Adapted from [68])

(57.47%) than in controls (44.12%); IMs are more frequent in controls (41.18%) than in AD (25.29%), especially the *1/*4 (C: 23.53%; AD: 12.64%) and *4/*10 genotypes (C: 5.88%; AD: 1.15%); the frequency of PMs is similar in AD (9.20%) and controls (8.82%); and UMs are more frequent among AD cases (8.04%) than in controls (5.88%); (iv) there is an accumulation of AD-related genes of risk in PMs and UMs; (v) PMs and UMs tend to show higher transaminase activities than EMs and IMs; (vi) EMs and IMs are the best responders, and PMs and UMs are the worst responders, to a combination therapy with cholinesterase inhibitors, neuroprotectants, and vasoactive substances; and (vii) the pharmacogenetic response in AD appears to be dependent upon the networking activity of genes involved in drug metabolism and genes involved in AD pathogenesis *(10–12, 68)*.

Taking into consideration the available data, it might be inferred that at least 15% of the AD population may exhibit an abnormal metabolism of cholinesterase inhibitors and/or other drugs which undergo oxidation via CYP2D6-related enzymes. Approximately 50% of this population cluster would show an ultrarapid metabolism, requiring higher doses of cholinesterase inhibitors to reach a therapeutic threshold, whereas the other 50% of the cluster would exhibit a poor metabolism, displaying potential adverse events at low doses. If we take into account that approximately 60–70% of therapeutic outcomes depend upon pharmacogenomic criteria (e.g., pathogenic mechanisms associated with AD-related genes), it can be postulated that pharmacogenetic and pharmacogenomic factors are responsible for 75–85% of the therapeutic response (efficacy) in AD patients treated with conventional drugs *(5, 10–12, 44, 68)*. Of particular interest are the potential interactions of cholinesterase inhibitors with other drugs in current use for patients with AD, such as antidepressants, neuroleptics, antiarrhythmics, analgesics, and antiemetics, which are metabolized by the cytochrome P450 CYP2D6 enzyme. Approximately 30–60% of drug failure or lack of therapeutic efficacy (and/or ADR manifestation) is not a matter of drug dosage but a problem of poor metabolizing capacity in PMs.

Additionally, inappropriate drug use is one of the risk factors for adverse drug reactions (ADRs) in the elderly. The prevalence of use of potentially inappropriate medications in patients older than 65 years of age admitted to a general medical or geriatric ward ranges from 16% to 20% *(82)*, and these numbers may double in ambulatory patients. Overall, the most prevalent inappropriate drugs currently prescribed to the elderly are amiodarone, long-acting benzodiazepines, and anticholinergic antispasmodics; however, the list of drugs with potential risk also includes antidepressants, antihistaminics, NSAIDs, amphetamines, laxatives, clonidine, indomethacin, and several neuroleptics *(82)*, most of which are processed via CYP2D6 and CYP3A5 enzymes *(5, 10–12, 83)*. Therefore, pretreatment CYP screening might be of great help to rationalize and optimize therapeutics in the elderly, by avoiding medications of risk in PMs and UMs.

5 APOE in Alzheimer's Disease Therapeutics

Polymorphic variants in the APOE gene (19q13.2) are associated with risk (APOE-4 allele) or protection (APOE-2 allele) for AD *(4, 12)*. For many years, alterations in ApoE and defects in the APOE gene have been associated with dysfunctions in lipid metabolism, cardiovascular disease, and atherosclerosis. During the past 25 years an enormous number of studies have clearly documented the role of APOE-4 as a risk factor for AD, and the accumulation of the APOE-4 allele has been reported as a risk factor for other forms of dementia and CNS disorders *(4, 12)*.

APOE-4 may influence AD pathology interacting with APP metabolism and ABP accumulation, enhancing hyperphosphorylation of tau protein and NFT formation, reducing choline acetyltransferase activity, increasing oxidative processes, modifying inflammation-related neuroimmunotrophic activity and glial activation, altering lipid metabolism, lipid transport, and membrane biosynthesis in sprouting and synaptic remodelling, and inducing neuronal apoptosis *(4, 12)*.

5.1 APOE-Related Phenotypic Profiles in Alzheimer's Disease

Different APOE genotypes confer specific phenotypic profiles to AD patients. Some of these profiles may add risk or benefit when the patients are treated with conventional drugs, and in many instances the clinical phenotype demands the administration of additional drugs which increase the complexity of therapeutic protocols. From studies designed to define APOE-related AD phenotypes *(4–8, 10–12, 36, 44, 68)*, several confirmed conclusions can be drawn: (i) the age-at-onset is 5–10 years earlier in approximately 80% of AD cases harbouring the APOE-4/4 genotype; (ii) the serum levels of ApoE are the lowest in APOE-4/4, intermediate in APOE-3/3 and APOE-3/4, and highest in APOE-2/3 and APOE-2/4; (iii) serum cholesterol levels are higher in APOE-4/4 than in the other genotypes; (iv) HDL-cholesterol levels tend to be lower in APOE-3 homozygotes than in APOE-4 allele carriers; (v) LDL-cholesterol levels are systematically higher in

APOE-4/4 than in any other genotype; (vi) triglyceride levels are significantly lower in APOE-4/4; (vii) nitric oxide levels are slightly lower in APOE-4/4; (viii) serum ABP levels do not differ between APOE-4/4 and the other most frequent genotypes (APOE-3/3, APOE-3/4); (ix) blood histamine levels are dramatically reduced in APOE-4/4 as compared with the other genotypes; (x) brain atrophy is markedly increased in APOE-4/4>APOE-3/4>APOE-3/3; (xi) brain mapping activity shows a significant increase in slow wave activity in APOE-4/4 from the early stages of the disease; (xii) brain hemodynamics, as reflected by reduced brain blood flow velocity and increase pulsatility and resistance indices, is significantly worse in APOE-4/4 (and in APOE-4 carriers, in general, as compared with APOE-3 carriers); (xiii) lymphocyte apoptosis is markedly enhanced in APOE-4 carriers; (xiv) cognitive deterioration is faster in APOE-4/4 patients than in carriers of any other APOE genotypes; (xv) occasionally, in approximately 3–8% of the AD cases, the presence of some dementia-related metabolic dysfunctions (e.g., iron, folic acid, vitamin B12 deficiencies) accumulate in APOE-4 carriers more than in APOE-3 carriers; (xvi) some behavioral disturbances (bizarre behaviors, psychotic symptoms), alterations in circadian rhythm patterns (e.g., sleep disorders), and mood disorders (anxiety, depression) are slightly more frequent in APOE-4 carriers; (xvii) aortic and systemic atherosclerosis is also more frequent in APOE-4 carriers; (xviii) liver metabolism and transaminase activity also differ in APOE-4/4 with respect to other genotypes; (xix) blood pressure (hypertension) and other cardiovascular risk factors also accumulate in APOE-4; and (xx) APOE-4/4 are the poorest responders to conventional drugs. These 20 major phenotypic features clearly illustrate the biological disadvantage of APOE-4 homozygotes and the potential consequences that these patients may experience when they receive pharmacological treatment *(1, 4–8, 10–12, 22, 23, 33, 36, 44, 68, 80)*.

5.2 APOE-Related Therapeutic Response to Cholinesterase Inhibitors and Multifactorial Treatments

Several studies indicate that the presence of the APOE-4 allele differentially affects the quality and size of drug responsiveness in AD patients treated with cholinergic enhancers (tacrine, donepezil, rivastigmine) *(84–86)*. For example, APOE-4 carriers show a less significant therapeutic response to tacrine (60%) than patients with no APOE-4 *(84)*. In another study the frequency of APOE-4 alleles was higher in responders to a single oral dose of tacrine *(86)*. It has been demonstrated that more than 80% of APOE-4(–) AD patients showed marked improvement after 30 weeks of treatment with tacrine, whereas 60% of APOE-4(+) carriers had a poor response *(84)*. Others found no differences after 6 months of treatment with tacrine among APOE genotypes, but after 12 months the CIBIC scores revealed that APOE-4 carriers had declined more than the APOE-2 and APOE-3 patients, suggesting that a faster rate of decline was evident in the APOE-4 patients, probably reflecting that APOE-4 inheritance is a negative predictor of treatment of tacrine in AD *(87)*. It has also been shown that the APOE genotype may influence the biological effect of donepezil on APP metabolism in AD *(88)*. Prospective studies with galantamine in large samples of patients in Europe *(89)* and in the U.S. *(90)* showed no effect of APOE genotypes on drug efficacy. APOE-4 noncarriers also exhibit cognitive and functional improvement to rosiglitazone, a PPARG agonist, whereas APOE-4 carriers show no improvement or some decline *(91)*. MacGowan et al. *(92)* reported that gender is likely to be a more powerful determinant of outcome of anticholinesterase treatment than APOE status in the short term. In contrast, other studies do not support the hypothesis that APOE and gender are predictors of the therapeutic response of AD patients to tacrine or donepezil *(93, 94)*. In a recent study, Petersen et al. *(95)* showed that APOE-4 carriers exhibited a better response to donepezil. Similar results have been found by Bizzarro et al. *(96)*; however, Rigaud et al. *(94)* did not find any significant difference between APOE-4-related responders and nonresponders to donepezil. An APOE-related differential response has also been observed in patients treated with other compounds devoid of acetylcholinesterase inhibiting activity (CDP-choline, anapsos) *(91, 97, 98)*, suggesting that APOE-associated factors may influence drug activity in the brain either directly acting on neural mechanisms or indirectly influencing diverse metabolic pathways *(99)*.

To date, few studies have addressed in a prospective manner the impact of pharmacogenetic and pharmacogenomic factors on AD therapeutics *(5–8, 10–12, 44, 68)*. Since APOE, PS1, and PS2 genes participate in AD pathogenesis regulating neuronal function and brain amyloidogenesis, in an attempt to envision the potential influence of major AD-associated genes on the therapeutic response in AD patients, we have performed the first pharmacogenomic study in AD using a genetic matrix model (trigenic haplotype-like model) to identify the response of a multifactorial therapy in different AD genotypes combining allelic associations of APOE+PS1+PS2 genes *(6)*. With this strategy we have demonstrated that the therapeutic response in AD is genotype-specific, with APOE-4/4 carriers as the worst responders, and that some polymorphic variants exert a dominant effect on treatment outcomes *(5–8, 10–12, 44)*. From these studies we can conclude the following: (i) Multifactorial treatments combining neuroprotectants, endogenous nucleotides, nootropic agents, vasoactive substances, cholinesterase inhibitors, and NMDA antagonists associated with metabolic supplementation on an individual basis adapted to the phenotype of the patient may be useful to improve cognition and slow down disease progression in AD. (ii) In our personal experience, the best results have been obtained combining (a) CDP-choline with piracetam and metabolic supplementation, (b) CDP-choline with piracetam and anapsos, (c) CDP-choline with piracetam and cholinesterase inhibitors (donepezil, rivastigmine), (d) CDP-choline with memantine, and (e) CDP-choline, piracetam, and nicergoline. (iii) Some of these combination therapies have proven to be effective, improving cognition during the first 9 months of treatment, and not showing apparent side effects. (iv) The therapeutic response in AD seems to be genotype-specific under different pharmacogenomic conditions. (v) In monogenic-related studies, patients with the APOE-2/3 and APOE-3/4 genotypes are the best responders, and APOE-4/4 carriers are the worst responders. (vi) PS1- and PS2-related genotypes do not

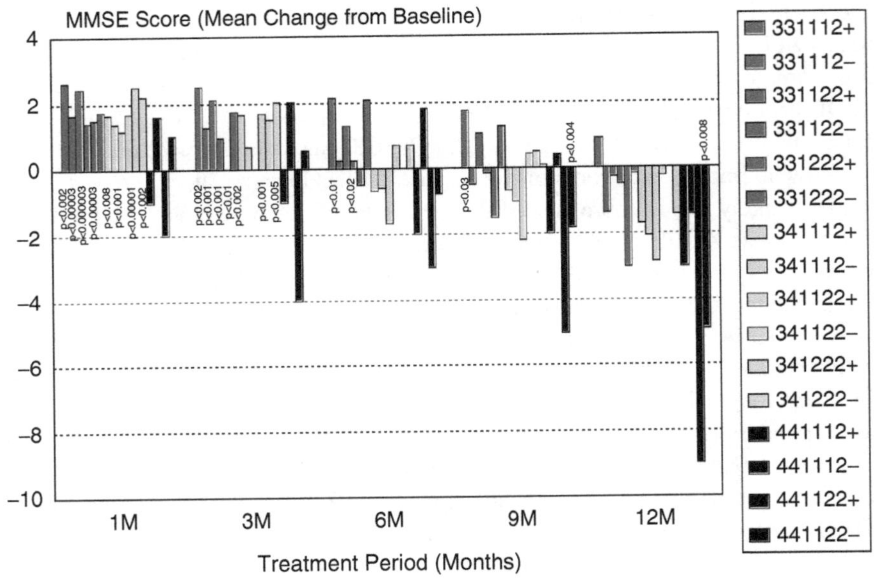

Fig. 16.7 Trigenic (APOE+PS1+PS2)-related therapeutic response to a combination therapy in patients with Alzheimer's disease (Adapted from [44])

appear to influence the therapeutic response in AD as independent genomic entities; however, APP, PS1, and PS2 mutations may drastically modify the therapeutic response to conventional drugs. (vii) In trigenic-related studies the best responders are those patients carrying the 331222–, 341122–, 341222–, and 441112–genomic clusters (Fig. 16.7). (viii) A genetic defect in the exon 5 of the PS2 gene seems to exert a negative effect on cognition, conferring upon PS2+ carriers in trigenic clusters the condition of poor responders to combination therapy. (ix) The worst responders in all genomic clusters are patients with the 441122+ genotype (Fig. 16.7). (x) The APOE-4/4 genotype seems to accelerate neurodegeneration, anticipating the onset of the disease by 5–10 years; and, in general, APOE-4/4 carriers show a faster disease progression and a poorer therapeutic response to all available treatments than any other polymorphic variant. (xi) Pharmacogenomic studies using trigenic, tetragenic, or polygenic clusters as a harmonization procedure to reduce genomic heterogeneity are very useful to widen the therapeutic scope of limited pharmacological resources *(4–8, 10–12, 44)*.

5.3 Influence of APOE-CYP2D6 Interactions on Alzheimer's Disease Therapeutics

APOE influences liver function and CYP2D6-related enzymes probably via regulation of hepatic lipid metabolism *(68, 80)*. It has been observed that APOE may influence liver function and drug metabolism by modifying hepatic steatosis and transaminase activity. There is a clear correlation between APOE-related TG levels and GOT, GPT, and GGT activities in AD *(80)*. Both plasma TG levels and transaminase activity are significantly lower in AD patients harbouring the APOE-4/4 genotype, probably indicating (a) that low TG levels protect against liver steatosis, and (b) that the presence of the APOE-4 allele influences TG levels, liver steatosis, and transaminase activity. Consequently, it is very likely that APOE influences drug metabolism in the liver through different mechanisms, including interactions with enzymes such as transaminases and/or cytochrome P450-related enzymes encoded in genes of the CYP superfamily *(68–80)*.

When APOE and CYP2D6 genotypes are integrated in bigenic clusters and the APOE+CYP2D6-related therapeutic response to a combination therapy is analyzed in AD patients after one year of treatment as in Fig. 16.6, it becomes clear that the presence of the APOE-4/4 genotype is able to convert pure CYP2D6*1/*1 EMs into full PMs (Fig. 16.8), indicating the existence of a powerful influence of the APOE-4 homozygous genotype on the drug metabolizing capacity of pure CYP2D6-EMs.

6 Angiotensin-Converting Enzyme (ACE) in Alzheimer's Disease

Angiotensin I-converting enzyme (EC 3.4.15.1) (Kininase II; Dipeptidyl carboxypeptidase 1, Carboxycathepsin, Dipeptide hydrolase, Peptidase P, Peptidyl dipeptidase-4(A), Pepdidyl-dipeptide hydrolase) is a zinc metallopeptidase with dipeptidyl carboxypeptidase activity that regulates blood pressure, the renin-angiotensin system, the kinin-kallikrein cascade, and electrolytic balance by hydrolyzing angiotensin I into angiotensinogen *(4)*. ACE is the target of the ACE inhibitor family of drugs (captopril, enalapril, fosinopril, imidapril, lisinopril) currently used as antihypertensive agents.

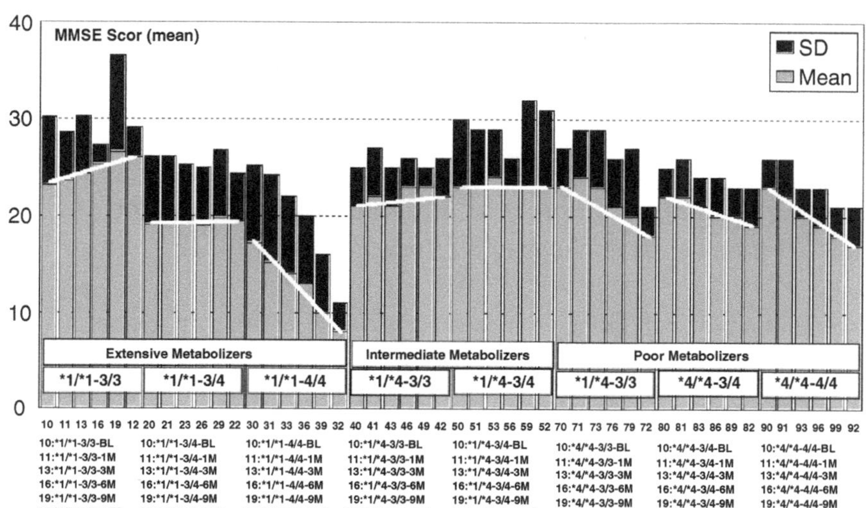

Fig. 16.8 Interaction of CYP2D6 and APOE in the pharmacogenetics of Alzheimer's disease (Adapted from [68])

The ACE gene maps on 17q23 and encodes a 732-residue preprotein with a 31-residue signal peptide and a mature molecular weight of 80,073. ACE contains two large homologous active domains, the N- and C-terminal domains. The ACE gene encodes two isozymes (somatic ACE isozyme and germinal ACE isozyme). ACE is a membrane-bound enzyme on the surface of vascular endothelial cells that also circulates in plasma, showing a great individual variability determined by an insertion (I)/deletion (D) polymorphism in intron 16 of the ACE gene (ACE-I/D polymorphism). More than 160 ACE polymorphisms have been reported, 34 of which are located in coding regions and 18 are missense mutations *(100)*. ACE-related polymorphic variants have been associated with hypertension, atherosclerosis, stroke, left ventricular hypertrophy, chronic renal failure in IgA nephropathy, Henoch-Schonlein purpura nephritis, mechanical efficiency of skeletal muscle, intracranial aneurysma, susceptibility to myocardial infarction, diabetic nephropathy, AD, and logevity *(4, 100)*.

Many studies have shown an association between ACE-I/D indel variants and AD *(4)*. The polymorphism at intron 16 of the ACE gene, consiting in an insertion/deletion (I/D) of 287 bp is associated with ACE concentrations, and the ACE-D/D genotype is associated with cardiovascular disorders and arterial occlusive disease. It has been proposed that ACE degrades ABP, retards ABP aggregation, deposition, and fibril formation, and inhibitis cytotoxicity, suggesting that ACE may affect susceptibility to AD by degrading ABP and preventing the accumulation of amyloid plaques in vivo *(101)*, and that treatment with ACE N-terminal domain-related peptides might be a potential therapeutic strategy in AD *(102)*. In a recent study, Eckman et al. *(103)* analyzed ABP accumulation in brains from ACE-deficient mice and in mice treated with ACE inhibitors and found that ACE deficiency did not alter steady-state ABP concentration. ABP levels are significantly elevated in endothelin-converting enzyme and neprilysin knockout mice, and inhibitors of these enzymes cause a rapid increase in ABP concentration in the brain *(103)*. In contrast, Hemming and Selkoe *(104)* have reported that ABP is degraded by ACE and elevated by ACE inhibitors, such as captopril, raising the question of whether currently prescribed ACE inhibitors could elevate brain ABP levels in humans.

6.1 ACE-Related Therapeutic Response to a Multifactorial Treatment in Alzheimer's Disease

No studies have been reported concerning the role of ACE in the therapeutic response to specific treatments in AD, with the exception of ACE inhibitors in hypertension and cardiovascular disorders. The positive effects of ACE inhibitors were thought to be the consequence of reducing angiotensin II levels and the degradation of bradykinin; however, some of the beneficial effects of ACE inhibitors can be attributed to novel mechanisms, including the accumulation of the ACE substrate N-acetyl-seryl-aspartyl-lysyl-proline, which blocks collagen deposition in the injured tissues, as well as the activation of an ACE signaling cascade that involves the activation of the kinase CK2 and the c-Jun N-terminal kinase in endothelial cells and leads to changes in gene expression *(105)*. Since hypertension, cardiovascular disorders, and alterations in cerebrovascular hemodynamics clearly affect brain perfusion, contributing to the acceleration of neuronal death in susceptible patients, it would be worthwhile to evaluate the effect of different ACE variants on cognition in AD patients treated with conventional antidementia drugs. It has also been observed for a long time that hypertensive and hypotensive patients are at risk of developing AD, and that the APOE-4 allele accumulates in hypertensive subjects *(4, 33, 34)*. In addition, patients treated with ACE inhibitors may show an increased rate of mood disorders, such as depression- and anxiety-like symptoms. Taking into consideration all these observations, the effects of ACE polymorphic variants, either alone or in conjunction with APOE-related genotypes, on cognitive performance and mood disorders have been studied, under pharmacogenomic protocols, in AD patients treated with a multifactorial therapy.

6.1.1 ACE-Related Cognitive Performance in Response to a Multifactorial Therapy in Alzheimer's Disease

Early- and late-onset AD patients (N=463; 257 females and 206 males; age: 63.51±13.12 years; range: 40–98 years) received for one year a multifactorial therapy (CNLA protocol) integrated by CDP-choline (500 mg/day, p.o.), nicergoline (5 mg/day, p.o.), E-SAR-94010 (LipoEsar®) (250 mg, t.i.d.), and Animon Complex® (2 capsules/day). E-SAR-94010 is a marine lipoprotein derivative extracted from *S. pilchardus*, with powerful anti-atherosclerotic and plasma lipid lowering activities, whose therapeutic properties exhibit an APOE-related profile *(11, 12, 68)* (Fig. 16.9). Animon Complex® is a nutraceutical compound integrated by a purified extract of *Chenopodium quinoa* (250 mg), ferrous sulphate (38.1 mg, equivalent to 14 mg of iron), folic acid (200 μg), and vitamin B12 (1 μg) per capsule (RGS: 26.06671/C). Patients with a chronic deficiency of iron (<35 μg/ml), folic acid (<2.5 ng/ml), or vitamin B12 (<150 pg/ml) received an additional supplementation of iron (80 mg/day), folic acid (5 mg/day), and B complex vitamins (B1, 15 mg/day; B2, 15 mg/day; B6, 10 mg/day; B12, 10 μg/day; nicotinamide, 50 mg/day) to maintain stable levels of serum iron (50–150 μg/ml), folic acid (5–20 ng/ml), and vitamin B12 levels (500–1000 pg/ml) in order to avoid the negative influence of all these metabolic factors on cognition *(11, 12, 68)*.

The distribution of ACE indel variants was the following: (a) ACE-D/D (35.64%) (N=165; 97 females, age: 64.86 ±13.08 yrs, range: 41–91 yrs; 68 males, age: 63.49±12.45 yrs, range: 44–96 yrs); (b) ACE-I/D (49.46%) (N=229; 122 females, age: 63.29±13.77 yrs, range: 42–91 yrs; 107 males, 63.35±13.10 yrs, range: 40–98 yrs); and (c) ACE-I/I (14.90%) (N=69; 38 females, age: 64.76±12.57 yrs, range: 45–90; 31 males, age: 59.22±13.06 yrs, range: 40–84 yrs). All ACE-I/D variants showed no differences in weight, height, or heart rate. ACE-I/D carriers had the highest blood pressure levels (139.06±22.91 mmHg, $p<0.05$ vs ACE-D/D), and ACE-I/I males represented the youngest population *(68)*.

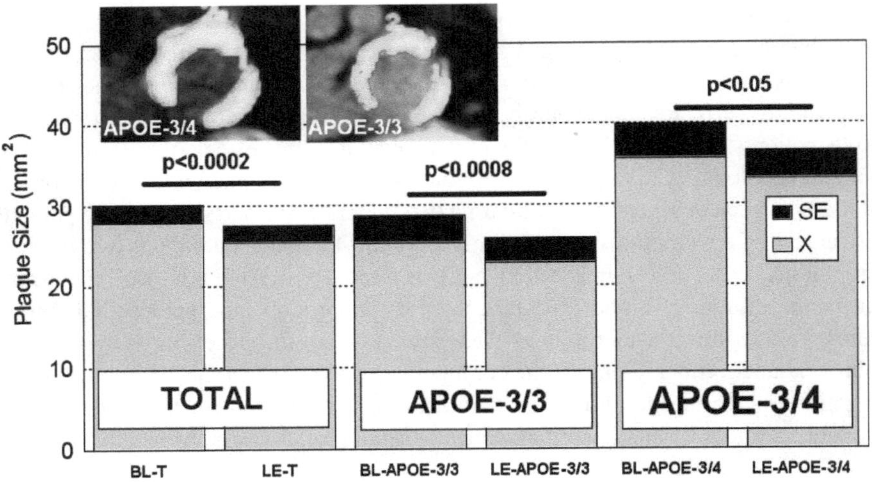

Fig. 16.9 APOE-related therapeutic efficacy of E-SAR-94010 on atheroma plaques in the abdominal aorta of patients with chronic hyperlipidemia (Adapted from *[68]*)

The therapeutic response of AD patients with variable degrees of cognitive deterioration (baseline MMSE score = 23.35 ± 7.51; range: 0–24) to the CNLA protocol showed a clear tendency to the stabilization of mental decline after one-year treatment (MMSE score = 22.32 ± 8.60; r = −0.09, a coef.: 22.90, a coef.: −0.02). Among ACE-I/D variants, ACE-D/D were the worst responders (r = −0.58, a coef.: 23.03, b coef.: −0.17), and ACE-I/D were the best responders (r = +0.26, a coef.: 22.7, b coef.: +0.12), with ACE-I/I showing an intermediate positive response (r = +0.01, a coef.: 23.11, b coef.: +0.007) *(68)* (Fig. 16.10).

6.1.2 Effect of ACE-APOE Interactions on the Therapeutic Response in Alzheimer's Disease

Since synergistic effects of APOE with many other genes have been documented in the international literature *(4)*, including ACE, AGT, NOS3, FOS, APP, PS1, PS2, MAPT, GTS, and others, we have characterized bigenic clusters integrating APOE and ACE genotypes in AD patients to evaluate the impact of different APOE genotypes on the ACE-related therapeutic response to a multifactorial therapy in AD. In classical studies, the association of ACE-D and APOE-4 alleles was found to be more frequent in AD than in controls, and the association of ACE-D/D genotypes and the APOE-4 allele may confer higher risk for cerebrovascular damage.

As previously reported *(1, 4–8, 10–12, 44)*, APOE-2/4 (r=+0.79, a coef.: 14.05, b coef.: +1.19) > APOE-3/4 (r = +0.64, a coef.: 21.12, b coef.: +0.70) > APOE-2/3 (r = +0.01, a coef.: 23.06, b coef.: +0.02) were the best responders, whereas APOE-4/4 patients were the worst responders (r = −0.98, a coef.: 25.15, b coef.: −1.30) *(68)* (Fig. 16.11). The integration of ACE and APOE genotypes in bigenic clusters yielded 18 different genotypes. The most frequent bigenic genotypes were 33ID

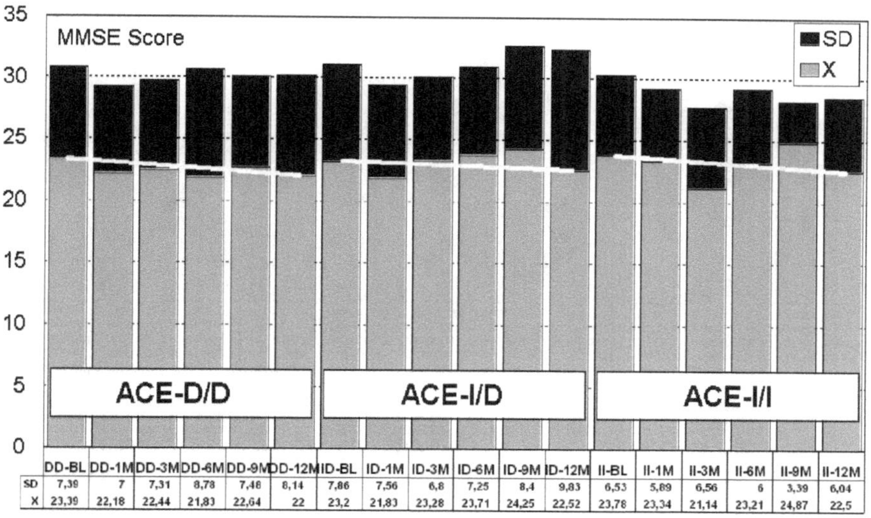

Fig. 16.10 ACE-related therapeutic response to a multifactorial treatment in Alzheimer's disease (Adapted from *[68]*)

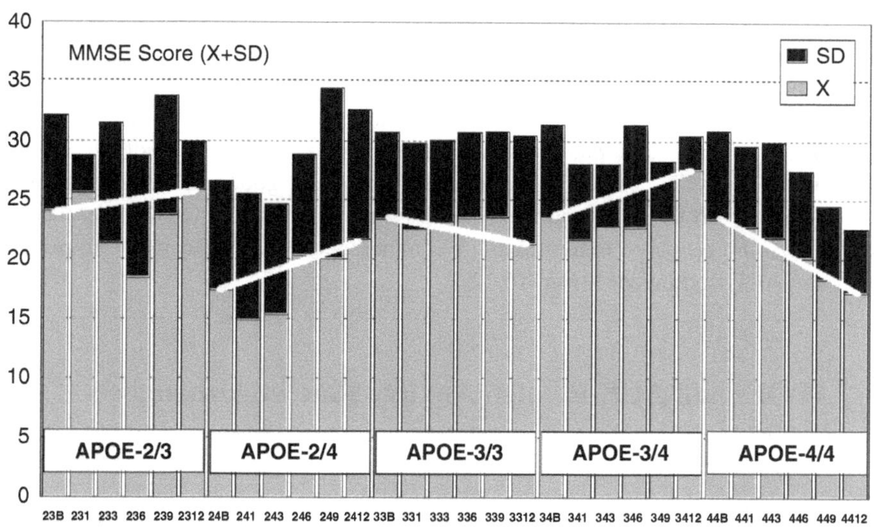

Fig. 16.11 APOE-related cognitive performance in patients with Alzheimer's disease treated with a combination therapy for one year (Adapted from *[68]*)

(33.74%), 33DD (22.68%), and 33II (9.29%). The frequencies of bigenic clusters integrated by APOE-4/4 and ACE variants were 0.86% 44DD, 1.51% 44ID, and 0% 44II. Among ACE-APOE bigenic genotypes, the best responders were ID34 (r = + 0.74, a coef.: 23.95, b coef.: +0.49) > ID23 (r = +0.50, a coef.: 23.85, b coef.: + 0.45) > II33 (r = +0.49, a coef.: 24.06, b coef.: +0.24) > DD34 (r=+0.35, a coef.:

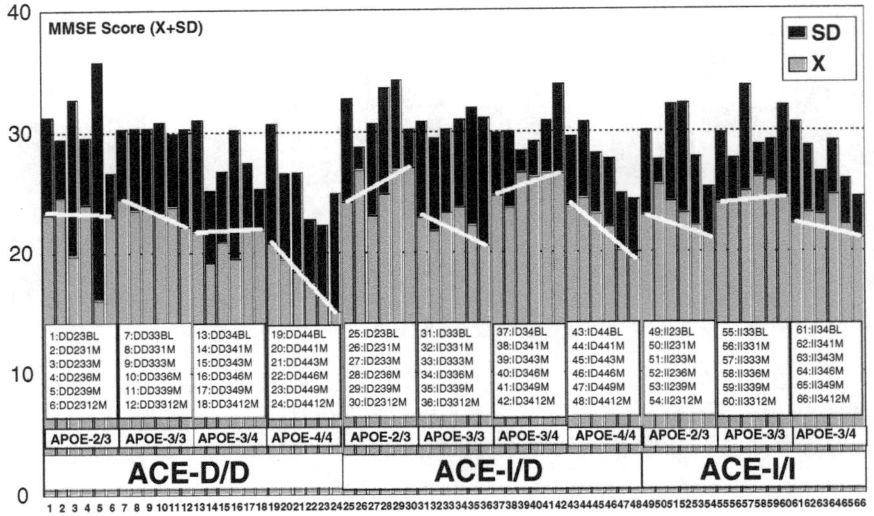

Fig. 16.12 ACE+APOE-related therapeutic response to a multifactorial treatment in Alzheimer's disease (Adapted from [68])

19.96, b coef.: +0.23) and the worst responders were DD44 (r=–0.99, a coef.: 21.75, b coef.: –1.11) > DD33 (r = –0.77, a coef.: 24.54, b coef.: –0.32) > II23 (r = – 0.71, a coef.: 25.21, b coef.: –0.58) > ID33 (r=– 0.46, a coef.: 23.37, b coef.: –0.29) > II34 (r = – 0.32, a coef.: 23.45, b coef.: –0.58) > DD23 (r = – 0.35, a coef.: 23.92, b coef.: –0.62) *(68)* (Fig. 16.12). These results clearly show that (a) the worst responders are those AD patients harbouring the DD44 bigenic genotype, (b) the presence of the ACE-D/D variant transforms potentially good (APOE-2/3) or moderately good (APOE-3/3) responders into poor responders, and (c) the presence of the APOE-4/4 genotype determines a poor therapeutic response when combined with any ACE variant *(68)* (Fig. 16.12).

7 APOE- and ACE-Related Anxiety Rate in Alzheimer's Disease

Behavioral disturbances and mood disorders are intrinsic components of dementia associated with memory disorders. The apperarance of anxiety, depression, psychotic symptoms, verbal and physical aggressiveness, agitation, wandering, and sleep disorders complicate the clinical picture of dementia and add important problems to the therapeutics of AD, and the daily management of patients as well. Under these conditions, psychotropic drugs (antidepressants, anxyolitics, hypnotics, and neuroleptics) are required, and most of these substances contribute to deteriorate cognition and psychomotor function. Both APOE- and ACE-related polymorphic variants have been associated with mood disorders and panic disorder *(106)*.

Differences in anxiety-related behavior have been detected between APOE-deficient C57BL/6 and wild-type C57BL/6 mice, suggesting that APOE variants may affect emotional state *(107)*. APOE-4 carriers with deep white matter hyperintesities in MRI show association with depressive symptoms and vascular depression *(108)*. Reduced caudate nucleus volumes and genetic determinants of homocysteine metabolism accumulate in patients with psychomotor slowing and cognitive deficits *(109)*, and older depressed subjects have persisting cognitive impairments associated with hippocampal volume reduction *(110, 111)*. Depressive symptoms are also associated with stroke and atherogenic lipid profile *(112)*. During the past two decades, antipsychotic, antianxiety and cognitive-enhancing effects have been attributed to ACE inhibitors. Some ACE inhibitors (captopril, SQ29,852) display similar effects to benzodiazepines in dealing with anxiety-related behaviors in animals, and another ACE inhibitor (ceronapril) might share with neuroleptic drugs an ability to enhance latent inhibition in learning tasks. One SNP (rs4291) located in the promoter region of the ACE gene has been recently associated with unipolar major depression *(106)*.

In order to understand whether or not cognitive function and mood disorders are cooperatively influenced by genetic factors in AD, and also to know the potential impact that conventional neuroprotection can exert on mood disorders, we have studied the effect of the therapeutic CNLA protocol on anxiety in AD and the differential APOE- and ACE-related responses, distinguishing the influence of monogenic and bigenic variants on emotional conditions.

Surprisingly, the CNLA protocol was extremely effective in reducing anxiety progressively from the first month to the twelfth month of treatment. The anxiety rate declined from a baseline HRS-A score of 10.90 ± 5.69 to 9.07 ± 4.03 ($p<0.0000000001$) at 1 month, 9.01 ± 4.38 ($p<0.000006$) at 3 months, 8.90 ± 4.47 ($p<0.005$) at 6 months, 7.98 ± 3.72 ($p<0.00002$) at 9 months, and 8.56 ± 4.72 ($p<0.01$) at 12 months of treatment ($r=-0.82$, a coef.: 10.57, b coef.: -0.43) *(68)*. From a global perspective, these data might suggest that improvement in mood conditions can contribute to stabilize cognitive function or that neuroprotection (with the consequent stabilization or improvement in mental performance) can enhance emotional equilibrium.

7.1 *APOE-Related Anxiety Rate*

At baseline, all APOE variants showed a similar anxiety rate, except the APOE-4/4 carriers, who differed from the rest in a significantly lower anxiety rate ($p<0.05$). Remarkable changes in anxiety were found among different APOE genotypes (Fig. 16.13). Practically all APOE variants responded with a significant diminution of anxiogenic symptoms, except patients with the APOE-4/4 genotype, who showed only a slight improvement. The best responders were APOE-2/4 ($r=-0.87$, a coef.: 14.80, b coef.: -1.03) > APOE-2/3 ($r=-0.77$, a coef: 11.04, b coef.: -0.45) > APOE-3/3 ($r=-0.69$, a coef.: 10.8, b coef.: -0.39) > APOE-3/4 carriers

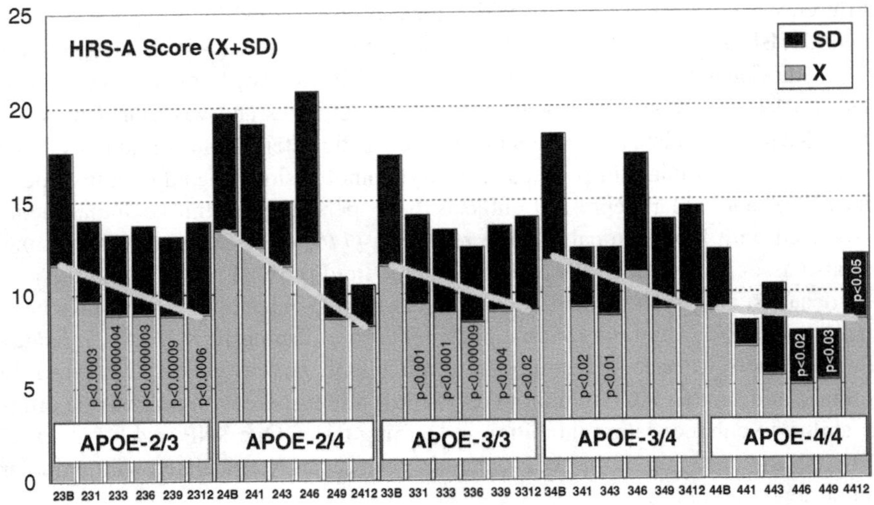

Fig. 16.13 APOE-related anxiety rate in patients with Alzheimer's disease treated with a combination therapy (Adapted from [68])

(r = –0.45, a coef.: 10.93, b coef.: -0.30) (68) (Fig. 16.13). The modest anxiolytic effect observed in APOE-4/4 patients (r = –0.25, a coef.: 7.53, b coef.: –0.23) might be due to the very low anxiety rate observed at baseline. In any case, APOE-4/4 carriers are the worst responders, with results similar to those obtained in cognitive performance; however, the potential influence of APOE variants on anxiety and cognition in AD does not show a clear parallelism, suggesting that other more complex mechanisms are involved in the onset of anxiety in dementia.

7.2 ACE-Related Anxiety Rate

Patients with each one of the three ACE-I/D indel variants are equally anxiogenic at baseline, and all of them favourably respond to the CNLA protocol by gradually reducing anxiety symptoms throughout the 12-month treatment period (Fig. 16.14). The best responders are ACE-I/D (r = –0.89, a coef.: 10.83, b coef.: –0.46), followed by ACE-D/D (r = – 0.68, a coef.: 10.49, b coef.: –0.45) and ACE-I/I (r = –0.08, a coef.: 10.57, b coef.: –0.06), the latter exhibiting the least significant change in anxiogenic parameters *(68)* (Fig. 16.14); in ACE-D/D carriers the anxiolytic response is faster and more sustainable during the treatment period (1M, $p<0.0003$ vs BL; 3M, $p<0.007$; 6M, $p<0.005$; 9M, $p<0.0007$; 12M, $p<0.03$) than in the other genotypes, whereas in ACE-I/D the response gradually reaches significant values after 9 months of treatment ($p<0.05$); in contrast, ACE-I/I patients show a very positive response during the first trimester of treatment (1M, $p<0.04$

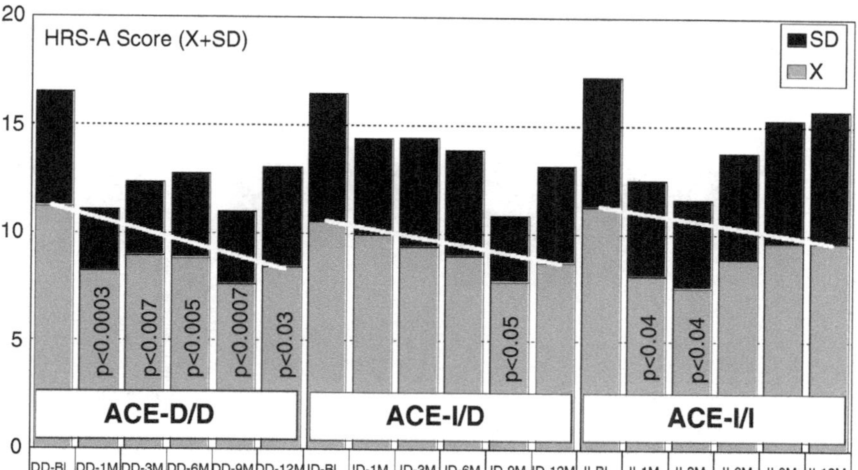

	DD-BL	DD-1M	DD-3M	DD-6M	DD-9M	DD-12M	ID-BL	ID-1M	ID-3M	ID-6M	ID-9M	ID-12M	II-BL	II-1M	II-3M	II-6M	II-9M	II-12M
SD	5,28	2,88	3,41	3,95	3,42	4,66	5,92	4,45	5,09	4,92	3,1	4,48	5,98	4,46	4,14	4,94	5,68	6,13
X	11,25	8,24	8,97	8,84	7,62	8,44	10,53	9,95	9,38	8,97	7,77	8,68	11,28	8,05	7,5	8,86	9,62	9,62

Fig. 16.14 ACE-related anxiety rate in patients with Alzheimer's disease treated with a combination therapy (Adapted from Cacabelos, 68)

vs BL; 3M, $p<0.04$), with an apparent relapse of anxiogenic symptomatology thereafter (Fig. 16.14). This differential ACE-related anxiety pattern might suggest some influence of ACE-I/D variants on mood disorders in AD *(68)*.

7.3 *Effect of APOE-ACE Interactions on Anxiety*

The combination of APOE and ACE polymorphic variants in bigenic clusters yields a quite different anxiety pattern (Figs. 16.15–16.16). The most anxiogenic patients at baseline are those with the DD23, ID44, and II34 genotypes, and the least anxiogenic patients are those harbouring the II23, DD44, and ID23 genotypes (Fig. 16.15). All bigenic clusters show a positive anxiolytic response to the CNLA protocol, except DD44 which exhibits the worst response by far ($r=+0.38$, a coef.: 8.16, b coef.: +0.19). The sequence of good responders from better to worse is the following: ID33 ($r=-0.89$) > DD23 ($r=-0.85$) > ID44 ($r=-0.79$) > DD34 ($r=-0.69$) > DD33 ($r=-0.63$) > ID34 ($r=-0.47$) > II33 ($r=-0.29$) > ID23 ($r=-0.19$ > II23 ($r=-0.13$) = II34 ($r=-0.13$) *(68)* (Fig. 16.16). Once again, as in the case of cognition, DD44 patients represent the poorest responders, clearly indicating that the association of the APOE-4/4 and ACE-D/D genotypes has a severely deleterious effect on mental performance, at least in cognition and anxiety. Another interesting conclusion from these results is that the association of ACE-I/D with APOE-4/4 is beneficial in terms of mood improvement, neutralizing the negative influence of APOE-4/4.

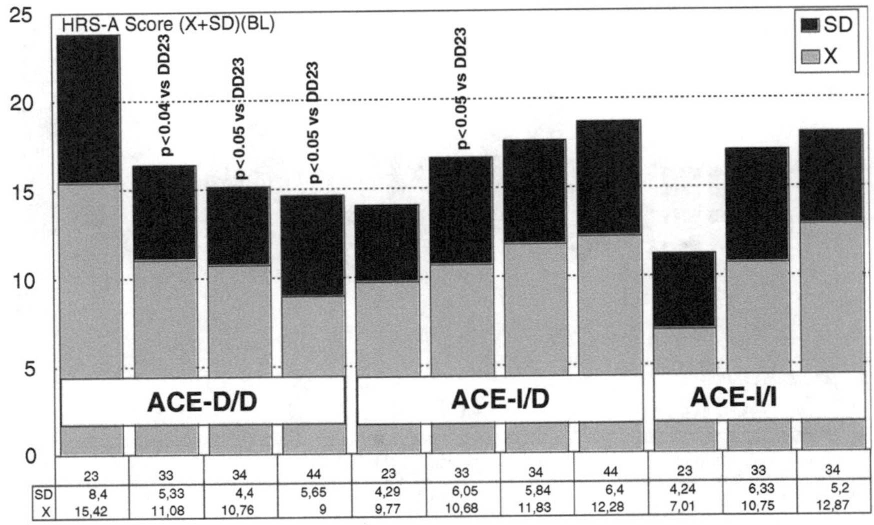

Fig. 16.15 APOE+ACE-related anxiety rate in patients with Alzheimer's disease (Adapted from Cacabelos, *68*)

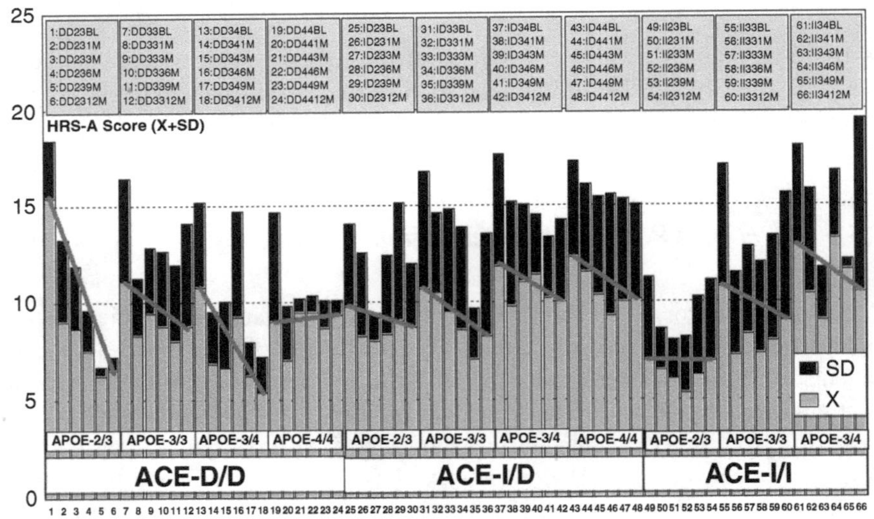

Fig. 16.16 ACE+APOE-related antianxiety effect of a multifactorial treatment in patients with Alzheimer's disease (Adapted from Cacabelos, *68*)

8 Optimization of Alzheimer's Disease Therapeutics

The optimization of AD therapeutics requires the establishment of new postulates regarding (a) the costs of medicines, (b) the assessment of protocols for global treatment in dementia, (c) the implementation of novel therapeutics addressing causative factors, and (d) the setting up of pharmacogenetic/pharmacogenomic strategies for drug development *(4–8, 10–12, 68)*.

The cost of medicines is a very important issue in many countries because of (i) the aging of the population (>5% disability), (ii) AD patients (5–15%>65 years) being an unproductive sector of the population with low income, and (iii) the high cost of health care systems in developed countries. Despite the effort of the pharmaceutical industry to demonstrate the benefits and cost-effectiveness of available drugs, the general impression in the medical community and in some governments is that the antidementia drugs present in the market are not cost-effective *(3)*. Conventional drugs for AD are relatively simple (and some of them are also very old) compounds with unreasonable prices *(2)*. There is an urgent need to assess the costs of new trials with pharmacogenetics and pharmacogenomics strategies, and to implement pharmacogenetic procedures to predict drug-related adverse events *(9–14)*.

Cost-effectiveness analysis has been the most commonly applied framework for evaluating pharmacogenetics. Pharmacogenetic testing is potentially relevant to large populations that incur high costs. For instance, the most common drugs metabolized by CYP2D6 account for 189 million prescriptions and US$12.8 billion in expenditures annually in the U.S., which represents 5–10% of total utilization and expenditures for outpatient prescription drugs *(113)*. Pharmacogenomics offer great potential to improve patients' health in a cost-effective manner; however, pharmacogenetics/pharmacogenomics will not be applied to all drugs available in the market, and careful evaluations should be done on a case-by-case basis prior to investing resources in R&D of pharmacogenomic-based therapeutics and making reimbursment decisions.

In performing pharmacogenomic studies in AD, it is necessary to rethink the therapeutic expectations of novel drugs, redesign the protocols for drug clinical trials, and incorporate biological markers as assessable parameters of efficacy and prevention *(10–12)*. In addition to the characterization of genomic profiles, phenotypic profiling of responders and nonresponders to conventional drugs is also important (and currently neglected). Brain imaging techniques, computerized electrophysiology, and optical topography, in combination with genotyping of polygenic clusters, can help in the differentiation of responders and nonresponders. For instance, brain mapping shows a good imaging correlation with APOE-related genotypes in AD patients *(11, 12)*. Age and AChE- and BuChE-related genotypes can also influence the therapeutic response to donepezil and rivastigmine *(114)*. The early identification of predictive risks requires genomic screening and molecular diagnosis, and individualized preventive programs will be achieved only when pharmacogenomic/pharmacogenetic protocols are incorporated into the clinical armamentarium with powerful bioinformatics support.

Another important issue in AD therapeutics is that antidementia drugs should be effective in covering the clinical spectrum of dementia symptoms represented by memory deficits, behavioural changes, and functional decline. It is difficult (or impossible) for a single drug to meet these criteria. A potential solution to this problem is the implementation of cost-effective, multifactorial (combination) treatments, taking into consideration that traditional neuroleptics and novel antipsychotics (and many other psychotropics) deteriorate both cognitive and psychomotor functions in the elderly and may also increase the risk of stroke. Few studies with combination treatments have been reported and most of them are poorly designed. We also have to realize that the vast majority of dementia cases in people older than 75–80 are of a mixed type, in which the cerebrovascular component associated with neurodegeneration cannot be therapeutically neglected. In most cases of dementia, the multifactorial (combination) therapy appears to be the most effective strategy *(5–8, 10–12, 44, 68)*. The combination of several drugs (neuroprotectants, vasoactive substances, AChEIs, metabolic supplementation) increases the direct costs (e.g., medication) by 5–10%, but in turn annual global costs are reduced by approximately 18–20%, and the average survival rate increases about 30% (from 8 to 12 years postdiagnosis).

There are major concerns regarding the validity of clinical trials in patients with severe AD. Despite the questionable experience with memantine, similar strategies have been used to demonstrate the utility of donepezil in severe AD. This kind of study has some important pitfalls, including (a) short duration (<1 yr), (b) institutionalized patients, (c) patients receiving many different types of drugs, (d) nonevaluated drug-drug interactions, (e) side effects (e.g., hallucinations, gastrointestinal disorders) that may require the administration of additional medication, (f) lack of biological parameters demonstrating actual benefits, and (e) no cost-effectiveness assessment, among many other possible technical criticisms. Some of these methodological (and costly) problems might be overcome with the introduction of pharmacogenetic/pharmacogenomic strategies to identify good responders who might obtain some benefit by taking expensive (or risky) medications.

Major impact factors associated with drug efficacy and safety include the following: (i) the mechanisms of action of drugs, (ii) drug-specific adverse reactions, (iii) drug-drug interactions, (iv) nutritional factors, (v) vascular factors, (vi) social factors, and (vii) genomic factors (nutrigenetics, nutrigenomics, pharmacogenetics, pharmacogenomics). Among genomic factors, nutrigenetics/nutrigenomics and pharmacogenetics/pharmacogenomics account for more than 80% of efficacy-safety outcomes in current therapeutics *(10–12, 68)*.

Some authors consider that the priority areas for pharmacogenetic research are to predict serious adverse reactions (ADRs) and to establish variation in efficacy (115). Both requirements are necessary in AD to cope with efficacy and safety issues associated with either conventional AD-related drugs, new drugs, and psychotropic drugs of current use in dementia. Since drug response is a complex trait, genome-wide approaches (oligonucleotide microarrays, proteomic profiling) may provide new insights into drug metabolism and drug response.

To achieve a mature discipline of pharmacogenetics and pharmacogenomics in CNS disorders and dementia, it would be convenient to accelerate the following processes: (a) educate physicians and the public on the use of genetic/genomic screening in daily clinical practice; (b) standardize genetic testing for major categories of drugs; (c) validate pharmacogenetic and pharmacogenomic procedures according to drug category and pathology; (d) regulate ethical, social, and economic issues; and (e) incorporate pharmacogenetic and pharmacogenomic procedures both to drugs in development and to drugs in the market in order to optimize therapeutics.

Acknowledgements. I am thankful to all my collaborators at EuroEspes Biomedical Research Center, Institute of CNS Disorders, especially Dr. Victor Pichel, Gladys Bahamonde, Ivan Tellado, Carmen Fraile, Lola Corzo, Verónica Couceiro, Margarita Alcaraz, Laura Nebril, Cristina Muiño, and Angela Casas, as well as Dr. Lucía Fernández-Novoa, Ruth Llovo, Francisco Rocha, Ramón Alejo, Juan Carlos Carril, and Dr. Valter Lombardi at Ebiotec, Coruña, Spain, for their technical assisstance. The Ebiotec Foundation provided financial support for studies of pharmacogenomics in Alzheimer's disease.

Bibliography

1. Cacabelos R, Alvarez XA, Lombardi V et al. Pharmacological treatment of Alzheimer disease: from psychotropic drugs and cholinesterase inhibitors to pharmacogenomics. Drugs Today 2000;36:415–99.
2. Giacobini E. Cholinesterases in the human brain: the effect of cholinesterase inhibitors on Alzheimer's disease and related disorders. In: Giacobini E, Pepeu G (ed). The brain cholinergic system in health and disease. Informa Healthcare, Oxford, 2006 pp 235–64.
3. Loveman E, Green C, Kirby J, et al. The clinical and cost-effectiveness of donepezil, rivastigmine, galantamine, and memantine for Alzheimer's disease. Health Technl Assess 2006;10:1–176.
4. Cacabelos R, Fernández-Novoa L, Lombardi V, Kubota Y, Takeda M. Molecular genetics of Alzheimer's disease and aging. Meth Find Exper Clin Pharmacol 2005;27 (Suppl. A):1–573.
5. Cacabelos R. The application of functional genomics to Alzheimer's disease. Pharmacogenomics 2003;4:597–621.
6. Cacabelos R, Alvarez A, Fernández-Novoa L, Lombardi VRM. A pharmacogenomic approach to Alzheimer's disease. Acta Neurol Scand 2000;176(Suppl.):12–9.
7. Cacabelos R. Pharmacogenomics in Alzheimer's disease. Min Rev Med Chem 2002;2:59–84.
8. Cacabelos R. Pharmacogenomics for the treatment of dementia. Ann Med 2002;34:357–79.
9. Roses AD. Pharmacogenetics and drug development: the path to safer and more effective drugs. Nature Rev Genet 2004;5:645–56.
10. Cacabelos R. Pharmacogenomics and therapeutic prospects in Alzheimer's disease. Exp Opin Pharmacother 2005;6:1967–87.
11. Cacabelos R. Pharmacogenomics, nutrigenomics and therapeutic optimization in Alzheimer's disease. Aging Health 2005;1:303–48.
12. Cacabelos R, Takeda M. Pharmacogenomics, nutrigenomics and future therapeutics in Alzheimer's disease. Drugs Future 2006;31(Suppl B):5–146.
13. Goldstein DB, Tate SK, Sisodiya SM. Pharmacogenetics goes genomic. Nature Rev Genet 2003;4:937–47.
14. Austin CP. The impact of the completed human genome sequence on the development of novel therapeutics for human disease. Annu Rev Med 2004;55:1–13.
15. Selkoe DJ, Podlisny MB. Deciphering the genetic basis of Alzheimer's disease. Annu Rev Genomics Hum Genet 2002;3:67–99.

16. Doshi JA, Shaffer T, Briesacher BA. National estimates of medication use in nursing homes: findings from 1997 Medicare current beneficiary survey and the 1996 medical expenditure survey. J Am Geriatr Soc 2005;53:438–43.
17. Fialová D, Topinková E, Gambassi G, et al. Potentially inappropriate medication use among elderly home care patients in Europe. JAMA 2005;293:1348–58.
18. Simon SR, Chan KA, Soumerai SB, et al. Potentially inappropriate medication use by elderly persons in U.S. health maintenance organizations, 2000–2001. J Am Geriatr Soc 2005;53:227–32.
19. Weinshilboum RM, Wang L. Pharmacogenetics and pharmacogenomics: development, science, and translation. Annu Rev Genomics Hum Genet 2006;7:223–45.
20. www.ncbi.nlm.nih.gov/OMIM
21. www.molgen.ua.ac.be/ADMutations/
22. Cacabelos R, Fernández-Novoa L, Corzo L, Pichel V, Lombardi V, Kubota Y. Genomics and phenotypic profiles in dementia: Implications for pharmacological treatment. Meth Find Exper Clin Pharmacol 2004;26:421–44.
23. Cacabelos R, Kubota Y, Isaza C, et al. Functional genomics and pharmacogenetics in Alzheimer's disease. In: Recent progress in Alzheimer's and Parkinson's disease. Hanin I, Cacabelos R, Fisher A. (eds) Taylor & Francis, London, 2005 pp 89–102.
24. www.mitomap.org/
25. Hunter DJ. Gene-environment interactions in human diseases. Nature Rev Genet 2005;6:287–98.
26. Teter B, Finch CE. Caliban's heritance and the genetics of neuronal aging. Trends Neurosci 2004;27:627–32.
27. Levenson JM, Sweatt JD. Epigenetic mechanisms in memory formation. Nature Rev Neurosci 2005;6:108–18.
28. Suh Y-H, Checler F. Amyloid precursor protein, presenilins, and α-synuclein: Molecular pahogenesis and pharmacological applications in Alzheimer's disease. Phamacol Rev 2002;54:469–525.
29. Sharp AJ, Cheng Z, Eichler EE. Structural variation of human genome. Annu Rev Genomics Hum Genet 2006;7:407–42.
30. Crawford DC, Akey DT, Nickerson DA. The patterns of natural variation in human genes. Annu Rev Genomics Hum Genet 2005;6:287–312.
31. Cacabelos R, Fernández-Novoa L, Lombardi V, Takeda M. Genetic variation and pharmacogenomics in Alzheimer disease. Psychiat Neurol Jap 2003;105:47–67.
32. Gregersen N, Bross P, Vang S, Christensen JH. Protein misfolding and human disease. Annu Rev Genomics Hum Genet 2006;7:103–24.
33. Cacabelos R, Fernández-Novoa L, Lombardi V, Corzo L, Pichel V, Kubota Y. Cerebrovascular risk factors in Alzheimer's disease: brain hemodynamics and pharmacogenomic implications. Neurol Res 2003;25:567–80.
34. Cacabelos R, Fernández-Novoa L, Corzo L, et al. Phenotypic profiles and functional genomics in dementia with a vascular component. Neurol Res 2004;26:459–80.
35. Cacabelos R, Lombardi V, Fernández-Novoa L, et al. A functional genomics approach to the analysis of biological markers in Alzheimer disease. In: Molecular neurobiology of Alzheimer disease and related disorders. Takeda M, Tanaka T, Cacabelos R (eds). Karger, Basel, 2004 pp 236–85.
36. Cacabelos R. Genomic characterization of Alzheimer's disease and genotype-related phenotypic analysis of biological markers in dementia. Pharmacogenomics 2004;5:1049–105.
37. Van Oijen M, Hofman A, Soares HD, Koudstaal PJ, Breteler MM. Plasma Aβ1–40 and Aβ1–42) and the risk of dementia: prospective case-cohort study. Lancet Neurol 2006;5:655–60.
38. Cacabelos R. The histamine-cytokine network in Alzheimer disease: Etiopathogenic and pharmacogenomic implications. In: Mapping Progress of Alzheimer's and Parkinson's diseases. Advances in behavioral biology, vol. 51. Mizuno Y, Fisher A, Hanin I (eds). Pergamon Press, New York, 2002 pp 59–64.
39. Fernández-Novoa L, Cacabelos R. Histamine function in brain disorders. Behav Brain Res 2001;124:213–33.

40. Hogan DB, Goldlist B, Naglie G, Patterson C. Comparison studies of cholinesterase inhibitors for Alzheimer's disease. Lancet Neurol 2004;3:622–8.
41. Emilien G, Ponchon M, Caldas C, Isacson O, Maloteux JM. Impact of genomics on drug discovery and clinical medicine. Q J Med 2000;93:391–423.
42. Verrils NM. Clinical proteomics: present and future prospects. Clin Biochem Rev 2006;27:99–116.
43. Meyer UA. Pharmacogenetics—five decades of therapeutic lessons from genetic diversity. Nature Rev Genet 2004;5:669–76.
44. Cacabelos R, Fernández-Novoa L, Pichel V, Lombardi V, Kubota Y, Takeda M. Pharmacogenomic studies with a combination therapy in Alzheimer's disease. In: Molecular neurobiology of Alzheimer disease and related disorders. Takeda M, Tanaka T, Cacabelos R (eds). Karger, Basel, 2004 pp 94–107.
45. Evans WE, McLeod HL. Pharmacogenomics-drug disposition, drug targets, and side effects. N Engl J Med 2003;348:538–49.
46. Arranz MJ, Collier D, Kerwin RW. Pharmacogenetics for the individualization of psychiatric treatment. Am J Pharmacogenomics 2001;1:3–10.
47. International Human Genome Sequencing Consortium. Finishing the euchromatic sequence of the human genome. Nature 2004;431:931–45.
48. Sink KM, Holden KF, Yaffe K. Pharmacological treatment of neuropsychiatric symptoms of dementia. A review of the evidence. JAMA 2005;293:596–608.
49. Tribut O, Lessard Y, Reymann JM, Allain H, Bentue-Ferrer D. Pharmacogenomics. Med Sci Monit 2002;8:152–63.
50. Saito S, Ishida A, Sekine A, et al. Catalog of 680 variants among eight cytochrome P450 (CYP) genes, nine esterase genes, and two other genes in the Japanese population. J Hum Genet 2003;48:249–70.
51. Van Dam D, De Deyn PP. Drug discovery in dementia: the role of rodent models. Nature Rev Drug Discov 2006;5:956–70.
52. Wooding SP, Watkins WS, Bamshad MJ, et al. DNA sequence variations in a 3.7-kb noncoding sequence 5-prime of the CYP1A2 gene: implications for human population history and natural selection. Am J Hum Genet 2002;71:528–42.
53. Mizutani T. PM frequencies of major CYPs in Asians and Caucasians. Drug Metab Rev 2003;35:99–106.
54. Gaikovitch EA, Cascorbi I, Mrozikiewicz PM, et al. Polymorphisms of drug-metabolizing enzymes CYP2C9;CYP2C19;CYP2D6;CYP1A1;NAT2 and of P-glycoprotein in a Russian population. Eur J Clin Pharmacol 2003;59:303–12.
55. Xie HG, Prasad HG, Kim RB, Stein CM. CYP2C9 allelic variants: ethnic ditribution and functional significance. Adv Drug Deliv Rev 2002;54:1257–70.
56. Xie HG, Kim RB, Wood AJ, Stein CM. Molecular basis of ethnic differences in drug disposition and response. Annu Rev Pharm Toxicol 2001;41:815–50.
57. Isaza CA, Henao J, López AM, Cacabelos R. Isolation, sequence and genotyping of the drug metabolizer CYP2D6 gene in the Colombian population. Meth Find Exp Clin Pharmacol 2000;22:695–705.
58. Madan A, Graham RA, Carroll KM, et al. Effects of prototypical microsomal enzyme inducers on cytochrome P450 expression in cultured human hepatocytes. Drug Metab Dispos 2003;31:421–31.
59. Pascussi JM, Gerbal-Chaloin S, Drocourt L, Maurel P, Vilarem MJ. The expression of CYP2B6, CYP2C9, and CYP2A4 genes: a tangle of networks of nuclear and steroid receptors. Biochim Biophys Acta 2003;1619:243–53.
60. Honkakoski P, Negishi M. Regulation of cytochrome P450 (CYP) genes by nuclear receptors. Biochem J 2000;347:321–37.
61. Hedlund E, Gustafsson JA, Warner M. Cytochrome P450 in the brain: a review. Curr Drug Metabol 2001;2:245–63.
62. www.icgeb.org/
63. www.imm.ki.se/CYPalleles/cyp2d6.htm.

64. Sachse C, Brockmoller J, Bauer S, Roots I. Cytochrome P450 2D6 variants in a Caucasian population: allele frequencies and phenotypic consequences. Am J Hum Genet 1997;60:284–95.
65. Bentue-Ferrer D, Tribut O, Polard E, Allain H. Clinically significant drug interactions with cholinesterase inhibitors: a guide for neurologists. CNS Drugs 2003;17:947–63.
66. Griese E-U, Zanger UM, Brudermanns U, et al. Assessment of the predictive power of genotypes for the in-vivo catalytic function of CYP2D6 in a German population. Pharmacogenetics 1998;8:15–26.
67. Bernal ML, Sinues B, Johansson I, et al. Ten percent of north Spanish individuals carry duplicated or triplicated CYP2D6 genes associated with ultrarapid metabolism of debrisoquine. Pharmacogenetics 1999;9:657–60.
68. Cacabelos R. Molecular pathology and pharmacogenomics in Alzheimer's disease: polygenic-related effects of multifactorial treatments on cognition, anxiety, and depression. Meth Find Exper Clin Pharmacol 2007;29(Suppl. B):1–91.
69. Bernard S, Neville KA, Nguyen AT, Flockhart DA. Interethnic differences in genetic polymorphisms of CYP2D6 in the U.S. population: clinical implications. Oncologist 2006;11:126–35.
70. Raimundo S, Fischer J, Eichelbaum M, Griese EU, Schwab M, Zanger. Elucidation of the genetic basis of the common intermediate metabolizer phenotype for drug oxidation by CYP2D6. Pharmacogenetics 2000;10:577–81.
71. Rasmussen JO, Christensen M, Svendsen JM, Skausig O, Hansen EL, Nielsen KA. CYP2D6 gene test in psychiatric patients and healthy volunteers. Scand J Clin Lab Invest 2006;66:129–36.
72. Yamada H, Dahl ML, Viitanen M, Winblad B, Sjoqvist F, Lannfelt L. No association between familial Alzheimer disease and cytochrome P450 polymorphisms. Alzheimer Dis Assoc Disord 1998;12:204–7.
73. Chen X, Xia Y, Alford M, et al. The CYP2D6B allele is associated with a milder synaptic pathology in Alzheimer's disease. Ann Neurol 1995;38 :653–8.
74. Cervilla JA, Russ C, Holmes C, et al. CYP2D6 polymorphisms in Alzheimer's disease, with and without extrapyramidal signs, showing no apolipoprotein E epsilon 4 effect modification. Biol Psychiatry 1999;45:426–9.
75. Atkinson A, Singleton AB, Steward A, et al. CYP2D6 is associated with Parkinson's disease but not with dementia with Lewy bodies or Alzheimer's disease. Pharmacogenetics 1999;9:31–5.
76. Nicholl DJ, Bennett P, Hiller L, et al. A study of five candidate genes in Parkinson's disease and related neurodegenerative disorders. European Study Group on Atypical Parkinsonism. Neurology 1999;53:1415–21.
77. Woo SI, Kim JW, Seo HG, et al. CYP2D6*4 polymorphism is not associated with Parkinson's disease and has no protective role against Alzheimer's disease in the Korean population. Psychiatry Clin Neurosci 2001;55 :373–7.
78. Furuno T, Kawanishi C, Iseki E, et al. No evidence of an association between CYP2D6 polymorphisms among Japanese and dementia with Lewy bodies. Psychiatry Clin Neurosci 2001;55:89–92.
79. Scordo MG, Dahl ML, Spina E, Cordici F, Arena MG. No association between CYP2D6 polymorphisms and Alzheimer's disease in an Italian population. Pharmacol Res 2006;53:162–5.
80. Cacabelos R. Pleiotropic effects of APOE in dementia: influence on functional genomics and pharmacogenetics. In: Advances in Alzheimer's and Parkinson's disease. Insights, progress, and perspectives. Fisher A, Memo M, Storchi F, Hanin I (eds), Springer, Secaucus, NJ, 2007 pp 355–367.
81. Varsaldi F, Miglio G, Scordo MG, et al. Impact of the CYP2D6 polymorphism on steady-state plasma concentrations and clinical outcome of donepezil in Alzheimer's disease patients. Eur J Clin Pharmacol 2006;62:721–6.
82. Egger SS, Bachmann A, Hubmann N, Schlienger RG, Krähenbühl S. Prevalence of potentially inappropriate medication use in elderly patients. Comparison between general medicine and geriatric wards. Drugs Aging 2006;23:823–37.

83. Schuetz EG, Relling MV, Kishi S, et al. PharGKB update: II. CYP3A5, cytochrome P450, family 3, subfamily A, polypeptide 5. Pharmacol Rev 2004;56:159.
84. Poirier J, Delisle M-C, Quirion R, et al. Apolipoprotein E4 allele as a predictor of cholinergic deficits treatment outcome in Alzheimer disease. Proc Natl Acad Sci U S A 1995;92: 12260–4.
85. Poirier J. Apolipoprotein E4; cholinergic integrity and the pharmacogenetics of Alzheimer's disease. J Psychiat Neurosci 1999;24:147–53.
86. Almkvist O, Jelic V, Amberla K, Hellstrom-Lindahl E, Meurling L, Nordberg A. Responder characteristics to a single oral dose of cholinesterase inhibitor: a double-blind placebo-controlled study with tacrine in Alzheimer patients. Dement Geriatr Cogn Disord 2001;12:22–32.
87. Sjögren M, Hesse C, Basun H, et al. Tacrine and rate of progression in Alzheimer's disease—relation to ApoE allele genotype. J Neural Transm 2001;108:451–8.
88. Borroni B, Colciaghi F, Pastorino L, et al. ApoE genotype influences the biological effects of donepezil on APP metabolism in Alzheimer disease: evidence from a peripheral model. Eur Neuropsychopharmacol 2002;12:195–200.
89. Aerssens J, Raeymaekers P, Lilienfeld S, Geerts H, Konings F, Parys W. APOE genotype: no influence on galantamine treatment efficacy nor on rate of decline in Alzheimer's disease. Dement Geriatr Cogn Disord 2001;2:69–77.
90. Raskind MA, Peskind ER, Wessel T, Yuan W. Galantamine in AD: a 6-month randomized, placebo-controlled trial with a 6-month extension. The Galantamine USA-1 Study Group. Neurology 2000;54:2261–2268.
91. Risner ME, Saunders AM, Altman JF, et al. Efficacy of rosiglitazone in a genetically defined population with mild-to-moderate Alzheimer's disease. Pharmacogenomics 2006;6:246–54.
92. MacGowan SH, Wilcock GK, Scott M. Effect of gender and apolipoprotein E genotype on response to anticholinesterase therapy in Alzheimer's disease. Int J Geriatr Psychiatry 1998;13:625–30.
93. Rigaud AS, Traykov L, Caputo L, et al. The apolipoprotein E epsilon 4 allele and the response to tacrine therapy in Alzheimer's disease. Eur J Neurol 2000;7 :255–8.
94. Rigaud AS, Traykov L, Latour F, et al. Presence of absence of least one epsilon 4 allele and gender are not predictive for the response to donepezil treatment in Alzheimer's disease. Pharmacogenetics 2002;12:415–20.
95. Petersen RC, Thomas RG, Grundman M, et al. Vitamin E and donepezil for the treatment of mild cognitive impairment. N Engl J Med 2005;352:2379–88.
96. Bizzarro A, Marra C, Acciarri A, et al. Apolipoprotein E epsilon-4 allele differentiates the clinical response to donepezil in Alzheimer's disease. Dement Geriatr Cogn Disord 2005;20:254–61.
97. Alvarez XA, Mouzo R, Pichel V, et al. Double-blind placebo-controlled study with citicoline in APOE genotyped Alzheimer's disease patients. Effects on cognitive performance, brain bioelectrical activity, and cerebral perfusion. Meth Find Exp Clin Pharmacol 1999;21:633–44.
98. Alvarez XA, Pichel V, Pérez PA, et al. Double-blind, randomized, placebo-controlled pilot study with anapsos in senile dementia: effects on cognition, brain bioelectrical activity and cerebral hemodynamics. Meth Find Exp Clin Pharmacol 2000;22:585–94.
99. Saunders AM, Trowers MK, Shimkets RA, et al. The role of apolipoprotein E in Alzheimer's disease: pharmacogenomic target selection. Biochem Biophys Acta 2000;1502:85–94.
100. Sayed-Tabatabaei FA, Oostra BA, Isaacs A, van Duijn CM, Witteman JC. ACE polymorphisms. Circ Res 2006;98:1123–33.
101. Hu J, Igarashi A, Kamata M, Nakagawa H. Angiotensin-converting enzyme degrades Alzheimer amyloid β-peptide (Aβ); retards Aβ aggregation, deposition, fibril formation; and inhibits cytotoxicity. J Biol Chem 2001;276:47863–8.
102. Oba R, Igarashi A, Kamata M, Nagata K, Takano S, Nakagawa H. The N-terminal active centre of human angiotensin-converting enzyme degrades Alzheimer amyloid beta-peptide. Eur J Neurosci 2005;21:733–40.

103. Eckman EA, Adams SK, Troendle FJ, et al. Regulation of steady-state beta-amyloid levels in the brain by neprilysin and endothelin-converting enzyme but not angiotensin-converting enzyme. J Biol Chem 2006;281:30471–8.
104. Hemming ML, Selkoe DJ. Amyloid β-protein is degraded by cellular angiotensin-converting enzyme (ACE) and elevated by an ACE inhibitor. J Biol Chem 2005;280:37644–50.
105. Fleming I. Signaling by the angiotensin-converting enzyme. Circ Res 2006;98:887–96.
106. Baghai TC, Binder EB, Schule C, et al. Polymorphisms in the angiotensin-converting enzyme gene are associated with unipolar depression, ACE activity and hypercortisolism. Mol Psychiatry 2006;11:1003–15.
107. McLachlan CS, Yi Xing Soh C. Differences in anxiety-related behaviour between apolipoprotein E-deficient C57BL/6 and wild type C57BL/6 mice. Physiol Res 2005;54 :701–4.
108. Nebes RD, Vora IJ, Meltzer CC, et al. Relationship of deep white matter hyperintensities and apolipoprotein E genotype to depressive symptoms in older adults without clinical depression. Am J Psychiatry 2001;158:878–84.
109. Naismith S, Hickie I, Ward PB, et al. Caudate nucleus volumes and genetic determinants of homocysteine metabolism in the prediction of psychomotor speed in older persons with depression. Am J Psychiatry 2002;159:2096–8.
110. O'Brien JT, Lloyd A, McKeith I, Gholkar A, Ferrier N. A longitudinal study of hippocampal volume, cortisol levels, and cognition in older depressed subjects. Am J Psychiatry 2004;161:2081–90.
111. Hickie I, Naismith S, Ward PB, et al. Reduced hippocampal volumes and memory loss in patients with early- and late-onset depression. Br J Psychiatry 2005;186:197–202.
112. Kim JM, Stewart R, Shin IS, Yoon JS. Vascular/risk and late-life depression in a Korean community population. Br J Psychiatry 2004;185:102–7.
113. Philips KA, Van Bebber SL. Measuring the value of pharmacogenomics. Nature Rev Drug Discovery 2005;4:500–9.
114. Bullock R, Bergman H, Touchon J, Gambina G, He Y, Nagel J, Lane R. Effect of age on response to rivastigmine or donepezil in patients with Alzheimer's disease. Curr Med Res Opin 2006;22:483–94.
115. Need AC, Motulsky AG, Goldstein DB. Priorities and standards in pharmacogenetic research. Nature Genet 2005;37:671–81.

Chapter 17
Pharmacogenomics Applications in Psychiatric Disorders

Todd Lencz and Anil K. Malhotra

Contents

Abstract Serious mental illnesses, including schizophrenia and major depressive disorder, result in considerable chronicity, morbidity, and mortality, and are amongst the leading causes of disability in the developed world. Despite advances in development of pharmacologic agents over the last two decades, only about one-third of patients with psychotic or affective disorders experience rapid or robust treatment response, while as many as 40–50% can be labeled as partially or completely treatment refractory. Pharmacogenetic studies offer the potential to enhance clinical prognosis, and ultimately to tailor individualized therapies; however, the psychiatric pharmacogenetic literature to date may give the appearance of diverse, unreplicated results of uncertain clinical significance. To overcome this impression, we review findings demonstrating a replicable role in clinical prediction—for both symptom response and side effect burden—of several polymorphisms in genes in the serotonin and dopamine systems. We also highlight the limitations in current research, including the role of ethnic heterogeneity, the need to study treatment-naïve patients, the lack of cost-benefit pharmacoeconomic studies, and the need for more comprehensive genotyping/haplotyping. We conclude by demonstrating the potential role of novel technologies, specifically whole genome association, in identifying robust, novel loci for pharmacogenomic prediction.

Keywords pharmacogenetics, pharmacogenomics, psychiatry, major depressive disorder, antidepressants, schizophrenia, antipsychotics, serotonin, dopamine

---

Todd Lencz
Department of Psychiatry Research, The Zucker Hillside Hospital, Glen Oaks, NY
lencz@lij.edu

N. Cohen (ed.) *Pharmacogenomics and Personalized Medicine*,

1 Introduction

Individual differences in clinical response to psychotropic drugs has long been recognized as a fundamental problem in the treatment of mental illness *(1, 2)*. As a generalization, only about one third of patients with psychotic or affective disorders experience rapid or robust treatment response, while as many as 40–50% can be labeled as partially or completely treatment refractory. There is also marked variability in susceptibility to adverse drug effects, which not only can lead to substantial excess morbidity, but also result in the considerable problem of treatment nonadherence. A priori identification of the patients who will respond well to a particular psychotropic drug, or be at a higher risk for development of side effects, has the potential to help clinicians avoid lengthy, ineffective medication trials and limit patients' exposure to adverse events. Moreover, enhanced predictability of treatment response early in the course of a patient's illness may result in enhanced medication adherence, a significant predictor of relapse *(3)*.

Since the mid 1990s, the field of pharmacogenetics has offered the potential for providing readily accessible, immutable biomarkers—DNA sequence variants—that might be predictive of an individual's propensity for both positive and adverse effects of drugs. However, to date, the promise of personalized medicine has remained unfulfilled. Because academic pharmacogenetic research is often limited to small and clinically heterogeneous samples, individual studies have been unable to provide compelling results. Additionally, the modest effect sizes which are common in complex genetics present an obstacle in the quest for valid biomarkers, which require high sensitivity and specificity for individual clinical prediction. Moreover, examination of disparate polymorphisms across a wide variety of candidate genes has created an impression of scattered, unreplicated findings. Recently, however, findings across multiple laboratories have begun to converge for genes related to serotonin and dopamine, the most prominent neurotransmitters targeted by drugs for major depressive disorder and schizophrenia.

The goal of the present chapter, then, is not to present an exhaustive review of all studies conducted in psychiatric pharmacogenetics. Rather, we will focus on the converging evidence implicating the most well-studied candidates in these two disorders. With additional focused research, it is possible that clinically useful predictions concerning the relative costs (side effects) and benefits (likelihood of response) of common serotonergic and dopaminergic treatments may soon be available to the individual patient and clinician. At the end of this chapter, we will consider future technological developments, including whole genome association and sequencing, which are likely to greatly accelerate the search for less obvious genes which may nevertheless have strong effects on phenotypes such as psychiatric drug response.

2 Major Depressive Disorder

Major depressive disorder (MDD) is one of the most common and disabling psychiatric disorders, with an estimated 12-month and lifetime prevalence of about 5% and 15%, respectively *(4, 5)*; similar prevalence rates have been observed in most

European countries *(6)*. The course of MDD is chronic and/or relapsing for a majority of patients *(7, 8)*, resulting in considerable morbidity and mortality. MDD is currently the fourth (and predicted to rapidly rise to the second) greatest medical cause of years lost to disability *(9)*, and it accounts for 20–35% of the nearly 30,000 annual suicides in the United States (10,11). Antidepressants represent the third largest pharmaceutical market worldwide, with sales well in excess of $10 billion. However, efficacy studies demonstrate that only slightly more than half of patients respond (defined as 50% reduction in symptoms) to currently available treatments *(2)*, and less than one third of patients experience full remission *(12)*. Because long-term quality of life, disability, and general health comorbidity are strongly correlated with ongoing levels of residual symptomatology *(13)*, optimizing response to treatment remains a pressing clinical concern.

2.1 Pharmacogenetic Studies of the Serotonin Transporter

Given that most currently used antidepressants operate either selectively or primarily on the inhibition of serotonin reuptake, it is perhaps not surprising the serotonin transporter gene (*SLC6A4*) has been the most common focus in pharmacogenetic studies. Located at chromosome 17q11.1-q12, *SLC6A4* contains a well-studied functional polymorphism (known as 5-HTTLPR) in a variable-repeat sequence in its promoter region *(14)*. The short ("*s*") allele, containing fewer repeats (a 44 base pair deletion) relative to the long ("*l*") allele, reduces transcription efficiency of the gene, resulting in reduced expression of the transporter protein *(15)*. The short allele has been associated with susceptibility to depressive traits, particularly in individuals with a history of major life stress *(16)*, although not necessarily to MDD itself *(17)*. Thus, MDD patients display the full range of genotypes at this locus, and both alleles are relatively common in the population, making this polymorphism an attractive candidate even for small pharmacogenetic studies.

2.2 Efficacy

In one of the first pharmacogenetic studies involving an SSRI, Smeraldi and colleagues *(18)* showed that the *s* allele form of 5HTTLPR was associated with reduced efficacy of fluvoxamine in a group of 53 patients with major depression. Since then, more than one dozen studies have examined the effect of this variant on response to SSRIs, albeit in relatively small samples of 50–130 subjects. Although sample characteristics, drug and dose selection, length of trial, and outcome criteria vary considerably, a recent meta-analysis of 15 studies (total n = 1435) indicates a robust effect consistent with the initial report *(19)*. Specifically, *ll* homozygotes were twice as likely as s carriers (odds ratio, OR = 2.01) to respond over the course of the trial, and were even more likely (OR = 2.57) to demonstrate early response (within the first 4 weeks of the trial). Moreover, *l* carriers were more likely to achieve remission criteria (OR = 2.21) compared to *ss* homozygotes. (Note that deleterious effects of the *s* allele were dominant with respect to response, but recessive with respect to remission.) While these odds ratios are modest and do not, of themselves, permit unambiguous classification of individual subjects, these effect sizes are relatively large in the context of complex genetics.

2.3 Side Effects

While efficacy studies demonstrate greater responsivity to SSRIs associated with the *l* allele, the *s* allele appears to confer greater sensitivity to adverse effects of antidepressants. In a study of depressed patients aged 65 or older, Murphy et al. *(20)* demonstrated that *s* allele carriers (n = 71) had greater severity of adverse events and higher rates of discontinuation relative to *ll* subjects (n = 40) taking paroxetine. These results were subsequently replicated in a smaller sample (n = 44) of patients taking a variety of antidepressants thought to act at the serotonin transporter *(21)*. Additionally, Smits et al. *(22)* recently reported that the rate of general adverse events (including dermatologic reactions, weight change, and fatigue) to SSRIs was significantly increased in subjects with one (OR = 1.77) or two (OR = 2.37) copies of the *s* allele. Extremely strong evidence for a role of 5HTTLPR in side effect burden was recently adduced in a pharmacogenetic investigation in the STAR*D effectiveness trial of citalopram *(2)*. Low activity allele carriers demonstrated significantly increased side effects in the full sample of >1650 subjects *(23)*. Although side effect ratings in this large and complex trial were limited, the data suggested that a major component of this side effect burden was treatment-emergent diarrhea, presumably related to abnormal gastrointestinal serotonin activity. Finally, it is intriguing that the first two studies above reported that deleterious effects of the *s* allele were not seen in subjects taking mirtazapine, which does not act upon the serotonin transporter. Murphy et al. *(20)* actually reported a *reverse* effect (greater adverse effects and discontinuation in *ll* patients taking mirtazapine).

Two studies have also demonstrated that *ss* homozygotes are at increased risk for anti-depressant induced mania *(24, 25)*. While both studies reported very strong effects (2.5<OR<4), both were retrospective studies of patients already diagnosed with bipolar disorder; no prospective studies of unipolar patients undergoing treatment have been reported. It should be noted that two additional studies reported no significant association between 5HTTLPR genotype and antidepressant-induced mania *(26, 27)*. A third study failed to find an overall association of the *s* allele to antidepressant-induced mania, but did report an association within subjects with rapid cycling *(28)*. A small study by Perlis and colleagues *(29)* suggests that medication-induced insomnia and agitation may be a mechanism underlying a "manic switch." Thirty-six outpatients with MDD were assessed prospectively over the course of a 12-week open-label trial of fluoxetine (up to 60 mg/day). Of nine subjects homozygous for the *s* allele, seven (78%) developed new or worsening insomnia and 6 (67%) developed agitation. By contrast, only 22% and 7% of *l* carriers developed insomnia or agitation, respectively. It should be noted that no data on manic switch were directly presented by these investigators.

2.4 Conclusions and Caveats

The results described above provide strong evidence that 5HTTLPR variation influences response to treatment SSRIs. Moreover, results converge in that *s* allele carriers, and particularly *ss* homozygotes, are less likely to achieve positive outcomes of response and remission, and are more likely to experience adverse events including a possibility of a switch into mania. Combined with evidence (reviewed in 30) that the *s* allele may be associated with increased risk for suicide (although treatment-induced suicidality has not been studied), it could be argued that SSRIs are indicated for *s* carriers only with caution. One "head-to-head" study comparing two SSRIs *(31)* indicated that paroxetine was significantly more effective than fluvoxamine in *ss* homozygotes. Further studies comparing SSRIs to treatments based on other mechanisms (e.g., mirtazapine, bupropion) would be extremely helpful to determine whether such medications would be significantly more efficacious or tolerable for *s* carriers. For example, it would be interesting to determine whether *s* carriers account for the notable additional efficacy (25–30%) of augmentation or switch strategies in nonresponders to conventional SSRI monotherapy *(32, 33)*.

Despite the relatively robust effects described above, several caveats must also be addressed. First, the (by far) largest single pharmacogenetic study to date, reported too recently for inclusion in the aforementioned meta-analytic study *(19)*, failed to find a significant effect of 5HTTLPR variation on symptom response or remission to citalopram *(23, 34)*. Examining >1300 Caucasian subjects as part of the STAR*D effectiveness trial *(2)*, the *s* allele was slightly overrepresented in nonresponders (OR=1.12), but results were far from statistically significant. However, since the direction of response is consistent with other studies, this result would attenuate, but not abolish, the effects reported in the meta-analysis. It is also possible that broader inclusion criteria of the STAR*D trial, including lower levels of depression at study entry as well as more permissive exclusion criteria, resulted in increased homogeneity of the sample and reduction of the power of genetic predictors. Still, it is likely that the STAR*D sample is more representative of patients seeking treatment with SSRIs; pharmacogenetic recommendations based on the results of more rarified efficacy trials should be considered provisional.

An additional limitation on the applicability of these pharmacogenetic data is the potential confound of ethnicity. The 5HTTLPR allelic frequencies are very sensitive to population of origin *(19)*, and this could lead to differing associations to treatment-relevant phenotypes. In Caucasians, the short form represents the minor allele, and is present on about 40% of all chromosomes. However, this rate is approximately doubled in Asian populations, for whom the short allele is predominant. By contrast, individuals of African descent (including African-Americans) exhibit only about a 20% *s* allele frequency. This latter group has been virtually unrepresented in pharmacogenetic research, with only the STAR*D study reporting any data; no significant association was observed in a sample of 251 patients taking citalopram *(34)*. Studies in Asian patients have revealed mixed results for 5HTTLPR. While the meta-analysis *(19)* demonstrated comparable (though more variable) results in Asian patients (i.e., reduced efficacy in *s* carriers), a recent large (n>200) Korean study of geriatric depression showed the reverse effect *(35)*; the *s* allele was associated with improved response to antidepressants, even in patients taking a norepinephrine reuptake inhibitor (nortriptyline). Two earlier studies (included in the meta-analysis) also showed a reverse relationship *(36, 37)*, and one study of adverse effects demonstrated no association in Asians *(38)*. Thus, pharmacogenetic recommendations are extremely limited for non-Caucasians at this time, and broader representation is required in future pharmacogenetic studies.

These interethnic differences, as well as the presence of other conflicting findings and failures to replicate, may be partially accounted for by other variations within the *SLC6A4* locus that may impact production of the serotonin transporter protein. Recent advances in genotyping technology, combined with more comprehensive understanding of genomic variation *(39)*, require that the next generation of pharmacogenetic studies of the serotonin transporter account for all major sources of variation at the gene. As shown in Figure 17.1, linkage disequilibrium structure and haplotypic frequencies differ dramatically across populations.

As an important example of the need for more comprehensive genotyping, it has recently been demonstrated that nucleotide substitutions within the long 5HTTLPR allele may result in lower expression of the transcript, comparable to the shorter allele *(40)*, and may affect reported associations to mood-related phenotypes *(41)*. Smeraldi et al. *(42)* demonstrated that response to fluvoxamine differed amongst *l* alleles carriers depending upon the specific nucleotide sequence of the full repeat region, yet no other studies to date have genotyped these subvariants. Similarly, the STAR*D side effects study demonstrated stronger effects, particularly in the Caucasian non-Hispanic subgroup, when *l* alleles carrying an activity-reducing A-to-G substitution were grouped with *s* alleles *(23)*. Two studies *(43, 44)* demonstrated a significant pharmacogenetic effect of a single nucleotide polymorphism (SNP, rs25531) which is in linkage disequilibrium with 5HTTLPR and may account for some of the phenotypic effects attributed to the repeat variant. Moreover, Kraft et al. *(44)* reported data indicating that rs25531 is functional, and affects binding of this segment of DNA to the activator protein 2 transcription factor, thus potentially mirroring transcription effects of 5HTTLPR. Finally, a trend-level effect on treatment response ($p = .02$, not significant when corrected for multiple comparisons) was reported in the STAR*D sample for rs140700, a SNP in intron 6 exhibiting modest LD with rs25531 and low LD with 5HTTLPR *(34)*.

2.5 Other Serotonin-Related Genes

A number other genes in the serotonin pathway have been investigated in pharmacogenetic studies of antidepressants; three such genes (*HTR2A, HTR1A,* and *TPH1*) have yielded significant associations that have been replicated at least once. Several studies have converged to indicate that variation in *HTR2A* (on chromosome 13q), encoding the postsynaptic serotonin receptor $5HT_{2A}$, may be associated with antidepressant response phenotypes. A promoter region SNP, rs6311 (also referred to

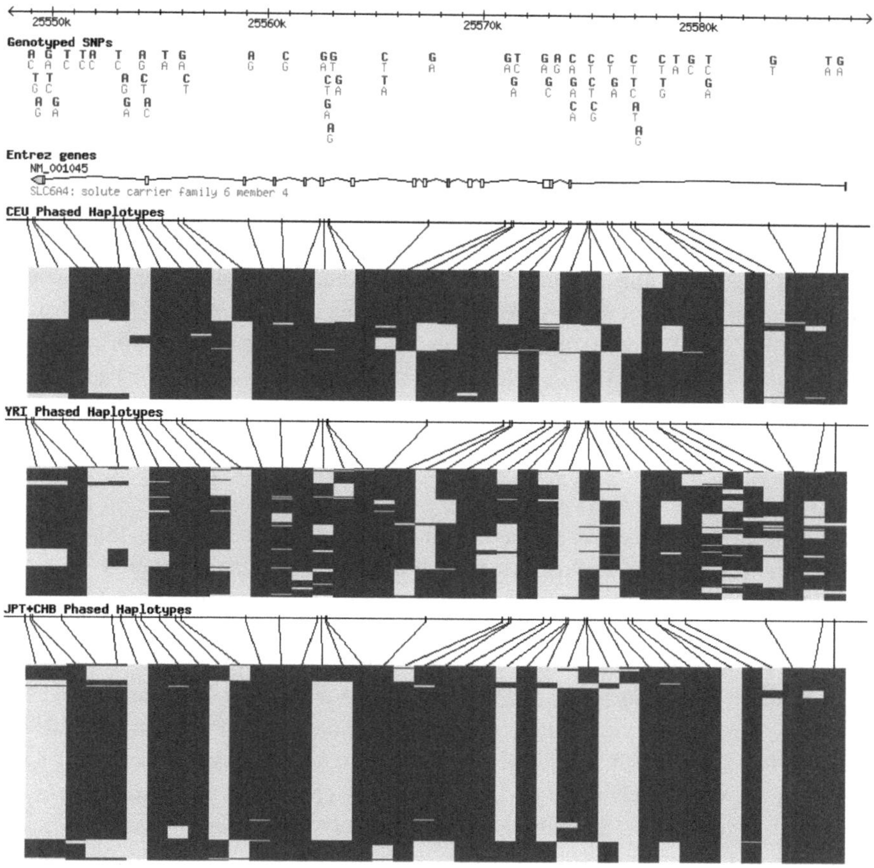

Fig. 17.1 Haplotype structure across the serotonin transporter gene (*SLC6A4*), based on Phase II HapMap genotypes (ref. 39) in three ethnic populations (CEU = Caucasian; YRI = African; JPT+CHB = Asian)

as -1438G/A), appears to affect transcription of the receptor (possibly in concert with an additional SNP, rs6312 [45]). Specifically, the G allele tends to be associated with reduced expression of the receptor *(46)*.

In a study of 77 Korean MDD patients receiving citalopram, GG homozygotes demonstrated more robust response to treatment; intriguingly, the G allele was also associated with the presence of MDD when this group was compared with healthy volunteers *(47)*. Similarly, Kato et al. *(38)* demonstrated better response in GG homozygotes (total n = 100 Japanese patients randomized to fluvoxamine or paroxetine). Virtually identical results were observed in a moderately large (n = 173) German sample undergoing various nonrandomized treatments, although a different (but functionally equivalent) SNP was assessed *(48)*; this SNP (rs6313, also designated T102C) is in perfect linkage disequilibrium with rs6311, thus providing identical information. The C allele at rs6313 corresponds to the low-activity G allele of rs6311.

Unfortunately, the same low-activity allele at rs6311 that is associated with good response has also been associated with increased rates of side effects in three studies. Bishop et al. *(49)* reported that GG homozygotes had increased sexual side effects in a primarily Caucasian sample on various SSRIs. Kato et al. *(38)* reported a greater total rate of adverse events, particularly nausea, associated with the G allele; increased gastrointestinal side effects were also reported in a subset of Japanese patients with both the G allele and low metabolizing genotypes at the *CYP2D6* gene *(50)*.

The studies listed above generally converge, demonstrating greater serotonergic sensitivity for G allele homozygotes in both Asians and Caucasians. As contrasted with the 5HTTLPR variant, allelic frequencies at rs6311 do not differ dramatically across populations, with each allele demonstrating roughly equal (~50%) population frequency. Still, two studies have reported no affect for rs6311 in both Asians and Caucasians *(51, 52)*. In the large STAR*D open trial of citalopram, McMahon et al. *(52)* failed to find an effect for rs6311 or rs6313, but did report a strongly significant effect ($p = 10^{-6}$) for rs7997012, a novel SNP at the other (3′) end of the gene. This SNP, near exon 3, was not in LD with rs6313/6311 in this sample. Despite the strong statistical significance of this finding, it is important to note that the clinical impact may be more modest. Even in the most robust subsample (Caucasian subjects), and comparing homozygotes only (excluding heterozygotes, which demonstrated intermediate response), the effect size was insufficient for individualized prediction (OR ~1.2). Finally, one additional study suggested that extremely rare homozygotes at a different promoter polymorphism (−1420 T/T homozygotes) demonstrated reduced response to antidepressant treatment *(53)*. Again, more work needs to be performed to fully characterize the functional consequences of haplotypic diversity at this moderately sized (62kb) gene.

In contrast to the postsynaptic $5HT_{2A}$ receptor, the $5HT_{1A}$ autoreceptor modulates the firing rate of dorsal raphe serotonergic neurons; the $5HT_{1A}$ protein is coded by the very small (<2kb) *HTR1A* gene at chromosome 5q11.2–q13. Some evidence from preclinical models has suggested that desensitization of the autoreceptor is implicated in the therapeutic mechanism of SSRIs *(54)*, and two functional SNPs have been identified in the gene. Receptor proteins carrying the G allele at a promoter region polymorphism (rs6295, C-1019G) are less responsive to the therapeutic desensitization effect in raphe neurons *(54)*. One PET study provides evidence that this results in greater 5-HT1A cortical binding potential in G allele carriers, perhaps due to greater gene expression *(55)*. At least four studies, with a combined sample of over 300 individuals, have demonstrated a relationship between antidepressant response and rs6295, with the alternate G allele associated with impaired response to antidepressants *(54–57)*. However, it should be noted that no effect was reported in the STAR*D study *(52)*, and one additional study reported an association in bipolar, but not unipolar depressed patients *(58)*. Additionally, one study has reported a nonsynonymous SNP in *HTR1A* (Gly272Asp, rs1800042), for which the substituted Asp allele is associated with significantly enhanced response to fluvoxamine *(59)*, although this effect was not replicated in one subsequent study *(57)*.

Relatedly, one SNP in the trytophan hydroxylase (*TPH1*) gene, A218C, has demonstrated a significant association to antidepressant efficacy, with carriers of the A allele exhibiting reduced response to paroxetine, fluvoxamine, and citalopram *(26, 43, 60, 61)*. Although the mechanism of this effect is unknown, and several studies have failed to replicate the association (e.g., *37, 52, 62*), TPH1 is the rate-limiting enzyme in the synthesis of serotonin, and this gene deserves further investigation.

3 Schizophrenia

Although their prevalence is slightly below 1% of the population *(63)*, schizophrenia (SCZ) and schizoaffective disorder together constitute the fifth leading cause of disability; in the United States, SCZ is responsible for more years of life lived with disability than all malignancies and HIV combined *(64, 65)*. In SCZ, disability typically persists throughout the person's lifetime and exacts a financial cost to society three to four times that of direct patient care *(66)*. Of the estimated 65 billion dollars spent in caring for individuals with SCZ in the USA (in 1991), $46 billion was attributed to lost productivity *(67)*. The introduction of second-generation antipsychotics did not substantially improve these figures 11 years later *(68)*. Although not often recognized, SCZ also carries substantial mortality; the disorder is associated with a doubling of mortality rates compared to the general population *(69)*, and a suicide rate that may be as high as 5% *(70)*.

Despite the introduction of several second-generation antipsychotics over the last decade, and the subsequent generation of a multibillion dollar market in such medications, a recent large-scale efficacy trial has yielded disappointing results *(71)*. This trial revealed that both old and new medications have only moderate long-term effectiveness, partially due to relatively high side effect burdens and extremely high rates of discontinuation (~75% discontinuation within 18 months). Even when taking medication, as many as 40% of patients fail to demonstrate adequate response on the hallmark positive symptoms of hallucinations and delusions *(72)*. Moreover, current treatments are, at best, only modestly effective in ameliorating negative symptoms and cognitive deficits associated with the illness *(73)*. The time course of treatment response has remained controversial, leaving clinicians without strong guidance for making decisions about when to switch medications *(74)*.

Given the compelling need for enhanced prognostic tools in clinical decision-making, it is perhaps surprising that pharmacogenetic predictors of antipsychotic response have been understudied to date. In a recent review *(75)*, we noted that most such studies have relied on small samples (often with $n < 100$) of convenience, often derived from open-label clozapine trials in which patients are already receiving frequent blood draws. Trial lengths have been generally short (4–8 weeks), with only a single endpoint rating. Negative symptom endpoints have only rarely been studied, and pharmacogenetic prediction of cognitive effects remains unexamined.

Only a few small studies have been conducted for first-line treatments such as risperidone and olanzapine *(76–80)*, and, to our knowledge, none for aripiprazole or ziprasidone. All studies have employed the candidate gene approach, examining one or a few SNPs primarily derived from genes encoding dopamine (*DRD2, DRD3*) or serotonin receptors (usually *HTR2A* and *HTR2C*); we will review these studies briefly below.

3.1 Dopamine Receptor Genes

Dopamine D_2 receptor blockade is a property of all known antipsychotics, as demonstrated in vitro *(81)* and in vivo *(82)*, yet a predictive relationship between variation in the *DRD2* gene (chromosome 11q22) and treatment response has not been firmly established. Most pharmacogenetic studies to date have examined the 3′ Taq1A polymorphism (rs1800497), which more recently has been determined to be a nonsynonymous coding SNP in a neighboring ankyrin repeat gene (ANKK1) *(83)*. Possibly due to linkage disequilibrium with another site within *DRD2*, the minor allele at rs1800497 has been associated with a 40% reduction in striatal D_2 receptor density based on in vivo imaging studies *(84)*. Carriers of the minor (A1) allele at this SNP have demonstrated enhanced antipsychotic efficacy, at least for positive symptoms, in three studies of first-generation antipsychotics *(85–87)*. However, opposite results were reported in African-American patients in one study of clozapine response *(88)*. This discrepancy may be due to different haplotypic structures observed across ethnicities, differing effects of clozapine and conventional neuroleptics, or ascertainment effects in the selection of treatment-refractory candidates for clozapine treatment. Consistent with the reports of enhanced efficacy for A1 carriers, several studies have also demonstrated increased sensitivity of A1 carriers to side effects associated with D_2 blockade, specifically prolactin elevation and extrapyramidal symptoms *(85, 89–92)*.

While these studies provide compelling evidence that A1 carriers may be more sensitive to both positive and negative effects of conventional antipsychotics, it is important to note that all of these studies were conducted in chronic patients with substantial prior exposure to antipsychotic medication. Both animal and human studies have demonstrated significant D_2 receptor upregulation subsequent to long-term administration of antipsychotics *(93, 94)*. It is therefore interesting that one study of antipsychotic-naïve first-episode patients demonstrated no effect of this polymorphism on treatment response *(78)*.

Beyond Taq1A, three functional missense polymorphisms have been identified within the *DRD2* coding region; while these are insufficiently common to have clinically useful predictive value *(95)*, one study suggests that carriers of the Cys allele at rs1801028 (Ser311Cys) demonstrated enhanced symptom response to risperidone *(79)*. On the other hand, SNPs in the 5' promoter region are likely candidates for alteration of transcriptional activity; there is evidence that alterations in this region may regulate *DRD2* expression through alteration of DNA methylation *(96)*.

To date, only two promoter region SNPs have been studied in *DRD2 (97)*: a substitution of guanine for adenine at position –241 (A-241G, rs1799978), and a deletion of cytosine at position –141 (–141C Ins/Del, rs1799732). Moreover, –141C Ins/Del has been found to alter gene expression in vitro, with the less common Del variant related to reduced transcription as well as reduced binding potential in postmortem cases. However, prior studies of chronically treated patients have not detected a relationship between these promoter variants and antipsychotic response *(88, 98, 99)*, and in vivo examination of receptor binding using PET imaging has demonstrated a puzzling *increase* in receptor density in -141C deletion carriers *(100)*.

In the first North American study of pharmacogenetics in first-episode schizophrenia, we reported that two SNPs in the promoter region of the D_2 receptor gene (*DRD2*) predicted positive symptom response to two first-line atypical antipsychotics *(101)*. First-episode patients were genotyped for two polymorphisms in the *DRD2* promoter region (A-241G and –141C Ins/Del) and treated for 16 weeks in a randomized trial of risperidone vs. olanzapine. Time until sustained response (two consecutive ratings without significant positive symptoms) for rare allele carriers vs. wildtypes was examined using Kaplan-Meier curves. Compared to wildtype homozygotes, -241G carriers showed significantly faster time until response ($p = .0038$); -141C Del carriers showed significantly longer time to respond ($p = 0.025$). The two SNPs were only weakly associated ($r^2 = 0.068$). Subjects possessing at least one G allele in their diplotype (N = 13) showed relatively high rates of sustained response (83% met criteria within 16 weeks). Subjects with the A-Ins/A-Ins diplotype (N = 21) were intermediate in their response rate (52%), and subjects whose diplotype contained at least one copy of the Del allele but zero copies of G (N = 27) were least likely to respond (30%) ($\chi^2 = 10.7$, df = 2, $p = 0.002$). Kaplan-Meier survival analysis performed on these three groups was significant (log-rank $\chi^2 = 11.4$, df = 2, $p < 0.004$, Figure 17.2).

To our knowledge, this is the first genetic study in schizophrenia examining time course of response, an important clinical parameter *(102)*. Moreover, this study demonstrates several potential strengths of our approach: 1) use of first-episode patients eliminated confounds of prior treatment, which could result in dopamine receptor upregulation *(94)*, potentially masking subtle genetic effects on dopamine receptor availability *(100)*; 2) use of a single, reliable rater team can substantially reduce noise related to phenotypic measurement error, thereby reducing sample size requirements *(103)*; and 3) all patients were recruited from a single geographic region, and treated by a unified team, reducing heterogeneity in application of the treatment algorithm. However, it should be noted that the opposite allele (–241A) was associated with improved response to risperidone in a study of previously treated Chinese patients *(77)*.

Like the D_2 receptor, the dopamine D_3 receptor is also selectively expressed in the basal ganglia and is considered to be a target of antipsychotic action *(104)*; consequently, several pharmacogenetic studies in schizophrenia have examined the *DRD3* gene, located on chromosome 3q13.3. To date, only one functional SNP (rs6280), a missense variant resulting in a Ser to Gly substitution at amino acid position 9, has been identified in *DRD3*. The Gly variant appears to represent an

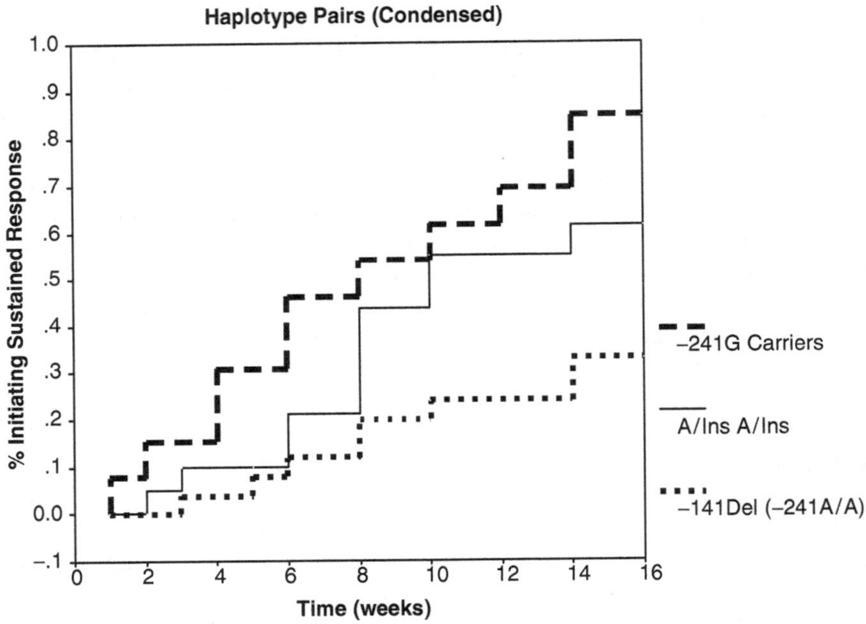

Fig. 17.2 Percentage of first-episode schizophrenia patients initiating a sustained response to risperidone or olanzapine, presented as a function of two polymorphisms in the *DRD2* promoter region (Subjects carrying the G allele at A-241G demonstrated the shortest time until response. By contrast, subjects carrying the deletion allele at -141C, in the absence of -241G, demonstrated the lowest (and slowest) response. For more details, see Lencz et al., 2006 *(101)*

unusual gain of function, in that it has been associated with fourfold greater dopamine binding affinity in vitro *(105)*, resulting in an increased dopamine-mediated cAMP response and a prolonged mitogen-associated protein kinase (MAPK) signal *(106)*. Several studies have indicated that subjects carrying the Gly variant exhibit enhanced symptom response to treatment with clozapine *(107, 108*; but see *109)* or risperidone *(78, 110, 111*; but see *76)*.

Concordant with the finding of heightened dopaminergic sensitivity for the Gly allele, multiple studies have demonstrated a significant increase in risk for tardive dyskinesia (TD) amongst Gly carriers *(112–114)*. Despite several failures to replicate, a recent meta-analysis *(115)* indicates that this effect is statistically significant across a large pooled sample, including patients of multiple ethnicities (12 individual samples, n = 695 with TD vs n = 915 without TD), although the effect size is modest (OR = 1.17) and evidence of a publication bias was detected. Consistent with these results, Eichammer et al. *(116)* reported increased incidence of akathisia amongst Gly carriers; however, two studies of extrapyramidal symptoms have been negative *(89, 117)*. Intriguingly, a recent study indicates a strong association of the Gly allele with familial essential tremor, the most common inherited movement disorder *(106)*. Additional studies with larger samples and more comprehensive genotyping *(76)* of this 50kb gene are needed.

3.2 Serotonin Receptor Genes

One of the common features of second generation antipsychotics is near-saturation binding of serotonin 5-HT_2 receptors, confirmed in vivo using PET imaging *(118, 119)*. This feature, which is less common amongst first-generation antipsychotics, may account for the increased liability to weight gain observed in the newer agents *(120)*. A survey of the literature of the regulation of feeding behavior points to a major role for serotonin, with both animal and human investigations showing, in general, that increasing serotonin results in decreased feeding, with the reverse also true. Pharmacologic agonists of 5-HT_{2C} lead to decreased feeding in animals *(121)*; it is logical to speculate that 5-HT_{2C} antagonists, including most second generation antipsychotics, might lead to increased food intake.

Perhaps the best evidence for a specific role of serotonin-related genetic factors in antipsychotic–induced weight gain is provided by studies of the promoter region polymorphism, –759 T/C (rs3813929), in the *HTR2C* gene (on the X chromosome). Reynolds and colleagues *(122)* studied 123 adult drug-naïve Han Chinese SCZ patients treated primarily with risperidone or chlorpromazine. Subjects with the T allele at this locus gained significantly less weight than subjects with the C allele in short-term (6- and 10-week) treatment; none of the 27 subjects with the T allele met criteria for severe (>7%) weight gain after 6 weeks, as compared to 28% of the 96 subjects without the T allele. Two studies (123, 124) also reported an association of the T allele with reduced weight gain in a small sample of clozapine-treated patients, although this effect was only significant in males in one of the studies. Ellingrod and colleagues *(125)* reported that the T allele is associated with less weight gain in Caucasian patients treated with olanzapine, and Templeman et al. *(126)* reported the same for weight gain associated with a mixed group of antipsychotics in a small Spanish first-episode cohort. Recently, Lane et al. *(127)* extended these findings to include risperidone (in 123 Han Chinese inpatients), and Ryu et al. *(128)* demonstrated the same effect for the T allele in 84 Korean inpatients treated on various antipsychotic monotherapies. A few studies, however, have not detected significant associations between –759 T/C and clozapine-induced weight gain *(129–131)*, but these studies were restricted to chronic patients with extensive prior treatment. Few pharmacogenetic studies have examined haplotypes within this large (>325kb) gene; in a cross-sectional study of 127 Caucasian patients taking antipsychotics, Mulder et al. *(132)* demonstrated an association between current obesity and a haplotype that included the T allele at position –759.

Surprisingly, the –759C/T variant has not been well-studied for effects on symptomatic response to antipsychotics, and studies examining other *HTR2C* variants in treatment response have been small and have yielded largely negative results *(133, 134)*. By contrast, several studies have reported associations between variants at *HTR2A* and antipsychotic response. In one of the earliest psychiatric pharmacogenetic studies, Arranz and colleagues *(135)* reported an association between the *HTR2A* T102C polymorphism and response to clozapine in a cohort of 149 patients with chronic schizophrenia who were retrospectively assessed with the Global Assessment Scale. Decreased likelihood of response to clozapine was associated with the C allele; recalling that the 102C allele is a perfect marker for the low activity G allele at rs6311, these results are in the opposite direction relative to the effects of the same allele on antidepressant response. This observation is congruent with the fact that antipsychotics have antagonistic effects at serotonin receptors, whereas antidepressants are designed to enhance serotonergic tone.

While these data were not replicated in a series of smaller, prospective clozapine studies from independent laboratories *(136)*, a meta-analysis of clozapine pharmacogenetic studies of 5-HT2A T102C revealed an excess of the 102C allele in clozapine nonresponders in each data set, with a significant effect of this variant on clozapine response in the combined sample *(137)*. Several more recent studies have also demonstrated a relationship between this SNP (or its counterpart, A-1438G) and response to various antipsychotics, including first-generation (typical) antispychotics *(138, 139)* and olanzapine *(140)* in Caucasian patients. While these studies generally converge to indicate a modestly deleterious effect of the C allele on symptom response, this same allele has been associated with modestly *increased* risk for tardive dyskinesia. In a recent meta-analysis, Lerer et al. *(141)* reported an odds ratio of about 1.6 for C allele carriers across 6 studies; effects were strongest in older patients (age > 47 years), and were specifically associated with limb-truncal (but not oro-facial) TD.

It should be noted that two studies in Asian patients taking risperidone *(79, 142)* demonstrated significant associations to symptom response in the opposite direction (C allele associated with better response). Whether this discrepancy is a function of ethnic difference in allelic frequency, choice of antipsychotics, history of TD, or other sample ascertainment characteristics remains unclear. Notably, both of these risperidone studies indicated improvement in general and/or negative symptoms, rather than positive symptoms per se. Relatedly, a few recent studies suggest that the effect of negative symptom response (or lack thereof) may play a role in interpretation of serotonin receptor studies in schizophrenia *(143–145)*.

4 Future Directions

4.1 Expanding Genotypes and Phenotypes

To date, the majority of pharmacogenetic studies in psychiatry have been limited to a few receptor-coding and neurotransmitter transporter genes. However, it is increasingly acknowledged that neurotransmitter signaling pathways are complex, with multiple potential regulatory bottlenecks *(146)*. For example, Xu et al. *(147)* interrogated the Kyoto Encyclopedia of Genes and Genomes (KEGG) database and identified 57 genes in the dopamine metabolic pathway alone; using multilocus data analytic techniques, three genotype combinations were found to increase susceptibility to schizophrenia. There are also numerous neurodevelopmental genes involved in the regulation of the dopaminergic system *(148)* and other CNS components.

Moreover, basic pharmacology research has placed attention on glutamatergic regulation *(149)*, as well as candidate genes that relate to more basic processes such as vesicular trafficking *(150)*.

Thus, candidate gene approaches to pharmacogenetics run a dual risk of either an overly restrictive search space, or a potentially overwhelming number of candidates. While initial pharmacogenetic studies have examined various genes in the broader pathways, the slow pace of individual candidate gene investigations has resulted in an appearance of scattered and isolated studies across investigators. On the other hand, the advent of whole genome association (WGA) technology *(151)* provides a hypothesis-free method of generating candidate genes for novel complex phenotypes; but this method carries statistical concerns, most notably limitations in statistical power (due to correction for multiple comparisons) in necessarily limited clinical trial samples. In our work on schizophrenia at the Zucker Hillside Hospital, we have therefore recently initiated a two-stage approach to address this problem. In the first stage, we use WGA to comprehensively genotype large numbers of patients with schizophrenia, characterized for treatment response and side effects history retrospectively and/or cross-sectionally. While such measures are necessarily limited, the reliability and validity of such measures is enhanced by the availability (with informed consent from the patient) of extensive inpatient and outpatient case records (mean treatment history of 13.52 +/– 8.91 years). Moreover, as noted above, a cross-sectional study of current obesity in 127 Caucasian patients taking antipsychotics demonstrated an association to the *HTR2C* –759T allele *(132)*; this finding supports an approach in which current patient phenotypes are considered reflective of historical treatment outcomes. Nevertheless, we seek to validate candidate genes/SNPs identified by WGA in a second-stage analysis: our ongoing, prospective controlled trials in antipsychotic-naïve first-episode patients *(101, 152)*.

In a proof-of-principle study, we have recently utilized the Affymetrix 500K microarray in several hundred of our retrospectively characterized patients with schizophrenia (and matched healthy controls). Initial analyses were published for data obtained from the first 322 Caucasian subjects (patient n = 178; control n = 144; ref. 153), demonstrating call rates in excess of 97% and call reproducibility in excess of 99%. All subjects self-identified as Caucasian non-Hispanic; testing of 210 ancestry informative markers (AIMs) revealed no evidence of population stratification, demonstrating an additional strength of our single-site recruitment strategy. Despite the relatively small sample, one SNP, rs4129148 (in pseudoautosomal region 1) demonstrated an association beyond the genomewide threshold ($p = 3.7*10^{-7}$). Homozygosity for the common allele at this SNP was significantly associated with SCZ (59% vs 31% of controls; OR = 3.23; 95% CI = 2.04–5.15). In an independent sample, we examined sequencing data from 71 Caucasian patients and 31 controls for two cytokine receptor genes (*CSF2RA* and *IL3RA*) neighboring this SNP. We identified 7 novel, rare missense mutations; 15 amino acid substitutions were detected in the cases, with only 1 detected in the controls (Fisher's exact p = 0.031). Additionally, 2 haplotype blocks composed of common SNPs were significantly associated with SCZ, yielding converging evidence for this novel susceptibility locus.

In this same sample, we have performed a preliminary analysis examining treatment responsiveness, using clozapine assignment as a proxy for poor response. Detailed chart reviews permitted classification of 97% of the sample. Approximately 35% of patients were assigned clozapine due to treatment nonresponsiveness, and groups were matched on key demographic variables including age, duration of illness, sex, and family history. Despite the small sample for this interim analysis, one SNP nearly obtained genomewide significance ($p = 4.3*10^{-7}$); this SNP neighbors the promoter region of a critical neuronal cell adhesion gene.

Initial examination of lifetime symptom data and cross-sectional cognitive data have also revealed a number of interesting potential targets. Notably, in previous candidate gene studies in our sample, we have accumulated increasing evidence that susceptibility genes for SCZ, including *DTNBP1* and *DISC1*, are associated with specific symptom and cognitive profiles *(154–159)*. A broader range of treatment outcomes (including persistent negative symptoms, cognitive impairment, and long-term functional disability) are often more important to psychiatric patients and their families than short-term response as measured by symptom rating scales. Thus, examination of these phenotypes will be critical for the next generation of pharmacogenetic studies in order to maximize both mechanistic clarity and clinical relevance, and to help clarify results. For example, Reynolds et al. *(78)* reported a double dissociation in which a SNP in *DRD3* predicted positive symptom response, while a SNP in *HTR2C* predicted negative symptom response over 10 weeks in 117 Han Chinese first-episode patients. However, treatment in that study was uncontrolled and variable, including a mixture of first-generation and second-generation antipsychotics.

4.2 Clinical Prediction and Personalized Medicine

The studies reviewed in this chapter begin to indicate the clinical utility for pharmacogenetic testing in psychiatry. For example, carriers of low-activity alleles at *SLC6A4* appear to be less likely to achieve symptomatic response to SSRIs, yet also have an increased side effects burden. However, three factors limit the ability of the field to deliver on the promise of personalized medicine at this time, and point to critical issues for the next generation of pharmacogenetic studies. First, a treating psychiatrist would be unable to use this information to offer a validated alternative, due to the lack of pharmacogenetic head-to-head comparisons of treatments with differing mechanisms. Second, even fairly consistent single-gene results, such as those observed for *SLC6A4*, are unlikely to provide large effect sizes. In order to provide a clinically useful test, with sufficient sensitivity and specificity to make confident individual predictions, a combination of SNPs across different loci will be required. In one of the few studies designed in this manner, Arranz and colleagues *(160)* created an index with 77% predictive accuracy for response to clozapine, but this index has not been replicated. The addition of pharmacokinetic markers, which have begun to provide replicable (and face valid) relationships to treatment-related phenotypes *(161)*, will likely enhance any such panel. Finally, the economics of conducting pharmacogenetic tests on a large clinical scale will need to be justified to payers, including the insurance companies and the federal government. In order to do so, pharmacogenetics researchers will need to quantify the beneficial economic impact of tailored prescription practices *(162)*.

References

1. Kane JM. Schizophrenia. New Engl J Med 1996 Jan 4;334*(1)*:34–41.
2. Rush AJ, Fava M, Wisniewski SR, Lavori PW, Trivedi MH, Sackeim HA, Thase ME, Nierenberg AA, Quitkin FM, Kashner TM, Kupfer DJ, Rosenbaum JF, Alpert J, Stewart JW, McGrath PJ, Biggs MM, Shores-Wilson K, Lebowitz BD, Ritz L, Niederehe G; STAR*D Investigators Group. Sequenced treatment alternatives to relieve depression (STAR*D): rationale and design. Control Clin Trials. 2004 Feb;25(1):119–42.
3. Robinson D, Woerner MG, Alvir JM, Bilder R, Goldman R, Geisler S, Koreen A, Sheitman B, Chakos M, Mayerhoff D, Lieberman JA. Predictors of relapse following response from a first episode of schizophrenia or schizoaffective disorder. Arch Gen Psychiatry. 1999 Mar; 56(3):241–7.
4. Hasin DS, Goodwin RD, Stinson FS, Grant BF. Epidemiology of major depressive disorder: results from the National Epidemiologic Survey on Alcoholism and Related Conditions. Arch Gen Psychiatry. 2005 Oct;62(10):1097–106.
5. Kessler RC, Berglund P, Demler O, Jin R, Koretz D, Merikangas KR, Rush AJ, Walters EE, Wang PS; National Comorbidity Survey Replication. The epidemiology of major depressive disorder: results from the National Comorbidity Survey Replication (NCS-R). JAMA. 2003 Jun 18;289(23):3095–105.
6. Weissman MM, Bland RC, Canino GJ, Faravelli C, Greenwald S, Hwu HG, Joyce PR, Karam EG, Lee CK, Lellouch J, Lepine JP, Newman SC, Rubio-Stipec M, Wells JE, Wickramaratne PJ, Wittchen H, Yeh EK. Cross-national epidemiology of major depression and bipolar disorder. JAMA. 1996 Jul 24–31;276(4):293–9.
7. Blier P, Keller MB, Pollack MH, Thase ME, Zajecka JM, Dunner DL. Preventing recurrent depression: long-term treatment for major depressive disorder. J Clin Psychiatry. 2007 Mar;68(3):e06.
8. Kennedy N, Abbott R, Paykel ES. Remission and recurrence of depression in the maintenance era: long-term outcome in a Cambridge cohort. Psychol Med. 2003 Jul;33(5):827–38.
9. Murray CJ, Lopez AD. Evidence-based health policy—lessons from the Global Burden of Disease Study. Science. 1996 Nov 1;274(5288):740–3.
10. Angst J, Angst F, Stassen HH. Suicide risk in patients with major depressive disorder. Journal of Clinical Psychiatry 1999; 60(supp. 2), 57–62.
11. Insel TR, Charney DS. Research on major depression:strategies and priorities. JAMA, 2003 Jun 18;289(23):3167–8.
12. Trivedi MH, Rush AJ, Wisniewski SR, Nierenberg AA, Warden D, Ritz L, Norquist G, Howland RH, Lebowitz B, McGrath PJ, Shores-Wilson K, Biggs MM, Balasubramani GK, Fava M; STAR*D Study Team. Evaluation of outcomes with citalopram for depression using measurement-based care in STAR*D: implications for clinical practice.Am J Psychiatry. 2006 Jan;163(1):28–40.
13. Judd LL, Akiskal HS, Zeller PJ, Paulus M, Leon AC, Maser JD, Endicott J, Coryell W, Kunovac JL, Mueller TI, Rice JP, Keller MB. Psychosocial disability during the long-term course of unipolar major depressive disorder. Arch Gen Psychiatry. 2000 Apr;57(4):375–80.
14. Heils A, Teufel A, Petri S, Stober G, Riederer P, Bengel D, Lesch KP. Allelic variation of human serotonin transporter gene expression. J Neurochem. 1996 Jun;66(6):2621–4.

15. Lesch KP, Bengel D, Heils A, Sabol SZ, Greenberg BD, Petri S, Benjamin J, Muller CR, Hamer DH, Murphy DL. Association of anxiety-related traits with a polymorphism in the serotonin transporter gene regulatory region. Science. 1996 Nov 9;274(5292):1527–31.
16. Caspi A, Sugden K, Moffitt TE, Taylor A, Craig IW, Harrington H, McClay J, Mill J, Martin J, Braithwaite A, Poulton R. Influence of life stress on depression: moderation by a polymorphism in the 5-HTT gene. Science. 2003 Jul 18;301(5631):386–9.
17. Levinson DF. The genetics of depression: a review. Biol Psychiatry. 2006 Jul 15;60(2): 84–92.
18. Smeraldi E, Zanardi R, Benedetti F, DiBella D, Perez J, Catalano M. Polymorphism within the promoter of the serotonin transporter gene and antidepressant efficacy of fluvoxamine. Mol Psychiatry. 1998 Nov;3(6):508–11.
19. Serretti A, Kato M, De Ronchi D, Kinoshita T. Meta-analysis of serotonin transporter gene promoter polymorphism (5-HTTLPR) association with selective serotonin reuptake inhibitor efficacy in depressed patients. Mol Psychiatry. 2007 Mar;12(3):247–57.
20. Murphy GM Jr, Hollander SB, Rodrigues HE, Kremer C, Schatzberg AF. Effects of the serotonin transporter gene promoter polymorphism on mirtazapine and paroxetine efficacy and adverse events in geriatric major depression. Arch Gen Psychiatry. 2004 Nov;61(11):1163–9.
21. Popp J, Leucht S, Heres S, Steiner W. Serotonin transporter polymorphisms and side effects in antidepressant therapy—a pilot study. Pharmacogenomics. 2006 Mar;7(2):159–66.
22. Smits K, Smits L, Peeters F, Schouten J, Janssen R, Smeets H, van Os J, Prins M. Serotonin transporter polymorphisms and the occurrence of adverse events during treatment with selective serotonin reuptake inhibitors. Int Clin Psychopharmacol. 2007 May;22(3):137–43.
23. Hu X-Z, Rush AJ, Charney D, Wilson AF, Sorant AJM, Papinacaolou GJ, Fava M, Trivedi MH, Wisniewski SR, Laje G, Paddock S, McMahon FJ, Manji H, Lipsky RH. Association between a functional serotonin transporter promoter polymorphism and citalopram treatment in adult outpatients with major depression. Arch Gen Psychiatry 2007 Jul;64(7):783–792.
24. Mundo E, Walker M, Cate T, Macciardi F, Kennedy JL. The role of serotonin transporter protein gene in antidepressant-induced mania in bipolar disorder: preliminary findings. Arch Gen Psychiatry. 2001 Jun;58(6):539–44.
25. Masoliver E, Menoyo A, Perez V, Volpini V, Rio ED, Perez J, Alvarez E, Baiget M. Serotonin transporter linked promoter (polymorphism) in the serotonin transporter gene may be associated with antidepressant-induced mania in bipolar disorder. Psychiatr Genet 2006 Feb:16(1):25–9.
26. Serretti A, Artioli P, Zanardi R, Lorenzi C, Rossini D, Cusin C, Arnoldi A, Catalano M. Genetic features of antidepressant induced mania and hypo-mania in bipolar disorder. Psychopharmacology (Berl). 2004 Aug;174(4):504–11.
27. Baumer FM, Howe M, Gallelli K, Simeonova DI, Hallmayer J, Chang KD. A pilot study of antidepressant-induced mania in pediatric bipolar disorder: Characteristics, risk factors, and the serotonin transporter gene. Biol Psychiatry. 2006 Nov 1;60(9):1005–12.
28. Rousseva A, Henry C, van den Bulke D, Fournier G, Laplanche JL, Leboyer M, Bellivier F, Aubry JM, Baud P, Boucherie M, Buresi C, Ferrero F, Malafosse A. Antidepressant-induced mania, rapid cycling and the serotonin transporter gene polymorphism. Pharmacogenomics J. 2003;3(2):101–4.
29. Perlis RH, Mischoulon D, Smoller JW, Wan YJ, Lamon-Fava S, Lin KM, Rosenbaum JF, Fava M. Serotonin transporter polymorphisms and adverse effects with fluoxetine treatment. Biol Psychiatry 2003 Nov 1;54(9):879–83.
30. Li D, He L. Meta-analysis supports association between serotonin transporter (5-HTT) and suicidal behavior. Mol Psychiatry. 2007 Jan;12(1):47–54.
31. Kato M, Ikenaga Y, Wakeno M, Okugawa G, Nobuhara K, Fukuda T, Fukuda K, Azuma J, Kinoshita T. Controlled clinical comparison of paroxetine and fluvoxamine considering the serotonin transporter promoter polymorphism. Int Clin Psychopharmacol. 2005 May;20(3):151–6.
32. Rush AJ, Trivedi MH, Wisniewski SR, Stewart JW, Nierenberg AA, Thase ME, Ritz L, Biggs MM< Warden D, Luther JF, Shores-Wilson K, Niederehe G, Fava M; STAR*D Study Team.

Bupropion-SR, sertraline, or venlafaxine-XR after failure of SSRIs for depression. N Engl J Med. 2006 Mar 23;354(12):1231–42.
33. Trivedi MH, Fava M, Wisniewski SR, Thase ME, Quitkin F, Warden D, Ritz L, Nierenberg AA, Lebowitz, BD, Biggs MM, Luther JF, Shores-Wilson K, Rush AJ, STAR*D Study Team. Medication augmentation after the failure of SSRIs for depression. N Engl J Med. 2006 Mar 23;354(12):1243–52.
34. Kraft JB, Peters EJ, Slager SL, Jenkins GD, Reinalda MS, McGrath PJ, Hamilton SP. Analysis of association between the serotonin transporter and antidepressant response in a large clinical sample. Biol Psychiatry 2007 Mar 15;61(6):734–42.
35. Kim H, Lim SW, Kim S, Kim JW, Chang YH, Carroll BJ, Kim DK. Monoamine transporter gene polymorphisms and antidepressant response in Koreans with late-life depression. JAMA. 2006 Oct 4;296(13):1609–18.
36. Kim DK, Lim SW, Lee S, Sohn SE, Kim S, Hahn CG, Carroll BJ. Serotonin transporter gene polymorphism and antidepressant response. Neuroreport. 2000 Jan 17;11(1):215–9.
37. Yoshida K, Ito K, Sato K, Takahashi H, Kamata M, Higuchi H, Shimizu T, Itoh K, Inoue K, Tezuka T, Suzuki T, Ohkubo T, Sugawara K, Otani K. Influence of the serotonin transporter gene-linked polymorphic region on the antidepressant response to fluvoxamine in Japanese depressed patients. Prog Neuropsychopharmacol Biol Psychiatry. 2002 Feb;26(2):383–6.
38. Kato M, Fukada T, Wakeno M, Fukada K, Okugawa G, Ikenaga Y, Yamashita M, Takekita Y, Nobuhara K, Azuma J, Kinoshita T. Effects of the serotonin type 2A, 3A and 3B receptor and the serotonin transporter genes on paroxetine and fluvoxamine efficacy and adverse drug reactions in depressed Japanese patients. Neuropsychobiology. 2006;53(4):186–95.
39. International HapMap Consortium A haplotype map of the human genome. Nature. 2005 Oct 27; 437(7063):1299–320.
40. Nakamura M, Ueno S, Sano A, Tanabe H. The human serotonin transporter gene linked polymorphism (5-HTTLPR) shows ten novel allelic variants. Mol Psychiatry. 2000 Jan;5(1):32–8.
41. Zalsman G, Huang YY, Oquendo MA, Burke AK, Hu XZ, Brent DA, Ellis SP, Goldman D, Mann JJ. Association of a triallelic serotonin transporter gene promoter region (5-HTTLPR) polymorphism with stressful life events and severity of depression. Am J Psychiatry. 2006 Sep;163(9):1588–93.
42. Smeraldi E, Serretti A, Artioli P, Lorenzi C, Catalano M. Serotonin transporter gene-linked polymorphic region: possible pharmacogenetic implications of rare variants.Psychiatr Genet. 2006 Aug;16(4):153–8.
43. Peters EJ, Slager SL, McGrath PJ, Knowles JA, Hamilton SP. Investigation of serotonin-related genes in antidepressant response. Mol Psychiatry. 2004 Sep;9(9):879–89.
44. Kraft JB, Slager SL, McGrath PJ, Hamilton SP. Sequence analysis of the serotonin transporter and associations with antidepressant response. Biol Psychiatry. 2005 Sep 1;58(5):374–81.
45. Myers RL, Airey DC, Manier DH, Shelton RC, Sanders-Bush E. Polymorphisms in the regulatory region of the human serotonin 5-HT2A receptor gene (HTR2A) influence gene expression. Biol Psychiatry. 2007 Jan 15;61(2):167–73. Epub 2006 May 12.
46. Parsons MJ, D'Souza UM, Arranz MJ, Kerwin RW, Makoff AJ. The -1438A/G polymorphism in the 5-hydroxytryptamine type 2A receptor gene affects promoter activity. Biol Psychiatry 2004;56(6):406–10.
47. Choi MJ, Kang RH, Ham BJ, Jeong HY, Lee MS. Serotonin receptor 2A gene polymorphism (-1438A/G) and short-term treatment response to citalopram. Neuropsychobiology. 2005;52(3):155–62. Epub 2005 Aug 25.
48. Minov C, Baghai TC, Schule C, Zwanzger P, Schwarz MH, Zill P, Rupprecht R, Bondy B. Serotonin-2A-receptor and -transporter polymorphisms: lack of association in patients with major depression. Neurosci Lett 2001;303(2):119–22.
49. Bishop JR, Moline J, Ellingrod VL, Schultz SK, Clayton AH. Serotonin 2A -1438 G/A and G-protein Beta3 subunit C825T polymorphisms in patients with depression and SSRI-associated sexual side-effects. Neuropsychopharmacol 2006;(10):2281–8.

50. Suzuki Y, Sawamura K, Someya T. Polymorphisms in the 5-hydroxytryptamine 2A receptor and cytochrome P450 2D6 genes synergistically predict fluvoxamine-induced side effects in Japanese depressed patients. Neuropsychopharmacol 2006;(4):825–31.
51. Sato K, Yoshida K, Takahashi H, Ito K, Kamata M, Higuchi H, Shimizu T, Itoh K, Inoue K, Tezuka T, Suzuki T, Ohkubo T, Sugawara K, Otani K. Association between -1438G/A promoter polymorphism in the 5-HT(2A) receptor gene and fluvoxamine response in Japanese patients with major depressive disorder. Neuropsychobiology 2002;46(3):136–40.
52. McMahon FJ, Buervenich S, Charney D, Lipsky R, Rush AJ, Wilson AF, Sorant AJ, Papanicolaou GJ, Laje G, Fava M, Trivedi MH, Wisniewski SR, Manji H. Variation in the gene encoding the serotonin 2A receptor is associated with outcome of antidepressant treatment. Am J Hum Genet 2006;78(5):804–14.
53. Cusin C, Serretti A, Zanardi R, Lattuada E, Rossini D, Lilli R, Lorenzi C, Smeraldi E. Influence of monoamine oxidase A and serotonin receptor 2A polymorphisms in SSRI antidepressant activity. Int J Neuropsychopharmacol 2002;5(1):27–35.
54. Lemonde S, Du L, Bakish D, Hrdina P, Albert PR. Association of the C(-1019)G 5-HT1A functional promoter polymorphism with antidepressant response. Int J Neuropsychopharmacol 2004;7(4):381–5.
55. Parsey RV, Olvet DM, Oguendo MA, Huang YY, Ogden RT, Mann JJ. Higher 5-HT1A receptor binding potential during a major depressive episode predicts poor treatment response: preliminary data from a naturalistic study. Neuropsychopharmacol 2006;31(8):1745–9.
56. Hong CJ, Chen TJ, Yu YW, Tsai SJ. Response to fluoxetine and serotonin 1A receptor (C-1019G) polymorphism in Taiwan Chinese major depressive disorder. Pharmacogenomics J 2006;6(1):27–33.
57. Yu YW, Tsai SJ, Liou YJ, Hong CJ, Chen TJ. Association study of two serotonin 1A receptor gene polymorphisms and fluoxetine treatment response in Chinese major depressive disorders. Eur Neuropsychopharmacol 2006;16(7):498–503.
58. Serretti A, Artioli P, Lorenzi C, Pirovano A, Tubazio V, Zanardi R. The C(-1019)G polymorphism of the 5-HT1A gene promoter and antidepressant response in mood disorders: preliminary findings. Int J Neuropsychopharmacol. 2004 Dec;7(4):453–60.
59. Suzuki Y, Sawamura K, Someya T. The effects of a 5-hydroxytryptamine 1A receptor gene polymorphism on the clinical response to fluvoxamine in depressed patients. Pharmacogenomics J 2004;4(4):283–6.
60. Serretti A, Zanardi R, Cusin C, Rossini D, Lorenzi C, Smeraldi E. Tryptophan hydroxylase gene associated with paroxetine antidepressant activity. Eur Neuropsychopharmacol 2001; 11(5):375–80.
61. Ham BJ, Lee BC, Paik JW, Kang RH, Choi MJ, Choi IG, Lee MS. Association between the tryptophan hydroxylase-1 gene A218C polymorphism and citalopram antidepressant response in a Korean population. Prog Neuropsychopharmacol Biol Psychiatry 2007;31(1):104–7.
62. Ham BJ, Lee MS, Lee HJ, Kang RH, Han CS, Choi MJ, Lee SH, Ryu SH. No association between the tryptophan hydroxylase gene polymorphism and major depressive disorders and antidepressant response in a Korean population. Psychiatr Genet 2005;15(4):299–301.
63. Saha S, Chant D, Welham J, McGrath J. A systematic review of the prevalence of schizophrenia. PLoS Med 2005;2(5):e141.
64. Moller HJ, Schmid-Bode W, Cording-Tommel C, Wittchen HU, Zaudig M, von Zerssen D. Psychopathological and social outcome in schizophrenia versus affective/schizoaffective psychoses and prediction of poor outcome in schizophrenia. Results from a 5–8 year follow-up. Acta Psychiatr Scand 1988;77(4):379–89.
65. Harrow M, Sands JR, Silverstein ML, Goldberg JF. Course and outcome for schizophrenia versus other psychotic patients: a longitudinal study. Schizophr Bull 1997;23(2):287–303.
66. Hall W, Goldstein G, Andrews G, Lapsley H, Bartels R, Silove D. Estimating the economic costs of schizophrenia. Schizophr Bull 1985;11(4):598–610.
67. Wyatt RJ, Henter I, Leary MC, Taylor E. An economic evaluation of schizophrenia—1991. Soc Psychiatry Psychiatr Epidemiol 1995;30(5):196–205.

68. Wu EQ, Birnbaum HG, Shi L, Ball DE, Kessler RC, Moulis M, Aggarwal J. The economic burden of schizophrenia in the United States in 2002. J Clin Psychiatry 2005;66(9):1122–9.
69. Laursen TM, Munk-Olsen T, Nordentoft M, Mortensen PB. Increased mortality among patients admitted with major psychiatric disorders: a register-based study comparing mortality in unipolar depressive disorder, bipolar affective disorder, schizoaffective disorder, and schizophrenia. J Clin Psychiatry 2007;68(6):899–907.
70. Palmer BA, Pankratz VS, Bostwick JM. The lifetime risk of suicide in schizophrenia: a reexamination. Arch Gen Psychiatry 2005;62(3):247–53.
71. Lieberman JA, Stroup TS, McEvoy JP, Swartz MS, Rosenheck RA, Perkins DO, Keefe RS, Davis SM, Davis CE, Lebowitz BD, Severe J, Hsiao JK; Clinical Antipsychotic Trials of Intervention Effectiveness (CATIE) Investigators. Effectiveness of antipsychotic drugs in patients with chronic schizophrenia. N Engl J Med 2005;353(12):1209–23.
72. Conley RR, Kelly DL. Management of treatment resistance in schizophrenia. Biol Psychiatry 2001;50(11):898–911.
73. Buckley PF, Stahl SM. Pharmacological treatment of negative symptoms of schizophrenia: therapeutic opportunity or cul-de-sac? Acta Psychiatr Scand 2007;115(2):93–100.
74. Leucht S, Busch R, Kissling W, Kane JM. Early prediction of antipsychotic nonresponse among patients with schizophrenia. J Clin Psychiatry. 2007 Mar;68(3):352–60.
75. Malhotra AK, Murphy GM, Kennedy JL. Pharmacogenetics of psychotropic drug response. Am J Psychiatry 2004;161(5):780–96.
76. Xuan J, Zhao X, He G, Yu L, Wang L, Tang W, Li X, Gu N, Feng G, Xing Q, He L. Effects of the dopamine D(3) receptor (DRD3) gene polymorphisms on risperidone response: a pharmacogenetic study. Neuropsychopharmacol 2007;[Epub ahead of print].
77. Xing Q, Qian X, Li H, Wong S, Wu S, Feng G, Duan S, Xu M, Gao R, Qin W, Gao J, Meng J, He L. The relationship between the therapeutic response to risperidone and the dopamine D2 receptor polymorphism in Chinese schizophrenia patients. Int J Neuropsychopharmacol. 2006 Nov 14:1–7 [Epub ahead of print].
78. Reynolds GP, Yao Z, Zhang X, Sun J, Zhang Z. Pharmacogenetics of treatment in first-episode schizophrenia: D3 and 5-HT2C receptor polymorphisms separately associate with positive and negative symptom response. Eur Neuropsychopharmacol 2005;15(2):143–51.
79. Lane HY, Lee CC, Chang YC, Lu CT, Huang CH, Chang WH. Effects of dopamine D2 receptor Ser311Cys polymorphism and clinical factors on risperidone efficacy for positive and negative symptoms and social function. Int J Neuropsychopharmacol 2004;7(4):461–70.
80. Lane HY, Chang YC, Chiu CC, Chen ML, Hsieh MH, Chang WH. Association of risperidone treatment response with a polymorphism in the 5-HT(2A) receptor gene. Am J Psychiatry. 2002 Sep;159(9):1593–5.
81. Seeman P, Lee T. Antipsychotic drugs: direct correlation between clinical potency and presynaptic action on dopamine neurons. Science 1975;188(4194):1217–9.
82. Kapur S, Barlow K, VanderSpek SC, Javanmard M, Nobrega JN. Drug-induced receptor occupancy: substantial differences in measurements made in vivo vs ex vivo. Psychopharmacology (Berl) 2001;157(2):168–71.
83. Neville MJ, Johnstone EC, Walton RT. Identification and characterization of ANKK1: a novel kinase gene closely linked to DRD2 on chromosome band 11q23.1. Hum Mutat. 2004 Jun;23(6):540–5.
84. Thompson J, Thomas N, Singleton A, Piggott M, Lloyd S, Perry EK, Morris CM, Perry RH, Ferrier IN, Court JA. D2 dopamine receptor gene (DRD2) Taq1A polymorphism: reduced dopamine D2 receptor binding in the human striatum associated with the A1 allele. Pharmacogenetics 1997;7(6):479–84.
85. Sakumoto N, Kondo T, Mihara K, Suzuki A, Yasui-Furukori N. Dopamine D2 receptor gene polymorphisms predict well the response to dopamine antagonists at therapeutic dosages in patients with schizophrenia. Psychiatry Clin Neurosci 2007;61(2):174–80.
86. Schafer M, Rujescu D, Giegling I, Guntermann A, Erfurth A, Bondy B, Moller HJ. Association of short-term response to haloperidol treatment with a polymorphism in the dopamine D(2) receptor gene. Am J Psychiatry. 2001 May;158(5):802–4.

87. Suzuki A, Mihara K, Kondo T, Tanaka O, Nagashima U, Otani K, Kaneko S. The relationship between dopamine D2 receptor polymorphism at the Taq1 A locus and therapeutic response to nemonapride, a selective dopamine antagonist, in schizophrenic patients. Pharmacogenetics 2000;10(4):335–41.
88. Hwang R, Shinkai T, De Luca V, Müller DJ, Ni X, Macciardi F, Potkin S, Lieberman JA, Meltzer HY, Kennedy JL. Association study of 12 polymorphisms spanning the dopamine D(2) receptor gene and clozapine treatment response in two treatment refractory/intolerant populations. Psychopharmacology (Berl) 2005;181(1):179–87.
89. Guzey C, Scordo MG, Spina E, Landsem VM, Spigset O. Antipsychotic-induced extrapyramidal symptoms in patients with schizophrenia: associations with dopamine and serotonin receptor and transporter polymorphisms. Eur J Clin Pharmacol. 2007 Mar; 63(3): 233–41.
90. Hedenmalm K, Guzey C, Dahl ML, Yue QY, Spigset O. Risk factors for extrapyramidal symptoms during treatment with selective serotonin reuptake inhibitors, including cytochrome P-450 enzyme, and serotonin and dopamine transporter and receptor polymorphisms. J Clin Psychopharmacol. 2006 Apr;26(2):192–7.
91. Young RM, Lawford BR, Barnes M, Burton SC, Ritchie T, Ward WK, Noble EP. Prolactin levels in antipsychotic treatment of patients with schizophrenia carrying the DRD2*A1 allele. Br J Psychiatry. 2004 Aug;185:147–51.
92. Mihara K, Kondo T, Suzuki A, Yasui N, Nagashima U, Ono S, Otani K, Kaneko S. Prolactin response to nemonapride, a selective antagonist for D2 like dopamine receptors, in schizophrenic patients in relation to Taq1A polymorphism of DRD2 gene. Psychopharmacology (Berl). 2000 Apr;149(3):246–50.
93. Lidow MS, Goldman-Rakic PS. Differential regulation of D2 and D4 dopamine receptor mRNAs in the primate cerebral cortex vs. neostriatum: effects of chronic treatment with typical and atypical antipsychotic drugs. J Pharmacol Exp Ther. 1997 Nov;283(2):939–46.
94. Silvestri S, Seeman MV, Negrete JC, Houle S, Shammi CM, Remington GJ, Kapur S, Zipursky RB, Wilson AA, Christensen BK, Seeman P. Increased dopamine D2 receptor binding after long-term treatment with antipsychotics in humans: a clinical PET study. Psychopharmacology (Berl). 2000 Oct;152(2):174–80.
95. Cravchik A, Sibley DR, Gejman PV. Functional analysis of the human D2 dopamine receptor missense variants. J Biol Chem. 1996 Oct 18;271(42):26013–7.
96. Popendikyte V, Laurinavicius A, Paterson AD, Macciardi F, Kennedy JL, Petronis A. DNA methylation at the putative promoter region of the human dopamine D2 receptor gene. Neuroreport. 1999 Apr 26;10(6):1249–55.
97. Arinami T, Gao M, Hamaguchi H, Toru M. A functional polymorphism in the promoter region of the dopamine D2 receptor gene is associated with schizophrenia. Hum Mol Genet. 1997 Apr;6(4):577–82.
98. Arranz MJ, Li T, Munro J, Liu X, Murray R, Collier DA, Kerwin RW. Lack of association between a polymorphism in the promoter region of the dopamine-2 receptor gene and clozapine response. Pharmacogenetics. 1998 Dec;8(6):481–4.
99. Mihara K, Kondo T, Suzuki A, Yasui N, Ono S, Otani K, Kaneko S. No relationship between--141C Ins/Del polymorphism in the promoter region of dopamine D2 receptor and extrapyramidal adverse effects of selective dopamine D2 antagonists in schizophrenic patients: a preliminary study. Psychiatry Res. 2001 Feb 14;101(1):33–8.
100. Jonsson EG, Nothen MM, Grunhage F, Farde L, Nakashima Y, Propping P, Sedvall GC. Polymorphisms in the dopamine D2 receptor gene and their relationships to striatal dopamine receptor density of healthy volunteers. Mol Psychiatry. 1999 May;4(3):290–6.
101. Lencz T, Robinson DG, Xu K, Ekholm J, Sevy S, Gunduz-Bruce H, Woerner MG, Kane JM, Goldman D, Malhotra AK. DRD2 promoter region variation as a predictor of sustained response to antipsychotic medication in first-episode schizophrenia patients. Am J Psychiatry 2006;163 (3):529–531.
102. Leucht S, Kane JM. Measurement-based psychiatry: definitions of response, remission, stability, and relapse in schizophrenia. J. Clin Psychiatry 2006;67(11):1813–1814.

103. Perkins DO, Wyatt RJ, Bartko JJ. Penny-wise and pound-foolish: the impact of measurement error on sample size requirements in clinical trials. Biol Psychiatry. 2000 Apr 15;47(8):762–6.
104. Schwartz JC, Diaz J, Pilon C, Sokoloff P. Possible implications of the dopamine D(3) receptor in schizophrenia and in antipsychotic drug actions. Brain Res Brain Res Rev 2000;31(2–3):277–287.
105. Lundstrom K, Turpin MP. Proposed schizophrenia-related gene polymorphism: expression of the Ser9Gly mutant human dopamine D3 receptor with the Semliki forest virus system. Biochem Biophys Res Commun1996; 23:225(3):1068–1072.
106. Jeanneteau F, Funalot B, Jankovic J, Deng H, Lagarde JP, Lucotte G, Sokoloff P. A functional variant of the dopamine D3 receptor is associated with risk and age-at-onset of essential tremor. Proc Natl Acad Sci USA 2006:11;103 (28):10753–10758.
107. Shaikh S, Collier DA, Sham PC, Ball D, Aitchison K, Vallada H, Smith I, Gill M, Kerwin RW. Allelic association between a Ser-9-Gly polymorphism in the dopamine D3 receptor gene and schizophrenia. Hum Genet 1996; 97(6):714–719.
108. Scharfetter J, Chaudhry HR, Hornik K, Fuchs K, Sieghart W, Kasper S, Aschauer HN. Dopamine D3 receptor gene polymorphism and response to clozapine in schizophrenic Pakastani patients. Eur Neuropsychopharmacol 1999; 10(1):17–20.
109. Malhotra AK, Goldman D, Buchanan RW, Rooney W, Clifton A, Kosmidis MH, Breier A, Pickar D. The dopamine D3 receptor (DRD3) Ser9Gly polymorphism and schizophrenia: a haplotype relative risk study and association with clozapine response. Mol Psychiatry 1998; 3(1):72–75.
110. Szekeres G, Kéri S, Juhász A, Rimanóczy A, Szendi I, Czimmer C, Janka Z. Role of dopamine D3 receptor (DRD3) and dopamine transporter (DAT) polymorphism in cognitive dysfunctions and therapeutic response to atypical antipsychotics in patients with schizophrenia. Am J Med Genet B Neuropsychiatr Genet 2004;124(1):1–5.
111. Lane HY, Hsu SK, Liu YC, Chang YC, Huang CH, Chang WH. Dopamine D3 receptor Ser9Gly polymorphism and risperidone response. J Clin Psychopharmacol. 2005 Feb;25(1):6–11.
112. Steen VM, Løvlie R, MacEwan T, McCreadie RG. Dopamine D3-receptor gene variant and susceptibility to tardive dyskinesia in schizophrenic patients. Mol Psychiatry 1997; 2(2):139–145.
113. Basile VS, Masellis M, Badri F, Paterson AD, Meltzer HY, Lieberman JA, Potkin SG, Macciardi F, Kennedy JL. Association of the MscI polymorphism of the dopamine D3 receptor gene with tardive dyskinesia in schizophrenia. Neuropsychopharmacology 1999; 21(1):17–27.
114. Lerer B, Segman RH, Fangerau H, Daly AK, Basile VS, Cavallaro R, Aschauer HN, McCreadie RG, Ohlraun S, Ferrier N, Masellis M, Verga M, Scharfetter J, Reitschel M, Lovlie R, Levy UH, Meltzer HY, Kennedy JL, Steen VM, Macciardi F. Pharmacogenetics of tardive dyskinesia: combined analysis of 780 patients supports association with dopamine D3 receptor gene Ser9Gly polymorphism. Neuropsychopharmacology 2002; 27(1):105–119.
115. Bakker PR, van Harten PN, van Os J. Antipsychotic-induced tardive dyskinesia and the Ser9Gly polymorphism in the DRD3 gene: a meta analysis. Schizophr Res 2006; 83(2–3):185–192.
116. Eichhammer P, Albus M, Borrmann-Hassenbach M, Schoeler A, Putzhammer A, Frick U, Klein HE, Rohrmeier T. Association of dopamine D3-receptor gene variants with neuroleptic induced akathisia in schizophrenic patients: a generalization of Steen's study on DRD3 and tardive dyskinesia. Am J Med Genet 2000; 96(2):187–191.
117. Gunes A, Scordo MG, Jaanson P, Dahl ML. Serotonin and dopamine receptor gene polymorphisms and the risk of extrapyramidal side effects in perphenazine-treated schizophrenic patients. Psychopharmacology (Berl) 2007; 190(4):479–484.
118. Farde L, Nyberg S, Oxenstierna G, Nakashima Y, Halldin C, Ericsson B. Positron emission tomography studies on D2 and 5-HT2 receptor binding in risperidone-treated schizophrenic patients. J Clin Psychopharmacol 1995; 15:19S-23S.

119. Kapur S, Zipursky RB, Remington G, Jones C, DaSilva J, Wilson AA, Houle S. 5-HT2 and D2 receptor occupancy of olanzapine in schizophrenia: a PET investigation. Am J Psychiatry 1998; 155(7):921–928.
120. Reynolds GP. Association of antipsychotic drug-induced weight gain with a 5-HT2C receptor gene polymorphism. J Psychopharmacol 2004; 18(3):340–345.
121. Davis R and Faulds D. Dexfenfluramine. An updated review of its therapeutic use in the management of obesity. Drugs 1996; 52(5):696–724.
122. Reynolds GP, Zhang ZJ, Zhang XB. Association of antipsychotic drug-induced weight gain with a 5-HT2C receptor gene polymorphism. Lancet 2002; 359:2086–2087.
123. Miller DD, Ellingrod VL, Holman TL, Buckley PF, Arndt S. Clozapine-induced weight gain associated with the 5HT2C receptor -759C/T polymorphism. 2005 133(1):97–100.
124. Reynolds GP, Zhang Z, Zhang X. Polymorphism of the promoter region of the serotonin 5-HT(2C) receptor gene and clozapine-induced weight gain. Am J Psychiatry 2003; 160(4):677–679.
125. Ellingrod VL, Perry PJ, Ringold JC, Lund BC, Bever-Stille K, Fleming F, Holman TL, Miller D. Weight gain associated with the -759C/T polymorphism of the 5HT2C receptor and olanzapine. Am J Med Genet B Neuropsychiatr Genet 2005;34(1):76–78.
126. Templeman LA, Reynolds GP, Arranz B, San L. Polymorphisms of the 5-HT2C receptor and leptin genes are associated with antipsychotic drug-induced weight gain in Caucasian subjects with a first-episode psychosis. Pharmacogenet Genomics 2005; 15(4):195–200.
127. Lane HY, Liu YC, Huang CL, Chang YC, Wu PL, Lu CT, Chang WH. Risperidone-related weight gain: genetic and nongenetic predictors. J Clin Psychopharmacol 2006; 26(2):128–134.
128. Ryu S, Cho EY, Park T, Oh S, Jang WS, Kim SK, Lee D, Hong KS. -759 C/T polymorphism of 5-HT2C receptor gene and early phase weight gain associated with antipsychotic drug treatment. Prog Neuropsychopharmacol Biol Psychiatry 2007; 31(3):673–677.
129. Tsai SJ, Hong CJ, Yu YW, Lin CH. -759C/T genetic variation of 5HT(2C) receptor and clozapine-induced weight gain. Lancet 2002; 360(9347):1790.
130. Basile VS, Masellis M, De Luca V, Meltzer HY, Kennedy JL. 759C/T genetic variation of 5HT(2C) receptor and clozapine-induced weight gain. Lancet 2002;360(9347):1790–1791.
131. Theisen FM, Hinney A, Brömel T, Heinzel-Gutenbrunner M, Martin M, Krieg JC, Remschmidt H, Hebebrand J. Lack of association between the -759C/T polymorphism of the 5-HT2C receptor gene and clozapine-induced weight gain among German schizophrenic individuals. Psychiatr Genet 2004; 14(3):139–142.
132. Mulder H, Franke B, Aart van der-Beek van der A, Arends J, Wilmink FW, Egberts AC, Scheffer H. The association between HTR2C polymorphisms and obesity in psychiatric patients using antipsychotics: a cross-sectional study. Pharmacogenomics J 2006; [Epub ahead of print]
133. Reynolds GP, Templeman LA, Zhang ZJ. The role of 5-HT2C receptor polymorphisms in the pharmacogenetics of antipsychotic drug treatment. Prog Neuropsychopharmacol Biol Psychiatry 2005; 29(6):1021–1028.
134. Malhotra AK, Goldman D, Ozaki N, Rooney W, Clifton A, Buchanan RW, Breier A, Pickar D. Clozapine response and the 5HT2C Cys23Ser polymorphism. Neuroreport 1996; 7(13): 2100–2102.
135. Arranz M, Collier D, Sodhi M, Ball D, Roberts G, Price J, Sham P, Kerwin R. Association between clozapine response and allelic variation in 5-HT2A receptor gene. Lancet 1995; 346(8970):281–282.
136. Malhotra AK, Goldman D, Ozaki N, Breier A, Buchanan R, Pickar D. Lack of association between polymorphisms in the 5-HT2A receptor gene and the antipsychotic response to clozapine. Am J Psychiatry 1996; 153(8):1092–1094.
137. Arranz MJ, Munro J, Sham P, Kirov G, Murray RM, Collier DA, Kerwin RW. Meta-analysis of studies on genetic variation in 5-HT2A receptors and clozapine response. Schizophr Res 1998; 32(2):93–99.
138. Joober R, Benkelfat C, Brisebois K, Toulouse A, Turecki G, Lal S, Bloom D, Labelle A, Lalonde P, Fortin D, Alda M, Palmour R, Rouleau GA. T102C polymorphism in the 5HT2A

gene and schizophrenia: relation to phenotype and drug response variability. J Psychiatry Neurosci 1999; 24(2):141–146.
139. Anttila S, Kampman O, Illi A, Rontu R, Lehtimäki T, Leinonen E. Association between 5-HT2A, TPH1 and GNB3 genotypes and response to typical neuroleptics: a serotonergic approach. BMC Psychiatry. 2007 May 23;7:22.
140. Ellingrod VL, Perry PJ, Lund BC, Bever-Stille K, Fleming F, Holman TL, Miller D. 5HT2A and 5HT2C receptor polymorphisms and predicting clinical response to olanzapine in schizophrenia. J Clin Psychopharmacol 2002; 22(6):622–624.
141. Lerer B, Segman RH, Tan EC, Basile VS, Cavallaro R, Aschauer HN, Strous R,Chong SA, Heresco-Levy U, Verga M, Scharfetter J, Meltzer HY, Kennedy JL, Macciardi F. Combined analysis of 635 patients confirms an age-related association of the serotonin 2A receptor gene with tardive dyskinesia and specificity for the non-orofacial subtype. Int J Neuropsychopharmacol 2005; 8(3):411–425.
142. Yamanouchi Y, Iwata N, Suzuki T, Kitajima T, Ikeda M, Ozaki N. Effect of DRD2, 5-HT2A, and COMT genes on antipsychotic response to risperidone. Pharmacogenomics J 2003; 3(6):356–361.
143. Ellingrod VL, Lund BC, Miller D, Fleming F, Perry P, Holman TL, Bever-Stille K. 5-HT2A receptor promoter polymorphism, -1438G/A and negative symptom response to olanzapine in schizophrenia. Psychopharmacol Bull 2003; 37(2):109–112.
144. Hamdani N, Bonnière M, Adès J, Hamon M, Boni C, Gorwood P. Negative symptoms of schizophrenia could explain discrepant data on the association between the 5-HT2A receptor gene and response to antipsychotics. Neurosci Lett 2005; 377(1):69–74.
145. Reynolds GP, Arranz B, Templeman LA, Fertuzinhos S, San L. Effect of 5-HT1A receptor gene polymorphism on negative and depressive symptom response to antipsychotic treatment of drug-naive psychotic patients. Am J Psychiatry 2006; 163(10):1826–9.
146. Svenningsson P, Nishi A, Fisone G, Girault JA, Nairn AC, Greengard P. DARPP-32: an integrator of neurotransmission. Annu Rev Pharmacol Toxicol. 2004;44:269–96.
147. Xu Q, Jia YB, Zhang BY, Zou K, Tao YB, Wang YP, Qiang BQ, Wu GY, Shen Y, Ji HK, Huang Y, Sun XQ, Ji L, Li YD, Yuan YB, Shu L, Yu X, Shen YC, Yu YQ, Ju GZ; Chinese Schizophrenia Consortium. Association study of an SNP combination pattern in the dopaminergic pathway in paranoid schizophrenia: a novel strategy for complex disorders. Mol Psychiatry. 2004 May;9(5):510–21.
148. Simeone A. Genetic control of dopaminergic neuron differentiation. Trends Neurosci. 2005 Feb;28(2):62–5.
149. Eastwood SL, Burnet PW, Harrison PJ. Decreased hippocampal expression of the susceptibility gene PPP3CC and other calcineurin subunits in schizophrenia. Biol Psychiatry. 2005 Apr 1;57(7):702–10.
150. Eastwood SL, Lyon L, George L, Andrieux A, Job D, Harrison PJ. Altered expression of synaptic protein mRNAs in STOP (MAP6) mutant mice. J Psychopharmacol. 2006 Oct 18; [Epub ahead of print]
151. Kennedy GC, Matsuzaki H, Dong S, Liu WM, Huang J, Liu G, Su X, Cao M, Chen W, Zhang J, Liu W, Yang G, Di X, Ryder T, He Z, Surti U, Phillips MS, Boyce-Jacino MT, Fodor SP, Jones KW. Large-scale genotyping of complex DNA. Nat Biotechnol. 2003 Oct;21(10):1233–7.
152. Robinson DG, Woerner MG, Napolitano B, Patel RC, Sevy SM, Gunduz-Bruce H, Soto-Perello JM, Mendelowitz A, Khadivi A, Miller R, McCormack J, Lorell BS, Lesser ML, Schooler NR, Kane JM. Randomized comparison of olanzapine versus risperidone for the treatment of first-episode schizophrenia: 4-month outcomes. Am J Psychiatry. 2006 Dec;163(12):2096–102.
153. Lencz T, Morgan TV, Athanasiou M, Dain B, Reed CR, Kane JM, Kucherlapati R, Malhotra AK. Converging evidence for a pseudoautosomal cytokine receptor gene locus in schizophrenia. Mol Psychiatry. 2007 Jun;12(6):572–80. Epub 2007 Mar 20.
154. Burdick KE, Goldberg TE, Funke B, Bates JA, Lencz T, Kucherlapati R, Malhotra AK. DTNBP1 genotype influences cognitive decline in schizophrenia. Schizophr Res. 2007 Jan;89(1–3):169–72. Epub 2006 Oct 30.

155. Burdick KE, Lencz T, Funke B, Finn CT, Szeszko PR, Kane JM, Kucherlapati R, Malhotra AK. Genetic variation in DTNBP1 influences general cognitive ability. Hum Mol Genet. 2006 May 15;15(10):1563–8. Epub 2006 Jan 13.
156. Burdick KE, Hodgkinson CA, Szeszko PR, Lencz T, Ekholm JM, Kane JM, Goldman D, Malhotra AK. DISC1 and neurocognitive function in schizophrenia. Neuroreport. 2005 Aug 22;16(12):1399–402.
157. DeRosse P, Hodgkinson CA, Lencz T, Burdick KE, Kane JM, Goldman D, Malhotra AK. Disrupted in schizophrenia 1 genotype and positive symptoms in schizophrenia. Biol Psychiatry. 2007 May 15;61(10):1208–10. Epub 2006 Oct 19.
158. DeRosse P, Funke B, Burdick KE, Lencz T, Goldberg TE, Kane JM, Kucherlapati R, Malhotra AK. COMT genotype and manic symptoms in schizophrenia. Schizophr Res. 2006 Oct;87(1–3):28–31. Epub 2006 Jul 7.
159. DeRosse P, Funke B, Burdick KE, Lencz T, Ekholm JM, Kane JM, Kucherlapati R, Malhotra AK. Dysbindin genotype and negative symptoms in schizophrenia. Am J Psychiatry. 2006 Mar;163(3):532–4.
160. Arranz MJ, Munro J, Birkett J, Bolonna A, Mancama D, Sodhi M, Lesch KP, Meyer JF, Sham P, Collier DA, Murray RM, Kerwin R. Pharmacogenetic prediction of clozapine response. Lancet. 2000 May 6;355(9215):1615–6.
161. de Leon J, Armstrong SC, Cozza KL. Clinical guidelines for psychiatrists for the use of pharmacogenetic testing for CYP450 2D6 and CYP450 2C19. Psychosomatics. 2006 Jan-Feb;47(1):75–85.
162. Perlis RH, Ganz DA, Avorn J, Schneeweiss S, Glynn RJ, Smoller JW, Wang PS. Pharmacogenetic testing in the clinical management of schizophrenia: a decision-analytic model. Clin Psychopharmacol. 2005 Oct;25(5):427–34.

Chapter 18
Pharmacogenomics in HIV Disease

Amalio Telenti

Contents

Abstract Pharmacogenetics holds promise in HIV treatment because of the complexity and potential toxicity of multidrug therapies that are prescribed for long periods. However, there has been limited success with the current approach, in which one or few candidate genes are examined for a limited number of allelic variants. A change in paradigm emerges from the availability of the HapMap, the wealth of data on less common genetic polymorphisms, and new genotyping technology. This chapter presents a comprehensive review of the existing literature on pharmacogenetic determinants of antiretroviral drug exposure and of drug toxicity, as well as on genetic markers associated with the rate of disease progression. In addition, this chapter discusses current opportunities in the clinical arena, as well as issues on genetics in HIV drug development. It is expected that larger-scale comprehensive genome approaches will profoundly change the landscape of knowledge in the future.

Keywords ADME, antiretroviral therapy, protease inhibitors, reverse transcriptase inhibitors, whole genome association studies

---

Amalio Telenti
Institute of Microbiology, University Hospital Center, University of Lausanne, Lausanne, Switzerland
Amalio.Telenti@chuv.ch

1 Introduction

Pharmacogenetics has considerable interest in HIV therapeutics because of the prevalence of toxicity *(1)*, the long term nature of the treatment program, and the complexity inherent to a multidrug therapy. In addition, there is a marked interindividual variation in plasma levels, and in susceptibility to adverse effects of antiretroviral drugs. Variable drug response likely reflects the combined influence of gender, environment, concurrent disease, concurrent drugs, and genetics *(2)*. Thus, this field would benefit from predictive tools to identify the drug combination most likely to be tolerated and effective. Work to date has been restricted to a reduced number of variants of a limited number of genes encoding metabolic enzymes and transporters, and to genes associated with drug toxicity. Moving from the current single candidate gene and single nucleotide polymorphism (SNP) approach requires the effective use of novel genotyping technologies that allow a more thorough, cost-effective genetic work *(3)*.

In addition to pharmacogenetics *sensu stricto*, genetic analysis holds promise for the study of HIV disease progression. This is of relevance for the understanding of pathogenesis and for vaccine development—through the investigation of mechanisms defining interindividual differences in susceptibility to HIV *(4)*. A number of genetic markers of susceptibility to HIV could be considered for guiding the decision to initiate treatment.

Finally, pharmacogenetic data are increasingly used to predict the efficacy and safety of new compounds and to guide decision making in the discovery and development of new drugs along the pharmaceutical pipeline *(5)*. In some situations, a gene, and its encoded protein, appears biologically dispensable because its absence in humans is not associated with a recognizable phenotype. This scenario may define an attractive pharmacological target, as it is assumed that "nature" has already done the necessary proof-of-concept experiment *(6)*. This reasoning greatly helped the development of CCR5 inhibitors—a new class of drugs in HIV therapeutics that targets the cellular receptor of HIV *(7)*.

2 Pharmacogenetics and Pharmacokinetics of ART

Current anti-HIV drugs are used in combinations usually referred to as antiretroviral therapy or ART. The three main drug classes are the nucleoside analogue reverse transcriptase inhibitors (NRTIs), the viral protease inhibitors (PIs), and the non-nucleoside reverse transcriptase inhibitors (NNRTIs). PIs and NNRTIs are extensively metabolized by cytochrome P450 enzymes such as CYP3A4, CYP2C19, CYP2D6, and CYP2B6 *(8, 9)*. In addition, most PIs have been shown to be substrates of the efflux transporter P-glycoprotein, and of other cellular transporters *(10)*. For NRTIs, it is essential to consider drug exposure in terms of intracellular NRTI triphosphate concentrations, because these are the moieties that exert antiretroviral and toxic activities. Host-cell-mediated sequential enzymatic phosphorylation steps are required for activating the nucleotide- and nucleoside-analogue reverse-transcriptase inhibitors *(11)*.

2.1 Single Gene Studies

Studies to date have identified a limited number of allelic variants of genes involved in metabolism and transport of ART (Table 18.1). The most solid associations are those of alleles of *CYP2B6* and efavirenz and nevirapine pharmacokinetics, *CYP3A5* and saquinavir, and *CYP2C19* and nelfinavir pharmacokinetics. Much less

Table 18.1 In herited differences in ADME of antiretroviral drugs. Only the most relevant associations are indicated. Compiled from www.hiv-pharmacogenomics.org

Gene or protein (*)	Allele or variant evaluated	Reported consequence for antiretroviral drugs
Metabolism		
CYP3A5	CYP3A5*3 (splice defect), and CYP3A5*6 (splice defect), CYP3A5*6 (Frameshift)—alleles associated with severely reduced enzyme activity	Higher saquinavir AUC and metabolite ratio. Reduction of oral indinavir clearance
CYP2C19	CYP2C19*2 (aberrant splice site, truncated protein, poor metabolizer)	Higher nelfinavir AUC and lower M8/nelfinavir AUC ratio, and less virological failure
CYP2B6	CYP2B6*6, *11, *18, *27, *28, *29 (alleles with diminished or loss function, associated with decreased expression, or decreased function, protein truncation, or gene deletion)	Higher efavirenz and nevirapine AUC. Associated with increased neuropsychological toxicity
Transport		
P-glycoprotein (*MDR1*, *ABCB1*)	3435C>T (synonymous I1145I, in linkage disequilibrium with *ABCB1*_1236, and 2677). Limited data on 61A>G (N21D), 1199G>A (S400N), other variants, or on haplotypes	Controversial data with a number of reports indicating an association of 3435T with decrease transport function resulting in increase protease inhibitor exposure. Recent data indicates that his synonymous SNP results in are codon usage for isoleucine, leads to a change in timing of cotranslational folding of the P-glycoprotein, and results in changes in substrate specificity *(12)*
MRP2 (ABCC2)	1249G>A (V417I)	Associated with risk of tenofovir-induced proximal tubulopathy in small study)
MRP4 (ABCC4)	3724G>A (A1203A), 4131T>G, 669C>T (I223I)	Elevated zidovudine- and 3TC-triphosphate concentration. Associated with risk of tenofovir-induced proximal tubulopathy (669C>T) in a small study
Protein binding		
α1-acid glycoprotein *(ORM1)*	F1 and S	Higher apparent clearance in F1F1 as compared to SS for indinavir and, weakly, for lopinavir/r

information is available on the role of transporter variants and drug exposure. Only *ABCB1 (MRP1)* variants, in particular *ABCB1*_3435C>T, have been extensively evaluated in HIV therapeutics (Table 18.1). This synonymous SNP (representing a rare codon usage for isoleucine) leads to a change in timing of cotranslational folding of the P-glycoprotein and results in changes in substrate specificity *(12)*. This novel mechanism explains to a large extent the controversial results or the lack of association of this variant, directly or through linkage disequilibrium, with causal variants or with changes in mRNA expression. In the larger scope of genetics, it opens a Pandora's box of biological consequences of silent polymorphisms *(13)*.

2.2 ADME Pathway Studies

Because of the limitations of single gene approaches, there has been increasing interest in establishing the basis for a more comprehensive approach through the use of comprehensive sets of SNPs *(14)*, or through the assessment of complete ADME (absorption, distribution, metabolism, and excretion) pathways *(15)*. Reconstitution of ADME pathways is a key step in establishing a frame of plausibility to select genes for study. For a given drug or drug class, the ADME proteins and their encoding genes can be classified according to their proven/proposed (existing evidence), putative (inferred evidence, e.g., from metabolites), or potential (rational basis, e.g., nuclear receptors and regulatory networks) role in transport, metabolism, and excretion. Overall, 126 ADME genes can be proposed as potentially relevant to current antiretroviral therapy *(15)*. This set does not include genes involved in phosphorylation, mitochondrial genes, mitochondrial transporters, or genes implicated in abacavir metabolism (alcohol and aldehyde dehydrogenases).

Similar to the process of establishing plausibility for genes involved in antiretroviral drug ADME pathways, a rational approach to genetic variation will integrate data from the literature on functionally relevant SNPs (e.g., nonsynonymous changes in the coding region, changes in expression, splicing, and general regulation of a gene), and for the prediction of functional consequences of a genetic variant by using bioinformatic tools. Proven/proposed functional polymorphisms represent the subset of SNPs for which there is experimental evidence for a functional effect of the substitution. Putative SNPs are defined by bioinformatic tools using programs like FastSNP *(16)* or TAMAL *(17)*, that score the likelihood of a functional effect according to predefined algorithms. These proven or putative functional SNPs will enrich a background of common human genetic variation as described by implementing data from the human HapMap. Progress in our understanding of the characteristics that define a SNP as functional will continue to evolve, and should be incorporated into future definitions of the minimum set of SNPs that characterize a gene. An estimate for the Caucasian population includes 175 proven and 470 putative functional variants in ADME genes that can be proposed for the study of current antiretroviral drugs (Table 18.2). In addition, common variation in these genes is captured by 1783 HapMap tSNPs (Table 18.2).

Table 18.2 Genetic variation in ADME pathways of anti-HIV drugs. Pr-fSNP = proven/proposed functional polymorphism, Pu-fSNP = putative functional polymorphism, Tag-SNP = HapMap tagging SNP. This set does not include genes involved in phosphorylation, mitochondrial genes, mitochondrial transporters, or genes implicated in abacavir metabolism (alcohol and aldehyde dehydrogenases). Adapted from Lubomirov et al. (15)

	SNP type			
Gene class (#)	Pr-fSNP	Pu-fSNP	Tag-SNP	Total SNPs (SNPs/gene)
Drug metabolism				
CYPs *(18)*	49	84	113	246 *(14)*
UGTs *(16)*	23	35	59	117 *(8)*
SULTs *(14)*	15	43	137	195 *(14)*
Transporters				
ABCs *(10)*	31	70	329	430 *(43)*
SLCs *(37)*	32	142	702	876 *(24)*
Other				
PBPs *(3)*	2	7	15	24 *(8)*
NRs *(23)*	23	77	400	500 *(22)*
PDZs *(5)*	0	12	28	40 *(8)*
Total *(126)*	**175**	**470**	**1783**	**2428 *(20)***

Overall, genetic variation can be captured by an average of 20 SNPs per candidate gene. As above, the resulting ranking of biological plausibility (i.e., proven, putative) can be used in the evaluation of results emanating from genetic association studies in sequential or in joint analysis.

3 Pharmacogenetics of ART Toxicity

The analysis of pharmacogenetic determinants of toxicity has been successful for the unequivocal identification of the genetic basis of hypersensitivity reactions to the NRTI abacavir, for the understanding of the genetic basis of PI-induced hyperlipidemia, and for defining associations of several PIs and unconjugated hyperbilirubinemia in the context of Gilbert syndrome. In addition, there is sparse information on the genetic bases for other recognized adverse effects of ART.

3.1 Drug Hypersensitivity Syndromes

The pathogenesis of a number of multisystem drug hypersensitivity reactions involves major histocompatibility complex (MHC)-restricted presentation of drug or drug metabolites to MHC molecules and/or haptenation to endogenous proteins prior to T cell presentation *(18–20)* Genetic loci within the MHC are determinants of hypersensitivity reactions to abacavir and to nevirapine. Only a subset of individuals exposed to abacavir develop hypersensitivity, typically within six weeks of initiating therapy, and those individuals who do not develop the syndrome within this time frame remain at low risk despite ongoing therapy *(21)*. Non-Caucasian racial origin also decreases risk of abacavir hypersensitivity, and familial predisposition has also been reported *(22)*. Specific MHC alleles are strongly associated with risk of abacavir hypersensitivity *(23, 24)*. The *HLA-B*5701* allele has an independent positive predictive value of greater than 70% and a negative predictive value of greater than 90% in Caucasians, suggesting that prospective testing for susceptibility to this syndrome may represent a useful clinical test in some populations *(25)*.

A cost-effectiveness study estimated that pretreatment screening of HLA-B*5701 in Caucasian (and Hispanic) populations would be a cost-effective use of healthcare resources *(26)*. The relevance of these findings to populations where presence of the HLA-B*5701 allele is at a significantly lower frequency (such as many Asian and African populations) is less certain *(27)*. These questions are currently being addressed by large-scale prospective international studies such as PREDICT-1 and SHAPE. There are practical considerations influencing the widespread implementation of a pharmacogenetic approach to abacavir prescription, because analysis is more complex than the analysis of simple SNPs. HLA-B*5701 diagnostic methods need high-resolution typing assays to resolve HLA alleles within the B17 serological family (e.g., HLA-B*5701, HLA-B*5702, HLA-B*5703, and HLA-B*5801) *(28)*.

Nevirapine hypersensitivity—manifesting as potentially life-threatening hepatotoxicity with or without rash—is also conferred by genetic factors. This syndrome is similar to abacavir hypersensitivity in that susceptible individuals develop symptoms within six weeks, whereas continuing therapy beyond this period is not associated with increased risk *(29)*. The protective effect of low CD4 T-cell count in the case of nevirapine hypersensitivity *(29, 30)* is consistent with a CD4 T-cell-dependent immune response to nevirapine-specific antigens and a participation of HLA Class II alleles *(31)*. Human cases involving combinations of hepatitis, fever, or rash have been associated with an interaction between HLA-DRB1*0101 and the percentage of CD4, whereas no associations were detected for isolated rash *(31)* (Table 18.3).

3.2 Metabolic Disorders

In considering the pharmacogenetics of ART-related dyslipidemia, it may be useful to evaluate factors that may influence lipid metabolism in the general population and may therefore potentiate the toxic effects of ART. Initial work identified the role of *APOE* and *APOC3* variants as risk factors for hyperlipoproteinemia (predominantly hypertriglycerdemia) *(32–34)*. In addition, there is a deleterious gene-drug interaction resulting in a high risk for extreme hypertriglyceridemia when ritonavir is prescribed to individuals with unfavorable genetic profiles. A recent analysis of selected allelic variants of 13 genes proposed in the literature as influencing plasma lipid levels in the general population validated five genes as contributing to ART-associated dyslipidemia (Table 18.3) *(35)*.

Table 18.3 Toxicogenetics of antiretroviral drugs. Only the most relevant associations are indicated. Compiled from www.hiv-pharmacogenomics.org

Gene or protein (*)	Allele or variant evaluated	Reported consequence for antiretroviral drugs
HLA-B	HLA-B*57.1 haplotype (defined by the presence of HLAB*5701, HLA-DR7 and HLA-DQ3)	Hypersensitivity reaction to abacavir
HLA-DR	*HLA-DRB1*0101*	High negative predictive value of hypersensitivity reactions to nevirapine (fever, rash, hepatitis)
TNFα	-238G/A TNF-α promoter polymorphism	Earlier onset of lipoatrophy
UGT1A1	*UGT1A1*28,* Promoter region (insertion at TATA box associated with reduction in bilirubin-conjugating activity)	Gilbert's syndrome. Hyperbilirubinemia, increased levels of bilirubin in presence of atazanavir or indinavir.
APOC3, APOE	APOC3 -482 C>T, -455 T>C, 3238 C>G. APOE ε2 and ε3 haplotypes.	Increased risk of hypertriglyceridemia associated with use of ritonavir. Including analysis of variants of APOA5, CETP, and ABCA1 may improve prediction and also help in identifying individuals at risk for low HDL-cholesterol.
SPINK1, CFTR	Multiple variants associated with cystic fibrosis and pancreatitis	Susceptibility to pancreatitis
Mitochondrial DNA	Tissue-specific mitochondrial DNA depletion may represent toxic effect of NRTI therapy on mitochondrial DNA synthesis. Possibility for accumulation of mutations in mtDNA due to gamma polymerase damage from nucleoside analogue reverse transcriptase inhibitors.	Certain human mtDNA haplotypes (haplotype T) may increase susceptibility to peripheral neuropathy. Depletion and mutation of mtDNA likely associated with lipodystrophy

The most favorable and unfavorable *APOE/APOC3/APOA5/CETP/ABCA1* genotypes resulted in median triglyceride levels of 2.6 and 4.1 mmol/l, respectively, when exposed to ritonavir. In contrast, the triglyceride levels for individuals with the most favorable and unfavorable genotypes were 1.37 and 2.3 mmol/l, respectively, in the absence of ritonavir exposure. The most favorable and unfavorable *CETP/APOA5* genotypes resulted in median HDL-cholesterol levels of 1.25 and 1.11 mmol/l, respectively, with no or NRTI-ART; and 1.5 and 1.17 mmol/l with NNRTI-ART. No genotype was significantly associated with non-HDL cholesterol levels. Thus, the contribution of any single SNP on lipid levels was modest. However, the magnitude of the genetic effects on dyslipidemia became apparent in the multigene analysis. A theoretical strategy of selecting the initial ART according to the results of genotyping would have the potential to reduce by 30% the number of patients with sustained hypertriglyceridemia; and even more for individuals with unfavorable genotypes (Table 18.3).

3.3 *Lipodystrophy and Mitochondrial Disorders*

Lipodystrophy has been described in 25–50% of ART-treated patients. The cumulative exposure to ART has been identified as the major risk factor in multiple studies. However, lipodystrophy affects some but not all patients, despite similar ART exposure, which suggests that genetic factors may be involved. A functional promoter polymorphism in *TNF-α* (-238A) has been associated with more rapid onset of lipoatrophy in some *(36, 37)* but not all studies *(34)*. The functional correlates of this effect have not been characterised, although higher TNF-α levels are described among individuals carrying the -238A *TNF-α* promoter variant *(36, 37)*.

Defects in either the quantity or quality of mitochondrial DNA have been associated with lipodystrophy, neuropathy, lactic acidosis, and with the associated complex metabolic disorders. In contrast to the nuclear genome, mitochondrial DNA may undergo quantitative and qualitative changes over an individual's lifetime, and may be influenced directly by environmental factors *(38)*. The effects are likely to be tissue-specific rather than general, reflecting the differing requirements of tissues for cellular energy and the differing availability of energy substrates. The putative mechanism that is invoked to explain mitochondrial toxicity of ART (and most prominently, NRTI), includes the inhibition of the gamma polymerase, the only enzyme that replicates mtDNA. Inhibition of gamma polymerase leads to depletion of mtDNA and inhibition of the transcription of proteins encoded by mitochondrial DNA, all of which represent enzymes of the electron transport system, which is involved in oxidative phosphorylation. Initiation of ART has triggered bilateral optic atrophy and blindness in HIV-infected individuals with unrecognized mitochondrial disorders, such as Leber's hereditary optic neuropathy *(38–42)*. Underlying human variation of mtDNA, represented by common haplotypes, has been associated with differences in susceptibility to ART-related neuropathy *(43)* (Table 18.3). In addition, the possible accumulation of mtDNA mutations during aging leads to mitochondrial dysfunction. Knock-in "mtDNA mutator mice" that expressed a exonuclease-deficient gamma polymerase developed a 3- to 5-fold increase in mtDNA mutations and deletions *(44)*. These mice presented subcutaneous fat loss, weight loss, osteoporosis, anemia, and cardiomegaly. Overall, the accumulation of mutations and reduction of mtDNA quantity associated with ART against a background of aging would be a plausible mechanism explaining the complex features of lipodystrophy and associated metabolic syndrome. Detailed analysis of the mtDNA genome may help identify individuals at risk of toxicity.

3.4 *Unconjugated Hyperbilirubinemia*

Unconjugated hyperbilirubinemia is an adverse event of therapy containing indinavir (IDV) or atazanavir (ATV) *(45, 46)*. Unconjugated bilirubin enters the hepatocyte by passive diffusion and may be facilitated through the human organic transporting polypeptide 1B1 (OATP1B1) encoded by *SLCO1B1 (47–49)*. Once in the hepatocyte, bilirubin is conjugated with glucuronic acid by the microsomal enzyme UDP-glucuronosyltransferase 1A1 (UGT1A1) and excreted in the bile by MRP2 (ABCC2) *(50)*. A polymorphism in the promoter TATA element of the gene encoding UGT1A1 (allele *UGT1A1*28*) decreases transcriptional activity; it is responsible for the unconjugated hyperbilirubinemia observed in the context of Gilbert syndrome *(51, 52)* (Table 18.3) and associates with the occurrence of jaundice upon initiation of PIs indinavir and atazanavir *(53, 54)*. Nonsynonymous polymorphisms in *SLCO1B1* have been associated with differences in the function of the transporter in vitro *(55–57)* and in vivo *(58–62)*.

The additive effect of the genes described above will influence the rates of hyperbilirubinemia upon the introduction of drugs such as atazanavir *(54, 63)*. There are ethnical/racial differences in the frequency of both *UGT1A1* and *OATP1B1* variants, such that hyperbilirubinemia may occur more frequently for African and less frequently for individuals of Japanese origin. The theoretical advantage of genotyping for *SLCO1B1* and *UGT1A1*28* before initiation of ART is that it would contribute to the reduction of bilirubin determinations in jaundice range from 22 to 5.0% *(63)*.

3.5 *Neurotoxicity of Efavirenz*

As described above, efavirenz and nevirapine are metabolized by CYP2B6. The best studied allele, 2B6*6 (516 G>T, Gln172His), is a pharmacogenetic marker of efavirenz neuropsychological toxicity. This allele predicts adverse neuropsychological scores during the first 12 weeks after initiation of efavirenz therapy *(64)*. The frequency of toxicity is expected to decrease thereafter *(65)*. However, genotyping can also identify individuals at risk for late or persistent neuropsychological toxicity while on long term efavirenz-containing therapy *(66)*. In the latter setting, the presence of the variant allele was two to three times more frequent among individuals describing sleep or mood disorders or fatigue.

3.6 *Pancreatitis*

Drug-induced pancreatitis in individuals with advanced HIV infection/AIDS has been attributed to the use of pentamidine, trimethoprim-sulfamethoxazole, or didanosine *(67)*. The drugs may be contributing to pancreatitis by potentiating other toxic agents, by a genetic predisposition, or by its action on a pancreas which was already diseased.*CFTR* (Cystic Fibrosis Transmembrane Conductance Regulator) mutations are associated with pancreatitis *(68, 69)*. *SPINK1* (Serine Protease Inhibitor Kazal-1), which encodes a trypsin inhibitor in the cytoplasm of pancreatic acinar cells, is also a genetic risk factor for pancreatitis *(70)*. Frossard et al. evaluated the frequency of *CFTR* and *SPINK1* mutations in HIV-positive patients with clinical pancreatitis or asymptomatic elevation of serum pancreatic enzymes *(71)*. Among 51 patients presenting with hyperamylasemia, there were 13 carriers of *CFTR* or *SPINK1* polymorphisms (12.7%). Four of ten patients (40%) with clinical acute pancreatitis had *CFTR* or *SPINK1* mutations.

4 When to Start ART—Predicting Disease Evolution

The rate of HIV disease progression reflects the influence of the genetic diversity of the virus as well as the variation in host factors *(72)*. Dominant host factors identified to date include diversity in the major histocompatibility complex class I, and alleles of chemokine, chemokine receptors, and cytokine genes. MHC homozygosity, as well as specific HLA class I alleles, are well documented modifiers of infection (Table 18.4). The most relevant alleles associated with protection are HLA-B*27 and B*57. In contrast, HLA-B*35Px, B*37, B*53, B*56, B*58, and A1-B8-DR3 have been associated with rapid progression *(73,74)*. Epistatic interactions between certain KIR (3DS1) and HLA-B alleles delay disease progression *(75)*. Following the discovery of the CCR5 Δ32 deletion, conferring a high level resistance to HIV infection *(76–78)*. extensive research has addressed the contribution of additional variants in the CCR5-CCR2 locus. Variants of the *CCR5* promoter region include a human haplotype HHE, that is associated with rapid disease progression *(79, 80)*. In contrast, haplotypes carrying the CCR2 64I allele are associated with a favorable prognosis *(81)*, and possibly with some degree of protection from infection. Duplication at the locus encoding the chemokine CCL3L1 leads to the gene dose effect, that alone or in association with genetic variants determining CCR5 expression or function, is proposed to modify the rate of disease progression *(82)*. Various cytokine variants have been reported to influence the course of HIV-1 disease through more general effects on HIV-1 pathogenesis and inflammatory homeostasis *(72)*. Variants in cellular host factors, and in antiviral defense genes have effect-sizes in the range of those of well-documented variants such as those in the CCR5/CCR 2 region *(83–85)*. However, the contribution of any genetic variant is limited, and genetic prediction needs to account for the influence of multiple alleles *(83, 86, 87)*.

As was discussed in earlier sections, there is great interest in going beyond single gene studies to more comprehensive approaches. The Center for HIV/AIDS Vaccine Immunology (CHAVI, www.chavi.org) launched whole-genome studies in the investigation of the control of the earlier phases of infection, focusing on viral set point (4). The first study has been recently completed and the results will be available in the near future. A second initiative, the HIV Elite Controller Study (www.massgeneral.org/aids/hiv_elite_controllers.asp), will apply genomic techniques to the investigation of HIV-1 infected people who have been able to maintain viral loads at or below the limits of detection. Analysis of data from whole-genome association studies remains a critical challenge because of the need to deal with an unprecedented quantity of genomic information *(88)*.

Table 18.4 Predictors of susceptibility to HIV and disease progression. Only the most relevant associations are indicated. Compiled from www.hiv-pharmacogenomics.org

Gene or protein (*)	Allele or variant evaluated	Reported consequence for HIV susceptibility
CCR5-CCR2 locus. Chemokine receptors; co-receptor of HIV-1 (CCR5)	CCR5 Δ32, CCR5 303T>A, CCR5 P1, CCR2 V64I, and derived haplotypes	Protection (CCR5 Δ32, CCR5 303T>A, CCR2 V64I) or progression (CCR5 P1)
HLA MHC; acquired immunity	HLA A, B, C homozygosity, or selected HLA B alleles:	HLA-B*27 and B*57 are associated with protection. In contrast, HLA-B*35Px, B*37, B*53, B*56, B*58, and A1-B8-DR3 have been associated with rapid progression
KIR Innate immunity; regulation of NK cell response.	Specific KIR–HLA associations	Epistatic interactions between certain KIR (3DS1) and HLA-B alleles delay disease progression
CXCL12 (SDF-1) Ligand of CXCR4	3′UTR SDF-3′A	Neutral or progression
TSG101 Vacuolar protein sorting; required for HIV-1 budding	Various haplotypes of promoter: −183T>C and intronic 181A>C	Protection or progression depending on haplotype
CCL5 (RANTES) Ligand of *CCR5*	Various haplotypes of promoter: −403G>A, −28C>G and intronic In1.1T>C	Protection or progression depending on haplotype
IL-10 Anti-inflammatory cytokine	Promoter −592C>A	Progression
CCL3L1 (MIP1αP), Ligand of CCR5	Variable gene copy number	Progression associated with low-copy number
CX3CR1, Fractalkine receptor; minor HIV-1 co-receptor	T280M	Progression
APOBEC3G, Intrinsic immunity; HIV-1 cDNA hypermutation *Cul5* (Cullin5)	APOBEC3G H186R or expression polymorphism. Various *Cul5*haplotypes.	Progression. Some haplotypes of Cul5 may have additive effect with APOBEC3G H186R. HIV-1 viral infectivity factor (Vif) suppresses Apobec3 activity through the Cullin 5-Elongin B-Elongin C E3 ubiquitin ligase complex
CCL3 (MIP1α) Ligand of CCR5	Intronic 459C>T	Progression

5 Issues in HIV Clinical Care

The number of genetic association studies is growing rapidly, and is likely to accelerate in the future. This requires attention to the need to establish the conditions for genetic testing, including its legal and ethical aspects. An important step in the area of pharmacogenomics and genetics has been the development of the Adult AIDS Clinical Trials Group (AACTG) Protocol A5128, approved in many U.S. states *(89)*. The A5128 protocol helps participants in past or present AACTG clinical trials contribute stored DNA for studies that were not planned when informed consent was provided. Extraction from whole blood is performed at a central laboratory, where the participants' unique identifiers are replaced by randomly assigned identifiers prior to DNA storage. Despite the negative perception of genetic research among the general public, recent studies indicate that this type of investigation is widely accepted by concerned parties: patients, relatives of patients, and healthy study volunteers *(90)*.

However, there is much work needed before genetic testing can be brought to routine clinical care. It is unlikely that the identification of multigene effects will change the management of HIV-1 disease in the near future, notwithstanding some pharmacogenetic and toxicogenetic applications which may soon contribute to patient care. In Figure 18.1 we present the estimated contribution of some of these markers to limiting the clinical toxicity of commonly used antiretroviral agents and to the prediction of disease progression.

a

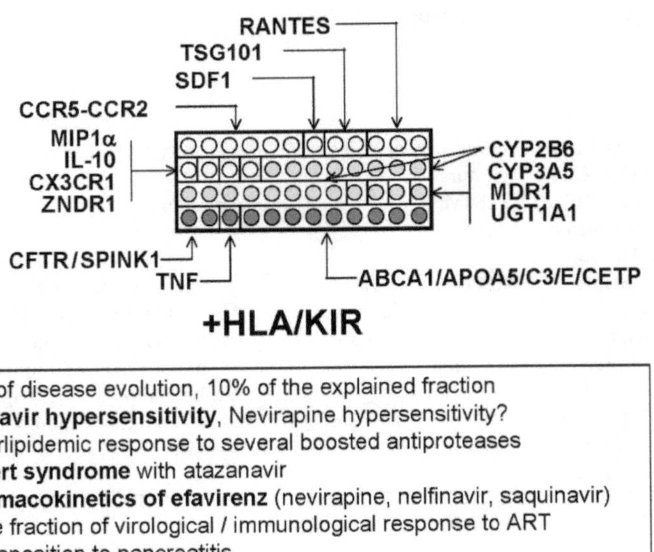

b

- 20% of disease evolution, 10% of the explained fraction
- **Abacavir hypersensitivity**, Nevirapine hypersensitivity?
- Hyperlipidemic response to several boosted antiproteases
- **Gilbert syndrome** with atazanavir
- **Pharmacokinetics of efavirenz** (nevirapine, nelfinavir, saquinavir)
- Some fraction of virological / immunological response to ART
- Predisposition to pancreatitis
- Predisposition to lipodystrophy?

Fig. 18.1 Current knowledge on HIV host genetics and ART pharmacogenetics. Panel A: The most relevant SNPs reported to date could be represented in a theoretical 50-well plate or array. In addition, HLA and KIR would need to be determined separately. Panel B: Listing of the estimated prediction and possible benefit that could be derived from the use of such a genotyping approach in the clinical setting

6 Issues in HIV Drug Development

As discussed in the introduction to this chapter, the situation in which a gene appears biologically dispensable because its absence in humans is not associated with a recognizable phenotype may define an attractive pharmacological target. This reasoning helped the development of CCR5 inhibitors.

Individuals that are homozygous CCR5 Δ32 have no apparent decrease in fitness. While this is reassuring for the purpose of a chemical or biological knockout of the protein, it does not provide sufficient evidence that such an intervention is safe in the general population. As a chemokine receptor, CCR5 helps to initiate immune responses and to distribute effector immune cells to sites of inflammation *(91)*. Several recent papers highlight the complex role of CCR5 in innate immunity against a number of pathogens, including *Toxoplama gondii (92)*, West Nile virus infection *(93)*, poxvirus *(94)*, tuberculosis *(95)*, and other infections *(96–98)*. According to the experimental data, genetic, biological, or chemical CCR5 knockout could be simultaneously protective against some pathogens (i.e., HIV), and deleterious for other processes involved in pathogen containment. The practical translation of these observations is that the immune system may have substantial redundancy and provide a good general protection to most pathogens, while hiding selective defects if exposed to a sufficient challenge of a particular pathogen. Pharmaceutical intervention on innate immunity may uncover selective immunodeficiency. This is illustrated by the experience with anti-TNFα therapy and the identification, during postmarketing surveillance, of an increased risk for reactivation of tuberculosis *(99)*.

To answer these concerns, Wheeler et al. *(100)* did a meta-analysis of studies in non-HIV infected populations in order to identify potential safety issues that may be relevant in the context of including patients co-infected with hepatitis C virus (HCV) and HIV in phase III clinical trials. They found little evidence for an association of CCR5 Δ32 with chronic HCV infection, with the response to treatment of chronic HCV, or with the risk of developing multiple sclerosis. CCR5 Δ32 may be protective against the development of rheumatoid arthritis. The conclusion is that treatment with a CCR5 inhibitor is unlikely to have related adverse effects due to CCR5 inhibition. This meta-analysis did not address recent reports on the association of CCR5 Δ32 with an increased risk of symptomatic West Nile virus infection *(101)*, and with improved recovery from HBV infection *(102)*.

7 Conclusions and Perspectives

HIV infection and treatment represent an important field of application and validation of pharmacogenetic knowledge. The field has excellent cohorts and well developed structures for clinical trials that could allow pharmacogenetic applications. Overall, five genes involved in metabolism, five in drug transporters, 23 in toxicity and treatment response, and 47 in HIV susceptibility and disease progression have been evaluated with more or less detail in recent years (www.hiv-pharmacogenomics.org).

Large scale approaches are expected to rapidly modify the landscape of knowledge. For pharmacogenetics *sensu stricto*, this represents the use of ADME arrays in studies with well defined pharmacokinetic, pharmacodynamic, or toxicity study endpoints (phenotypes) *(15)*. Pharmacogenetic data can be integrated into population pharmacokinetic modeling. On a larger scale, HIV disease is currently approached by using whole genome-wide association analysis *(4, 103)*. The proof of concept and the validity of the whole-genome approach is provided by recent publications on whole-genome association analysis in inflammatory bowel disease, diabetes, and leukemia *(104–106)*. Followup studies of candidate genes and gene variants will be needed to assess their functional role in vitro (4). In vivo validation studies should be performed with well defined study phenotypes, study design, and adequate power.

Resources

www.hiv-pharmacogenomics.org A public resource that presents host genetic information concerning HIV-1 susceptibility and treatment response.

References

1. Fellay J, Boubaker K, Ledergerber B et al. Prevalence of adverse events associated with potent antiretroviral treatment: Swiss HIV Cohort Study. Lancet 2001;358:1322–7.
2. Rotger M, Csajka C, Telenti A. Genetic, ethnic, and gender differences in the pharmacokinetics of antiretroviral agents. Curr HIV /AIDS Rep 2006;3:118–25.
3. Syvanen AC. Toward genome-wide SNP genotyping. Nat Genet 2005;37 Suppl:S5–10.
4. Telenti A, Goldstein DB. Genomics meets HIV. Nat Rev Microbiol 2006;4:9–18.
5. Roses AD. Pharmacogenetics and drug development: the path to safer and more effective drugs. Nat Rev Genet 2004;5:645–56.
6. Telenti A, Egger M. Identifying safety concerns from genetic data: lessons from the development of CCR5 inhibitors. Antivir Ther 2007;12:147–8.
7. Este JA, Telenti A. HIV entry inhibitors. Lancet 2007;370:81–8.
8. Eagling VA, Back DJ, Barry MG. Differential inhibition of cytochrome P450 isoforms by the protease inhibitors, ritonavir, saquinavir and indinavir. Br J Clin Pharmacol 1997;44:190–4.
9. Barry M, Mulcahy F, Merry C, Gibbons S, Back D. Pharmacokinetics and potential interactions amongst antiretroviral agents used to treat patients with HIV infection. Clin Pharmacokinet 1999;36:289–304.
10. Kim RB. Drug transporters in HIV Therapy. Top HIV Med 2003;11:136–9.
11. Anderson PL, Kakuda TN, Lichtenstein KA. The cellular pharmacology of nucleoside- and nucleotide-analogue reverse-transcriptase inhibitors and its relationship to clinical toxicities. Clin Infect Dis 2004;38:743–53.
12. Kimchi-Sarfaty C, Oh JM, Kim IW et al. A "silent" polymorphism in the MDR1 gene changes substrate specificity. Science 2007;315:525–8.
13. Komar AA. Genetics. SNPs, silent but not invisible. Science 2007;315:466–7.
14. Ahmadi KR, Weale ME, Xue ZY et al. A single-nucleotide polymorphism tagging set for human drug metabolism and transport. Nat Genet 2005;37:84–9.
15. Lubomirov R, Csajka C, Telenti A. An ADME pathway approach for pharmacogenetic studies of anti-HIV therapy. Pharmacogenomics 2007;8:623–33.

16. Yuan HY, Chiou JJ, Tseng WH et al. FASTSNP: an always up-to-date and extendable service for SNP function analysis and prioritization. Nucleic Acids Res 2006;34:W635–W641.
17. Hemminger BM, Saelim B, Sullivan PF. TAMAL: an integrated approach to choosing SNPs for genetic studies of human complex traits. Bioinformatics 2006;22:626–7.
18. Zanni MP, von Greyerz S, Schnyder B et al. HLA-restricted, processing- and metabolism-independent pathway of drug recognition by human alpha beta T lymphocytes. J Clin Invest 1998;102:1591–8.
19. Schnyder B, Burkhart C, Schnyder-Frutig K et al. Recognition of sulfamethoxazole and its reactive metabolites by drug-specific CD4+ T cells from allergic individuals. J Immunol 2000;164:6647–54.
20. Park BK, Naisbitt DJ, Gordon SF, Kitteringham NR, Pirmohamed M. Metabolic activation in drug allergies. Toxicology 2001;158:11–23.
21. Hewitt RG. Abacavir hypersensitivity reaction. Clin Infect Dis 2002;34:1137–42.
22. Peyrieere H, Nicolas J, Siffert M, Demoly P, Hillaire-Buys D, Reynes J. Hypersensitivity related to abacavir in two members of a family. Ann Pharmacother 2001;35:1291–2.
23. Mallal S, Nolan D, Witt C et al. Association between presence of HLA-B*5701, HLA-DR7, and HLA-DQ3 and hypersensitivity to HIV-1 reverse-transcriptase inhibitor abacavir. Lancet 2002;359:727–32.
24. Hetherington S, Hughes AR, Mosteller M et al. Genetic variations in HLA-B region and hypersensitivity reactions to abacavir. Lancet 2002;359:1121–2.
25. Nolan D, Gaudieri S, Mallal S. Pharmacogenetics: a practical role in predicting antiretroviral drug toxicity? J HIV Ther 2003;8:36–41.
26. Hughes DA, Vilar FJ, Ward CC, Alfirevic A, Park BK, Pirmohamed M. Cost-effectiveness analysis of HLA B*5701 genotyping in preventing abacavir hypersensitivity. Pharmacogenetics 2004;14:335–42.
27. Hughes AR, Mosteller M, Bansal AT et al. Association of genetic variations in HLA-B region with hypersensitivity to abacavir in some, but not all, populations. Pharmacogenomics 2004;5:203–11.
28. Lucas A, Nolan D, Mallal S. HLA-B*5701 screening for susceptibility to abacavir hypersensitivity. J Antimicrob Chemother 2007;59:591–3.
29. Stern JO, Robinson PA, Love J, Lanes S, Imperiale MS, Mayers DL. A comprehensive hepatic safety analysis of nevirapine in different populations of HIV infected patients. J Acquir Immune Defic Syndr 2003;34 Suppl 1:S21–S33.
30. Patel SM, Johnson S, Belknap SM, Chan J, Sha BE, Bennett C. Serious adverse cutaneous and hepatic toxicities associated with nevirapine use by non-HIV-infected individuals. J Acquir Immune Defic Syndr 2004;35:120–5.
31. Martin AM, Nolan D, James I et al. Predisposition to nevirapine hypersensitivity associated with HLA-DRB1*0101 and abrogated by low CD4 T-cell counts. AIDS 2005;19:97–9.
32. Behrens G, Schmidt HH, Stoll M, Schmidt RE. ApoE genotype and protease-inhibitor-associated hyperlipidaemia. Lancet 1999;354:76.
33. Fauvel J, Bonnet E, Ruidavets JB et al. An interaction between apo C-III variants and protease inhibitors contributes to high triglyceride/low HDL levels in treated HIV patients. AIDS 2001;15:2397–406.
34. Tarr PE, Taffe P, Bleiber G et al. Modeling the influence of APOC3, APOE, and TNF polymorphisms on the risk of antiretroviral therapy-associated lipid disorders. J Infect Dis 2005;191:1419–26.
35. Arnedo M, Taffé P, Sahli R et al. Evaluation of the contribution of 20 variants of 13 genes to dyslipidemia associated with antiretroviral therapy. Pharmacogenetics Genomics 2007;17:755–64.
36. Nolan D, Moore C, Castley A et al. Tumour necrosis factor-alpha gene -238G/A promoter polymorphism associated with a more rapid onset of lipodystrophy. AIDS 2003;17:121–3.
37. Maher B, Alfirevic A, Vilar FJ, Wilkins EG, Park BK, Pirmohamed M. TNF-alpha promoter region gene polymorphisms in HIV-positive patients with lipodystrophy. AIDS 2002;16:2013–8.

38. Wallace KB, Starkov AA. Mitochondrial targets of drug toxicity. Annu Rev Pharmacol Toxicol 2000;40:353–88.
39. Luzhansky JZ, Pierce AB, Hoy JF, Hall AJ. Leber's hereditary optic neuropathy in the setting of nucleoside analogue toxicity. AIDS 2001;15:1588–9.
40. Shaikh S, Ta C, Basham AA, Mansour S. Leber hereditary optic neuropathy associated with antiretroviral therapy for human immunodeficiency virus infection. Am J Ophthalmol 2001;131:143–5.
41. Warner JE, Ries KM. Optic neuropathy in a patient with AIDS. J Neuroophthalmol 2001;21:92–4.
42. Mackey DA, Fingert JH, Luzhansky JZ et al. Leber's hereditary optic neuropathy triggered by antiretroviral therapy for human immunodeficiency virus. Eye 2003;17:312–7.
43. Hulgan T, Haas DW, Haines JL et al. Mitochondrial haplogroups and peripheral neuropathy during antiretroviral therapy: an adult AIDS clinical trials group study. AIDS 2005;19: 1341–9.
44. Trifunovic A, Wredenberg A, Falkenberg M et al. Premature ageing in mice expressing defective mitochondrial DNA polymerase. Nature 2004;429:417–23.
45. Boffito M, Kurowski M, Kruse G et al. Atazanavir enhances saquinavir hard-gel concentrations in a ritonavir-boosted once-daily regimen. AIDS 2004;18:1291–7.
46. Hammer SM, Squires KE, Hughes MD et al. A controlled trial of two nucleoside analogues plus indinavir in persons with human immunodeficiency virus infection and CD4 cell counts of 200 per cubic millimeter or less. AIDS Clinical Trials Group 320 Study Team. N Engl J Med 1997;337:725–33.
47. Briz O, Serrano MA, MacIas RI, Gonzalez-Gallego J, Marin JJ. Role of organic anion-transporting polypeptides, OATP-A, OATP-C and OATP-8, in the human placenta-maternal liver tandem excretory pathway for foetal bilirubin. Biochem J 2003;371:897–905.
48. Cui Y, Konig J, Leier I, Buchholz U, Keppler D. Hepatic uptake of bilirubin and its conjugates by the human organic anion transporter SLC21A6. J Biol Chem 2001;276:9626–30.
49. Konig J, Cui Y, Nies AT, Keppler D. A novel human organic anion transporting polypeptide localized to the basolateral hepatocyte membrane. Am J Physiol Gastrointest Liver Physiol 2000;278:G156-G164.
50. Tukey RH, Strassburg CP. Human UDP-glucuronosyltransferases: metabolism, expression, and disease. Annu Rev Pharmacol Toxicol 2000;40:581–616.
51. Bosma PJ, Chowdhury JR, Bakker C et al. The genetic basis of the reduced expression of bilirubin UDP-glucuronosyltransferase 1 in Gilbert's syndrome. N Engl J Med 1995;333:1171–5.
52. Monaghan G, Ryan M, Seddon R, Hume R, Burchell B. Genetic variation in bilirubin UPD-glucuronosyltransferase gene promoter and Gilbert's syndrome. Lancet 1996;347:578–81.
53. Zucker SD, Qin X, Rouster SD et al. Mechanism of indinavir-induced hyperbilirubinemia. Proc Natl Acad Sci U S A 2001;98:12671–6.
54. Rotger M, Taffe P, Bleiber G et al. Gilbert syndrome and the development of antiretroviral therapy-associated hyperbilirubinemia. J Infect Dis 2005;192:1381–6.
55. Kameyama Y, Yamashita K, Kobayashi K, Hosokawa M, Chiba K. Functional characterization of SLCO1B1 (OATP-C) variants, SLCO1B1*5, SLCO1B1*15 and SLCO1B1*15+C1007G, by using transient expression systems of HeLa and HEK293 cells. Pharmacogenet Genomics 2005;15:513–22.
56. Nozawa T, Minami H, Sugiura S, Tsuji A, Tamai I. Role of organic anion transporter OATP1B1 (OATP-C) in hepatic uptake of irinotecan and its active metabolite, 7-ethyl-10-hydroxycamptothecin: in vitro evidence and effect of single nucleotide polymorphisms. Drug Metab Dispos 2005;33:434–9.
57. Tirona RG, Leake BF, Merino G, Kim RB. Polymorphisms in OATP-C: identification of multiple allelic variants associated with altered transport activity among European- and African-Americans. J Biol Chem 2001;276:35669–75.
58. Mwinyi J, Johne A, Bauer S, Roots I, Gerloff T. Evidence for inverse effects of OATP-C (SLC21A6) 5 and 1b haplotypes on pravastatin kinetics. Clin Pharmacol Ther 2004; 75:415–21.

59. Niemi M, Schaeffeler E, Lang T et al. High plasma pravastatin concentrations are associated with single nucleotide polymorphisms and haplotypes of organic anion transporting polypeptide-C (OATP-C, SLCO1B1). Pharmacogenetics 2004;14:429–40.
60. Niemi M, Backman JT, Kajosaari LI et al. Polymorphic organic anion transporting polypeptide 1B1 is a major determinant of repaglinide pharmacokinetics. Clin Pharmacol Ther 2005; 77:468–78.
61. Niemi M, Kivisto KT, Hofmann U, Schwab M, Eichelbaum M, Fromm MF. Fexofenadine pharmacokinetics are associated with a polymorphism of the SLCO1B1 gene (encoding OATP1B1). Br J Clin Pharmacol 2005;59:602–4.
62. Nishizato Y, Ieiri I, Suzuki H et al. Polymorphisms of OATP-C (SLC21A6) and OAT3 (SLC22A8) genes: consequences for pravastatin pharmacokinetics. Clin Pharmacol Ther 2003;73:554–65.
63. Rotger, M., Taffe, P., Bleiber, G., Günthard, H. F., Furrer, H., Vernazza, P., Drechsler, H., Bernasconi, E., Rickenbach, M., and Telenti, A. Contribution of genetic polymorphisms in UGT1A1 and SCLO1B1 to the development of antiretroviral therapy assocîated hyperbilirubinemia. 45th International Conference on Antimicrobial Agents and Chemotherapy, Washington. 2005.
64. Haas DW, Ribaudo HJ, Kim RB et al. Pharmacogenetics of efavirenz and central nervous system side effects: an Adult AIDS Clinical Trials Group study. AIDS 2004;18:2391–400.
65. Adkins JC, Noble S. Efavirenz. Drugs 1998;56:1055–64.
66. Lochet P, Peyriere H, Lotthe A, Mauboussin JM, Delmas B, Reynes J. Long-term assessment of neuropsychiatric adverse reactions associated with efavirenz. HIV Med 2003;4:62–6.
67. Dassopoulos T, Ehrenpreis ED. Acute pancreatitis in human immunodeficiency virus-infected patients: a review. Am J Med 1999;107:78–84.
68. Sharer N, Schwarz M, Malone G et al. Mutations of the cystic fibrosis gene in patients with chronic pancreatitis. N Engl J Med 1998;339:645–52.
69. Cohn JA, Friedman KJ, Noone PG, Knowles MR, Silverman LM, Jowell PS. Relation between mutations of the cystic fibrosis gene and idiopathic pancreatitis. N Engl J Med 1998;339:653–8.
70. Pfutzer RH, Barmada MM, Brunskill AP et al. SPINK1/PSTI polymorphisms act as disease modifiers in familial and idiopathic chronic pancreatitis. Gastroenterology 2000;119:615–23.
71. Frossard JL, Morris MA, Wonkam A et al. The role of CFTR and SPINK-1 mutations in pancreatic disorders in HIV-positive patients: a case control study. AIDS 2004;18:1521–7.
72. Telenti A, Bleiber G. Host genetics of HIV-1 susceptibility. Future Virol 2006;1:55–70.
73. Carrington M, Nelson G, O'Brien SJ. Considering genetic profiles in functional studies of immune responsiveness to HIV-1. Immunol Lett 2001;79:131–40.
74. Carrington M, O'Brien SJ. The influence of HLA genotype on AIDS. Annu Rev Med 2003;54:535–51.
75. Martin MP, Gao X, Lee JH et al. Epistatic interaction between KIR3DS1 and HLA-B delays the progression to AIDS. Nat Genet 2002;31:429–34.
76. Dean M, Carrington M, Winkler C et al. Genetic restriction of HIV-1 infection and progression to AIDS by a deletion allele of the CKR5 structural gene. Hemophilia Growth and Development Study, Multicenter AIDS Cohort Study, Multicenter Hemophilia Cohort Study, San Francisco City Cohort, ALIVE Study. Science 1996;273:1856–62.
77. Samson M, Libert F, Doranz BJ et al. Resistance to HIV-1 infection in caucasian individuals bearing mutant alleles of the CCR-5 chemokine receptor gene. Nature 1996;382:722–5.
78. Huang Y, Paxton WA, Wolinsky SM et al. The role of a mutant CCR5 allele in HIV-1 transmission and disease progression. Nat Med 1996;2:1240–3.
79. Gonzalez E, Bamshad M, Sato N et al. Race-specific HIV-1 disease-modifying effects associated with CCR5 haplotypes. Proc Natl Acad Sci U S A 1999;96:12004–9.
80. Mummidi S, Ahuja SS, Gonzalez E et al. Genealogy of the CCR5 locus and chemokine system gene variants associated with altered rates of HIV-1 disease progression. Nat Med 1998;4:786–93.
81. Smith MW, Dean M, Carrington M et al. Contrasting genetic influence of CCR2 and CCR5 variants on HIV-1 infection and disease progression. Hemophilia Growth and Development

Study (HGDS), Multicenter AIDS Cohort Study (MACS), Multicenter Hemophilia Cohort Study (MHCS), San Francisco City Cohort (SFCC), ALIVE Study. Science 1997;277:959–65.
82. Gonzalez E, Kulkarni H, Bolivar H et al. The Influence of CCL3L1 Gene-Containing Segmental Duplications on HIV-1/AIDS Susceptibility. Science 2005;307:1434–40.
83. Bleiber G, May M, Martinez R et al. Use of a combined ex vivo/in vivo population approach for screening of human genes involved in the human immunodeficiency virus type 1 life cycle for variants influencing disease progression. J Virol 2005;79:12674–80.
84. Telenti A. Host polymorphism in post-entry steps of the HIV-1 life cycle and other genetic variants influencing HIV-1 pathogenesis. Curr Opin HIV/AIDS 2006;1:232–40.
85. Bashirova A, Bleiber G, Hutcheson H et al. Consistent effects of variation in the tumor susceptibility gene 101 on multiple outcomes to HIV-1 exposure. J Virol 2006;80:6757–63.
86. O'Brien SJ, Nelson GW. Human genes that limit AIDS. Nat Genet 2004;36:565–74.
87. Nelson GW, O'Brien SJ. Using mutual information to measure the impact of multiple genetic factors on AIDS. J Acquir Immune Defic Syndr 2006;42:347–54.
88. Evans DM, Cardon LR. Genome-wide association: a promising start to a long race. Trends Genet 2006;22:350–4.
89. Haas DW, Wilkinson GR, Kuritzkes DR et al. A multi-investigator/institutional DNA bank for AIDS-related human genetic studies: AACTG Protocol A5128. HIV Clin Trials 2003;4:287–300.
90. Chen DT, Rosenstein DL, Muthappan P et al. Research with stored biological samples: what do research participants want? Arch Intern Med 2005;165:652–5.
91. Lederman MM, Penn-Nicholson A, Cho M, Mosier D. Biology of CCR5 and its role in HIV infection and treatment. JAMA 2006;296:815–26.
92. Khan IA, Thomas SY, Moretto MM et al. CCR5 is essential for NK cell trafficking and host survival following Toxoplasma gondii infection. PLoS Pathog 2006;2:e49.
93. Glass WG, Lim JK, Cholera R, Pletnev AG, Gao JL, Murphy PM. Chemokine receptor CCR5 promotes leukocyte trafficking to the brain and survival in West Nile virus infection. J Exp Med 2005;202:1087–98.
94. Rahbar R, Murooka TT, Hinek AA et al. Vaccinia virus activation of CCR5 invokes tyrosine phosphorylation signaling events that support virus replication. J Virol 2006;80:7245–59.
95. Floto RA, MacAry PA, Boname JM et al. Dendritic cell stimulation by mycobacterial Hsp70 is mediated through CCR5. Science 2006;314:454–8.
96. Ank N, Petersen K, Malmgaard L, Mogensen SC, Paludan SR. Age-dependent role for CCR5 in antiviral host defense against herpes simplex virus type 2. J Virol 2005;79:9831–41.
97. Machado FS, Koyama NS, Carregaro V et al. CCR5 plays a critical role in the development of myocarditis and host protection in mice infected with Trypanosoma cruzi. J Infect Dis 2005;191:627–36.
98. Belnoue E, Kayibanda M, Deschemin JC et al. CCR5 deficiency decreases susceptibility to experimental cerebral malaria. Blood 2003;101:4253–9.
99. Gardam MA, Keystone EC, Menzies R et al. Anti-tumour necrosis factor agents and tuberculosis risk: mechanisms of action and clinical management. Lancet Infect Dis 2003;3:148–55.
100. Wheeler J, McHale M, Jackson V, Penny M. Assessing theoretical risk and benefit suggested by genetic association studies of CCR5: experience in a drug development programme for maraviroc. Antivir Ther 2007;12:233–45.
101. Glass WG, McDermott DH, Lim JK et al. CCR5 deficiency increases risk of symptomatic West Nile virus infection. J Exp Med 2006;203:35–40.
102. Thio CL, Astemborski J, Bashirova A et al. Genetic protection against HBV conferred by CCR5{Delta}32: evidence that CCR5 contributes to viral persistence. J Virol 2006.
103. Fellay J, Shianna KV, Ge D et al. Identification of major determinants of the host control of HIV-1 through a whole genome association study. Science 2007;317:944–7.
104. Sladek R, Rocheleau G, Rung J et al. A genome-wide association study identifies novel risk loci for type 2 diabetes. Nature 2007;445:881–5.
105. Duerr RH, Taylor KD, Brant SR et al. A genome-wide association study identifies IL23R as an inflammatory bowel disease gene. Science 2006;314:1461–3.
106. Mullighan CG, Goorha S, Radtke I et al. Genome-wide analysis of genetic alterations in acute lymphoblastic leukaemia. Nature 2007;446:758–64.

Chapter 19
Pharmacogenomics and Cardiovascular Drugs

Gérard Siest, Hind Berrahmoune, Jean-Brice Marteau, and Sophie Visvikis-Siest

Contents

Abstract Cardiovascular diseases are a large group of multifactorial pathologies. Thus, it is not surprising that more than 13 classes and many subclasses of drugs have been developed in this field. However, the responses to these drugs differ significantly between patients.
Five groups of genes are involved in these different responses:

1. The genes regulating the pharmacokinetics phase of the drug. Cytochromes P450, 2D6, and C9-C19 are the most frequently involved. However, transporters like ABC families also have to be taken into account.
2. The genes related to the pharmacodynamics phase. The enzymes inhibited by the drugs (angiotensine converting enzyme, HMG CoA reductase) the receptors involved in their actions (β-adrenergic receptors, angiotensine I and II receptors) and the lipoproteins modified in their expression levels in plasma (apolipoprotein E, apolipoprotein B, apolipoprotein CIII, CETP) are also important pharmacogenomic targets.
3. Pathologies and metabolic pathways related to gene polymorphisms from the patients under treatment introduce a third range of pharmacological variability, i.e., inflammation pathway genes.
4. Health and physiological mechanisms (i.e., age, gender, ethnicity, weight) could modify the gene polymorphisms' effects.
5. Finally, genes environmentally sensitive to diet, tobacco, pollutants, etc., are important and interfere in the pharmacogenomic response of many drugs.

Gérard Siest
Inserm, University Henri Poincaré, Nancy, France
Gerard.Siest@pharma.uhp-nancy.fr

N. Cohen (ed.) *Pharmacogenomics and Personalized Medicine*,

The development of new cardiovascular drugs and the survey of some existing ones should take into account some of these polymorphisms in order to adapt the drug dosage to each individual and to avoid drug side effects.

Keywords cardiovascular drugs, cardiovascular diseases, environmental interaction, physiological variability, antihypertensive drugs, lipid lowering drugs, inflammation

Cardiovascular diseases (CVD) are a large group of disorders with varying pathologies. They are in general multifactorial, with environmental components, and can be grouped together under two categories: diseases of the circulatory system, and metabolic disorders. Examples of diseases of the circulatory system include hypertensive disease, hypertensive heart and renal disease, ischemic heart disease, acute myocardial infarction, cardiac dysrhythmias, chronic rheumatic heart disease, cerebrovascular disease, atherosclerosis, arterial embolism and thrombosis, phlebitis and thrombophlebitis, and varicose veins. Examples of metabolic disorders include diabetes mellitus and metabolic syndrome. It is not unexpected that many different classes of drugs are used to treat such a complex group of diseases. Cardiovascular (CV) drug classes include antianginals, antihypertensives, antiarrhythmics, cardiotonics, vasodilators, anticoagulants, antiaggregating agents, antidiabetics, antiinflammatories, and lipid-lowering drugs; these are often further divided into subclasses. As CVD also affect organs and functions other than heart and blood vessels, the list of drugs can be expanded to include thyroid therapies, antismoking agents, contraceptives, and hormonal replacement therapies, all of which affect the functioning of the CV system.

In view of such numerous pathologies and the corresponding drugs, we have proposed a five-step pharmacogenomic approach *(1)* for a new cardiovascular drug, successively taking into account the genes involved in:

- pharmacokinetics (absorption, distribution, metabolism, transport);
- pharmacodynamics (enzyme inhibitors, receptors);
- specific cardiovascular disorders and related metabolic pathways deviations;
- biological variability in gene responses, including their physiological regulation; and
- environmental effects.

However, given the current existing pharmacogenomic tools and the development of the pharmacoproteomic field, a complete strategy needs the integration of gene products measured in laboratory medicine *(2)*.

We will be discussing successively all the five sets of genes able of modifying individual responses to cardiovascular drugs.

1 Pharmacokinetics-Related Genes

A large number of CV drugs are lipophilic and are influenced by the four pharmacokinetic processes: absorption, distribution, metabolism, and elimination. Genes encoding for drug-metabolizing enzymes and, more recently, drug and metabolite transporter genes, are the most extensively characterized genes in the field of pharmacogenetics. Although the enzymes involved in drug metabolism are primarily found in the liver, they are also expressed in other tissues. The large number of environmental chemicals metabolized by these enzymes likely explains why these enzymes have evolved into multigene families with both unique and overlapping substrate specificity.

1.1 Phase I Enzymes: Cytochromes P450

Recent reports estimate that there are ~60 distinct cytochrome P450 (CYP) genes in human (57 functional genes and 58 pseudogenes) *(3)*. An up-to-date list of CYP gene polymorphisms can be obtained online *(85)*. Interestingly, although many of these enzymes have the capacity to metabolize drugs, the majority of CYP-mediated drug metabolism in humans is catalyzed by the CYP enzyme subfamilies CYP3A, CYP2D6, and CYP2C.

CYP1A, CYP2A6, CYP2B6, and CYP2E1 also show a relative importance. The impact of genetic variation in these enzymes on drug metabolism differs among the enzymes. Polymorphic CYP activity is of great interest in the exploration of adverse drug reactions, especially during drug development. Indeed, if a CYP isoform is involved in the metabolism of a new drug candidate, health authorities may request *in vivo* information on its metabolic pathway(s). If genetic variation in metabolism is reported to be of *in vivo* clinical significance, then this would alter the course of drug development *(4)*. A cardiovascular drug, perhexiline, marked the beginning of the pharmacogenetics era, after the death of many patients having a CYP2D6-deficient enzyme.

1.1.1 Cytochrome P450 Isoenzyme 2D6

CYP2D6 is not a major CYP enzyme in terms of quantity in the liver. However, it metabolizes one quarter of all drugs, and many of them are used in the treatment of CVD (Table 19.1). Individuals with genetically determined low or no CYP2D6 enzyme activity are referred to as poor metabolizers, whereas individuals with fully functional enzymes are known as extensive metabolizers. Poor metabolizers display an exaggerated response and may be at greater risk for toxicity if a drug is either principally metabolized by CYP2D6 or presents a narrow therapeutic index. In contrast, some individuals have been observed to display excessive enzyme activity and are known as ultrarapid metabolizers. These ultrarapid metabolizers may not achieve therapeutically active plasma concentrations of certain drugs. The CYP2D6 metabolizer status of an individual can be largely explained by the many different mutations (Table 19.2) that exist in the *CYP2D6* gene. Details can be found in a review by Zanger et al. *(5)*. An individual's metabolizer status can be safely determined using a specific (probe) substrate that has a large therapeutic index; for example, dextromethorphan or debrisoquine for CYP2D6. The phenotyping approach commonly involves

Table 19.1 Major phase I enzymes, phase II enzymes, and transporters implicated in cardiovascular drugs metabolism and transport

Substrates	Enzymes (CYP450 & phase II)	Transporters
Aldosterone antagonists		
Spironolactone		ABCB1
Angiotensin II receptor antagonists		
Candesartan	2C9	
Irbesartan	2C9	
Losartan	3A - 2C9	ABCB1
Valsartan	2C9	
Angiotensin-converting enzyme inhibitors		
Captopril	2D6	OATP, PEPT
Enalapril	3A	OATP, PEPT
Losartan	3A	
Antihypertensives (others)		
Clonidine	2D6	OCT1
Debrisoquine	2D6 –2D7P2 – 2D8P1/P2	ABCB1
Guanoxan	2D6	
Prazosin		ABCB1, ABCG2, OCT1
Reserpine		ABCB1
Spironolactone		ABCB1
Appetite suppressants		
Amphetamine	2D6	
Dexfenfluramine	2D6	
Fenfluramine	2D6	
Antiaggregating		
Clopidogrel	3A	
Dipyridamole		ABCB1
Ticlopidine	2C19	
Antiarrythmics		
Amidarone	3A - 2D6 – 2C8	ABCB1
Disopyramide	3A	
Encainide	2D6	
Flecainide	3A - 2D6	
Lidocaine	1A2 - 2A6 – 3A4 - 2D6	ABCB1
Mexiletine	1A2 - 2D6	
N-Propylajmaline	2D6	
Procainamide	2D6	OCT
Propafenone	1A2 - 3A - 2D6	ABCB1
Quinidine	3A	ABCB1, OATP, OCT
Sparteine	2D6	
Verapamil	3A - 2C8	
Anti-vitamin K		
Acenocoumarol	1A2 - 2C9 – 2C19	
Warfarin	1A2 – 3A - 2C8 – 2C9 – 2C19	
Antidiabetic drugs		
Glimepride	2C9	
Glipizide	2C9	
Glyburide/glibenclamide	3A - 2C9	

(continued)

Table 19.1 (continued)

Substrates	Enzymes (CYP450 & phase II)	Transporters
Nateglinide	3A - 2C9 – 2D6	
Phenformin	2D6	
Repaglinide	3A - 2C8	
Rosiglitazone	2C8 – 2C9	
Tolbutamide	2C8 – 2C9 – 2C19	
Troglitazone	3A - 2C8	
β-Blockers		
Acebutolol		ABCB1
Alprenolol	2D6	
Atenolol		ABCB1
Bisoprolol	3A - 2D6	
Bufuralol	1A2 – 3A – 2C19 - 2D6	
Bunitrolol		ABCB1
Bupranolol	2D6	
Carvedilol	1A2 – 2C9 - 2D6 – 2E1	ABCB1
Celiprolol	3A	ABCB1
Labetalol	2D6	
Metroprol	2C19 - 2D6	ABCB1
Nadolol		ABCB1
Pindolol	2D6	
Propanolol	1A2 – 3A – 2D6- 2C19	ABCB1, OCT2
Talinolol		ABCB1
Timolol	2D6	ABCB1
Calcium channel blockers		
Amlodipine	3A	
Bepridil	3A	ABCB1
Cinnarizine	2D6	
Diltiazem	3A – 2C9 – 2D6	ABCB1
Felodipine	3A	
Flunarizine	2D6	
Isradipine	3A	
Lercanidipine	3A	
Mibefradil	1A2 - 3A – 2D6	ABCB1
Nevirapine	3A	
Nicardipine	3A – 2C9 – 2D6	ABCB1
Nifedipine	3A – 2C9 – 2D6	ABCB1
Niludipine	3A	
Nimodipine	3A - 2D6	
Nisoldipine	3A	
Nitrendipine	3A - 2D6	ABCB1
Perhexiline	2D6	
Verapamil	1A2 - 3A – 2C8	ABCB1, OCT1
Cardiotonics (digitalis)		
Digitoxine	3A	ABCB1
Digoxin	3A	ABCB1, OATP
Contraceptives		
Ethinylesteradiol	3A - 2D6	
Estradiol	3A	
Estrogens	3A	
Progesterone	3A	

(continued)

Table 19.1 (continued)

Substrates	Enzymes (CYP450 & phase II)	Transporters
Corticosteroids		
Dexamethasone	3A	ABCB1
Methylprednisolone	3A	ABCB1
Prednisone	3A	ABCB1
Diuretics		
Amiloride		OCT2
Bumetanide		OAT4
Furosemide	UGT1A8	
Indapamide	3A - 2D6 – 2C9	
Triamterene	Sulfotransferase	OCT2
Tienilic acid	2C9	
Torasemide	2C9	
Lipid-lowering drugs		
Atorvastatin	3A	ABCB1
Cerivastatin	3A - 2C8	
Fluvastatin	2C9	
Lovastatin	3A	ABCB1
Pravastatin	3A	ABCB1, MCT, OATP
Simvastatin	3A	
Rosuvastatin	3A	
Nonsteroidal antiinflammatory drugs		
Aceclofenac	2C9	
Celecoxib	3A4 - 2C9	
Diclofenac	3A4 - 2C8 – 2C9 – 2C19	
Flurbiprofen	2C9	
Ibuprofen	2C9 – 2C19	
Indometacin	2C9 – 2C19	
Lornoxicam	2C9	
Mefenamic acid	2C9	
Meloxicam	3A4 - 2C9	
Naproxen	1A2 - 2C9	
Phenylbutazone	2C9	
Piroxicam	2C9	
Suprofen	2C9	
Tenoxicam	2C9	
Tobacco		
Bupropion (tobacco cessation)	3A - 2C9	
Nicotine	2A6 - 2D6	
Tobacco (polycyclic hydrocarbones)	1A1 - 1A2	
Others		
Caffeine	3A	
Dextrometorphan	2D6	

ABC = ATP-binding cassette transporter; MCT = monocarboxylate transporter; OAT = organic anion transporter; OCT = organic cation transporter; PEPT = dipeptide transporter

Table 19.2 Functional consequences of the CYP2D6 gene mutations

Allele	Nucleotide change	Effect	Predicted enzyme activity
*1	None		Normal
*2ABD	**C-1584G**, C1039T, G1661C, **C2850T**, **G4180C**	**R296C; S486T**	Normal
*3	**2549A del**	**Frameshift**	None
*4ABDJK	C100T, C1039T, G1661C, **G1846A**, C2850T, G4180C	P34S, **Splicing defect**; R296C; S486T	None
*5	**Entire CYP2D6 deleted**	***CYP2D6* deleted**	None
*6ABC	**1707T del**, G1976A, G4180C	**Frameshift**	None
*7	**A2935C**	**H324P**	None
*8	G1661C, **G1758T**, C2850T, G4180C	**Stop codon**	None
*9	**2613–2615delAGA**	**K281del**	Reduced
*10AB	**C100T**, C1039T, G1661C, G4180C	**P34S**; S486T	Reduced
*11	**G883C**, G1661C, C2850T, G4180C	**Splicing defect**; R296C; S486T	None
*14A	C100T, **G1758A**, C2850T, G4180C	P34S; **G169R**; R296C; S486T	None
*14B	G1661C, **G1758A**, C2850T, G4180C	**G169R**; R296C; S486T	Unknown
*15	**T138ins**	**Frameshift**	None
*17	**C1023T**, G1661C, C2850T, G4180C	**T107I**; R296C; S486T	Reduced
*19	G1661C, **2539–2542delAACT**, C2850T, G4180C	**Frameshift**	None
*20	G1661C, **1973insG**, C1978T, T1979C, C2850T, G4180C	**Frameshift**	None
*25	**C3198G**	**R343G**	Unknown
*26	**T3277C**	**I369T**	Unknown
*29	**G1659A**, G1661C, C2850T, **G3183A**, G4180C	**V136M**; R296C; **V338M**; S486T	Reduced
*30	G1661C, **1855–1863ins(TTTCGCCCC) repeat**, C2850T, G4180C	**174_175insFRP**; R296C; S486T	Unknown
*31	G1661C, C2850T, **G4042A**, G4180C	R296C; **R440H**; S486T	Unknown
*35	C-1584G, **G31A**, G1661C, C2850T, G4180C	**V11M**; R296C; S486T	Normal
*36	**C100T**, C1039T, G1661C, G4180C, **gene conversion to CYP2D7 in exon 9**	**P34S**; P469A; T470A; H478S; G479A; F481V; A482S; S486T	Reduced
*40	**C1023T**, G1661C, **1863ins(TTT CGC CCC)2**; C2850T, G4180C	**T107I; 174_175ins(FRP)2**; R296C; S486T	None
*41	**C-1584G**, G1661C, **C2850T**, **G4180C**	R296C; S486T	Reduced
*1XN	Duplicated active *1 genes (n is not determined-range 2–13)		Increased
*2XN	Duplicated active *2 genes (n is not determined-range 2–13)		Increased
*4XN	Duplicated inactive *4 genes (n is not determined)		None

(continued)

Table 19.2 (continued)

Allele	Nucleotide change	Effect	Predicted enzyme activity
*10XN	Duplicated partially active *10 genes (n is not determined)		Reduced
*17XN	Duplicated partially active *17 genes (n is not determined)		Reduced
*35XN	Duplicated active *35 genes (n is not determined)		Increased
*41XN	Duplicated partially active *41 genes (n is not determined)		Reduced

Adapted from Roche AmpliChip CYP450 Test worksheet

the calculation of the urine metabolic ratio, which is the ratio of the unchanged drug to the drug metabolite, and is measured in the urine within a defined time frame following the administration of a single dose of the probe drug. As a practical alternative, genotyping by PCR methods can also be used to predict the metabolizer status, and a specific DNA chip is now on the market (Roche Diagnostics' AmpliChip™ CYP450) (Table 19.2). Genotyping has many advantages over phenotyping and is the preferred approach for metabolizer status assessment, particularly during ongoing therapy due to the risk of drug-drug interactions *(5)*.

1.1.2 Cytochrome P450 2C Subfamily

Members of the CYP2C subfamily of drug-metabolizing enzymes share a high degree of sequence similarity, making it difficult to separate different isoforms, both molecularly and functionally. There is also overlapping substrate specificity among members of the CYP2C family, but CYP2C9 is the isoform expressed in the highest concentration in the human liver and is likely to be responsible for the majority of drug-drug interactions in this subfamily *(6)*. Like CYP2D6, CYP2C enzymes are under the influence of genetic variation. CYP2C9 polymorphisms seem to be able to initiate adverse side reactions with CYP2C9 substrates. Among these allelic variants, *CYP2C9*2* and *CYP2C9*3* have been shown to be responsible for the poor metabolizer phenotype *(7)*. Thus, individuals harboring these polymorphisms, particularly homozygous variant individuals, often require lower doses of drugs, especially compounds with narrow therapeutic index, such as warfarin and other CYP2C9 substrates. In the case of warfarin, individualization of the therapy is a standard procedure, but the initial dose can be better predicted by knowing the *CYP2C9* genotype before initiating treatment. For drugs with large therapeutic indices, such as propranolol, genetic polymorphisms in *CYP2C9* are of negligible clinical consequence. Of the other polymorphic CYP2C family enzymes, CYP2C19 contributes minimally to the metabolism of some CV drugs, such as metoprolol or warfarin, and CYP2C8 is primarily important in the metabolism of some antidiabetic drugs (Table 19.1) that can have indirect consequences for the CV system.

1.1.3 Cytochrome P450 3A Subfamily

CYP3A enzymes metabolize almost 50% of all drugs on the market. As such, they are often implicated in adverse drug reactions or drug-drug interactions. The most clinically relevant occurrence with CYP3A is inhibition by drugs or dietary components *(8)*. In this chapter CYP3A4 is considered to be the main enzyme contributing to total CYP3A activity for CV drugs in most individuals (Table 19.1). Although there is interindividual variability in the expression of the CYP3A4 and CYP3A5, and variant alleles for these isozymes have been described, variability in expression is not quantitatively important *(4)*. But in the revue of Schmitz and Langhmann *(9)*, differential effects of CYP3A4 and CYP3A5 are described. Interindividual variation in expression is more likely to be multifactorial and multiallelic, and it may be linked to transcription factors.

1.1.4 Other Cytochrome P450s

Some minor polymorphic CYP enzymes, such as CYP1A1, CYP2A6, and CYP2B6, are also responsible for the metabolism of CV drugs. Genetic variation in CYP2A6 has been reported to be responsible in decreased enzyme activity and drug metabolism; for example, nicotine or coumarin metabolism (Table 19.1).

1.2 Phase II Enzymes

Genetic polymorphisms have been described in many phase II drug-metabolizing enzymes. However, they seem to be less important to the pharmacogenomics of CV drugs. Nevertheless, some clinical consequences of phase II enzyme polymorphism have been reported. For example, procainamide acetylation is affected by the N-acetyltransferase 2 (NAT-2) metabolizer status. Slow acetylators have been proposed to be more susceptible to develop a drug-induced lupus-like syndrome than rapid acetylators. However, this remains controversial *(10)*. For the UDP-glucuronosyl-transferases (UGTs), only one drug, tranilast (which was developed for stent reaction stabilization but failed to reach the market), revealed a genetically influenced clinical outcome. Individuals who are (TA)7 homozygous for the *UGT1A1* gene have been shown to have higher serum bilirubin levels when compared with individuals who carry the (TA)6 allele. The (TA)7 homozygous genotype is associated with Gilbert's syndrome and with an increased risk of tranilast-induced hyperbilirubinemia, which occurs in ~2% of Caucasian patients, but is less frequent in Asian patients *(11)*. Genetic polymorphisms in sulfotransferase enzymes have not been appreciably investigated *(12)*. Glutathione *S*-transferases are involved in tobacco-related metabolite detoxification, and this seems to have CV consequences *(1)*.

1.3 Phase III Drug Transporters

Drug metabolism is not the sole determinant of drug pharmacokinetics. Drug transporter systems, which can be subdivided into uptake and efflux systems, have received increased attention for their role in determining drug disposition, intestinal absorption, and renal drug elimination. There are five classes of uptake carrier systems:

- organic anion transporters (OATPs),
- organic cation transporters (OCTs),
- dipeptide transporters (PEPTs),
- nucleoside transporters (CNTs), and
- monocarboxylate transporters (MCTs).

For efflux of drugs and metabolites, the most studied is the ATP-binding cassette (ABC) transporter. The ABC superfamily can be divided into seven subfamilies. The *ABCB1* gene (also named multi-drug resistance 1 [*MDR1*]), which is responsible for resistance of cancerous cells to cytotoxic drugs via a drug efflux mechanism, is a member of the ABC-B subfamily of transporters. This gene encodes for the major drug transporter P-glycoprotein (P-gp), which is expressed in the gut, kidneys, brain, liver, and other organs. P-gp transports diverse drugs across renal and intestinal cells, thus playing a role in the distribution and elimination processes. Many drugs have been shown to be substrates, inducers, or inhibitors of drug transporters (Table 19.1). Some drugs are both substrates and inhibitors of P-gp, while other drugs are only inhibitors (e.g., nifedipine) or substrates (e.g., digoxin). CYP3A and P-gp have many substrates (e.g., digoxin) and modulators (e.g., the inhibitor verapamil) in common. Consequently, this enzyme family and transporters are often considered in tandem. In some cases, their effects on pharmacokinetics can be complementary *(13)*. Notably, mibefradil, a calcium channel inhibitor, is both a substrate and an inhibitor of both CYP3A and P-gp. It is not surprising that this drug was withdrawn from the market due to serious adverse effects. Altered P-gp expression has been associated with genetic polymorphisms and altered drug exposure. Specifically, the polymorphism 3435C/T in the *ABCB1* gene has been associated with reduced intestinal expression of P-gp and a corresponding exposure to digoxin. Patients carrying this genetic polymorphism may require the lowest doses of CV drugs that are substrates of P-gp *(1)*. Further characterization of this gene is required. It is worthwhile to mention that endogenous substances like cholesterol, or endogenous-like substances, such as phytoestrogens, are also transported by these systems. Finally, a large study on 2735 individuals on statin therapy (half on atorvastatin, and the other half devided among fluvastatin, lovastatin, pravastatin, and simvastatin) showed an effect of the *ABCB1* 5893A polymorphism: a differential 3% response for lowering LDL-cholesterol *(14)*.

In summary, it is necessary, as reported in Table 19.1, to determine simultaneously the polymorphisms of cytochromes P450 and transporters.

2 Pharmacodynamics-Related Genes

In the context of pharmacogenomics, the evaluation of variations in gene sequence of pharmacological targets is a task important to achieve. There are several pharmacological targets, including receptors, enzymes, ion channels, lipoproteins, coagulation factors, and signal transduction pathways. They are localized or expressed differently in tissues and cells. These targets exhibit genetic variability that can, for example, alter the binding affinity of a drug or its metabolites, and thus modulate drug response. For CV drugs, the main described polymorphisms influencing pharmacodynamics are in:

- α-adducin (*ADD1*) (Gly460Trp),
- angiotensinogen (*AGT*) (Met235Thr),
- angiotensin-II receptor type 1 (*AGTR1*) (*A1166C*),
- angiotensin-converting enzyme (*ACE*) (insertion/deletion [*I/D*]),
- apolipoprotein E (*APOE*) (*ε2/ε4*),
- β2-Adrenoreceptor (*ADRB2*) (Arg16Gly),
- bradykinin receptor B2 (*BDKRB2*) (C-58T),
- cholesteryl ester transfer protein (*CETP*) (*B1/B2*),
- factor V Leiden (*F5*) (Arg506Gln),
- hepatic lipase (*LIPC*) (C-514T),
- HMG CoA reductase (*HMGCR*) (SNPs 12 and 29),
- glycoprotein IIIa (*ITGB3*) (PlA*1/A2*), and
- potassium channel (*KCNE2*) (T8 in MiRP1).

The impact of genetic polymorphisms in these genes has been reviewed in detail elsewhere *(15–17)* (Table 19.3).

We will report successively examples of antiaggregants, anticoagulants, lipid lowering, antihypertensive, and antidiabetic drugs.

2.1 Antiaggregants

2.1.1 Aspirin

Platelets play an important role in acute thrombotic events, including myocardial infarction. This is supported by the efficacy of antiplatelet therapy in preventing and reducing mortality and morbidity in large randomized trials. Antiplatelet therapy is based on the inhibition of several pathways of platelet aggregation, such as thromboxane A2 production, ADP activation, or GPIIb/IIIa fibrinogen binding. Aspirin is widely used as an antiplatelet drug to prevent arterial thrombosis events. This drug blocks the thromboxane A2 pathway through the ireversible acetylation of platelet cyclooxygenase-1 (COX-1) *(1)*. However, 10% of cardiac patients are resistant to aspirin, as determined by measures of platelet aggregation. Similar findings

Table 19.3 Polymorphic genes influencing pharmacodynamic actions of cardiovascular drugs

Gene (polymorphism)	Name	Example	Clinical consequences
ADRB2 (Arg16Gly)	B2-Adenoreceptor	Albuterol, Isoproterenol	Variable effects in treatment of heart failure
KCNE2 (T8A in MiRO1)	Potassium channel	Sulfamethoxazole, trimethoprim	Drug-induced long QT syndrome in carriers of the variant
α-Adducin (Gly460Trp)	α-Adducin	Hydrochlorothiazide	Greater reduction in blood pressure in response to salt restriction and to HCT treatment in 460Gly/Trp carriers
CETP (B1/B2)	Cholesteryl ester transfer protein	Pravastatin	Slowing of coronary atherosclerosis progression by pravastatin in B1B1 carriers only
APOE (E2/E4)	Apolipoprotein E	Statins, HRT, vitamin K	Differential decrease in cholesterol or apolipoprotein modulation
ACE (I/D)	Angiotensin-I-converting enzyme	Hydrochlorothiazide, enalaprilat	Greater and longer drug response in ACE II allele carriers
GPIIIa (PlA1/A2)	Glycoprotein IIIa	Antiplatelet drugs (aspirin, abciximab)	Drug response lower in PlA2 carriers
Factor V Leiden (Arg506Gln)	Factor V	Estrogen, oral contraceptives	Increased venous thromboenbolism risk
AGT (Met235Thr)	Angiotensinogen	Antihypertensive drugs	Reduction of blood pressure and decrease in left ventricular mass with antihypertensive treatment
AGTR1 (A1166C)	Angiotensin-II receptor type 1	Angiotensin-II receptor antagonists	Increase arterial responsiveness to angiotensin II in ischemic heart disease and inreased aortic stiffness in hypertension
BDKRB2 (C-58T)	Bradykinin receptor B2	ACE inhibitors	ACE inhibitor-related cough
LIPC (C-514T)	Hepatic lipase	Statins	Influences serial changes in HDL cholesterol levels
HMGCR (SNPs 12 and 29)	3-hydroxy-3-methylglutaryl -coenzyme A reductase	Pravastatin	Smaller reduction in total cholesterol and LDL cholesterol

D = deletion, HCT = Hydrochlorothiazide; HDL = high-density-lipoprotein; HRT = hormone replacement therapy; I = insertion; LDL = low-density lipoprotein; MiRP1 = MinK-related peptide 1

have also been observed in stroke patients receiving aspirin therapy. The *COX1* polymorphisms don't seem to play a role in "aspirin resistance" *(18)*.

Moreover, the PlA2 polymorphism in the gene encoding the GPIIIa portion of GPIIb/IIIa (a receptor for fibrinogen), *ITGB3,* increases platelet aggregation, and was described as a risk factor for patients with acute coronary disease who initially received aspirin, among other therapies. It was shown that the inhibition of the PlA*1/A2* platelet with aspirin was greater than with the PlA*1/A1*, and bleeding time both pre- and post-treatment was associated with the PlA*1/A2* polymorphism, with shorter bleeding times being reported in carriers of the PlA*2* allele. The mechanism(s) by which genetic variation in *ITGB3* influences the anticoagulant effect of aspirin remain(s) to be elucidated *(1)*. However, it is known that thromboxane A2 induces the expression of the high-affinity receptor molecule (GPIIb/IIIa) for fibrinogen on the surface of platelets. Wheeler et al. have studied the antiplatelet effect of abciximab (a Fab fragment of a monoclonal antibody antagonist of GPIIb/IIIa) in association with the PlA*2* polymorphism. They found that PlA*1/A2* platelets were less completely inhibited with abciximab than PlA*1/A1* *(19)*. It was also reported that orbofiban, another GPIIb/IIIa antagonist, increased bleeding in a dose-dependent manner in PlA2 noncarriers, but did not increase bleeding events in PlA2 carriers *(20)*. Moreover, Feng et al. *(21)* reported an interaction between the PlA genotype and fibrinogen levels on platelet aggregability. This group showed increased fibrinogen levels only in the PlA*1/A1* genotype and suggested that plasma fibrinogen levels might modulate the platelet reactivity associated with the PlA polymorphism. Finally, the superior binding ability of fibrinogen to the PlA*2* variant receptor upon stimulation of platelets with ADP *(22)* suggests that therapies (including aspirin and a thienopyridine—either ticlopidine or clopidogrel) may be more effective in PlA*2* subjects, particularly since the thienopyridines clopidogrel and ticlopidine block the ADP purinoceptor subtype P2Y12 by acting on the adenylyl cyclase pathway of this receptor.

2.2 *Anticoagulants*

Warfarin, a coumarin anticoagulant, is used worldwide for the treatment and prevention of thromboembolic disease. Warfarin acts as a vitamin K antagonist, by inhibiting the regeneration of reduced vitamin K, an essential cofactor for the clotting cascade. The target enzyme for warfarin, vitamin K epoxide reductase complex 1 (VKORC1), catalyzes the rate-limiting step of the vitamin K cycle. It is now well established that common polymorphisms in regulatory regions of the *VKORC1* gene correlate strongly with warfarin response across the normal dosing range. In Caucasian and Asian populations, the *VKORC1* genotype predicts 25% of the variability in warfarin dose *(23)*.

2.3 *Lipid-Lowering Drugs*

2.3.1 Statins

An excellent example of the large range of drug responses induced by statins (or 3-hydroxy-3-methyl-glutaryl coenzyme A reductase [HMG CoA reductase] inhibitors) that can be found in individuals is given by the results of the study of Pedra-Botet et al. *(24)*. Their study investigated 328 men and women who participated in a multicentric, double-blind clinical trial and were treated by atorvastatin at the dosage of 10 mg/day. The majority of individuals presented a mean percentage change in low-density lipoprotein (LDL)-cholesterol, triglycerides, and high-density lipoprotein (HDL)-cholesterol relatively consistently. However, several patients did not respond or had an increase in LDL-cholesterol. The broad range of response obtained is a good example of the need for personalized therapy. Genetics' contribution to the variability of drug disposition and effects is estimated to 20–95% *(25)*. For pharmacokinetics, *CYP3A1*, *CYPC2D6*, *CYP2C9*, *ABCB1*, and *ABC* polymorphisms could explain part of this variability *(9)*.

When considering pharmacodynamics targets, two major systems can be assessed, namely specific target genes and pleiotropic target genes.

2.3.1.1 Specific Target Genes

By the term *specific target genes*, we refer to the genes which belong either to the drug's mechanism of action or, more generally, to the metabolic pathway aimed at by the drug. Therefore, in our examples, we will consider target genes of hypolipemic drugs, and more specifically, target genes of statins. Here we deal with genes of lipid pathways implicated directly/indirectly in the mechanism of action of statins. A large list of other genes was described recently *(9)* (Table 19.4).

- **APOE**

Detailed information on *APOE* and its pharmacogenomics can be found in more specific reviews *(15, 26)*. The *APOE* genotype appears to be the single most important genotype influencing the LDL-cholesterol-lowering response to statins. In the longitudinal Scandinavian Simvastatin Survival Study (4S), which investigated data from myocardial infarction survivors, the mortality risk ratio of 1.8 in carriers of the *APOE* ε4 allele was more appreciably reduced with simvastatin treatment than in noncarriers *(27)*. The identification of particular subgroups, such as these *APOE* ε4 coronary patients, may eventually allow for tailored statin therapy. Another genetic polymorphism of the *APOE* gene, *-491A/T*, has been found to modulate the response of atorvastatin and bezafibrate in patients suffering from combined hyperlipidemia *(28)*.

- **CETP**

In a pharmacogenetic study led by the Regression Growth Evaluation Statin Study (REGRESS) group, administration of pravastatin therapy was found to attenuate the progression of coronary atherosclerosis in *CETP B1B1* genotype subjects, but not in *B2B2* genotype subjects. A reduction in CV events by statins was also shown to be substantially enhanced by the presence of the *B2* allele *(29)*. The *Taq*IB and A629C genetic variants of the *CETP* gene appeared to modify the effect of atorvastatin on HDL-cholesterol elevation, with a better response to the treatment observed in *B1B1* and *CC* individuals *(30)*.

Table 19.4 Candidate genes and their respective encoded proteins for an integrative study of the pharmacogenomics of statins

HUGO gene nomenclature of **candidate genes involved in the lipid pathway** (cholesterol synthesis, absorption, transport, etc.) that may affect hypolipemic drugs' efficacy by modifying lipid concentration regulation
ABCA1 (ATB-binding cassette transporter A1)
ABCG8 (ATB-binding cassette transporter G8)
ACAT/ACAT1 (mitochondrial acetyl-CoA acetyltransferase)
APOA1 (apolipoprotein A-I)
APOA2 (apolipoprotein A-II)
APOC3 (apolipoprotein A-III)
APOA4 (apolipoprotein A-IV)
APOA1-C3-A4 cluster
APOA5 (apolipoprotein A-V)
APOB (apolipoprotein B)
APOE (apolipoprotein E)
CETP (cholesteryl ester transfer protein)
CYP7A1 (cholesterol 7α hydroxylase)
EL (endothelial lipase)
FABPL/FABP1 (liver fatty acid-binding protein)
FATP (fatty acid transport protein)
FDFT1 (farnesyldiphosphate farnesyltransferase 1, squalene synthase)
HL/LIPC/LIPH (hepatic triglyceride lipase)
HMGCR (3-hydroxy-3-methylglutaryl coenzyme A reductase)
INSIG1 (insulin-induced gene 1)
INSIG2 (insulin-induced gene 2)
LCAT (lecithin cholesterol acyltransferase)
LDLR (LDL receptor)
LEPR (leptin receptor)
Lp(a) (lipoprotein (a))
LPL (lipoprotein lipase)
MTP (microsomial triglyceride transfer protein)
PON1 (paraoxonase 1)
PPARA (peroxisome proliferator-activated receptor alpha)
PPARD (peroxisome proliferator-activated receptor delta)
PPARG (peroxisome proliferator-activated receptor gamma)
S1P (site-1 protease)
S2P (site-2 protease)
SCAP (SREBP cleavage activating protein)
SRBP1 (sterol regulatory element-binding protein 1)
SRBP2 (sterol regulatory element-binding protein 2)
SCARB1 (scavenger receptor class B, member 1)
Candidate genes not involved in the lipid pathway
ACE (angiotensin-converting enzyme)
FBG (beta fibrinogen)
MMP3/STMY1 (Stromelysin 1)
GPIIIA (glycoprotein III A)
Cd36/GP IIIb (Cd36 antigen, glycoprotein 3b, fatty acid translocase)
ESR1 (estrogen receptor alpha)
IL6 (interleukin 6)
IL1B (interleukin 1B)
TLR4 (Toll-like receptor 4)
F XII (factor XII)
eNOS (endothelial nitric oxide synthase)

• HMGCR

Two common and tightly linked SNPs in the 3-hydroxy-3-methyl-glutaryl coenzyme A reductase gene (*HMGCR*) (a A > T substitution at position 74726928 and a T > G substitution at position 74739571) were related to the response to pravastatin treatment *(31)*. Individuals with a single copy of the minor allele of these SNPs had their overall efficacy for modifying total cholesterol concentration reduced by 22%. These effects were largely due to differences in LDL cholesterol: individuals heterozygous for the SNP experienced approximately 19% less LDL-cholesterol reduction after pravastatin treatment. On the contrary, no significant difference was found between genotypes concerning the change in HDL-cholesterol with pravastatin. The differences observed in total cholesterol reduction by genotype were also true when studying men and women separately, even if these were more significant in men.

Among 43 SNPs in 16 genes, Thompson et al. *(14)*, aside from ABCB1 polymorphisms, found a significant effect only for ApoE2. Carriers of the rare allele who took atorvastatin lowered their LDL-cholesterol by 3.5% more than those homozygous for the common allele.

Finally, the polymorphisms of the transcription factors, e.g., PPARs *(32)*, should be studied in more detail for statin response.

2.3.1.2 Pleiotropic Target Genes

These genes, which concern other metabolic pathways, have generally been proposed previously to be candidates for cardiovascular diseases. The pleiotropic genes, variations of which have been studied with statins, are for example the angiotensin-converting enzyme (*ACE*) gene, the β-fibrinogen (*FGB*) gene, the glycoprotein IIIa (*ITGB3*) gene, the stromelysin-1 (*MMP3*) gene, the *CD36* gene, and the estrogen receptor alpha (*ESR1*) gene *(9)*.

This last gene is a good example of the pleiotropic target genes that can alter the lipid response to statin. The *ESR1 Pvu*II(–) *Xba*I(+) haplotype was significantly and independently associated with a greater HDL-cholesterol raising in women, but not in men, in 338 hypercholesterolemic patients treated by atorvastatin. Thus, the estrogen receptor-mediated pathway may play a role in HDL-cholesterol response to statin treatment *(33)*.

2.3.2 Fibrates

Fibrates, another class of lipid-lowering drugs, produce a stronger reduction in triglyceride levels and more efficiently increase HDL-cholesterol, which may be of equal importance for the prevention of CVD in patient subsets.

Concerning the common *APOE* gene polymorphisms, the response to probucol in familial hypercholesterolemic patients was first reported stronger in ε4 carriers. However, ε2 patients seem to be better responders to gemfibrozil or bezafibrate, two drugs of the fibrates family. In contradiction, two independent studies showed that ε4 carriers exhibited the strongest response to gemfibrozil, or that the *APOE* genotype did not at all influence the response to the same drug. In addition, it was observed that the relationship between *APOE* genotype and gemfibrozil response depends on the type of hyperlipoproteinemia under scrutiny *(26)*.

Brousseau ME et al. *(34)* explored the role of *LPL* variants in coronary heart diseases risk, and examined their associations with plasma lipid and lipoprotein levels, in response to gemfibrozil therapy. They found that carriers of the *LPL* N9 allele had significantly higher plasma concentrations of small, dense LDL during gemfibrozil therapy than did noncarriers. This is in contrast to baseline values, in which significant differences in LDL subclass levels were not observed among the genotypes. Thus, carriers of the *LPL* N9 allele experienced an increase in small, dense LDL in response to gemfibrozil, whereas noncarriers experienced a decrease.

For fibrates, PPARs transcription factors are very important as specific genes intervening in this class of drugs: *PPARA* Leu162Val differentiates the HDL2C response to gemfibrozil, while *PPARA* Intron 7G>C differentiates triglyceride response to fenofibrate.

2.4 Antihypertensive Drugs

Major pharmacogenetic studies involving hypertensive drugs are well described in the review written by Arnett DK et al. *(35)*. An up-to-date list of the linked polymorphisms can be obtained online *(87)*.

2.4.1 The Renin-Angiotensin System

Tremendous efforts have been made to understand the renin-angiotensin system (RAS) and its role in the control of blood pressure and sodium balance. Genetic variations corresponding to this system were shown to be associated with a tendency to high blood pressure. These observations make the RAS genes the subject of intense investigation, and they represent a major target for antihypertensive drugs, mainly represented by angiotensin receptor blockers (ARBs), vasopeptidase inhibitors (VPIs), and beta adrenoceptor blockers.

2.4.1.1 Angiotensin Converting Enzyme Inhibitors

The *ACE* insertion/deletion (I/D) polymorphism is one of the most famous polymorphisms of the RAS known that is linked to hypertension. The deletion allele of the polymorphism is strongly associated with an increased level of circulating ACE; and serum ACE activity has been recently correlated with measured adherence with ACE inhibitor treatment in congestive heart failure, suggesting that more investigations should be done in other diseases, such as hypertension *(2)*.

As with the ACE locus, several publications aim to predict patient response to antihypertensive drugs using genetic polymorphisms at the angiotensinogen locus (*AGT*). Carriers of the T allele genotyped for the angiotensinogen Met235Thr variation tend to have higher plasma levels of angiotensinogen *(2)*. The association of the Met235Thr polymorphism and blood pressure response to antihypertensives is confused. It seems that the Met235Thr variant may be important as a predictor of patient response to ACE inhibitor therapy *(36)*, illustrating the potential use of SNP genotyping as a pharmacogenetic tool in antihypertensive treatment. However, a meta-analysis of more than 45,000 subjects *(37)* revealed that genotype did not predict plasma angiotensinogen levels in Asian and black subjects, hypertension in black subjects, or systolic or diastolic blood pressure in either ethnic group. Measurements of AGT levels and genotyping of *AGT polymorphisms* are highly dependent on ethnicity.

In conclusion, interest in individual genotyping for *AGT* polymorphisms to predict blood pressure response is clear; however, which *AGT* polymorphism could be taken into consideration is unclear, particularly since the association of angiotensinogen gene haplotypes with hypertension is discussed *(38, 39)*.

2.4.1.2 Angiotensin-Receptor Blockers (ARBs) or Sartans

Angiotensin receptor blockers (ARBs) provide a complete and specific suppression of the renin-angiotensin-aldosterone system. ARBs decrease blood pressure by blocking the binding of Angiotensin II (Ang II) to the angiotensin type I (AT_1) receptor, independent of the pathway of Ang II generation *(40)*. In addition, ARB administration indirectly activates the AT_2 receptor by blocking feedback inhibition of renin release and shunting the angiotensin II generated from AT1 to AT2. ARBs have already proven to be successful treatments for hypertension and heart failure. The first angiotensin receptor blocker to be approved in the United States for the treatment of heart failure was valsartan. At present, many ARBs are available.

The A1166C polymorphism of the angiotensin II type I receptor (*AT1R*) gene was investigated in relation with AT1R blockade. Blood pressure responses to an active metabolite of losartan were significantly blunted in CC genotype patients compared to patients with the AA genotype *(41)*, suggesting that hemodynamic responses to AT1R blockade depend in part on this polymorphism. The relationship between the *AT1R* A1166C polymorphism and the therapeutic response to losartan was also supported by Sookoian et al. *(42)* in patients with cirrhosis and portal hypertension. Although more investigations are needed, present results could suggest that genetic testing may be used as a predictive factor of response to losartan.

2.4.1.3 Renin Inhibitors

Renin is a protease that is synthesized by the kidney and splits angiotensinogen to produce the decapeptide angiotensin I. Overexpression of renin and its metabolic products predisposes individuals to develop hypertension and related target organ damage. In this regard, efforts have been made to produce renin inhibitors for clinical use. Old peptidic and peptidomimetic renin inhibitors had problems with oral bioavailability and high costs of synthesis. Fortunately, recent work has led to the synthesis of a potent nonpeptidic inhibitor of renin, aliskiren (SPP-100), which has acceptable oral bioavailability *(43)*, and which has been shown in early trials to be similar in effectiveness and tolerability to losartan *(44)* and irbesartan *(45)*. Aliskiren seems to offer the prospect of highly effective RAS inhibition for the treatment of hypertension and could be a promising drug. However, the lack of pharmacogenetic studies investigating aliskiren effects in carriers of the most prominent renin polymorphism (Arg387→term) requires further attention, although this polymorphism failed to predict BP response to 25 mg-hydrochlorothiazide diuretics *(46)*.

2.4.2 Aldosterone Antagonists

The prevalence of primary aldosteronism is less than 2% within the hypertensive population and is characterized by an excess production of the normal adrenal hormone, aldosterone, low serum potassium, and also a suppressed plasma renin. Tests looking at other adrenal steroid hormones can be very useful, as well as tests looking for the normal physiologic changes in hormones in the morning and evening, and responses to sodium challenge or sodium restriction. Body sodium has been established to change with age in hypertensive patients and to be correlated with blood pressure. In the same manner, the aldosterone-renin ratio was positively related to age and plasma sodium concentration in hypertensives, relationships that could not be detectable using plasma aldosterone levels, and to blood pressure in hypertensives *(2)*. As suggested, the aldosterone-renin ratio might help to isolate patients with inappropriate aldosterone activity who would respond favourably to aldosterone antagonists. However, although several studies have shown the favourable blood pressure-lowering effects of aldosterone antagonists, these results need to be investigated in large cohorts. As previously suggested, the aldosterone-renin ratio seems to have a greater predictive power with respect to blood pressure response to diuretics than with respect to aldosterone levels. This could also explain why the aldosterone C-344T polymorphism that could influence aldosterone levels is not found to be associated with a greater blood pressure reduction in response to diuretics *(2)*.

2.4.3 β-Blockers

Beta-blockers are used frequently for CVD. They are first-line therapy for the treatment of hypertension, heart failure, and angina in post-myocardial infarction patients.

From a pharmacodynamic point of view, adrenergic receptors (subtypes alpha 1, alpha 2, beta 1, and beta 2) are components of a prototypic family of guanine nucleotide-binding regulatory protein-coupled receptors that mediate the physiological effects of the hormone epinephrine and the neurotransmitter norepinephrine. Two major polymorphisms encoded by the beta-1 adrenergic receptor gene are commonly used in both hypertension and heart failure pharmacogenetic studies of beta-blockers. These polymorphisms result in an amino acid substitution at codon 389 (Arg389Gly) (C1165G polymorphism) that codes for the intracellular part of the receptor and at codon 49 (Ser49Gly) (A145G polymorphism) that codes for the extracellular part of the receptor.

Several studies, but not all, have reported a greater effect of beta-blockers in 1165C homozygotes *(12–14)*. Consideration of haplotypes could explain approximately 40% more of the variability in blood pressure response to metoprolol monotherapy than consideration of the codon 389 polymorphism alone *(47)*. These polymorphisms could not, however, explain the changes in heart rate and blood pressure linked to treatment with atenolol (50–100 mg) *(48)*.

Two recent studies investigate the local vascular responses in humans triggered by a highly selective alpha 2-adrenergic agonist *(49, 50)*. Responses to azepexole (B-HT 933) show prominent differences in function of age and gender, but appear not to depend on common allelic variations at the ADRA2B receptor *(50)*. In contrast, the *ADRA1A* Arg347Cys polymorphism seems to be associated with the BP therapeutic response in patients with 150 mg of irbesartan *(49)*.

Studies using microarray genotyping have also reported significant pharmacogenetic effects with beta-blockers in G-protein subunit genes, the adducin or endothelin gene. Thus, a pharmacogenetic effect of the *GNB3* (C825T polymorphism) with atenolol was shown in males *(51)*. Liljedahl *(52)* reported that the *ADRA2* A1817G polymorphism predicted the change in left ventricular mass during antihypertensive therapy with atenolol. Kurland *(36)* found that carriers of the *ADD1*–6A and 1198C alleles produce a significant decrease in blood pressure with atenolol. Finally, men carrying the T-allele of the G5665T gene polymorphism of the preproendothelin-1 gene responded with an average reduction twice as large as in those with the G/G genotype (–21.9 mmHg [13.9] vs. –8.9 [2.3], $p = 0.007$) *(53)*.

2.4.4 Diuretics

Other genes are predictive of blood pressure response to drugs, and prediction of the effect of medication on blood pressure is highly dependent on the drug taken into consideration. Thus, the C825T polymorphism of the G-protein β3gene (*GNB3*) appears to predict patient response to thiazide diuretics *(2)*, while CA repeat length of the 11-β-hydroxysteroid dehydrogenase type 2 (*HSD11B2*) gene was strongly associated with the BP response to hydrochlorothiazide *(54)*. The *HSD11B2* G534A polymorphism can cause a rare form of salt-sensitive monogenic hypertension and is proposed as a "salt-sensitive" marker. Interestingly, a microsatellite CA repeat marker in intron 1 of the *HSD11B2* gene was associated with the urinary cortisol metabolites ratio, reflecting a mild reduction in 11-β-hydroxysteroid dehydrogenase type 2 activity, which in turn was significantly related to plasma renin activity levels *(2)*.

2.4.5 Calcium Channel Blockers

Identification of sequence variability in the genes for calcium pathways, i.e., Ca^{2+}-sensitive K^+ channel beta 1 subunit, recently defined as protective against hypertension *(55)*, needs to be improved. In this regard, *in vitro* studies to test the functional significance of polymorphisms (patch-clamp studies, in the case of calcium channels) and to determine the association between a drug's antihypertensive effects and genetic polymorphisms are of interest. The E65K polymorphism in the $[beta]_1$-subunit of the large-conductance, Ca^{2+}-dependent K^+ (BK) channel, a key element in the control of arterial tone, has recently been associated with low prevalence of diastolic hypertension *(56)*. However, antihypertensive treatment with dibutyril cGMP was not able to modify the K allele effect on DBP *(57)*.

2.5 *Antidiabetic Drugs*

Glitazones have been described as potential therapeutics for metabolic syndrome. At present, little is known about the pharmacogenomics of this drug family *(58)*. Using *in vitro* studies, Qi et al. *(59)* demonstrated that administration of pioglitazone was associated with significantly lower circulating levels of fatty acids, triglycerides, and insulin in spontaneously hypertensive rats (SHR) that expressed the wild-type *Cd-36* allele, compared with those harboring a deletion mutation in *Cd-36*. PPARγ are involved in the response of thiazolidinediones. PPARG Pro12Ala modifies glucose and hemoglobin A1C (HBA1C) reductions. Biguanides are another class of antidiabetics that have demonstrated efficacy in type 2 diabetes treatment and may have implications for CVD. The administration of metformin, either as monotherapy or in combination with a sulfonylurea, was found to improve glycemic control and to lead to a decrease in several CVD risk factors in patients with type 2 diabetes *(60)*. The sulfonylurea glibenclamide, another antidiabetic drug, has both pharmacokinetic and pharmacodynamic genetic considerations. Glibenclamide was shown to be metabolized by CYP2C9, since oral clearances of homozygous carriers of the *CYP2C9*3* allele were 47% lower than those of homozygous wild-type carriers. Moreover, the elimination half-lifes were significantly longer in *CYP2C9*3/*3* carriers *(61)*. Therefore, treated individuals are at a higher risk of developing hypoglycemia, since poor metabolizers for this drug-metabolizing enzyme have more pronounced increases in insulin levels than the intermediate or extensive metabolizers *(16, 61)*.

3 Pathology-Related Genes

The third set of genes involved in the personal response to drugs consists of the genes linked to the CV pathologies. We have chosen inflammation, which is a physiopathological state and a subclinical cause of several CV risk factors (e.g., metabolic syndrome, diabetes, obesity). Thus the pharmacogenomics of cardiovascular drugs should take into account this metabolic deviation.

3.1 Inflammation

More than 100 genes are related to inflammation, if we take into account those regulated by nuclear factor-κB (NF-κB), activator protein-1 (AP-1), peroxisomal proliferation-activating receptor-α (PPAR-α), etc. Inflammation biomarkers, which are measurable in blood, could be divided in five groups: acute phase reactants (e.g., C-reactive protein, serum amyloid A protein, and fibrinogen); cytokines (e.g., interleukin-1 beta [IL-1β], interleukin-6 [IL-6], and tumor necrosis factor-α [TNF-α]); chemokines (e.g., monocyte chemoattractant protein-1 [MCP-1]); adhesion molecules (soluble forms) and proteases; and lipoprotein-associated phospholipase A2 (Lp-PLA_2) and CD40 ligand *(2)*.

Many polymorphisms could influence their level in circulation *(62)*. Some of them have been studied in relation to cardiovascular risk. Indeed, they could affect the balance of the cytokine network, which can lead in addition to some environmental risk factors, to disrupting cytokine equilibrium, and to improving atherogenesis *(63)*. Finally, they could also have an impact on cardiovascular therapy.

The Cholesterol and Recurrent Events (CARE) trial and the Air Force/Texas Coronary Atherosclerosis Prevention Study (AFCAPS/TexCAPS) suggest that statin therapy may be differentially effective among those with inflammation, compared to those without.

Irbesartan-treated patients, who were carriers of the C-allele at position 915 in the *TGFB1* gene, which is associated with low expression of TGF-β1, responded with a markedly greater decrease in the left ventricular mass index than subjects with the G/G genotype, independent of blood pressure reduction *(2)*. Indeed, angiotensin-converting enzyme inhibitors drugs have been known for a long time to have an antiinflammatory effect *(2)*. Considerable evidence now supports a role for angiotensin II as a proinflammatory mediator, elevating it to the category of an "honorary" cytokine. It can, for example, elicit vascular cell adhesion molecule 1 (VCAM1) and MCP-1 expression by endothelial cells, and IL-6 production by smooth muscle cells *(64)*.

Another study on the effect of *IL1B*-511 C/T polymorphism on treatment by pravastatin indicates that, after 6 months of treatment, in men with the *IL1B* C allele, levels of IL-1β decreased, while in men with the T allele, it increased; however, this difference is not very significant ($p = 0.061$). In addition, researchers found that changes in adenosine-stimulated flow and coronary flow reserve with pravastatin were significantly dependent on *IL1B* genotype. They explained their results by the fact that statin treatment decreased IL-1β level more effectively in subjects with the CC genotype, thus leading to a lower endothelial inflammatory response, and better endothelial function as indicated by increased adenosine-stimulated flow and coronary flow reserve *(65)*.

The *IL6*-174G/C genotype is a much studied one, as it is correlated with IL-6 level in circulation *(66)*. It is related to carotid intima-media thickness (IMT), peripheral artery occlusive disease, and retinal artery occlusion *(2)*.

IL6 polymorphism also interacts with pravastatin, as men carrying the GG + GC genotype treated with this drug for one year had a 25% lower risk (OR = 1 reduced to OR = 0.75), compared with the GG + GC placebo group; whereas in the CC group, risk was 77% lower than that in the CC placebo men (OR reduced from 1.19 to 0.42). In addition, the reduction in LDL cholesterol was greater in the CC group than in the GG + GC group. Larger declines in fibrinogen and C-reactive protein and a larger elevation in HDL levels in the CC group were found, compared with the GG + GC group; these latter differences were, however, statistically not significant. Researchers hypothesized that the protective effect of the CC genotype in the treated group was likely to be due to either a greater pravastatin lipid-lowering effect or a greater inflammation-lowering effect in this genotype group. Analysis of the WOSCOPS (West of Scotland Coronary Prevention Study) data suggests that both of these effects may be involved *(67)*. In addition, in randomized men awaiting coronary artery bypass graft, enalapril produced a highly significant decrease of 51% in the release of IL-6 in patients identified as high producers of IL-6 by the -174 G/C polymorphism, whereas losartan has a similar but less marked effect *(68)*.

On the other hand, results from the Physicians Heart Study showed that the benefit of aspirin treatment was greatest in subjects with elevated baseline C-reactive protein levels. This finding is confirmed by other results indicating that the effect of aspirin in preventing a first myocardial infarction was greatest among men with the highest baseline C-reactive protein concentrations, and that the benefit diminished significantly with decreasing concentrations of this inflammatory marker *(2)*.

These results suggest that the benefit of antiinflammatory treatment may be greatest in those with highest inflammation and so, in part, in individuals who carry alleles of polymorphisms that contribute to increased gene expression.

4 Health and Physiology

Despite variability in the genome, fundamental pharmacologic processes may also be affected by other biological factors that characterize health or environmental status. Nongenetic biological factors can be divided into two categories: constitutive factors (e.g., gender, age, and ethnicity) and acquired factors (e.g., drug exposure, diet, alcohol use, tobacco use, exposure to industrial/environmental pollutants, and exercise).

Thus, the variability in an individual's response to drugs is now best understood as an integrated complex interplay between genetics and various biological factors that can influence pharmacologic mechanisms. In this context, physiologically-based pharmacogenomics emerges as a preferred model to describe interindividual drug response. This section examines the impact of specific biological variables on the therapeutic outcome of CV drug treatment. We present components of health status as determinants of therapeutic outcome, which may include numerous traits and conditions, such as ethnicity, age, gender, and body weight.

4.1 Ethnicity

Ethnicity is a population trait that combines both genetic and behavioral influences. Physiologic and pharmacologic responses may be influenced by ethnicity as a result of genetic factors, environmental factors, or interactions between them. The difference in drug metabolism and response to antihypertensive agents between Caucasian and Black populations is one of several examples. In general, the pharmacologic treatment of hypertension in Blacks is most consistently achieved through diuretics and calcium channel blockers, whereas ACE inhibitors and β-blockers are more efficient in Caucasians. These patterns are consistent with the higher prevalence of salt sensitivity, stress-induced vasoconstriction, slower natriuresis and α-adrenoceptor-mediated vascular reactivity observed in Blacks compared with Caucasians. Most of the published data on interethnic differences in CV drug response have focused on the genetic component of ethnicity. Different ethnic groups vary in their allele distribution, some of which can have an effect on drug metabolism and efficacy. Pronounced differences were commonly observed in drug-metabolizing enzymes when ethnically defined groups, such as Caucasians and Asians, are compared. This has been demonstrated for the CYP isozymes, in particular CYP2D6 and CYP2C19, both of which are key metabolizing enzymes of numerous CV agents. A number of *CYP2D6* alleles have been identified that are associated with abnormal metabolism. For example, interethnic differences in the incidence of the "poor metabolizer" phenotype of CYP2D6 range from 0% in the Cuna Indians to 19% in San Bushmen *(5)*. For *CYP2C19*, the *CYP2C19*2* allele occurs in 25% of the Asian population and 13% of Caucasians, while the *CYP2C19*3* allele occurs in 8% of Asians and only 1% of Caucasians. Individuals who are homozygous for the "null" allele of *CYP2C19* are highly responsive to substrates, such as propranolol *(69)*. Information derived from 42 studies of interindividual variability in drug-metabolizing enzymes indicates that in 28 such cases, the frequency of the variant differed between ethnic groups *(70)*. In a similar vein, the heterogeneity of the *APOE* allele distribution in the general population is another useful example of interethnic differences. Three major alleles of the *APOE* gene have been described, namely ε*2*, ε*3*, and ε*4*. The distribution of these alleles is highly variable among populations throughout the world. The ε*3* is the most frequent allele, displaying > 60% occurrence in all populations studied to date. The ε*2* allele frequency does not exceed 10% on any continent and has not been detected in American Indians. The ε*4* allele frequency ranges from ~5–7% in Chinese populations to ~10% in other Asian and American Indian groups; it approaches ~37% in Papua New Guineans. The ε*4* allele frequency is also elevated in African-American and African groups with a frequency of ~20% and 30%, respectively *(71)*. There is a clear decreasing north-to-south gradient of the ε*4* allele frequency throughout European countries, ranging from 22% in Scandinavia and Scotland to 7% in Mediterranean populations *(72, 73)*. Of particular interest is the observation that interindividual variation in response to many CV drugs may depend, in part, on *APOE* genotype (see above). Differences between ethnically dissimilar subpopulations are due to a variety of genetic (as described above) and nongenetic factors. The environmental (nongenetic) component of ethnicity will be addressed in a later section (see the section discussing environmental status).

4.2 Age and Gender

A broad body of evidence suggests that clinically relevant differences between gender and age groups exist in the pharmacological processes and are also influenced by genetics. There are a variety of physiological and biochemical reasons that explain why sensitivity to chemicals varies with age. Among the most important differences are the physiological changes that occur with aging. The aging organism undergoes changes at the molecular, cellular, and organic levels. In the elderly, the combination of reduced organ function and the increased prevalence of risk factors, as well as disease, influences the drug response. The impact of age is, therefore, a net result of the interaction between age-related and concomitant disease-associated changes in organ function. Nevertheless, even in the absence of overt coexisting disease, some of the age-related changes in organ function alone can affect drug response. The pharmacokinetic parameters most consistently affected by age are the volume of distribution, clearance, and the half-life of the drug. The renal drug clearance is consistently diminished with age. However, aging does not eliminate the gender-related differences. Major differences in pharmacokinetic parameters between the genders are, on average, lower weight, volume of distribution, and renal drug clearance in women when compared to men *(1)*. Gender has been identified as a significant source of interindividual variation in the oral clearance of nifedipine and verapamil, which are both CYP3A substrates. Accordingly, clearance was significantly more rapid in women versus men, without a detectable age effect. Hepatic clearance is also more variably affected by gender. Pharmacodynamic changes, although present, have not been as extensively examined for gender- and age-related effects, but do include a higher rate of adverse CV drug effects in women compared to men *(1)*. The importance of accounting for (patho)physiologic changes related to aging when investigating the impact of genetic variation on phenotype was emphasized by the study of the *ADRB2* gene, which encodes the β2-adrenoceptor *(74)*. This receptor acts as a mediator of the vasodilatory response to adrenergic agonists in the vasculature. Variants of the *ADRB2* gene, especially the Gly16Arg and Gln27Glu polymorphisms or their haplotypes, may have varying effects on the functional responses to adrenergic stimulation, and may thereby modulate CV and metabolic phenotypes. Some studies reported enhanced desensitization of ADRB2 in Arg16-Gln27 homozygotes *(74)*. The desensitization appeared to be related to Arg16 rather than to Gln27; on the other hand, Gly16-Glu27 homozygotes had the significantly highest maximal vasodilatory response to isoprenaline. A key qualification of these findings is that the effect of Arg16-Gln27 haplotype is limited to the youngest individuals. This is consistent with the hypothesis of an age-related decline of the receptor-mediated activity, which may help obscure the influence of the *ADRB2* polymorphisms on blood pressure regulation in older individuals.

Overall evidence suggests that gender- and age-specific differences in drug metabolism may occur as general traits in CV pharmacology. The relative role of gender and aging on CV pharmacology as compared to genetics and illness, environmental factors (such as co-medications, diet, and social habits), and their potential interactions in the clinical setting is not yet fully known, but should be routinely acknowledged and studied further *(1)*.

4.3 Obesity

In the case of obesity, there has been a rapid increase in recent years in the understanding of biochemical events thought to be causative factors, resulting in the development of new therapeutic approaches. The new generation of drugs targeting obesity focuses on (1) reducing energy intake (leptin and leptin receptors, pro-opiomelanocortin and melanocortin receptors, neuropeptide Y and its receptors, endocannabinoids and cannabinoid CB1 receptors, etc.); (2) increasing energy expenditure (uncoupling protein 1, β_3-adrenoceptors, PPAR-γ modulators); and (3) producing thermogenic effects (β_3-adrenoceptors, PPAR-δ agonists) *(75, 76)*. In clinical practice, the current drugs for long-term treatment of obesity are sibutramine and orlistat, which are designed to reduce food intake and the utilization of ingested energy, respectively. Sibutramine is a serotonin, norepinephrine, and dopamine reuptake inhibitor; while orlistat inactivates pancreatic lipase, thereby inhibiting hydrolysis and absorption of dietary triacylglycerol. The use of orlistat has successfully achieved modest long-term reductions in body weight. Recently, the effect of weight reduction with orlistat treatment on lipid peroxidation levels, which is found to be associated with obesity, was investigated.

The fact that many genes are implicated in obesity gives rise to new drug targets, but also verifies the complexity of this phenomenon and underlines the importance of considering the genetic variants of these genes for evaluating the outcomes of drug therapeutic interventions. To date, there exist 426 findings of positive associations between obesity phenotypes and genetic variations of 127 candidate genes *(77)*. The latest version of the list is available online *(86)*.

Genetic variants of leptin, an adipocytokine secreted by the adipose tissue, and its receptor are related to obesity and increased body mass index, while polymorphisms in the gene of adiponectin result in phenotypes such as insulin resistance and type 2 diabetes, in additional to obesity and increased adiposity. Interestingly, variations in both genes can result in altered circulating levels of these two proteins *(78)*, signalling the importance of taking the polymorphisms into account when using these molecules as biomarkers. Finally, there are cited polymorphisms of dopamine receptors (DRD2, DRD4) related to obesity, and of hepatic lipase related to abdominal visceral fat and to body mass index *(79)*, suggesting possible variations in drug response in the case of sibutramine and orlistat.

5 Environmentally Interfering Genes

5.1 Diet

Dietary recommendations are the first therapeutic approach in cardiovascular diseases. A diet low in total fats (particularly those of animal origin), low in cholesterol, and high in antioxidant elements has showed favorable outcomes in patients and an improved quality of life in healthy subjects. The responses to diet and the interactions between diet and disease depend on genetic polymorphisms (nutrigenetics). In the case of cardiovascular disease, the most established gene-nutrient interactions concern the dietary fats and genes involved in lipid metabolism (apolipoproteins, lipoprotein lipase, and hepatic lipase, among others). The *APOE* gene remains the locus most consistently reported with respect to gene environment. In subjects carrying the apoε4 allele, a low-fat and low-cholesterol strategy may be particularly beneficial in terms of lowering plasma cholesterol levels *(80)*. The same strategy can possibly be applied in altering the HDL concentrations, after dietary intake of polyunsaturated fatty acids (PUFA). It has been reported recently that their effect on HDL-cholesterol concentrations is modulated by a common genetic polymorphism in the promoter region of the *APOA1* gene. Thus, subjects carrying the A allele at the -75G/A polymorphism show an increase in HDL-cholesterol concentrations with increased intakes of PUFA, whereas those homozygotes for the more common G allele have the expected lowering of HDL-cholesterol levels as the intake of PUFA increases. Subsequently, it could be predicted that subjects with low levels of HDL-cholesterol and carriers of the A allele may benefit from diets containing higher percentages of PUFA. A third very interesting example has been recently reported, focusing on the interaction between the intake of animal-origin fat and variability at the hepatic lipase gene, encoding a key enzyme involved in reverse cholesterol transport. It has been shown that subjects carrying the CC genotype (the most common among Caucasian subjects) "react" to high contents of fat in their diets by increasing the concentrations of HDL-cholesterol, which could be interpreted as a "defense mechanism" to maintain the homeostasis of lipoprotein metabolism. Conversely, carriers of the TT genotype experience decreases in HDL-cholesterol levels *(80)*. Beyond citing these interesting examples, it is important to note that there have been studies extensively on other genetic variants, concerning mostly the *APOAI*, the *APOAIV*, the *APOCIII*, the *APOB*, and the *APOE*, some examples of which are cited in Table 19.5 *(81)*.

Table 19.5 Examples of apolipoprotein polymorphisms modifying diet response

Polymorphism and study	Subjects	Genotype groups	Intervention	Response			
				Cholesterol	LDL	HDL	TG
Apolipoprotein AI –75(G/A)	89 males	G/G, 58	NCEP-I vs. high fat, high MUFA diet	S		NS	NS
Lopez-Miranda et al.		G/G, 31					
Apolipoprotein CIII C1100T	55 males and females	C/C, 38	High SFA vs. high PUFA diet	NS	NS	NS	NS
Humphries et al.		C/T and T/T, 17					
Apolipoprotein AIV Thr347Ser	41 males	Thr/Thr, 25	NCEP-I vs. high MUFA diet	S	NS	NS	NS
Jansen et al.		Ser (Thr/Ser and Ser/Ser), 16					
Apolipoprotein B Asn1887Ser	54 females	Asn/Asn, 52	Low fat, low cholesterol, high P/S diet	NS	NS		
Ilmonen et al.		Asn/Ser, 2					
Apolipoprotein E ε2, ε3, ε4	29 males	ApoE2 (2/2, 3/2 and 4/2), 8	Low vs. high cholesterol diet	S	S	NS	NS
Miettinen et al.		ApoE3 (3/3), 9 ApoE4 (4/4), 12					

Adapted from Masson et al. (83) HDL = high-density lipoprotein; LDL = low-density lipoprotein; MUFA = monounsaturated fatty acid; NCEP = National Cholesterol Education Program; P/S = polyunsaturated to saturated acid ratio; PUFA = polyunsaturated fatty acids; SFA = saturated fatty acids; TG = triglycerides; NS = nonsignificant; S = significant.

5.2 *Environmental Pollutants*

5.2.1 Tobacco

It is well known that smoking is an important CV risk factor. However, it was reported in numerous studies that the risk of developing cardiovascular disease is different, according to some genetic polymorphisms. Indeed, a large list of genes was described which interact with smoking in the development of these diseases. This list includes apolipoprotein E gene (*APOE*), paraoxonase 1 (*POX1*), lipoprotein lipase (*LPL*), NO synthase (*NOS*), tumor protein p53 (*TP53*), cluster of differentiation 14 (*CD14*), interleukin 6 (*IL6*), metalloproteinase 3 (*MMP3*), gluthation-S-transferase (*GST*), angiotensin converting enzyme (*ACE*), and factor V (*FV*).

Large interindividual differences occur in human nicotine disposition, and it has been proposed that genetic polymorphism in nicotine metabolism may be a major determinant of an individual's smoking behaviour. Hepatic cytochrome P4502A6 (CYP2A6) catalyses the major route of nicotine metabolism: C-oxidation to cotinine, followed by hydroxylayion to trans-3'-hydroxycotinine. Polymorphims of CYP2D6 are associated with differences in nicotine C-oxidation in vitro, and with plasma cotinine levels after experimental administration of nicotine and voluntary smoking. Moreover, kinetic studies with Japanese and Chinese volunteers confirm that the presence of the CYP2A6*4A deletion allele, as well as the CYP2A6*7 and CYP2A6*10 alleles, is associated with reduced in vivo nicotine metabolism to cotinine. However, concerning effects on smoking behavior, associations were reported for polymorphisms of CYP2A6 *(82)*. This observation could explain the differential response to nicotine substitutes. CYP2D6, hepatic flavin-containing monooxygenase form 3 (FMO3), and uridine diphosphate-glucuronosyltransferase (UGT) enzymes are also responsible for nicotine metabolism. However, current evidence does not consistently and conclusively support the hypothesis that genetic polymorphisms in these genes are determinants of an individual's smoking behaviour *(83)*. A recent article summarized the current state of knowledge for the effect of genes altering nicotine metabolism, and also of genes involved in the neurotransmitter pathways for the brain reward system on smoking behaviors and therapeutic outcomes for drugs used to assist smoking cessation *(84)*.

Conclusion

In summary, the goal of CV pharmacogenomics is to guide CV drug development and therapy toward optimizing therapeutic benefit and minimizing the potential for toxicity. Genetics-based differences in drug metabolism have long been recognized but are only just beginning to achieve clinical application.

- A large majority of CV drugs are metabolized through CYP2D6, -2C, and -3A.
- The clinical problems for CV drugs are actually only related to CYP2D6 and -2C.

- Polymorphisms in the transporters are becoming more and more important to follow.
- More than 20 relevant cardiovascular drug targets have been identified from the pharmacogenomics point of view.
- Pharmacogenomics cannot be limited to the drug actions themselves. It is necessary to integrate the genetic variations into the corresponding cardiovascular pathologies or, better, to the metabolic pathway involved.
- The biological variability also has to be integrated by studying healthy subjects and healthy families to determine the main functions involved, including the environmental effects.

Pharmacogenomics may enable clinicians to identify patients who are most likely to derive benefit from a drug, with minimal likelihood of adverse events.

In the near future, a pharmacoproteomics approach should be used also. Numerous enzymes, proteins, peptides, and receptors can be used as phenotypes to enter into the pharmacoproteomic followup of cardiovascular drugs. Proteomics approaches are clearly very useful during the development of new drugs to control some toxicities, including drug interactions in different pathological states. However, for a more specific use of pharmacoproteomics in the cardiovascular field, we need to better know the proteome profile of the organs involved: heart, vessels, and specific blood cells, including lymphocytes. For such multifactorial chronic diseases as cardiovascular ones, we have to dissect them into separate metabolic entities for selecting the genes and gene products involved in each pathway.

Genomic and proteomic markers for cardiovascular drugs should be used to pinpoint individuals at high risk for the disease and at risk for drug side effects or a probability of nonresponse. The practice of personalized medicine should use the huge amount of genomic, proteomic, and metabolomic data which will be developed during the next few years with powerful array technologies. However, we should not forget that humans are living in special environments regulating the expression of genes and gene products. Nutrition, tobacco, alcohol, obesity, and other drugs such as contraceptives, have been particularly linked to the pharmacogenomic strategy for cardiovascular drugs.

References

1. Siest G, Jeannesson E, Berrahmoune H, Maumus S, Marteau JB, Mohr S et al. Pharmacogenomics and drug response in cardiovascular disorders. Pharmacogenomics 2004;5:779–802.
2. Siest G, Marteau JB, Maumus S, Berrahmoune H, Jeannesson E, Samara A et al. Pharmacogenomics and cardiovascular drugs: need for integrated biological system with phenotypes and proteomic markers. Eur J Pharmacol 2005;527:1–22.
3. Nelson DR, Zeldin DC, Hoffman SM, Maltais LJ, Wain HM, Nebert DW. Comparison of cytochrome P450 (CYP) genes from the mouse and human genomes, including nomenclature recommendations for genes, pseudogenes and alternative-splice variants. Pharmacogenetics 2004;14:1–18.

4. Pirmohamed M, Park BK. Cytochrome P450 enzyme polymorphisms and adverse drug reactions. Toxicology 2003;192:23–32.
5. Zanger UM, Raimundo S, Eichelbaum M. Cytochrome P450 2D6: overview and update on pharmacology, genetics, biochemistry. Naunyn Schmiedebergs Arch Pharmacol 2004;369:23–37.
6. Nakagawa K, Ishizaki T. Therapeutic relevance of pharmacogenetic factors in cardiovascular medicine. Pharmacol Ther 2000;86:1–28.
7. Takahashi H, Echizen H. Pharmacogenetics of warfarin elimination and its clinical implications. Clin Pharmacokinet 2001;40:587–603.
8. Burk O, Wojnowski L. Cytochrome P450 3A and their regulation. Naunyn Schmiedebergs Arch Pharmacol 2004;369:105–124.
9. Schmitz G, Langmann T. Pharmacogenomics of cholesterol-lowering therapy. Vascul Pharmacol 2006;44:75–89.
10. Zschieschang P, Hiepe F, Gromnica-Ihle E, Roots I, Cascorbi I. Lack of association between arylamine N-acetyltransferase 2 (NAT2) polymorphism and systemic lupus erythematosus. Pharmacogenetics 2002;12:559–563.
11. Danoff TM, Campbell DA, McCarthy LC, Lewis KF, Repasch MH, Saunders AM et al. A Gilbert's syndrome UGT1A1 variant confers susceptibility to tranilast-induced hyperbilirubinemia. Pharmacogenomics J 2004;4:49–53.
12. Glatt H, Meinl W. Pharmacogenetics of soluble sulfotransferases (SULTs). Naunyn Schmiedebergs Arch Pharmacol 2004;369:55–68.
13. Shapiro LE, Shear NH. Drug interactions: Proteins, pumps, and P-450s. J Am Acad Dermatol 2002;47:467–484.
14. Thompson JF, Man M, Johnson KJ, Wood LS, Lira ME, Lloyd DB et al. An association study of 43 SNPs in 16 candidate genes with atorvastatin response. Pharmacogenomics J 2005;5:352–358.
15. Siest G, Ferrari L, Accaoui MJ, Batt AM, Visvikis S. Pharmacogenomics of drugs affecting the cardiovascular system. Clin Chem Lab Med 2003;41:590–599.
16. Meisel C, Gerloff T, Kirchheiner J, Mrozikiewicz PM, Niewinski P, Brockmoller J et al. Implications of pharmacogenetics for individualizing drug treatment and for study design. J Mol Med 2003;81:154–167.
17. Mukherjee D, Topol EJ. Pharmacogenomics in cardiovascular diseases. Curr Probl Cardiol 2003;28:317–347.
18. Hillarp A, Palmqvist B, Lethagen S, Villoutreix BO, Mattiasson I. Mutations within the cyclooxygenase-1 gene in aspirin non-responders with recurrence of stroke. Thromb Res 2003;112:275–283.
19. Wheeler GL, Braden GA, Bray PF, Marciniak SJ, Mascelli MA, Sane DC. Reduced inhibition by abciximab in platelets with the PlA2 polymorphism. Am Heart J 2002;143:76–82.
20. O'Connor FF, Shields DC, Fitzgerald A, Cannon CP, Braunwald E, Fitzgerald DJ. Genetic variation in glycoprotein IIb/IIIa (GPIIb/IIIa) as a determinant of the responses to an oral GPIIb/IIIa antagonist in patients with unstable coronary syndromes. Blood 2001;98:3256–3260.
21. Feng D, Lindpaintner K, Larson MG, O'Donnell CJ, Lipinska I, Sutherland PA et al. Platelet glycoprotein IIIa Pl(a) polymorphism, fibrinogen, and platelet aggregability: The Framingham Heart Study. Circulation 2001;104:140–144.
22. Goodall AH, Curzen N, Panesar M, Hurd C, Knight CJ, Ouwehand WH et al. Increased binding of fibrinogen to glycoprotein IIIa-proline33 (HPA-1b, PlA2, Zwb) positive platelets in patients with cardiovascular disease. Eur Heart J 1999;20:742–747.
23. Rettie AE, Tai G. The pharmocogenomics of warfarin: closing in on personalized medicine. Mol Interv 2006;6:223–227.
24. Pedro-Botet J, Schaefer EJ, Bakker-Arkema RG, Black DM, Stein EM, Corella D et al. Apolipoprotein E genotype affects plasma lipid response to atorvastatin in a gender specific manner. Atherosclerosis 2001;158:183–193.
25. Evans WE, McLeod HL. Pharmacogenomics—drug disposition, drug targets, and side effects. N Engl J Med 2003;348:538–549.

26. Siest G, Bertrand P, Herbeth B, Vincent-Viry M, Schiele F, Sass C et al. Apolipoprotein E polymorphisms and concentration in chronic diseases and drug responses. Clin Chem Lab Med 2000;38:841–852.
27. Gerdes LU, Gerdes C, Kervinen K, Savolainen M, Klausen IC, Hansen PS et al. The apolipoprotein epsilon4 allele determines prognosis and the effect on prognosis of simvastatin in survivors of myocardial infarction : a substudy of the Scandinavian simvastatin survival study. Circulation 2000;101:1366–1371.
28. Garcia-Otin AL, Civeira F, Aristegui R, Diaz C, Recalde D, Sol JM et al. Allelic polymorphism -491A/T in apo E gene modulates the lipid-lowering response in combined hyperlipidemia treatment. Eur J Clin Invest 2002;32:421–428.
29. Carlquist JF, Muhlestein JB, Horne BD, Hart NI, Bair TL, Molhuizen HO et al. The cholesteryl ester transfer protein Taq1B gene polymorphism predicts clinical benefit of statin therapy in patients with significant coronary artery disease. Am Heart J 2003;146:1007–1014.
30. van Venrooij FV, Stolk RP, Banga JD, Sijmonsma TP, van Tol A, Erkelens DW et al. Common cholesteryl ester transfer protein gene polymorphisms and the effect of atorvastatin therapy in type 2 diabetes. Diabetes Care 2003;26:1216–1223.
31. Chasman DI, Posada D, Subrahmanyan L, Cook NR, Stanton VP, Jr., Ridker PM. Pharmacogenetic study of statin therapy and cholesterol reduction. JAMA 2004;291:2821–2827.
32. Cresci S. The PPAR genes, cardiovascular disease and the emergence of PPAR pharmacogenetics. Expert Opin Pharmacother 2005;6:2577–2591.
33. Kajinami K, Brousseau ME, Lamon-Fava S, Ordovas JM, Schaefer EJ. Gender-specific effects of estrogen receptor alpha gene haplotype on high-density lipoprotein cholesterol response to atorvastatin: interaction with apolipoprotein AI gene polymorphism. Atherosclerosis 2005;178:331–338.
34. Brousseau ME, Goldkamp AL, Collins D, Demissie S, Connolly AC, Cupples LA et al. Polymorphisms in the gene encoding lipoprotein lipase in men with low HDL-C and coronary heart disease: the Veterans Affairs HDL Intervention Trial. J Lipid Res 2004;45:1885–1891.
35. Arnett DK, Claas SA, Glasser SP. Pharmacogenetics of antihypertensive treatment. Vascul Pharmacol 2006;44:107–118.
36. Kurland L, Liljedahl U, Karlsson J, Kahan T, Malmqvist K, Melhus H et al. Angiotensinogen gene polymorphisms: relationship to blood pressure response to antihypertensive treatment. Results from the Swedish Irbesartan Left Ventricular Hypertrophy Investigation vs Atenolol (SILVHIA) trial. Am J Hypertens 2004;17:8–13.
37. Sethi AA, Nordestgaard BG, Tybjaerg-Hansen A. Angiotensinogen gene polymorphism, plasma angiotensinogen, and risk of hypertension and ischemic heart disease: a meta-analysis. Arterioscler Thromb Vasc Biol 2003;23:1269–1275.
38. Brand-Herrmann SM, Kopke K, Reichenberger F, Schmidt-Petersen K, Reineke T, Paul M et al. Angiotensinogen promoter haplotypes are associated with blood pressure in untreated hypertensives. J Hypertens 2004;22:1289–1297.
39. Renner W, Nauck M, Winkelmann BR, Hoffmann MM, Scharnagl H, Mayer V et al. Association of angiotensinogen haplotypes with angiotensinogen levels but not with blood pressure or coronary artery disease: the Ludwigshafen Risk and Cardiovascular Health Study. J Mol Med 2005;83:235–239.
40. Birkenhager WH, de Leeuw PW. Non-peptide angiotensin type 1 receptor antagonists in the treatment of hypertension. J Hypertens 1999;17:873–881.
41. Spiering W, Kroon AA, Fuss-Lejeune MJ, de Leeuw PW. Genetic contribution to the acute effects of angiotensin II type 1 receptor blockade. J Hypertens 2005;23:753–758.
42. Sookoian S, Castano G, Garcia SI, Viudez P, Gonzalez C, Pirola CJ. A1166C angiotensin II type 1 receptor gene polymorphism may predict hemodynamic response to losartan in patients with cirrhosis and portal hypertension. Am J Gastroenterol 2005;100:636–642.
43. Stanton A, Jensen C, Nussberger J, O'Brien E. Blood pressure lowering in essential hypertension with an oral renin inhibitor, aliskiren. Hypertension 2003;42:1137–1143.
44. Stanton A. Therapeutic potential of renin inhibitors in the management of cardiovascular disorders. Am J Cardiovasc Drugs 2003;3:389–394.

45. Gradman AH, Schmieder RE, Lins RL, Nussberger J, Chiang Y, Bedigian MP. Aliskiren, a novel orally effective renin inhibitor, provides dose-dependent antihypertensive efficacy and placebo-like tolerability in hypertensive patients. Circulation 2005;111:1012–1018.
46. Frazier L, Turner ST, Schwartz GL, Chapman AB, Boerwinkle E. Multilocus effects of the renin-angiotensin-aldosterone system genes on blood pressure response to a thiazide diuretic. Pharmacogenomics J 2004;4:17–23.
47. Johnson JA, Zineh I, Puckett BJ, McGorray SP, Yarandi HN, Pauly DF. Beta 1-adrenergic receptor polymorphisms and antihypertensive response to metoprolol. Clin Pharmacol Ther 2003;74:44–52.
48. Karlsson J, Lind L, Hallberg P, Michaelsson K, Kurland L, Kahan T et al. Beta 1-adrenergic receptor gene polymorphisms and response to beta1-adrenergic receptor blockade in patients with essential hypertension. Clin Cardiol 2004;27:347–350.
49. Jiang S, Mao G, Zhang S, Hong X, Tang G, Li Z et al. Individual and joint association of alpha1A-adrenergic receptor Arg347Cys polymorphism and plasma irbesartan concentration with blood pressure therapeutic response in Chinese hypertensive subjects. Clin Pharmacol Ther 2005;78:239–248.
50. King D, Etzel JP, Chopra S, Smith J, Cadman PE, Rao F et al. Human response to alpha2-adrenergic agonist stimulation studied in an isolated vascular bed in vivo: Biphasic influence of dose, age, gender, and receptor genotype. Clin Pharmacol Ther 2005;77:388–403.
51. Filigheddu F, Reid JE, Troffa C, PinnaParpaglia P, Argiolas G, Testa A et al. Genetic polymorphisms of the beta-adrenergic system: association with essential hypertension and response to beta-blockade. Pharmacogenomics J 2004;4:154–160.
52. Liljedahl U, Kahan T, Malmqvist K, Melhus H, Syvanen AC, Lind L et al. Single nucleotide polymorphisms predict the change in left ventricular mass in response to antihypertensive treatment. J Hypertens 2004;22:2321–2328.
53. Hallberg P, Karlsson J, Lind L, Michaelsson K, Kurland L, Kahan T et al. Gender-specific association between preproendothelin-1 genotype and reduction of systolic blood pressure during antihypertensive treatment—results from the Swedish Irbesartan Left Ventricular Hypertrophy Investigation versus Atenolol (SILVHIA). Clin Cardiol 2004;27:287–290.
54. Williams TA, Mulatero P, Filigheddu F, Troffa C, Milan A, Argiolas G et al. Role of HSD11B2 polymorphisms in essential hypertension and the diuretic response to thiazides. Kidney Int 2005;67:631–637.
55. Nelson MT, Bonev AD. The beta1 subunit of the Ca2+-sensitive K+ channel protects against hypertension. J Clin Invest 2004;113:955–957.
56. Fernandez-Fernandez JM, Tomas M, Vazquez E, Orio P, Latorre R, Senti M et al. Gain-of-function mutation in the KCNMB1 potassium channel subunit is associated with low prevalence of diastolic hypertension. J Clin Invest 2004;113:1032–1039.
57. Senti M, Fernandez-Fernandez JM, Tomas M, Vazquez E, Elosua R, Marrugat J et al. Protective effect of the KCNMB1 E65K genetic polymorphism against diastolic hypertension in aging women and its relevance to cardiovascular risk. Circ Res 2005;97:1360–1365.
58. Bluher M, Lubben G, Paschke R. Analysis of the relationship between the Pro12Ala variant in the PPAR-gamma2 gene and the response rate to therapy with pioglitazone in patients with type 2 diabetes. Diabetes Care 2003;26:825–831.
59. Qi N, Kazdova L, Zidek V, Landa V, Kren V, Pershadsingh HA et al. Pharmacogenetic evidence that cd36 is a key determinant of the metabolic effects of pioglitazone. J Biol Chem 2002;277:48501–48507.
60. Abbasi F, Chu JW, McLaughlin T, Lamendola C, Leary ET, Reaven GM. Effect of metformin treatment on multiple cardiovascular disease risk factors in patients with type 2 diabetes mellitus. Metabolism 2004;53:159–164.
61. Kirchheiner J, Brockmoller J, Meineke I, Bauer S, Rohde W, Meisel C et al. Impact of CYP2C9 amino acid polymorphisms on glyburide kinetics and on the insulin and glucose response in healthy volunteers. Clin Pharmacol Ther 2002;71:286–296.
62. Berrahmoune H, Lamont J, Fitzgerald P, Visvikis-Siest S. Inter-individual variation of inflammatory markers of cardiovascular risks and diseases. Clin Chem Lab Med 2005;43:671–684.

63. Alam SE, Nasser SS, Fernainy KE, Habib AA, Badr KF. Cytokine imbalance in acute coronary syndrome. Curr Opin Pharmacol 2004;4:166–170.
64. Libby P. Inflammation in atherosclerosis. Nature 2002;420:868–874.
65. Lehtimaki T, Laaksonen R, Janatuinen T, Vesalainen R, Nuutila P, Mattila K et al. Interleukin-1B genotype modulates the improvement of coronary artery reactivity by lipid-lowering therapy with pravastatin: a placebo-controlled positron emission tomography study in young healthy men. Pharmacogenetics 2003;13:633–639.
66. Haddy N, Sass C, Maumus S, Marie B, Droesch S, Siest G et al. Biological variations, genetic polymorphisms and familial resemblance of TNF-alpha and IL-6 concentrations: STANISLAS cohort. Eur J Hum Genet 2005;13:109–117.
67. Basso F, Lowe GD, Rumley A, McMahon AD, Humphries SE. Interleukin-6 -174G>C polymorphism and risk of coronary heart disease in West of Scotland coronary prevention study (WOSCOPS). Arterioscler Thromb Vasc Biol 2002;22:599–604.
68. Trevelyan J, Brull DJ, Needham EW, Montgomery HE, Morris A, Mattu RK. Effect of enalapril and losartan on cytokines in patients with stable angina pectoris awaiting coronary artery bypass grafting and their interaction with polymorphisms in the interleukin-6 gene. Am J Cardiol 2004;94:564–569.
69. Evans WE, Johnson JA. Pharmacogenomics: the inherited basis for interindividual differences in drug response. Annu Rev Genomics Hum Genet 2001;2:9–39.
70. Kalow W. Interethnic variation of drug metabolism. Trends Pharmacol Sci 1991;12:102–107.
71. Siest G, Schlenck A, Starck M, Vincent-Viry M, Schiele F, Visvikis S. Apolipoprotein E: laboratory determinations and clinical interest. In: Rifai N, Warnick GR, Dominiczak MH, editors. Handbook of Lipoprotein Testing. 2000: 401–440.
72. Gerdes LU, Klausen IC, Sihm I, Faergeman O. Apolipoprotein E polymorphism in a Danish population compared to findings in 45 other study populations around the world. Genet Epidemiol 1992;9:155–167.
73. Tiret L, de Knijff P, Menzel HJ, Ehnholm C, Nicaud V, Havekes LM. ApoE polymorphism and predisposition to coronary heart disease in youths of different European populations. The EARS Study. European Atherosclerosis Research Study. Arterioscler Thromb 1994;14:1617–1624.
74. Castellano M, Rossi F, Giacche M, Perani C, Rivadossi F, Muiesan ML et al. Beta(2)-adrenergic receptor gene polymorphism, age, and cardiovascular phenotypes. Hypertension 2003;41:361–367.
75. Jandacek RJ, Woods SC. Pharmaceutical approaches to the treatment of obesity. Drug Discov Today 2004;9:874–880.
76. Nisoli E, Carruba MO. Emerging aspects of pharmacotherapy for obesity and metabolic syndrome. Pharmacol Res 2004;50:453–469.
77. Rankinen T, Zuberi A, Chagnon YC, Weisnagel SJ, Argyropoulos G, Walts B et al. The human obesity gene map: the 2005 update. Obesity (Silver Spring) 2006;14:529–644.
78. Cancello R, Tounian A, Poitou C, Clement K. Adiposity signals, genetic and body weight regulation in humans. Diabetes Metab 2004;30:215–227.
79. Perusse L, Rankinen T, Zuberi A, Chagnon YC, Weisnagel SJ, Argyropoulos G et al. The human obesity gene map: the 2004 update. Obes Res 2005;13:381–490.
80. Ordovas JM, Mooser V. Nutrigenomics and nutrigenetics. Curr Opin Lipidol 2004;15:101–108.
81. Masson LF, McNeill G, Avenell A. Genetic variation and the lipid response to dietary intervention: a systematic review. Am J Clin Nutr 2003;77:1098–1111.
82. Gambier N, Batt AM, Marie B, Pfister M, Siest G, Visvikis-Siest S. Association of CYP2A6*1B genetic variant with the amount of smoking in French adults from the Stanislas cohort. Pharmacogenomics J 2005;5:271–275.
83. Tricker AR. Nicotine metabolism, human drug metabolism polymorphisms, and smoking behaviour. Toxicology 2003;183:151–173.
84. HO MK, Tyndale RF. Overview of the pharmacogenomics of cigarette smoking. The Pharmacogenomics journal 2007.
85. http://www.imm.ki.se/CYPalleles/
86. http://obesitygene.pbrc.edu/
87. http://www.pharmgkb.org/

Chapter 20
Pharmacogenomic Applications in Children

Struan F.A. Grant and Hakon Hakonarson

Contents

Abstract Genetic diversity, together with specific environmental exposures, contributes to both disease susceptibility and interindividual variability in response to drugs. It has proven difficult to isolate disease genes that confer susceptibility to complex disorders, and as a consequence even fewer genetic variants that influence clinical response to drugs have been uncovered. As such, the candidate gene approach has largely failed to deliver and, although the family-based linkage approach has certain theoretical advantages in dealing with common/complex disorders, progress has been slower than was hoped. More recently, genome-wide association (GWA) studies have increasingly gained popularity and been found to be highly robust in identifying variants that associate with and predispose to complex disease, such as age-related macular degeneration, type 2 diabetes, and coronary artery disease. While these diseases dominantly affect adults, more recent studies have unveiled significant association of novel genes predisposing to Type 1 diabetes and autism, and replicated associations to IBD and obesity genes in children. In this regard, the Children's Hospital of Philadelphia recently founded a large-scale high-throughput genotyping

---

Hakon Hakonarson
The Children's Hospital of Philadelphia of the University of Pennsylvania School of Medicine
Philadelphia, PA
hakonarson@chop.edu

N. Cohen (ed.) *Pharmacogenomics and Personalized Medicine*,

program aimed at resolving the pathogenic mechanisms of complex pediatric disorders, through GWA studies of over 100,000 children. This has stirred new hope for the mapping of genes that regulate drug response related to pediatric conditions. Collectively, these studies support the notion that modern high-throughput SNP genotyping technologies, when applied to large and comprehensively phenotyped patient cohorts, capture the most clinically relevant disease-modifying and drug response genes. This review addresses both recent advances in the genotyping field, and some highlights from GWA studies, focusing on pediatric disorders, which have conclusively uncovered variants that underlie disease susceptibility and/or variability in drug response in common disorders.

Keywords Genetics, Pharmacogenomics, Pediatrics, Single Nucleotide Polymorphism, Copy Number Variation, Genome Wide Association

1 Introduction

Pharmacogenomics is a discipline that seeks to examine the genetic basis for individual variation in response to a given therapeutic *(1–3)*. All genes harbor variants termed single nucleotide polymorphisms (SNPs); however, identification of those that are most relevant with respect to their influence on disease susceptibility or drug response traits remains a challenge. At present, there are no good biomarkers that can predict which group of patients will respond positively, which patients are nonresponders, and which will experience an adverse reaction for the same medication and dose *(4–7)*.

The candidate gene approach has been widely used to study the genetic basis of pharmacogenomic traits. Success has been most forthcoming in cancer, where the ability to determine sensitivity to drugs such as trastuzumab (Herceptin; Genentech) and imatinib mesylate (Gleevec [USA], Glivec; Novartis) has made a significant positive impact on patient care and has prompted enthusiasm among investigators to find new opportunities of comparable relevance. Indeed, recent discoveries have unveiled the roles of variants that are pertinent for other drugs demonstrating variable efficacy or adverse effect profiles, which are explained by specific alleles in the metabolizing enzyme gene classes *(7–10)*. However, for most drugs, the genetic variants that determine response remain elusive, and clinicians are being forced to determine dosage regimen for individual patients by a trial-and-error method. Most drugs result in adverse reactions in a subset of patients, with such reactions occurring in more than two million cases annually in the U.S., and accounting for a significant number of deaths and hospital admissions *(11)*.

Since interindividual differences in genetic makeup are found to underlie both disease susceptibility and variability in drug response, better understanding of the genetic information that regulates these processes is needed to elucidate the molecular mechanisms involved and allow for new and more effective therapeutic strategies to be developed *(2, 3, 12)*. However, it must not be forgotten either that drug response is also influenced by numerous nongenetic factors, including dietary factors, sex, disease status, and multiple drug therapy. While clinicians take every measure to avoid adverse reactions, the combinations of interindividual variability as it relates to the disease determinants themselves, genetic and environmental factors, and variability in drug target response via pharmacokinetic, pharmacodynamic, or other idiosyncratic measures, are too complex for any meaningful prediction of drug selection to be made currently.

Notwithstanding the important contribution of the environment, inherited determinants remain the major cause of interindividual differences in drug response *(13)*, underpinning the important need to understand the distribution of genetic variations in the context of the building blocks of the human genome (i.e., linkage disequilibrium [LD] structure) and how ethnic and sex-related differences may influence gene-gene and gene-environment interactions. Variants within the drug metabolizing enzymes, the transporters, or the drug target/pathway members themselves may only be expressed to the extent that they become influential in the context of specific environmental exposures. Ethnic differences may also have a profound impact on drug clearance, thereby affecting safety, efficacy, and dosing regimen. Accordingly, all these factors, either alone or in combination, may influence how drugs are absorbed and distributed in the human body, and also how they are metabolized and excreted *(14)*. In order to improve drug safety and efficacy, a better understanding of these factors and how they interact is required. While traditional linkage and association studies have been highly successful in uncovering variants that underlie monogenetic disorders, and delivering a degree of success in the field of multigenic disorders, the sequencing of the human genome and the completion of the International HapMap Project mark the start of a new and more systematic approach in human genetics. The HapMap project provides an unprecedented resource to investigators with the characterization of the patterns of genetic variation and LD structure across four geographical populations. This has facilitated the design of genome-wide association (GWA) studies and has been a key factor in the unveiling of some of the complexity of human genetic diversity.

This review provides an overview of genetic/genomic discoveries made in IBD, diabetes, asthma, obesity, and cancer. We highlight the studies that have uncovered variants that predispose to these conditions, and discuss how they may influence the observed variability in drug response pertaining to these disorders.

2 Inflammatory Bowel Disease

Inflammatory bowel disease (IBD) is a relatively common inflammatory disorder affecting the gastrointestinal tract, which is resistant to most available therapies. The two common forms of IBD, Crohn's disease (CD) and ulcerative colitis

(UC) have been linked to specific variants in the caspase recruitment domain-containing protein 15 (*CARD15*) gene on chromosome 16q12; the *IBD5* haplotype spanning the organic cation transporter, *SLC22A4*; and genes on chromosome 5q31 *(15–19)*. CD and UC are thought to be related disorders that share some genetic susceptibility loci but differ at others.

Treatment options for IBD have improved considerably in recent years, most notably with the introduction of the TNFα-inhibitor drug. However, anti-TNF therapy is expensive and the response rate is highly variable, with at least one third of the eligible patients failing to show a clinically measurable response. Finding a means to predict those who will respond and exclude those who won't would be beneficial to IBD patients. T helper-type 1 lymphocytes orchestrate much of the inflammation in Crohn's disease, mainly via production of TNFα and IL1β both of which appear to play a pivotal role as proinflammatory cytokines that synergize with each other. A considerably greater effort has been focused on pharmacogenetic approaches to the TNFα pathway, addressing its receptor family (TNFR1 and TNFR2) and signaling events via c-Jun N-terminal kinase/stress-activated protein kinase (JNK/SAPK) activation and NFκB activation that leads to apoptosis. Activated NFκB enters the nucleus and induces transcription of genes associated with inflammation, host defense, and cell survival. The promoter region of the TNF gene lies between nucleotides -1 and -1300, and encompasses numerous polymorphic sites associated with potential binding sites for various transcription factors. Carriers of the TNF allele 2 (TNF2), which contains a single base-pair polymorphism at the -308 promoter position, produce slightly more TNFα in their intestinal mucosa than non-TNF2 carriers. TNF polymorphisms also appear to influence the nature and frequency of extraintestinal manifestations of IBD. A number of routes of inhibition of TNF are being investigated. Among the most extensively evaluated is the use of monoclonal antibodies against TNFα (e.g., infliximab). Several large controlled trials indicate that infliximab has a role in treating patients with moderate to severely active Crohn's disease and with fistulating Crohn's disease. Although it would be useful to genetically differentiate "responders" from "nonresponders," currently there are very few published studies addressing TNF polymorphisms in IBD. Small studies have shown possible associations between poor response to infliximab and increasing mucosal levels of activated NFκB, homozygosity for the polymorphism in exon 6 of TNFR2 (genotype Arg196Arg), positivity for perinuclear antineutrophil cytoplasmic antibodies (ANCA) and the presence of increased numbers of activated lamina propia mononuclear cells producing interferon-gamma and TNFα.

Apart from biotechnology agents targeted against TNFα and IL-1β, others are now being evaluated that are targeted against leukocyte adhesion, T-helper cell (T(h))-1 polarization, T-cell activation, or nuclear factor NFκB. Lymphocyte-endothelial interactions mediated by adhesion molecules are important in leukocyte migration and recruitment to sites of inflammation, and selective blockade of these adhesion molecules is a novel and promising strategy to treat CD. Therapeutic agents that inhibit leukocyte trafficking include natalizumab, MLN-02, and alicaforsen (ISIS 2302). Other agents being investigated for the treatment of Crohn's disease include inhibitors of T-cell activation, peroxisome proliferator-activated receptors, proinflammatory cytokine receptors, and T(h)1 polarization, plus growth hormones and growth factors. Agents being investigated for treatment of UC include many of those mentioned for Crohn's disease. These new therapies will be most meaningful if they carry sufficient horsepower to halt the biomolecular processes that underlie disease progression, an exciting prospect towards development of individualized therapies for IBD.

In late 2006, Duerr et al. made major progress towards our understanding of the pathogenesis of IBD, where they reported highly significant associations between CD and the *IL23R* gene on chromosome 1p31, using the HumanHap 317K gene chip from Illumina *(20)*. Specifically, an uncommon coding variant, rs11209026 (c.1142G>A, p.Arg381Gln), was shown to confer a strong protective effect against the disease and was then replicated in independent cohorts of patients with CD or UC. This innovative genetic study in people, together with two other recent studies in mice, have uncovered a key factor in the pathogenesis of IBD *(21–23)*. The research highlights the proinflammatory cytokine interleukin IL23 *(24, 25)* for prioritizing this molecule and associated signaling pathways as therapeutic targets in IBD and other autoimmune and chronic inflammatory diseases.

IL-23 initiates and perpetuates both innate and T cell–mediated intestinal inflammation. What are the implications of the new findings for the clinic? Active CD is associated with increased IL12 and IL23 production, and IL12 may still have value as a drug target. Indeed, a controlled trial of patients with CD showed that an antibody to the p40 subunit of IL12/IL23 results in higher rates of clinical responses and remissions compared to placebo therapy. These results suggested that targeting both IL12 and IL23 reduces proinflammatory cytokine production by mucosal immune cells. However, selective targeting of IL23 is now emerging as an attractive concept—not only with the new findings, but also because IL12 mediates protective systemic antimicrobial immunity. Thus, blockade of IL23 may be as effective as blocking both cytokines—but may result in fewer infection problems. Yet other observations suggest that selective neutralization of IL23 may not be beneficial under all circumstances. p19-deficient mice are highly susceptible to T cell–mediated colitis induced by a hapten reagent. It seems that in the absence of IL23, gut dendritic cells produced excessive amounts of IL12 (IL23 normally crossregulates IL12). Thus, in the absence of IL23, mice develop enhanced IL12-driven mucosal immunopathology; whether such crossregulation is relevant in patients with IBD remains to be determined. The strong effect of the protective allele identified by Duerr et al. *(20)* could potentially be exploited to define desired functional outcomes. A genetic prediction of responsiveness to anti-IL23 therapy would open the door toward an individualized therapy of IBD patients. Studies are underway addressing how IL23 signaling affects gut inflammation in individual patients, as selective inhibitors and appropriate genetic tools are forthcoming. It is likely that blockade of IL23 function in selected patients will be a breakthrough for clinical therapy. It seems that IL23 plays a unique function for the initiation and perpetuation of innate and T cell–mediated forms of IBD, which genotype-directed pharmacotherapy is about to exploit.

Our laboratory has replicated the findings of Duerr and colleagues in a pediatric study cohort *(23)*, lending further support for the protective role of the *IL23R* gene in CD, and for the first time in pediatric CD, suggesting that interventions at the IL23 pathway level may be of value in both pediatric and adult patients who suffer from this devastating disease. It would seem likely that the culprit variant may influence the therapeutic response of patients to pharmacologic intervention at this biological pathway.

Notwithstanding the potentially important role of IL23, earlier this year, through the genotyping of 16,360 nonsynonymous SNPs, a highly significant association was reported between CD and the autophagy-related 16-like 1 gene (*ATG16L1*) gene *(26)*. Specifically, a common coding variant, rs2241880 (T300A), was shown to confer strong risk for the disease and was then replicated in the same study in separate cohorts of patients with CD but not UC. Since independent replication efforts are now considered mandatory for GWA findings *(27)*, it is pertinent to note that we have also replicated the association of the variant, rs2241880, in the *ATG16L1* gene with CD, and demonstrated for the first time that the effects of this variant are also seen in the childhood form of CD *(28)*. Thus, here is another novel signaling pathway that presents a therapeutic target in IBD and potentially also in other autoimmune or chronic inflammatory diseases. Again, it would seem likely that the culprit variant may influence the therapeutic response of patients to pharmacologic intervention at this biological pathway.

3 Diabetes

Diabetes affects almost 200 million people worldwide and more than 18 million in the United States, with approximately 90 percent of those affected having type 2 diabetes (T2D).

Type 1 diabetes (T1D) risk is strongly influenced by multiple genetic loci and environmental factors. The disease is heritable, with first-degree relatives of cases being at 15-fold greater risk than the general population. Variation in several loci has already been established to account for a significant proportion of the familial clustering of T1D. The major histocompatibility complex (MHC) region on 6p21 (mostly residing in the *HLA-DRB1*, *-DQA1*, and *-DQB1* genes *(29–31)*) is the most influencial locus in T1D. Other loci include the insulin locus (*INS*) on 11p15 *(32–34)*, the protein tyrosine phosphatase-22 (*PTPN22*) gene on 1p13 *(35, 36)*, and the gene encoding the cytotoxic T-lymphocyte-associated protein 4 (*CTLA4*) on 2q31 *(37–39)*. The interleukin-2 receptor alpha (*CD25*) locus on 10p15 *(40)* has also been implicated, while a report of association with a nonsynonymous variant in the innate immunity gene, *IFIH1(41)*, remains to be independently replicated. Several other reported associations *(42–44)* have not been convincingly replicated and remain controversial.

Recently, two independent studies *(45–47)* reported several new T1D loci. Among the genes localized, the *KIAA0350* presents a prime candidate for harboring the causative variant. *KIAA0350* encodes a protein of unknown function and its genomic location is next to the suppressor of cytokine signaling 1 (*SOCS1*) gene. The almost exclusive expression specificity of *KIAA0350* in immune cells (http://symatlas.gnf.org/SymAtlas), including dendritic cells, B lymphocytes, and natural killer (NK) cells, all known to be pivotal in the pathogenesis of T1D *(48, 49)*, suggests that the variant contributes to the disease by modulating immunity. The predicted protein product of *KIAA0350* is a C-type lectin, which belongs to a family of molecules that are known for their recognition of a diversity of carbohydrates, and are critical for a variety of processes ranging from cell adhesion to pathogen recognition. In light of the critical role of the MHC genetic repertoire in antigen presentation involving sugar groups such as lectin, it is plausible that a genetic variant in the binding site for such a molecule on the activating cytotoxic T-cell could elicit an autoimmune response that results in destruction of the islet cells of the pancreas, as seen in T1D. This presents a compelling pharmacogenetic target for T1D intervention, directed at disease prevention.

T2D is also a serious and costly disease that represents approximately $132 billion per year in direct and indirect medical expenses in the U.S. Typically it is a late onset disease (>40 years) and is on the increase due to an aging population and increasing obesity; most concerning is the fact that an increasing number of children and young adults are now developing T2D, a trend that correlates with increased weight gain in these age groups *(50)*. The chronic complications of diabetes include accelerated development of cardiovascular and microvascular disease. T2D is the consequence of hyperglycemia through two possible mechanisms: insulin resistance in skeletal, muscle, liver, and adipose tissue; or abnormal insulin secretion due to pancreatic β-cell defects.

Sulfonylureas stimulate insulin secretion, while metformin addresses insulin resistance through the suppression of glucose production by the liver and increasing skeletal muscle glucose metabolism. Insulin resistance can also be counteracted with thiazolidinediones or glitazones, such as rosiglitazone, that act as insulin sensitizers through the targeting of peroxisomal proliferator-activated receptor-γ. In addition, α-glucosidase inhibitors, such as acarbose, can be utilized to compromise the inhibition of carbohydrate breakdown in the gut. Glucagon-like peptide-1 (GLP-1) is a major physiologic incretion that exerts critical effects on blood glucose homeostasis *(51)*; there is great promise in the extensive clinical developments currently underway of GLP-1 analogs, such as exenatide (synthetic exendin-4) and inhibitors of dipeptidyl peptidase IV. However, successful glycemic control often requires a combination of several oral agents, together with intravenous insulin for more severe cases. The use of currently available therapeutics can often lead to side effects, including increase in body weight, risk of hypoglycemia, and gastrointestinal problems. In addition, the efficacy of these drugs is limited to the early stages of T2D, when fasting blood glucose levels are relatively low, with approximately 40% of T2D patients on oral antidiabetics failing to control their blood glucose and having to supplement with insulin.

There is now clear evidence of a strong genetic component to the disease due to prevalence differences between racial groups, a higher concordance rate among monozygotic than dizygotic twins, and a sibling risk ratio of approximately 3.5 *(52)*. Maturity-onset diabetes of the young (MODY) is the autosomal dominantly inherited form of diabetes without insulin dependency, characterized by β-cell dysfunction, and is diagnosed relatively young (<25 yrs) *(53, 54)*; it is made up of subtypes defined on the basis of genetic etiology. These genetic subtypes have aided the identification of patients who will respond to a given therapy from those who are unlikely to respond. As such, this opens the possibility of tailored drug therapy, both at the individual level for MODY and for the general treatment of type 1 and type 2 diabetics as a whole. Identifying further forms of this monogenic diabetes will provide crucial insights into patterns of β-cell dysfunction and the associated therapeutic response. Of the seven MODY genes identified to date, the most common forms present as a consequence of mutations in the genes encoding the glycolytic enzyme, glucokinase, and the transcription factor, hepatic nuclear factor-1α (HNF1α) *(55, 56)*.

Those MODY patients with glucokinase mutations do not require treatment, as they have only mild hyperglycemia; however, these cases are often incorrectly treated, as they are regularly misdiagnosed as having type 1 or type 2 diabetes. Indeed, when they are given either insulin or oral hypoglycemic medication, there is little impact on their glycemia *(57)*; treating glucose-sensing defects with insulin and oral agents will have minimal impact. Recently, a novel hypoglycemic therapy, which acts as a glucokinase activator *(58, 59)*, has been developed for T2D as a consequence of the genetic characterization of this monogenic form of the disease *(60, 61)*. On the other hand, patients with MODY as a consequence of HNF1α mutations are extremely sensitive to the hypoglycemic effects of sulfonylureas *(62–64)*, representing clear evidence for a pharmacogenetic effect. With such patients, even after a mean of 20 years of insulin treatment, they were able to discontinue insulin therapy and be treated with sulfonylureas without risk of ketoacidosis *(65)*.

The pancreatic ß-cell ATP-sensitive potassium channel (K_{ATP}) is composed of two distinct subunits, an inwardly rectifying ion channel forming the pore (Kir6.2) and a regulatory subunit, the sulfonylurea receptor-1 (SUR1), which binds sulfonylureas. It is well established that loss of function mutations in the *KCNJ11* gene, which encodes Kir6.2, and the *ABCC8* gene, which encodes SUR1, can lead to the oversecretion of insulin and thus hyperinsulinemia. The mutations make the K_{ATP} channel less likely to close in the presence of ATP. Prior to the genetics of this phenotype being resolved, all these patients were treated with insulin and responded like type 1 patients, as they had negligible endogenous insulin secretion. As such, these subjects might secrete insulin in response to sulfonylureas; in fact, in initial physiological studies these patients had no insulin secretory response to glucose or glucagon, but did secrete insulin in response to tolbutamide *(66)*. Sulfonylurea therapy has been tried in many patients with *KCNJ11* mutations; in all reported studies there has been an improvement in glycemic control *(67–70)*.

There is strong evidence that novel T2D genes will potentially be exciting pharmaceutical targets. There is no doubt that the next few years will result in novel susceptibility genes for T2D being identified. There is strong evidence in favor of this already, as the most established T2D susceptibility genes are also well known drug targets, namely the peroxisomal proliferator-activated receptor-γ (*PPARG*) gene, and thiazolidinediones *(71)* and the *KCNJ11* gene, encoding Kir6.2, and sulfonylurea therapy *(72, 73)*.

From the first GWA study of T2D, very recently published in *Nature (74)*, the strongest association observed was with a gene already established as playing a role in the disease, namely the Wnt-signaling pathway member, transcription factor 7-like 2 (*TCF7L2*)*(75)*, which has already been extensively replicated independently *(76–85)*. This association has now been refined utilizing a West African patient cohort *(86)*; this is because in this cohort the associated SNP is contained in a smaller LD block due to higher haplotype diversity in populations of African ancestry, and thus the region most likely to contain the functional variant was narrowed down. The precise mechanism of action for this variant and its influence on the susceptibility to T2D is still to be elucidated; but it is speculated that it could operate through the alteration of levels of the insulinotropic hormone, glucagon-like peptide 1 (GLP-1), one of the peptides encoded by the proglucagon gene whose expression in enteroendocrine cells is transcriptionally regulated by TCF7L2 *(51)*. In tandem with insulin, GLP-1 has a strong influence on blood glucose homeostasis *(51)*. GLP-1 analogs and inhibitors of dipeptidyl peptidase IV are indeed currently in clinical development. It has been noted that individuals with both impaired glucose tolerance and the at-risk *TCF7L2* variant are more likely to go on to develop T2D *(76)*, with the effect reported to be stronger in a placebo group than in metformin and lifestyle-intervention groups. The variant is also associated with decreased insulin secretion, but not increased insulin resistance at baseline *(76)*. The risk-conferring genotypes in *TCF7L2* are thus associated with impaired β-cell function, but not with insulin resistance; and may, therefore, give some indication on optimal therapeutic intervention for the one in five T2D cases this variant impacts.

At least three other variants determined in the GWA study *(74)*, including in the *SLC30A8* and insulin-degrading enzyme (*IDE*) genes, have held up in large-scale independent studies *(87–89)*, and it's likely that they may also interplay with known therapeutic agents. As such, *SLC30A8* encodes a zinc transporter expressed specifically in the secretory vesicles of β-cells, and is thus implicated in the final stages of insulin biosynthesis, which involves co-crystallization with zinc. This may have possible dietary implications and therapeutic approaches through zinc supplementation or, more plausibly, pharmacological manipulation of its transport. Reduction of insulin-degrading enzyme (IDE) activity by a pharmacological inhibitor increases islet amyloid polypeptide (amylin) accumulation and amylin-mediated cytotoxicity in cultured β-cells *(90)*, whereas IDE ablation causes glucose intolerance in knockout mice *(91)*. Three other loci, *CDKAL1*, *CDKN2A/CDKN2B*, and *IGF2BP2*, were also identified by all three studies independently, suggesting that these genes are involved in the pathogenesis of T2D *(87–89)*.

4 Obesity

Obesity is an important risk factor for T2D, cardiovascular disease, and overall mortality *(92, 93)*. Weight-lowering drugs have been developed to facilitate weight reduction in obese individuals who experience difficulties in their efforts to lose weight. A study examining response to the centrally acting noradrenaline and serotonine reuptake inhibitor sibutramine reported a dramatic difference in response to both pharmacological and nonpharmacological programs to reduce weight, a difference attributed to the C825T polymorphism in the guanine nucleotide-binding protein beta-3 (*GNB3*) gene *(94)*. Thus, genotyping of the *CNB3* C825T polymorphism may help predict outcome and identify obese individuals who may benefit from sibutramine therapy. The effort devoted to studying obesity and potential therapeutic interventions is very high, and numerous studies are about to deliver new targets and pharmacogenomic approaches to this much too common medical problem in the coming years. One such target is summarized below.

There is strong evidence for a genetic component to the risk of obesity *(95, 96)*, including prevalence differences between racial groups, from 5% or less in Caucasian and Asian populations to 50% or more among Pima Indians *(97)* and south sea island populations *(98)*. The familial occurrences of obesity have been long noted, with the concordance for fat mass among monozygotic twins reported to be 70–90%, higher than the 35–45% concordance in dizygotic twins *(99, 100)*; as such the estimated heritability of BMI ranges from 30 to 70% *(101–104)*.

A common genetic variant with modest relative risk (RR = ~1.2), located 10 kb upstream of insulin-induced gene 2 (*INSIG2*), has been recently described in *Science* to be associated with both adult and childhood obesity, from the first GWA published for this phenotype, employing a 100,000 SNP genotyping platform *(105)*. In the same study, the investigators presented replication in four out of five separate samples of different ethnicity; in the fifth sample, a large cohort of the Nurses Health Study (NHS), no such association was detectable.

However, this reported association to *INSIG2* has proven controversial, with three subsequent technical reports sent to *Science* refuting the observation. The U.K. group found no evidence of association between this variant and obesity risk in two large ethnically homogeneous population-based cohorts (n = 6599) *(106)*; indeed, they found a trend in the opposite direction. The French study similarly found no effect on the risk of adult obesity or childhood obesity, either in case-control or family-based settings *(107)*; while the German study, although also observing no association in their overall cohort, found an increased risk for obesity in a subgroup analysis of already overweight subjects *(108)*. Therefore, the relative merits of *INSIG2*, plus the newly described Fatso (*FTO*) gene (also in *Science*) *(109)*, with respect to the pathogenesis of obesity, have still to be fully elucidated.

5 Osteoporosis

Osteoporosis is characterized by diminished bone mass and increased bone fragility, leading to the development of fractures, which may be spontaneous or occur as the result of minimal trauma. Osteoporosis has traditionally been defined to exist when a fracture occurs in an individual with low bone mineral density (BMD) i.e., osteopaenia. Osteopaenia in turn is defined as a reduction in bone density when compared with normal values in young healthy individuals; thus, osteopaenic patients may or may not have osteoporotic fractures. During their lifetime, women lose about 30–50% of peak bone mass, and men lose 20–30%, with trabecular bone loss greater than cortical bone loss *(110)*. As a result, both men and women can go on to develop osteoporosis, and the process often starts in childhood.

Calcium and vitamin D intake, together with regular weight-bearing exercises, are important for skeletal health, but are not adequate treatments for osteoporosis. Therapies for the treatment and/or prevention of osteoporosis include bisphosphonates (alendronate, etidronate, ibandronate, and risedronate), calcitonin, estrogens, teriparatide, and raloxifene. For most patients, oral bisphosphonates are the treatment of choice; they are currently the most widely used antiresorptive therapies for the treatment of postmenopausal osteoporosis, mainly because they are usually well tolerated long term. Bisphosphonates are potent antiresorptive agents which, when embedded in the bone matrix, are taken up by osteoclasts engaged in bone resorption, leading to osteoclast apoptosis. Bone resorption subsequently decreases, leading to improved mechanical properties of the bone and a reduced risk of fracture.

BMD is a classic example of a complex trait resulting from the interplay between behavioral, environmental, and genetic factors influencing an individual outcome. There is strong evidence for a genetic component in the predisposition to osteoporosis, with an estimated 60–80% of the variability in the risk explained by heritable factors *(111–113)*. Twin studies also suggest that genetic predisposition determines up to 80% of peak bone mass, whereas the remaining 20% is modulated by environmental factors and sex hormone levels during puberty *(114)*. This genetic influence is consistent with the findings that BMD is reduced in the daughters of osteoporotic women *(115)* and in men and women with first-degree relatives who have osteoporosis *(116)*.

Several studies have examined the influence of variants in the vitamin D receptor (*VDR*) gene on BMD in children. In adult women, *VDR* polymorphisms contribute to a relatively small variation in BMD *(117, 118)*; by contrast, in children, *VDR* polymorphisms account for a greater difference when femoral and vertebral BMD are compared to those with homozygous recessive (bb) and dominant genotypes (BB) *(119, 120)*, suggesting that these polymorphisms have a greater influence on BMD during childhood. In a study of prepubertal girls, dietary calcium intake also correlated with change in BMD in those with homozygous dominant and heterozygous *VDR* (BB and Bb) genotypes, but not in those with the homozygous (bb) genotype *(120)*. Investigation of *VDR* genotype response to 1αOHD$_3$ treatment (1 μg/day) in a one-year retrospective trial among Japanese women found that the common bb genotype was associated with a higher 1αOHD$_3$ response than the Bb genotype *(121)*. In a U.K. twin study, using 800 IU vitamin D3/day, there was a more modest trend toward a positive treatment effect for total hip BMD *(122)*. Furthermore, in a study among Australian women, a greater parathyroid hormone (PTH) response was observed with the *VDR* bb genotype versus the BB genotype with short-term calcitriol administration *(123)*.

A polymorphism in the regulatory region of the collagen 1 alpha 1 (*COL1A1*) gene affects the binding site for the transcription factor Sp1 *(124)*. This polymorphism was shown to be associated with reduced BMD and osteoporotic fracture in pre- and postmenopausal women *(124, 125)*; subsequent meta-analyses of published studies of this polymorphism's association with BMD and fracture incidence have confirmed this initial observation *(126, 127)*. Qureshi et al. *(128)* sought to determine if the *COLIA1* Sp1 polymorphism might act as a predictor of the response to treatment of osteoporosis with bisphosphonate therapy. There was no association between *COLIA1* genotype and response of lumbar spine BMD during cyclical etidronate treatment. However, the response of femoral neck BMD differed significantly between the genotype groups throughout the study period, in which femoral neck BMD increased by 0.56%, 2.36%, 1.82%, and 1.32% after 1, 2, 2.5, and 3 years, respectively, in the SS genotype group; compared with –1.56%, –0.62%, –0.37%, and –0.66% in the Ss/ss genotype groups. Their data raise the possibility that *COLIA1* genotyping could be used to target etidronate therapy to those most likely to respond in terms of femoral neck BMD.

More recently, human genetics has pointed out the role of the Wnt signaling pathway as a major regulator of bone mass accrual *(129)*. A family study of an unusual autosomal dominant inherited high bone mass phenotype was used to map a mutation in the gene encoding the low-density lipoprotein receptor-related protein 5 (*LRP5*) gene *(130, 131)*. The LRP5 protein normally mediates the binding of a growth factor, Wnt, to its receptor, which allows activation of intracellular signaling to promote osteoblastic differentiation. Osteoporosis-pseudoglioma syndrome, characterized by low bone mass with childhood fractures and abnormal eye development, is the result of an inherited loss of function of the *LRP5* gene *(132)*, leading to inhibition of Wnt signaling. Wnts are secreted glycoproteins that bind to receptor complexes, including low-density lipoprotein receptor-related protein (LRP)-5/6 and frizzled proteins. A subsequent intracellular cascade of events stabilizes β-catenin, leading to its translocation into the nucleus, where, associated with Tcf/Lef transcription factors, it triggers gene expression. The existence of many potential pharmacological targets in this pathway makes it attractive for bone anabolic drug discovery, but further work is required on this interesting target in order to potentially reveal pharmacogenetic properties.

6 Asthma

Asthma is a complex genetic disorder with a heterogeneous phenotype affecting approximately 20 million individuals in the United States and over 300 million worldwide *(133, 134)*. Asthma is attributed to the interactions between many genes and the environment, and it has been suggested that genetics may contribute to as much as 60–80% of the interindividual variability in therapeutic response to asthma medications. Numerous genetic studies have reported linkage or association with asthma and the asthma-associated phenotypes, atopy, elevated immunoglobulin E (IgE) levels, and bronchial hyperresponsiveness. In addition, specific alleles tagging cytokine/chemokine, remodeling, or IgE regulating genes have been shown to confer risk to these phenotypes.

Although many studies reporting these observations are compelling, only a handful of genes have been uncovered that confer a meaningful risk of asthma. Moreover, the clinical implications of genetic variation reported within the numerous candidate asthma genes with respect to therapeutic response to drugs remain largely undetermined. Although progress has been slow, the asthma research community has benefited tremendously from recent developments, including the cloning of the *ADAM 33* (a disintegrin and metalloproteinase domain 33), *PHF11* (PHD finger protein 11) and *GPRA* (G protein-coupled receptor 154) genes *(135–137)*. These discoveries reveal how genetic/genomic factors may influence the pathobiology underlying complex disease. They have also stimulated interest in the study of gene-gene and gene-environment interactions, where LD structure can be leveraged to pinpoint mutations. In addition, these variants may well influence asthma susceptibility and treatment response, which has implications for the next step, namely individualized therapy.

Common diseases, such as asthma, that have a strong but complex genetic component, together with variable drug response, present an ideal challenge for pharmacogenomic research *(138–141)*. Currently used drugs are not effective in all individuals, with relapse in a high percentage of patients, and severe adverse effects also observed. The ability to analyze SNP patterns and expression levels of thousands of genes using oligonucleotide microarrays allows for a powerful screen of multiple molecular pathways simultaneously that may elucidate genes that determine drug response *(142, 143)*. Generally, several genes are involved which, in conjunction with specific environmental factors, influence the efficacy of the drug response in certain individuals and the potential for adverse events in others. In addition, the allelic interactions of the respective variants (i.e., SNP pattern) of the genes or gene pathways involved are highly complex, and the resulting gene-gene and gene-environment interactions remain for the most part unexplained. Thus, it is no surprise that as many as 2/3 of patients with asthma may not attain full control of their symptoms despite modern therapies *(144, 145)*. It also appears that about 1/3 of patients treated with inhaled corticosteroids (ICSs) may not achieve objective improvements in airway function or measures of airway reactivity *(146)*. A similar number of patients using oral corticosteroids develop osteoporosis *(147–149)*; cataracts and glaucoma are also reported side effects from ICS use *(150–152)*. In addition, approximately 5000 asthma deaths occur in the US every year, which in large part is due to the use of long-acting beta-agonists *(153)*.

Drug responses vary widely between different populations and are also highly variable among individuals within the same population. A representative example is the observed variability between asthma patients to beta$_2$-agonist therapy, where up to ¾ of the variability is genetically based, albeit the proportion is different among different ethnic groups *(13)*. Homozygosity for arginine at position 16 (the Arg/Arg genotype) of the beta-adrenergic receptor predicts therapeutic response to beta$_2$-agonists in Puerto Ricans, but not in Mexicans *(154)*. There is also evidence suggesting that variants in the ß$_2$-adrenergic receptor may explain differences in airway responsiveness in smokers versus nonsmokers *(155)*; this phenomenon is also evident in subjects using both ICSs and cigarettes *(156)*. Numerous candidate gene studies have been conducted in an attempt to unravel this mystery, although the hunt for polymorphisms in candidate genes has not been productive thus far; but the results from ongoing GWA studies in asthma are likely to fuel the interest of asthma investigators in the near future.

Polymorphisms can occur in coding and noncoding regions of genes, with their mechanism of action with respect to altered gene function generally remaining poorly understood. SNPs are by far the most commonly studied variants in pharmacogenetic/genomic studies *(157)*. Most disease-associated variants are not expected to be directly functional themselves, but instead are more likely to be in LD with the functional "smoking gun" mutations. Approximately 10 million SNPs are known to exist in the human genome, and they are stable over time *(158, 159)*. A different set of variants, known as "microsatellites," constitute variable numbers of tandem repeats that may also produce functional changes or serve as markers for other changes in the genome. Examining haplotypes, defined as varying combinations (similar to a barcode) of SNPs and/or variable numbers of tandem repeats over a linked region on a single chromosome, is also considered an informative way of studying disease susceptibility or drug response in pharmacogenomic association studies.

6.1 Pharmacogenomic Overview of Beta$_2$-Agonists, Leukotriene Modifiers and Corticosteroids

The classes of antiasthma medications that are available to patients include the bronchodilators, such as beta$_2$-adrenergic agonists, and the antiinflammatory agents, glucocorticoids and leukotriene modifiers, with other drugs being rarely used. Pharmacogenomic studies on asthma are typically designed to determine whether the variations under study influence function with respect to these drugs. Most of these studies have been hypothesis driven and are based on a relatively small number of patients, thereby lacking the power to assess factors that can confound genetic associations. A more broad-based nonhypothesis driven genome-wide approach requires many more patients and is more costly; but it is more likely to uncover novel variants in genes that influence or modify drug response. Thus, the GWA approach extends beyond the gene or pathway of interest and is used to screen for unknown disease or drug response variants. While these studies are in their infancy, it should be noted that a somewhat comparable approach was used to identify the association between the metalloproteinase gene, *ADAM 33*, and asthma *(135)*. To the extent that drug response is heritable, pharmacogenomics seeks to define the relationship between variability in the human genetic code and variability in response to pharmacologic interventions. Most studies to date have dealt with the signaling pathway from the receptor drug targets themselves to the drug transporters and metabolizing enzyme cascades, focusing on the pharmacokinetic and pharmacodynamic characteristics of the drug in terms of clinical response measures. The following section addresses the genetic diversity among individuals as it pertains to the receptor signaling pathways of the major drug classes used in asthma therapy.

6.2 Beta$_2$-Agonists

Signaling through the beta$_2$-adrenergic receptor (beta$_2$AR) mediates numerous airway functions that are beneficial for subjects with asthma. As a result, beta$_2$-agonists are considered the first line of therapy for bronchodilation and rapid relief from asthma symptoms *(160)*. The beta$_2$AR is also considered a putative candidate gene in the pathogenesis of asthma and related traits. Numerous studies have highlighted the important role of the airway smooth muscle in asthma, mediating not only the bronchoconstrictor effects of agents, such as histamine and cholinergic agonists, but also the bronchodilator effects of beta$_2$-agonists through the beta$_2$-AR *(161, 162)*. The sequence of the beta$_2$-AR has been known for many years, and the effect of gene polymorphisms on receptor function has been thoroughly investigated *(163–169)*. At least nine different point mutations have been found in the gene at nucleotide positions 46, 79, 100, 252, 491, 523, 1053, 1098, and 1239 *(164)*. Four of these were found to cause changes in the encoded amino acids at residues at positions 16, 27, 34, and 164, with Arg16Gly and Gln27Glu being the most frequent and showing the most effect. Several studies have investigated the role of the beta$_2$-AR in asthma, including both bronchial hyperreactivity and modulation of the response to acute or chronic beta$_2$-agonist therapy *(165–167)*. As a result, bronchodilator desensitization was found to be much higher with homozygous Gly-16 than with homozygous Arg-16 for maximal forced expiratory volume in 1s (FEV1) response *(168)*. Another group studying the effects of beta$_2$-AR genotypes on responsiveness to beta$_2$-agonist therapy in children reported that asthmatic patients who were homozygous for Arg-16 had a significantly greater (>5 fold) bronchodilator response to albuterol than homozygous Gly-16 individuals *(165)*. Similar results have been reported in multiple other populations, suggesting they are real *(166, 167, 169)*. However, replication attempted in the Indian population reported exactly the opposite effect of these genotypes *(170)*, and others have found either no difference between Gly-16 and Arg-16 receptor variants *(161)* or a decrease in response in mild asthmatics carrying the homozygous Arg-16 genotype *(171)*.

Interestingly, regular use of beta-agonist drugs has been reported to have detrimental effects on symptoms and lung function in double-blinded placebo-controlled studies *(172)*. Moreover, asthma patients carrying the Arg/Arg form may benefit by minimizing the use of both short-acting and long-acting beta$_2$-agonists; and Arg/Arg patients do not get any benefit from the use of salmeterol, even when used concurrently with inhaled corticosteroids, and may develop worse airway function with chronic use of long-acting beta$_2$-agonists *(173)*. Salmeterol may even provoke a proinflammatory effect in Arg/Arg patients *(173, 174)*. Studies also suggest that the genotype-phenotype correlations may differ significantly across different ethnic groups, such as in the Study of African-Americans, Asthma, Genes, and Environments (SAGE), in which the authors reported a significant association of the SNP at position –47 (Arg-19Cys) with bronchodilator drug responsiveness in certain groups and not others *(175)*. Replication studies are needed to validate the differential role of this SNP on drug response in subjects of different ethnic backgrounds.

Reports suggest that 60% of asthma children who are homozygous for arginine at position 16 (Arg^{16}/Arg^{16}) may respond favorably to albuterol, compared with only 13% in individuals homozygous for glycine at that position *(176, 177)*. Others have not found such a striking difference, in studies including both pediatric *(170)* and adult patients *(154)*. In a study addressing haplotype diversity based on 13 SNPs in the $beta_2$-AR gene, haplotypes were detected at the 5-prime end that differed significantly among different ethnic populations *(163)*. Interestingly, a relatively common haplotype that captured the Arg16 variant that was found to associate with decreased response to $beta_2$-agonists, showed the opposite effect in other cohorts *(154, 177)*, illustrating the important differences among subjects of different ethnic backgrounds. It is important to test for these variants in subjects who do not respond well to standard therapies, particularly if the patients are using high doses of $beta_2$-agonists and controller medications, and their asthma remains poorly controlled. It is less clear if the long-acting $beta_2$-agonists are affected the same way by these pharmacogenetic variants, and studies investigating the effects of these polymorphisms on the response to long-acting $beta_2$-agonists are currently underway. Thus, the genetics of drug response traits is complex *(178, 179)*, and broader genomics approaches are needed to provide new insights into the molecular mechanisms of complex diseases and how to optimize therapy for the individual patient.

6.3 Leukotriene Modifiers

The cysteinyl-leukotrienes, LTC_4, LTD_4, and LTE_4, are lipoxygenase-derived eicosanoids and potent proinflammatory mediators that regulate contractile and inflammatory responses through G protein-coupled receptors. Pharmacological studies have identified two classes of cysteinyl leukotriene receptors, CysLT1 and CysLT2, and additional subtypes are likely to exist. Molecular cloning of the human CysLT1 and CysLT2 receptors has confirmed their structural differences. Cysteinyl-LTs have been causatively implicated in asthma and allergic rhinitis, and have also been shown to play a role in other inflammatory conditions, such as cardiovascular diseases, cancer, and dermatitis. The leukotriene pathway genes have been examined for functional variants in the form of SNPs or other changes that may account for disease susceptibility or differences in therapeutic responses to leukotriene modifier drugs. In this regard, variations of the promoter region of the 5-lipoxygenase (*ALOX5*) gene and the leukotriene C_4 (LTC_4) synthase gene have been characterized best, and both have been associated with functional changes of these genes that affect drug response. Genetic variants have also been identified for the CysLT1 and CysLT2 receptors and are being examined in the context of asthma and atopy. Although several studies addressing the effects of variations in the LT pathway genes on responses to leukotriene modifier therapy have reported effects on drug response that may have clinical relevance, there are as many studies that have reported negative findings. Better powered studies are needed, since meta-analysis on existing data is unlikely to sort this out.

6.4 *ALOX5*

The first committed enzyme in the leukotriene biosynthetic pathway is 5-lipoxygenase (ALOX5). Several naturally occurring mutations are known to exist in the *ALOX5* gene, including a variable number of tandem repeats in the promoter region of the gene that can modify transcription factor binding and reporter gene transcription. These microsatellites have been shown to code for the binding motif of the Sp1 and Egr1 transcription factors, thereby affecting the transcription rate of the gene *(180)*. Alterations in the number of tandem repeats have been shown to alter the efficiency of gene transcription such that any variation from the wild type decreased gene transcription, at least in subjects with asthma *(13)*. Patients with mild-to-moderate asthma who were treated with an ALOX5 inhibitor and who carried at least one wild-type allele of the *ALOX5* promoter locus were shown to have greater improvement in FEV_1 than those without any wild-type alleles *(181)*. These data suggest that the absence of at least one copy of the wild-type allele creates a phenotype that is less responsive to leukotriene modifiers. While these results may sound intriguing with respect to pharmacogenetic applications, the variations account for only about 5% of the variability in response to leukotriene modifier therapy.

6.5 *Leukotriene C_4 (LTC4) Synthase*

The LTC_4 synthase enzyme converts LTA_4 to LTC_4. The latter molecule is a critical mediator of the adverse reactions in aspirin-sensitive patients with asthma *(182)*. Substitution of A to C at the -444 site of the promoter of the gene is associated with three times the eosinophil-mediated LTC_4 production in individuals with the wild-type genotype *(183)*. Patients possessing the variant LTC_4 synthase, enhanced leukotriene synthesis, may contribute disproportionately to asthma pathophysiology, potentially making these patients a good target group for leukotriene modifier therapy. In a study of patients with asthma, those with variant LTC_4 synthase genotypes receiving the leukotriene receptor antagonist zafirlukast for two weeks had a 9% increase in FEV_1, whereas patients with the wild-type genotype conversely had a 12% decrease *(183)*. In contrast, no genotype effects were shown on airway hyperresponsiveness in patients on leukotriene modifier therapy *(184)*. As a result, the observed differential response in FEV1 to leukotriene modifier therapy with respect to LTC_4 synthase polymorphisms suggests that this locus may help determine those who may benefit more from this therapy. Because variant LTC_4 synthase genotypes are prevalent in patients with both aspirin-tolerant and -intolerant asthma *(185)*, if the effects of this polymorphism are confirmed, its high prevalence may make it a useful predictor of response to this class of agents.

Leukotriene-modifer drugs are widely used to treat asthma; however, there is growing evidence that the vast majority of asthma patients may not benefit from leukotriene antagonists when administered in combination with other therapies *(186, 187)*. LTC_4 receptor antagonist drugs have been found to be safe and well tolerated. In contrast, up to 5% of patients using 5-lipoxygenase inhibitors develop increases in liver function enzymes *(188)*.

6.6 Corticosteroids

Glucocorticoids (GCs) are the most effective drugs available in asthma therapy *(189)*. In sensitive individuals, inhalation of GCs at doses <1,000 μg per day has been shown to have relatively little capacity to activate transcription within PBMC at concentrations found in plasma, and their action is thought to occur mainly within the lung *(190)*. This finding is in keeping with their relatively restricted systemic side effects at low or intermittent doses, whereas their repression of transcription factor activities, such as AP-1 and NF-κB, in the airways concurs with their clinical efficacy in glucocorticoid-sensitive (GC-S) patients *(190)*. In contrast, glucocorticoid resistant (GC-R) patients may suffer serious side effects because of escalation of drug dose caused by hyporesponsiveness. GC resistance has been defined as the lack of a response to a prolonged course of high-dose (0.5–1.0 mg/kg per day) oral GC *(191, 192)*. Two forms of GC-R asthma have been reported, primary and acquired types *(193–195)*. The acquired form (type I) has been associated with abnormally reduced GC receptor ligand and DNA binding affinity, whereas type II GC-R asthma has been associated with primary GC receptor binding abnormality. In both forms, there is lack of GC-mediated inhibition of expression and release of molecules in PBMC, including the cytokines, interleukin (IL)-13 and IL-4 *(193–195)*.

Modern asthma therapy is largely centered on inhaled corticosteroids (ICSs) with the vast majority of patients demonstrating a favorable response to therapy *(196)*. ICSs have been shown to mediate multiple beneficial effects in individuals with asthma, but are also associated with multiple adverse effects. The mechanisms of action of ICSs are complex and remain incompletely characterized, and only a few pharmacogenomic studies have been reported. A candidate gene study in three study populations suggested a relationship between the response to ICSs and a polymorphism in the corticotropin-releasing hormone receptor 1 (*CRHR1*) gene *(197)*. Polymorphisms in *CRHR1* were positively associated with significantly improved lung function after eight weeks of ICS therapy. A haplotype in 27% frequency (GAT) showed modest increase in FEV_1 in response to ICSs in homozygous subjects in two out of the three populations, whereas a single SNP correlated with similar improvement in the third population. The association of different SNPs in the same gene with changes in lung function suggests that the actual causal variant in *CRHR1* remains to be discovered, but that the three variants studied are imperfectly correlated markers in LD with a causal polymorphism. However, it is too early to tell whether the *CRHR1* polymorphisms will be useful clinical predictors of response to ICSs.

A functional variant in the gene coding for transcription factor T-bet (T-box expressed in T-cells) was recently reported by the same group *(197)*, a finding that may be able to predict responsiveness to ICSs. A variant in the *TBX21* gene associates with significant improvement in methacholine responsiveness in children with asthma who are being treated with ICSs. However, the minor allele frequency for this mutation (H33Q) is only 4.5%, suggesting that although the effect of the mutation may be large, it may only affect a small number of individuals.

In a study applying a high-density oligonucleotide microarray approach to search for differences in mRNA expression profiles in peripheral blood mononuclear cells (PBMC) from GC-S and GC-R asthma patients, gene expression was examined at baseline (resting PBMCs) and following treatment with a combination of IL-1β and TNFα *(198)*. In an attempt to further unveil genes that contribute to the responsiveness of GC, in vitro effects of GC treatment on gene expression were compared in cells that were activated with IL-1β and TNFα. The rationale for this strategy was based on the concepts that the manifestations of asthma are, at least in part, channeled through the actions of IL-1β and TNFα *(199, 200)*, and that the efficacy of GCs in asthma is, at least in part, through its effect on the expression of genes that are modulated by proinflammatory cytokines *(199)*. The authors showed that GC responders could be separated from nonresponders with over 80% accuracy, by using the expression levels of only a few genes. The gene encoding the NFκB DNA binding subunit (*NFKB1*) was shown to confer the best predictive ability. A large number of genes are being translated after NFκB activation, including cytokines, chemokines, growth factors, cellular ligands, and adhesion molecules, many of which have been strongly associated with asthma, and most of which react briskly to glucocorticoid therapy in sensitive individuals. Indeed, the efficacy of GC drugs in asthma is, at least in part, related to their efficacy in inhibiting transcription factors such as NFκB. Thus NFκB is an exciting pharmacogenetic candidate, and a growing body of evidence suggests that it may be among the key culprit candidates in asthma *(201, 202)*.

7 Genome-Wide Association Studies and Pediatric Biorepository Efforts

The Children's Hospital of Philadelphia (CHOP) recently completed a pediatric genomic center, the Center for Applied Genomics (CAG), which is directed at high-throughput genetic analyses in children, allowing for a genotyping rate of hundreds of DNA samples per day, and aiming at genotyping over 100,000 children in 3–4 years. The facility is coupled to electronic medical records within the health care network at CHOP for those patients that volunteer to participate. All personal information and data, including both phenotypes and genotypes, are thoroughly encrypted to ensure deidentification of the research. The CAG has currently genotyped over 25,000 subjects at a SNP density of 550,000 per sample. The diseases that are being examined include some of the most common complex pediatric disorders, such as asthma, obesity, IBD, T1D, attention deficit hyperactivity disorder, autism, SLE, JIA, SLE, atopic dermatitis, and neuroblastoma, to name a few. In addition, extensive effort has been devoted towards high-resolution mapping of copy number variations (CNVs) in "healthy" individuals, wherein several thousand subjects and family trios have been examined, in order to better define the "normal" CNVs of the genome. This will render it easier to assess both de novo alterations, as well as novel heritable CNVs, based on the family trios analysis, and addressing the role these variaions play in disease.

Since several of the diseases under study manifest themselves as inflammatory disorders (i.e., asthma, IBD, JIA, T1D, SLE, AD), where the same cells are involved in the pathogenesis, albeit in different organ systems, the notion that there may be a final common pathway involved that underlies the cellular perturbation in these disorders is highly compelling. Thus an effort is underway directed at addressing the genetic factors involved in these disorders "collectively." This is likely to bear fruit, given recent advances in the technology platforms that have made gene discovery highly robust. Thus, by applying a GWA approach to address the causes of some of these most common and complex diseases that we are challenged with every day, and that we currently treat empirically, discovery can be made not only of those genetic factors that are disease specific, but more importantly also on those factors that are common among these related genetic disorders. Moreover, apart from unveiling the mechanisms of these diseases themselves, a project of this size and scope is also in an ample position to dissect out the environmental factors that interact with the disease genes and constitute the gene-environment network that underlies complex diseases, as well as to address the pharmacogenomic opportunities for those subjects who harbor these variants and who are most likely to benefit from a given therapy.

8 Summary

Pharmacogenetics is the study of genetic variation underlying differential responses to drugs. Examples of pharmacogenetic markers discovered through a hypothesis-driven approach in which polymorphisms were identified in a plausible candidate gene remain few. Pharmacogenomics is charged with applying large-scale systematic approaches that expedite the discovery of drug response markers, whether they act at the level of the drug target, drug metabolism, or disease pathways. The Human Genome Project, together with various commercial efforts, has largely driven this effort by their successful release of the human genome DNA sequence. While pharmacogenomics is a developing field with the principal objective of dissecting the effects of genetic variations on human drug responses, it is also likely to play a key role in identifying novel drug targets that may lead to improved and more effective therapies. Until recently, pharmacogenetic studies were usually limited to investigations of a single polymorphism/gene in small groups of individuals in research settings. With the development of GWA studies, a technology using hundreds of thousands of SNPs in a search for variants that contribute to complex diseases, the linkage and candidate gene approach has been replaced with high-throughput genotyping methods that allow for examination of multiple genetic loci, spanning the entire human genome, in large pools of individuals simultaneously. This is likely to deliver a new generation of drugs and diagnostics and lead to a major paradigm shift from conventional medicine to efficient predictive medicine.

In light of the observations that interindividual differences in the efficacy and toxicity of medication are common among patients, knowledge of an individual genetic variability in drug response becomes clinically and economically important. Pharmacogenetics and pharmacogenomics approaches are tailored towards investigating interindividual variations and their effects on drug response. Genetic profiling of a population has the potential of providing benefits for future medical care by predicting drug response phenotypes using DNA-based tests. The rapid development of new technology platforms in recent years is now enabling investigators to conduct high-throughput experiments scanning the whole genome in search of genes and variants that underlie many of the common diseases that affect human beings, as well as of therapeutic responses to drugs used to treat these conditions. In contrast to "candidate gene" approaches, GWA studies have a key advantage: they offer a relatively unbiased survey of the genome and make no a priori assumptions about where the risk variants reside. The powerful combination of GWA, coupled with ultra-high-throughput microarray genotyping platforms, gene expression technologies, and innovative bioinformatic and computational biology approaches, is bringing such knowledge closer to reality, as these integrative strategies enable scientists to pinpoint disease-causing gene pathways that may also influence differential responses to drugs. While several genes that confer disease susceptibility have been uncovered, the genetic causes of most common diseases remain unresolved. Optimal use of the HapMap dataset in future genome-wide association studies, conducted on large cohorts and replicated in different populations, presents a major challenge for gene hunters in the coming years. The incorporation of pharmacogenetic data into clinical practice will guide risk assessment and treatment decisions, thereby revolutionizing the practice of medicine in the future.

With the successful completion of genome-wide association (GWA) studies, numerous loci have been identified, most of which will require resequencing. For gene mutation identification, resequencing is the natural extension of high-resolution genotyping and must be carried out for both quality control and discovery purposes. Ultra-high throughput bidirectional resequencing of the corresponding linkage disequilibrium (LD) blocks (averaging 50kb in Caucasians) for all candidate loci in genomic DNA, derived from both cases and controls harboring the key SNP alleles and/or haplotypes established to be associated with the disease phenotype under study, will enhance the chances that causal variants are identified. Ultra-high throughput sequencing of all candidate LD blocks in parallel will provide unprecedented information to fully understand and interpret the regions under study and to identify the underlying causative mutations. Validation of SNP genotypes via direct sequencing will verify any newly discovered sequence variants directly by sequencing in both directions. New single nucleotide insertion or deletion alterations discovered during resequencing need to be analyzed in the context of the existing SNP data. The high-throughput sequencing systems available from Illumina, Roche, and ABI allow for the sequencing of billion(s) of bases (1Gb) per run in a matter of weeks. This represents a major advance in sequencing technologies, as more established methodologies, such as capillary-based platforms, require many years to generate the same amount of data. No doubt, the whole genome sequencing approach will have a stunning impact on the practice of medicine within the next five years.

References

1. Cartwright CP (2001) Pharmacogenetics: the Dx perspective. Expert Rev Mol Diagn 1(4):371–376.
2. Roses AD (2002) Pharmacogenetics place in modern medical science and practice. Life Sci 70(13):1471–1480.
3. Roses AD (2000) Pharmacogenetics and the practice of medicine. Nature 405(6788):857–865.
4. Lin M, Aquilante C, Johnson JA, Wu R (2005) Sequencing drug response with HapMap. Pharmacogenomics J 5(3):149–156.
5. Stoughton RB, Friend SH (2005) How molecular profiling could revolutionize drug discovery. Nat Rev Drug Discov 4(4):345–350.
6. Phillips KA, Van Bebber SL (2005) Measuring the value of pharmacogenomics. Nat Rev Drug Discov 4(6):500–509.
7. Wilkinson GR (2005) Drug metabolism and variability among patients in drug response. N Engl J Med 352(21):2211–2221.
8. Voora D, Eby C, Linder MW et al (2005) Prospective dosing of warfarin based on cytochrome P-450 2C9 genotype. Thromb Haemostasis 93(4):700–705.
9. Totah RA, Rettie AE (2005) Cytochrome P450 2C8: substrates, inhibitors, pharmacogenetics, and clinical relevance. Clin Pharmacol Ther 77(5):341–352.
10. de Leon J, Susce MT, Pan RM et al (2005) The CYP2D6 poor metabolizer phenotype may be associated with risperidone adverse drug reactions and discontinuation. J Clin Psychiat 66(1):15–27.
11. Lazarou J, Pomeranz BH, Corey PN (1998) Incidence of adverse drug reactions in hospitalized patients: a meta-analysis of prospective studies. JAMA 279(15):1200–1205.
12. Hakonarson H, Thorvaldsson S, Helgadottir A et al (2005) Effects of a 5-lipoxygenase-activating protein inhibitor on biomarkers associated with risk of myocardial infarction: a randomized trial. JAMA 293(18):2245–2256.
13. Drazen JM, Silverman EK, Lee TH (2000) Heterogeneity of therapeutic responses in asthma. Brit Med Bull 56(4):1054–1070.
14. Xie HG, Kim RB, Wood AJ, Stein CM (2001) Molecular basis of ethnic differences in drug disposition and response. Ann Rev Pharmacol Toxicol 41, 815–850.

15. Vermeire S, Pierik M, Hlavaty T et al (2005) Association of organic cation transporter risk haplotype with perianal penetrating Crohn's disease but not with susceptibility to IBD. Gastroenterology 129(6):1845–1853.
16. Hugot JP, Chamaillard M, Zouali H et al (2001) Association of NOD2 leucine-rich repeat variants with susceptibility to Crohn's disease. Nature 411(6837):599–603.
17. Ogura Y, Bonen DK, Inohara N et al (2001) A frameshift mutation in NOD2 associated with susceptibility to Crohn's disease. Nature 411(6837):603–606.
18. Rioux JD, Daly MJ, Silverberg MS et al (2001) Genetic variation in the 5q31 cytokine gene cluster confers susceptibility to Crohn disease. Nat Genet 29(2):223–228.
19. Peltekova VD, Wintle RF, Rubin LA et al (2004) Functional variants of OCTN cation transporter genes are associated with Crohn disease. Nat Genet 36(5):471–475.
20. Duerr RH, Taylor KD, Brant SR et al (2006) A genome-wide association study identifies IL23R as an inflammatory bowel disease gene. Science 314(5804):1461–1463.
21. Hue S, Ahern P, Buonocore S et al (2006) Interleukin-23 drives innate and T cell-mediated intestinal inflammation. J Exp Med 203(11):2473–2483.
22. Kullberg MC, Jankovic D, Feng CG et al (2006) IL-23 plays a key role in Helicobacter hepaticus-induced T cell-dependent colitis. J Exp Med 203(11):2485–2494.
23. Baldassano RN, Bradfield JP, Monos DS et al (2007) Association of variants of the interleukin-23 receptor (IL23R) gene with susceptibility to pediatric Crohn's disease. Clin Gastroenterol Hepatol (in press).
24. Oppmann B, Lesley R, Blom B et al (2000) Novel p19 protein engages IL-12p40 to form a cytokine, IL-23, with biological activities similar as well as distinct from IL-12. Immunity 13(5):715–725.
25. Becker C, Wirtz S, Blessing M et al (2003) Constitutive p40 promoter activation and IL-23 production in the terminal ileum mediated by dendritic cells. The J Clin Invest 112(5):693–706.
26. Hampe J, Franke A, Rosenstiel P et al (2007) A genome-wide association scan of nonsynonymous SNPs identifies a susceptibility variant for Crohn disease in ATG16L1. Nat Genet 39(2):207–211.
27. Patterson M, Cardon L (2005) Replication publication. PLoS Biol 3(9):e327.
28. Baldassano RN, Bradfield JP, Monos DS et al (2007) Association of the T300A non-synonymous variant of the ATG16L1 gene with susceptibility to pediatric Crohn's disease. Gut (in press).
29. Cucca F, Lampis R, Congia M et al (2001) A correlation between the relative predisposition of MHC class II alleles to type 1 diabetes and the structure of their proteins. Human Mol Genet 10(19):2025–2037.
30. Nerup J, Platz P, Andersen OO et al (1974) HL-A antigens and diabetes mellitus. Lancet 2(7885):864–866.
31. Noble JA, Valdes AM, Cook M et al (1996) The role of HLA class II genes in insulin-dependent diabetes mellitus: molecular analysis of 180 Caucasian, multiplex families. Am J Human Genet 59(5):1134–1148.
32. Bell GI, Horita S, Karam JH (1984) A polymorphic locus near the human insulin gene is associated with insulin-dependent diabetes mellitus. Diabetes 33(2):176–183.
33. Bennett ST, Lucassen AM, Gough SC et al (1995) Susceptibility to human type 1 diabetes at IDDM2 is determined by tandem repeat variation at the insulin gene minisatellite locus. Nat Genet 9(3):284–292.
34. Vafiadis P, Bennett ST, Todd JA et al (1997) Insulin expression in human thymus is modulated by INS VNTR alleles at the IDDM2 locus. Nat Genet 15(3):289–292.
35. Bottini N, Musumeci L, Alonso A et al (2004) A functional variant of lymphoid tyrosine phosphatase is associated with type I diabetes. Nat Genet 36(4):337–338.
36. Smyth D, Cooper JD, Collins JE et al (2004) Replication of an association between the lymphoid tyrosine phosphatase locus (LYP/PTPN22) with type 1 diabetes, and evidence for its role as a general autoimmunity locus. Diabetes 53(11):3020–3023.

37. Kristiansen OP, Larsen ZM, Pociot F (2000) CTLA-4 in autoimmune diseases—a general susceptibility gene to autoimmunity? Genes Immun 1(3):170–184.
38. Ueda H, Howson JM, Esposito L et al (2003) Association of the T-cell regulatory gene CTLA4 with susceptibility to autoimmune disease. Nature 423(6939):506–511.
39. Anjos SM, Tessier MC, Polychronakos C (2004) Association of the cytotoxic T lymphocyte-associated antigen 4 gene with type 1 diabetes: evidence for independent effects of two polymorphisms on the same haplotype block. The J Clin Endocr Metab 89(12):6257–6265.
40. Vella A, Cooper JD, Lowe CE et al (2005) Localization of a type 1 diabetes locus in the IL2RA/CD25 region by use of tag single-nucleotide polymorphisms. Am J Human Genet 76(5):773–779.
41. Smyth DJ, Cooper JD, Bailey R et al (2006) A genome-wide association study of nonsynonymous SNPs identifies a type 1 diabetes locus in the interferon-induced helicase (IFIH1) region. Nat Genet 38(6):617–619.
42. Guo D, Li M, Zhang Y et al (2004) A functional variant of SUMO4, a new I kappa B alpha modifier, is associated with type 1 diabetes. Nat Genet 36(8):837–841.
43. Mirel DB, Valdes AM, Lazzeroni LC et al (2002) Association of IL4R haplotypes with type 1 diabetes. Diabetes 51(11):3336–3341.
44. Biason-Lauber A, Boehm B, Lang-Muritano M et al (2005) Association of childhood type 1 diabetes mellitus with a variant of PAX4: possible link to beta cell regenerative capacity. Diabetologia 48(5):900–905.
45. Wellcome Trust Case Control Consortium (2007) Genome-wide association study of 14,000 cases of seven common diseases and 3,000 shared controls. Nature 447(7145):661–678.
46. Todd JA, Walker NM, Cooper JD et al (2007) Robust associations of four new chromosome regions from genome-wide analyses of type 1 diabetes. Nat Genet 39(7):857–864.
47. Hakonarson H, Grant SF, Bradfield JP et al(2007). A Genome-Wide Association Study Identifies KIAA0350 as a Type 1 Diabetes Gene. Nature 448:591–594.
48. Poirot L, Benoist C, Mathis D (2004) Natural killer cells distinguish innocuous and destructive forms of pancreatic islet autoimmunity. Proc Natl Acad Sci U S A 101(21):8102–8107.
49. Rodacki M, Svoren B, Butty V et al (2007) Altered natural killer cells in type 1 diabetic patients. Diabetes 56(1):177–185.
50. Zimmet P, Alberti KG, Shaw J (2001) Global and societal implications of the diabetes epidemic. Nature 414(6865):782–787.
51. Yi F, Brubaker PL, Jin T (2005) TCF-4 mediates cell type-specific regulation of proglucagon gene expression by beta-catenin and glycogen synthase kinase-3beta. J Biol Chem 280(2):1457–1464.
52. Rich SS (1990) Mapping genes in diabetes. Genetic epidemiological perspective. Diabetes 39(11):1315–1319.
53. Tattersall RB (1974) Mild familial diabetes with dominant inheritance. The Q J Med 43(170):339–357.
54. Tattersal RB, Fajans SS (1975) Prevalence of diabetes and glucose intolerance in 199 offspring of thirty-seven conjugal diabetic parents. Diabetes 24(5):452–462.
55. Froguel P, Zouali H, Vionnet N et al (1993). Familial hyperglycemia due to mutations in glucokinase. Definition of a subtype of diabetes mellitus. N Engl J Med 328(10):697–702.
56. Frayling TM, Bulamn MP, Ellard S et al (1997). Mutations in the hepatocyte nuclear factor-1alpha gene are a common cause of maturity-onset diabetes of the young in the U.K. Diabetes 46(4):720–725.
57. Hattersley AT, Beards F, Ballantyne E et al (1998). Mutations in the glucokinase gene of the fetus result in reduced birth weight. Nat Genet 19(3):268–270.
58. Grimsby J, Sarabu R, Corbett WL et al (2003). Allosteric activators of glucokinase: potential role in diabetes therapy. Science 301(5631):370–373.
59. Matschinsky FM, Magnuson MA, Zelent D et al (2006). The network of glucokinase-expressing cells in glucose homeostasis and the potential of glucokinase activators for diabetes therapy. Diabetes 55(1):1–12.
60. Hattersley AT, Turner RC, Permutt MA et al (1992). Linkage of type 2 diabetes to the glucokinase gene. Lancet 339(8805):1307–1310.

61. Njolstad PR, Sovik O, Cuesta-Munoz A et al (2001). Neonatal diabetes mellitus due to complete glucokinase deficiency. N Engl J Med 344(21):1588–1592.
62. Heiervang E, Folling I, Sovik O et al (1989). Maturity-onset diabetes of the young. Studies in a Norwegian family. Acta Paediatr Scand 78(1):74–80.
63. Sovik O, Njolstad P, Folling I et al (1998). Hyperexcitability to sulphonylurea in MODY3. Diabetologia 41(5):607–608.
64. Pearson ER, Liddell WG, Shepherd M, Corrall RJ, Hattersley AT (2000). Sensitivity to sulphonylureas in patients with hepatocyte nuclear factor-1alpha gene mutations: evidence for pharmacogenetics in diabetes. Diabet Med 17(7):543–545.
65. Shepherd M, Pearson ER, Houghton J et al (2003). No deterioration in glycemic control in HNF-1alpha maturity-onset diabetes of the young following transfer from long-term insulin to sulphonylureas. Diabet Care 26(11):3191–3192.
66. Gloyn AL, Pearson ER, Antcliff JF et al (2004). Activating mutations in the gene encoding the ATP-sensitive potassium-channel subunit Kir6.2 and permanent neonatal diabetes. N Engl J Med 350(18):1838–1849.
67. Codner E, Flanagan S, Ellard S, Garcia H, Hattersley AT (2005). High-dose glibenclamide can replace insulin therapy despite transitory diarrhea in early-onset diabetes caused by a novel R201L Kir6.2 mutation. Diabet Care 28(3):758–759.
68. Klupa T, Edghill EL, Nazim J et al (2005). The identification of a R201H mutation in KCNJ11, which encodes Kir6.2, and successful transfer to sustained-release sulphonylurea therapy in a subject with neonatal diabetes: evidence for heterogeneity of beta cell function among carriers of the R201H mutation. Diabetologia 48(5):1029–1031.
69. Sagen JV, Raeder H, Hathout E et al (2004). Permanent neonatal diabetes due to mutations in KCNJ11 encoding Kir6.2: patient characteristics and initial response to sulfonylurea therapy. Diabetes 53(10):2713–2718.
70. Zung A, Glaser B, Nimri R, Zadik Z (2004). Glibenclamide treatment in permanent neonatal diabetes mellitus due to an activating mutation in Kir6.2. The J Clin Endocr Metab 89(11):5504–5507.
71. Altshuler D, Hirschhorn JN, Klannemark M et al (2000). The common PPARgamma Pro12Ala polymorphism is associated with decreased risk of type 2 diabetes. Nat Genet 26(1):76–80.
72. Gloyn AL, Weedon MN, Owen KR et al (2003). Large-scale association studies of variants in genes encoding the pancreatic beta-cell KATP channel subunits Kir6.2 (KCNJ11) and SUR1 (ABCC8) confirm that the KCNJ11 E23K variant is associated with type 2 diabetes. Diabetes 52(2):568–572.
73. Florez JC, Burtt N, de Bakker PI et al (2004). Haplotype structure and genotype-phenotype correlations of the sulfonylurea receptor and the islet ATP-sensitive potassium channel gene region. Diabetes 53(5):1360–1368.
74. Sladek R, Rocheleau G, Rung J et al (2007). A genome-wide association study identifies novel risk loci for type 2 diabetes. Nature.
75. Grant SF, Thorleifsson G, Reynisdottir I et al (2006). Variant of transcription factor 7-like 2 (TCF7L2) gene confers risk of type 2 diabetes. Nat Genet 38(3):320–323.
76. Florez JC, Jablonski KA, Bayley N et al (2006). TCF7L2 polymorphisms and progression to diabetes in the Diabetes Prevention Program. N Engl J Med 355(3):241–250.
77. Damcott CM, Pollin TI, Reinhart LJ et al (2006). Polymorphisms in the Transcription Factor 7-Like 2 (TCF7L2) Gene Are Associated With Type 2 Diabetes in the Amish: Replication and Evidence for a Role in Both Insulin Secretion and Insulin Resistance. Diabetes 55(9):2654–2659.
78. Groves CJ, Zeggini E, Minton J et al (2006). Association Analysis of 6,736 U.K. Subjects Provides Replication and Confirms TCF7L2 as a Type 2 Diabetes Susceptibility Gene With a Substantial Effect on Individual Risk. Diabetes 55(9):2640–2644.
79. Scott LJ, Bonnycastle LL, Willer CJ et al (2006). Association of Transcription Factor 7-Like 2 (TCF7L2) Variants With Type 2 Diabetes in a Finnish Sample. Diabetes 55(9):2649–2653.
80. Zhang C, Qi L, Hunter DJ et al (2006). Variant of Transcription Factor 7-Like 2 (TCF7L2) Gene and the Risk of Type 2 Diabetes in Large Cohorts of U.S. Women and Men. Diabetes 55(9):2645–2648.

81. Cauchi S, Meyre D, Dina C et al (2006). Transcription Factor TCF7L2 Genetic Study in the French Population: Expression in Human {beta}-Cells and Adipose Tissue and Strong Association With Type 2 Diabetes. Diabetes 55(10):2903–2908.
82. Saxena R, Gianniny L, Burtt NP et al (2006). Common Single Nucleotide Polymorphisms in TCF7L2 Are Reproducibly Associated With Type 2 Diabetes and Reduce the Insulin Response to Glucose in Nondiabetic Individuals. Diabetes 55(10):2890–2895.
83. Chandak GR, Janipalli CS, Bhaskar S et al (2006). Common variants in the TCF7L2 gene are strongly associated with type 2 diabetes mellitus in the Indian population. Diabetologia.
84. Humphries SE, Gable D, Cooper JA et al (2006). Common variants in the TCF7L2 gene and predisposition to type 2 diabetes in UK European Whites, Indian Asians and Afro-Caribbean men and women. J Mol Med 84(12):1–10.
85. van Vliet-Ostaptchouk JV, Shiri-Sverdlov R, Zhernakova A et al (2006). Association of variants of transcription factor 7-like 2 (TCF7L2) with susceptibility to type 2 diabetes in the Dutch Breda cohort. Diabetologia.
86. Helgason A, Palsson S, Thorleifsson G et al (2007). Refining the impact of TCF7L2 gene variants on type 2 diabetes and adaptive evolution. Nat Genet.
87. Saxena R, Voight BF, Lyssenko V et al (2007). Genome-wide association analysis identifies loci for type 2 diabetes and triglyceride levels. Science 316(5829):1331–1336.
88. Zeggini E, Weedon MN, Lindgren CM et al (2007). Replication of genome-wide association signals in UK samples reveals risk loci for type 2 diabetes. Science 316(5829):1336–1341.
89. Scott LJ, Mohlke KL, Bonnycastle LL et al (2007). A genome-wide association study of type 2 diabetes in Finns detects multiple susceptibility variants. Science 316(5829): 1341–1345.
90. Bennett RG, Hamel FG, Duckworth WC (2003). An insulin-degrading enzyme inhibitor decreases amylin degradation, increases amylin-induced cytotoxicity, and increases amyloid formation in insulinoma cell cultures. Diabetes 52(9):2315–2320.
91. Farris W, Mansourian S, Chang Y et al (2003). Insulin-degrading enzyme regulates the levels of insulin, amyloid beta-protein, and the beta-amyloid precursor protein intracellular domain in vivo. Proc Natl Acad Sci U S A 100(7):4162–4167.
92. Rennert NJ, Charney P (2003). Preventing cardiovascular disease in diabetes and glucose intolerance: evidence and implications for care. Primary Care 30(3):569–592.
93. Dominiczak MH (2003). Obesity, glucose intolerance and diabetes and their links to cardiovascular disease. Implications for laboratory medicine. Clin Chem Lab Med 41(9):1266–1278.
94. Hauner H, Meier M, Jockel KH, Frey UH, Siffert W (2003). Prediction of successful weight reduction under sibutramine therapy through genotyping of the G-protein beta3 subunit gene (GNB3) C825T polymorphism. Pharmacogenetics 13(8):453–459.
95. Friedman JM (2004). Modern science versus the stigma of obesity. Nat Med 10(6):563–569.
96. Lyon HN, Hirschhorn JN (2005). Genetics of common forms of obesity: a brief overview. Am J Clin Nutr 82(1 Suppl):215S-217S.
97. Knowler WC, Pettitt DJ, Saad MF, Bennett PH (1990). Diabetes mellitus in the Pima Indians: incidence, risk factors and pathogenesis. Diabetes Metab Rev 6(1):1–27.
98. Zimmet P, Dowse G, Finch C, Serjeantson S, King H (1990). The epidemiology and natural history of NIDDM—lessons from the South Pacific. Diabetes Metab Rev 6(2):91–124.
99. Stunkard AJ, Foch TT, Hrubec Z (1986). A twin study of human obesity. JAMA 256(1):51–54.
100. Borjeson M (1976). The aetiology of obesity in children. A study of 101 twin pairs. Acta Paediatr Scand 65(3):279–287.
101. Hebebrand J, Friedel S, Schauble N, Geller F, Hinney A (2003). Perspectives: molecular genetic research in human obesity. Obes Rev 4(3):139–146.
102. Farooqi IS, O'Rahilly S (2005). New advances in the genetics of early onset obesity. Int J Obes (Lond) 29(10):1149–1152.

103. Bell CG, Walley AJ, Froguel P (2005). The genetics of human obesity. Nat Rev 6(3):221–234.
104. Schousboe K, Willemsen G, Kyvik KO et al (2003). Sex differences in heritability of BMI: a comparative study of results from twin studies in eight countries. Twin Res 6(5):409–421.
105. Herbert A, Gerry NP, McQueen MB et al (2006). A common genetic variant is associated with adult and childhood obesity. Science 312(5771):279–283.
106. Loos RJ, Barroso I, O'Rahilly S, Wareham NJ (2007). Comment on "A common genetic variant is associated with adult and childhood obesity". Science 315(5809):187; author reply 187.
107. Dina C, Meyre D, Samson C et al (2007). Comment on "A common genetic variant is associated with adult and childhood obesity". Science 315(5809):187; author reply 187.
108. Rosskopf D, Bornhorst A, Rimmbach C et al (2007). Comment on "A common genetic variant is associated with adult and childhood obesity". Science 315(5809):187; author reply 187.
109. Frayling TM, Timpson NJ, Weedon MN et al (2007). A common variant in the FTO gene is associated with body mass index and predisposes to childhood and adult obesity. Science.
110. Riggs BL, Melton LJ, 3rd (1986). Involutional osteoporosis. N Engl J Med 314(26):1676–1686.
111. Heaney RP, Abrams S, Dawson-Hughes B et al (2000). Peak bone mass. Osteoporos Int 11(12):985–1009.
112. Mora S, Gilsanz V (2003). Establishment of peak bone mass. Endocrin Metab Clin 32(1):39–63.
113. Krall EA, Dawson-Hughes B (1993). Heritable and life-style determinants of bone mineral density. J Bone Miner Res 8(1):1–9.
114. Gueguen R, Jouanny P, Guillemin F et al (1995). Segregation analysis and variance components analysis of bone mineral density in healthy families. J Bone Miner Res 10(12):2017–2022.
115. Seeman E, Hopper JL, Bach LA et al (1989). Reduced bone mass in daughters of women with osteoporosis. N Engl J Med 320(9):554–558.
116. Soroko SB, Barrett-Connor E, Edelstein SL, Kritz-Silverstein D (1994). Family history of osteoporosis and bone mineral density at the axial skeleton: the Rancho Bernardo Study. J Bone Miner Res 9(6):761–769.
117. Morrison NA, Qi JC, Tokita A et al (1994). Prediction of bone density from vitamin D receptor alleles. Nature 367(6460):284–287.
118. Cooper GS, Umbach DM (1996). Are vitamin D receptor polymorphisms associated with bone mineral density? A meta-analysis. J Bone Miner Res 11(12):1841–1849.
119. Sainz J, Van Tornout JM, Loro ML et al (1997). Vitamin D-receptor gene polymorphisms and bone density in prepubertal American girls of Mexican descent. N Engl J Med 337(2):77–82.
120. Ferrari SL, Rizzoli R, Slosman DO, Bonjour JP (1998). Do dietary calcium and age explain the controversy surrounding the relationship between bone mineral density and vitamin D receptor gene polymorphisms? J Bone Miner Res 13(3):363–370.
121. Matsuyama T, Ishii S, Tokita A et al (1995). Vitamin D receptor genotypes and bone mineral density. Lancet 345(8959):1238–1239.
122. Hunter D, Major P, Arden N et al (2000). A randomized controlled trial of vitamin D supplementation on preventing postmenopausal bone loss and modifying bone metabolism using identical twin pairs. J Bone Miner Res 15(11):2276–2283.
123. Howard G, Nguyen T, Morrison N et al (1995). Genetic influences on bone density: physiological correlates of vitamin D receptor gene alleles in premenopausal women. The J Clin Endocr Metab 80(9):2800–2805.
124. Grant SF, Reid DM, Blake G et al (1996). Reduced bone density and osteoporosis associated with a polymorphic Sp1 binding site in the collagen type I alpha 1 gene. Nat Genet 14(2):203–205.

125. Uitterlinden AG, Burger H, Huang Q et al (1998). Relation of alleles of the collagen type Ialpha1 gene to bone density and the risk of osteoporotic fractures in postmenopausal women. N Engl J Med 338(15):1016–1021.
126. Lohmueller KE, Pearce CL, Pike M, Lander ES, Hirschhorn JN (2003). Meta-analysis of genetic association studies supports a contribution of common variants to susceptibility to common disease. Nat Genet 33(2):177–182.
127. Mann V, Hobson EE, Li B et al (2001). A COL1A1 Sp1 binding site polymorphism predisposes to osteoporotic fracture by affecting bone density and quality. J Clin Invest 107(7):899–907.
128. Qureshi AM, Herd RJ, Blake GM, Fogelman I, Ralston SH (2002). COLIA1 Sp1 polymorphism predicts response of femoral neck bone density to cyclical etidronate therapy. Calcified Tissue Int 70(3):158–163.
129. Little RD, Carulli JP, Del Mastro RG et al (2002). A mutation in the LDL receptor-related protein 5 gene results in the autosomal dominant high-bone-mass trait. Am J Human Genet 70(1):11–19.
130. Boyden LM, Mao J, Belsky J et al (2002). High bone density due to a mutation in LDL-receptor-related protein 5. N Engl J Med 346(20):1513–1521.
131. Johnson ML, Gong G, Kimberling W et al (1997). Linkage of a gene causing high bone mass to human chromosome 11 (11q12–13). Am J Human Genet 60(6):1326–1332.
132. Gong Y, Slee RB, Fukai N et al (2001). LDL receptor-related protein 5 (LRP5) affects bone accrual and eye development. Cell 107(4):513–523.
133. Worldwide variations in the prevalence of asthma symptoms: the International Study of Asthma and Allergies in Childhood (ISAAC) (1998). Eur Respir J, 12(2):315–335.
134. Eder W, Ege MJ, von Mutius E (2006). The asthma epidemic. N Engl J Med 355(21):2226–2235.
135. Van Eerdewegh P, Little RD, Dupuis J et al (2002). Association of the ADAM33 gene with asthma and bronchial hyperresponsiveness. Nature 418(6896):426–430.
136. Zhang Y, Leaves NI, Anderson GG et al (2003). Positional cloning of a quantitative trait locus on chromosome 13q14 that influences immunoglobulin E levels and asthma. Nat Genet 34(2):181–186.
137. Laitinen T, Polvi A, Rydman P et al (2004). Characterization of a common susceptibility locus for asthma-related traits. Science 304(5668):300–304.
138. Hakonarson H, Gulcher JR, Stefansson K (2003). deCODE Genetics, Inc. Pharmacogenomics 4(2):209–215.
139. McLeod HL (2001). Pharmacogenetics: more than skin deep. Nat Genet 29(3):247–248.
140. Fenech A, Hall IP (2002). Pharmacogenetics of asthma. Brit J Clin Pharmacol 53(1):3–15.
141. Hall IP (2002). Pharmacogenetics, pharmacogenomics and airway disease. Resp Res 3:10.
142. Roses AD (2000). Pharmacogenetics and future drug development and delivery. Lancet 355(9212):1358–1361.
143. Hakonarson H, Wjst M (2001). Current concepts on the genetics of asthma. Curr Opin Pediatr 13(3):267–277.
144. Bateman ED (2001). Measuring asthma control. Curr Opin Allergy Clin Immun 1(3):211–216.
145. Bateman ED, Boushey HA, Bousquet J et al (2004). Can guideline-defined asthma control be achieved? The Gaining Optimal Asthma ControL study. Am J Resp Crit Care 170(8):836–844.
146. Szefler SJ, Martin RJ, King TS et al (2002). Significant variability in response to inhaled corticosteroids for persistent asthma. J Allergy Clin Immun 109(3):410–418.
147. Ledford D, Apter A, Brenner AM et al (1998). Osteoporosis in the corticosteroid-treated patient with asthma. J Allergy Clin Immun 102(3):353–362.
148. Wong CA, Walsh LJ, Smith CJ et al (2000). Inhaled corticosteroid use and bone-mineral density in patients with asthma. Lancet 355(9213):1399–1403.
149. Baylink DJ (1983). Glucocorticoid-induced osteoporosis. N Engl J Med 309(5):306–308.

150. Garbe E, LeLorier J, Boivin JF, Suissa S (1997). Inhaled and nasal glucocorticoids and the risks of ocular hypertension or open-angle glaucoma. JAMA 277(9):722–727.
151. Garbe E, Boivin JF, LeLorier J, Suissa S (1998). Selection of controls in database case-control studies: glucocorticoids and the risk of glaucoma. J Clin Epidemiol 51(2):129–135.
152. Cumming RG, Mitchell P, Leeder SR (1997). Use of inhaled corticosteroids and the risk of cataracts. N Engl J Med 337(1):8–14.
153. Chinchilli VM (2007).General principles for systematic reviews and meta-analyses and a critique of a recent systematic review of long-acting beta-agonists. J Allergy Clin Immun 119(2):303–306.
154. Choudhry S, Ung N, Avila PC et al (2005). Pharmacogenetic differences in response to albuterol between Puerto Ricans and Mexicans with asthma. Am J Resp Crit Care 171(6):563–570.
155. Litonjua AA, Silverman EK, Tantisira KG et al (2004). Beta 2-adrenergic receptor polymorphisms and haplotypes are associated with airways hyperresponsiveness among nonsmoking men. Chest 126(1):66–74.
156. Chalmers GW, Macleod KJ, Little SA et al (2002). Influence of cigarette smoking on inhaled corticosteroid treatment in mild asthma. Thorax 57(3):226–230.
157. Palmer LJ, Cookson WO (2001). Using single nucleotide polymorphisms as a means to understanding the pathophysiology of asthma. Respir Res 2(2):102–112.
158. Gray IC, Campbell DA, Spurr NK (2000). Single nucleotide polymorphisms as tools in human genetics. Human Mol Genet 9(16):2403–2408.
159. Schork NJ, Fallin D, Lanchbury JS (2000). Single nucleotide polymorphisms and the future of genetic epidemiology. Clin Genet 58(4):250–264.
160. Sears MR (1998). Asthma treatment: inhaled beta-agonists. Can Respir J 5(Suppl A):54A–59A.
161. Hancox RJ, Sears MR, Taylor DR (1998). Polymorphism of the beta2-adrenoceptor and the response to long-term beta2-agonist therapy in asthma. Eur Respir J 11(3):589–593.
162. Billington CK, Penn RB (2003). Signaling and regulation of G protein-coupled receptors in airway smooth muscle. Respir Res 4, 2.
163. Drysdale CM, McGraw DW, Stack CB et al (2000). Complex promoter and coding region beta 2-adrenergic receptor haplotypes alter receptor expression and predict in vivo responsiveness. Proc Natl Acad Sci U S A 97(19):10483–10488.
164. Reihsaus E, Innis M, MacIntyre N, Liggett SB (1993). Mutations in the gene encoding for the beta 2-adrenergic receptor in normal and asthmatic subjects. Am J Respir Cell Mol 8(3):334–339.
165. Martinez FD, Graves PE, Baldini M, Solomon S, Erickson R (1997). Association between genetic polymorphisms of the beta2-adrenoceptor and response to albuterol in children with and without a history of wheezing. The J Clin Invest 100(12):3184–3188.
166. Kotani Y, Nishimura Y, Maeda H, Yokoyama M (1999). Beta2-adrenergic receptor polymorphisms affect airway responsiveness to salbutamol in asthmatics. J Asthma 36(7):583–590.
167. Lima JJ, Thomason DB, Mohamed MH et al (1999). Impact of genetic polymorphisms of the beta2-adrenergic receptor on albuterol bronchodilator pharmacodynamics. Clin Pharmacol Ther 65(5):519–525.
168. Tan S, Hall IP, Dewar J, Dow E, Lipworth B (1997). Association between beta 2-adrenoceptor polymorphism and susceptibility to bronchodilator desensitisation in moderately severe stable asthmatics. Lancet 350(9083):995–999.
169. Cho SH, Oh SY, Bahn JW et al (2005). Association between bronchodilating response to short-acting beta-agonist and non-synonymous single-nucleotide polymorphisms of beta-adrenoceptor gene. Clin Exp Allergy 35(9):1162–1167.
170. Kukreti R, Bhatnagar P, C BR et al (2005). Beta(2)-adrenergic receptor polymorphisms and response to salbutamol among Indian asthmatics*. Pharmacogenomics 6(4):399–410.
171. Israel E (2000). Assessment of therapeutic index of inhaled steroids. Lancet 356(9229): 527–528.

172. Israel E, Chinchilli VM, Ford JG et al (2004). Use of regularly scheduled albuterol treatment in asthma: genotype-stratified, randomised, placebo-controlled cross-over trial. Lancet 364(9444):1505–1512.
173. Jackson CM, Lipworth B (2004). Benefit-risk assessment of long-acting beta2-agonists in asthma. Drug Saf 27(4):243–270.
174. Abramson MJ, Walters J, Walters EH (2003). Adverse effects of beta-agonists: are they clinically relevant? Am J Respir Med 2(4):287–297.
175. Tsai HJ, Shaikh N, Kho JY et al (2006). Beta 2-adrenergic receptor polymorphisms: pharmacogenetic response to bronchodilator among African American asthmatics. Human Genet 119(5):547–557.
176. Snyder EM, Beck KC, Dietz NM et al (2006). Influence of beta2-adrenergic receptor genotype on airway function during exercise in healthy adults. Chest 129(3):762–770.
177. Silverman EK, Kwiatkowski DJ, Sylvia JS et al (2003). Family-based association analysis of beta2-adrenergic receptor polymorphisms in the childhood asthma management program. J Allergy Clin Immun 112(5):870–876.
178. Shah RR (2005). Pharmacogenetics in drug regulation: promise, potential and pitfalls. Philos T Roy Soc 360(1460):1617–1638.
179. Goldstein DB (2005). The genetics of human drug response. Philos T Roy Soc 360(1460):1571–1572.
180. Silverman ES, Du J, De Sanctis GT et al (1998). Egr-1 and Sp1 interact functionally with the 5-lipoxygenase promoter and its naturally occurring mutants. Am J Respir Cell Mol 19(2):316–323.
181. Drazen JM, Silverman ES (1999). Genetic determinants of 5-lipoxygenase transcription. Int Arch Allergy Immun 118(2–4):275–278.
182. Sampson AP, Cowburn AS, Sladek K et al (1997). Profound overexpression of leukotriene C4 synthase in bronchial biopsies from aspirin-intolerant asthmatic patients. Int Arch Allergy Immun 113(1–3):355–357.
183. Sampson AP, Siddiqui S, Buchanan D et al (2000). Variant LTC(4) synthase allele modifies cysteinyl leukotriene synthesis in eosinophils and predicts clinical response to zafirlukast. Thorax 55 Suppl 2, S28–31.
184. Currie GP, Lima JJ, Sylvester JE et al (2003). Leukotriene C4 synthase polymorphisms and responsiveness to leukotriene antagonists in asthma. Brit J Clin Pharmacol 56(4):422–426.
185. Sanak M, Simon HU, Szczeklik A (1997). Leukotriene C4 synthase promoter polymorphism and risk of aspirin-induced asthma. Lancet 350(9091):1599–1600.
186. Deykin A, Wechsler ME, Boushey HA et al (2007). Combination therapy with a long-acting beta-agonist and a leukotriene antagonist in moderate asthma. Am J Resp Crit Care 175(3):228–234.
187. (2007).Clinical trial of low-dose theophylline and montelukast in patients with poorly controlled asthma. Am J Resp Crit Care 175(3):235–242.
188. Lazarus SC, Lee T, Kemp JP et al (1998). Safety and clinical efficacy of zileuton in patients with chronic asthma. Am J Manag Care 4(6):841–848.
189. Barnes PJ (1998). Efficacy of inhaled corticosteroids in asthma. J Allergy Clin Immun 102(4 Pt 1):531–538.
190. Gagliardo R, Chanez P, Vignola AM et al (2000). Glucocorticoid receptor alpha and beta in glucocorticoid dependent asthma. Am J Resp Crit Care 162(1):7–13.
191. Sher ER, Leung DY, Surs W et al (1994). Steroid-resistant asthma. Cellular mechanisms contributing to inadequate response to glucocorticoid therapy. J Clin Invest 93(1):33–39.
192. Chan MT, Leung DY, Szefler SJ, Spahn JD (1998). Difficult-to-control asthma: clinical characteristics of steroid-insensitive asthma. J Allergy Clin Immun 101(5):594–601.
193. Chikanza LC, Panayi GS (1993). The effects of hydrocortisone on in vitro lymphocyte proliferation and interleukin-2 and -4 production in corticosteroid sensitive and resistant subjects. Eur J Clin Invest 23(12):845–850.
194. Sousa AR, Lane SJ, Cidlowski JA, Staynov DZ, Lee TH (2000). Glucocorticoid resistance in asthma is associated with elevated in vivo expression of the glucocorticoid receptor beta-isoform. J Allergy Clin Immun 105(5):943–950.

195. Lane SJ, Lee TH (1997). Mechanisms of corticosteroid resistance in asthmatic patients. Int Arch Allergy Immun 113(1–3):193–195.
196. Leung DY, Chrousos GP (2000). Is there a role for glucocorticoid receptor beta in glucocorticoid-dependent asthmatics? Am J Resp Crit Care 162(1):1–3.
197. Tantisira KG, Lake S, Silverman ES et al (2004). Corticosteroid pharmacogenetics: association of sequence variants in CRHR1 with improved lung function in asthmatics treated with inhaled corticosteroids. Human Mol Genet 13(13):1353–1359.
198. Hakonarson H, Bjornsdottir US, Halapi E et al (2005). Profiling of genes expressed in peripheral blood mononuclear cells predicts glucocorticoid sensitivity in asthma patients. Proc Natl Acad Sci U S A 102(41):14789–14794.
199. Hakonarson H, Halapi E, Whelan R et al (2001). Association between IL-1beta/TNF-alpha-induced glucocorticoid-sensitive changes in multiple gene expression and altered responsiveness in airway smooth muscle. Am J Respir Cell Mol 25(6):761–771.
200. Kim MH, Agrawal DK (2002). Effect of interleukin-1beta and tumor necrosis factor-alpha on the expression of G-proteins in CD4+ T-cells of atopic asthmatic subjects. J Asthma 39(5):441–448.
201. Roth M, Black JL (2006). Transcription factors in asthma: are transcription factors a new target for asthma therapy? Curr Drug Targets 7(5):589–595.
202. D'Acquisto F, Ianaro A (2006). From willow bark to peptides: the ever widening spectrum of NF-kappaB inhibitors. Curr Opin Pharmacol 6(4):387–392.

Chapter 21
Pharmacogenomics of Rare and Monogenic Disorders

Paul D. Maher

Contents

Abstract The rare monogenic diseases provide the most clearly evident examples of pathology resulting from a single genetic lesion. As such, they are in some sense the "low hanging fruit" for the application of pharmacogenomic therapeutic approaches. These quite often serious diseases, while still not fully understood, have seen a revolution in both disease classification as well as therapeutic approaches. Advances in genomic understanding of rare diseases both challenge traditional disease classifications as well as reveal, in many instances, a complex interplay of the host genome with its environment. Therapeutic approaches initially developed as "orphan" products, including molecular chaperones, agents to promote or stop codon skipping, various gene therapy techniques, substrate reduction therapies, and other novel therapies, have all either recently seen market approval or show clear promise as potential future treatment approaches.

Keywords rare disease, pharmacogenomics, orphan products, monogenic, disease classification, sickle cell anemia, DNA, genomics, human genome, recombinant, gene therapy, therapy

---

Paul D. Maher
Medical Reviewer, Office of Orphan Products Development, Food and Drug Administration, LCDR, United States Public Health Service, Rockville, MD
paul.maher@fda.hhs.gov

N. Cohen (ed.) *Pharmacogenomics and Personalized Medicine*,

1 Background

The concept of a monogenic disease is a relatively new addition to the medical terminology. Its roots may be seen to extend back to the pea plants of Gregor Mendel and the formulation of the statistical rules of inheritance and of recessive and dominant traits *(1)*. In the 1940s Avery Oswald first demonstrated that a relatively overlooked cellular substance, deoxyribonucleic acid (DNA) was capable of transforming the phenotype of bacteria and was therefore a likely candidate for the cellular genetic material *(2)*. Some 100 years after Mendel's pea plants, James Watson, Francis Crick, and Rosalind Franklin determined the molecular structure of DNA. In 1953, in the subsequent landmark paper in the journal *Nature*, the double helix and the physical mechanism behind the generational inheritance of traits was made known to the world *(3)*.

Even prior to Avery's work, however, the scientist who most presciently foresaw the concept of a monogenic disease was English physician Archibald Garrod. Garrod's groundbreaking turn of the 19th century work in alkaptonuria, a disease which leads to darkened urine upon exposure to air, led to the concept of the "inborn error of metabolism" and his formulation of the hypothesis "one gene, one disease" *(4)*. Through careful data collection and application of Mendel's principles, Garrod correctly hypothesized that alkaptonuria was inherited in an autosomal recessive fashion. More importantly, however, he was also able to generalize the significance of these findings, stating,

> "While the signs of alkaptonuria aere highly visible, many more disorders of metabolism undoubtedly exist with more subtle manifestations" *(5)*.

Garrod's theory in alkaptonuria went well beyond generalized speculation. He clearly recognized that there was an error in the metabolism of tyrosine and phenylalanine and correctly deduced,

> "the splitting of the benzene ring in normal metabolism is the work of a special enzyme, that in congenital alkaptonuria this enzyme is wanting" *(6)*.

It would be many decades before scientists were able to confirm that patients with this disease indeed lack a functional homgenistate oxidase enzyme and even longer till the genetic source of this error was mapped to a specific locus on the short arm of the third chromosome *(7)*. The concepts put forth in Garrod's 1923 seminal work "Inborn Errors of Metabolism," though refined by additional discovery, remain central to the concept of rare monogenic diseases.

Most recently, some of the most interesting and groundbreaking work to come about in genomics has come out of the National Institutes of Health (NIH) in Bethesda, Maryland. In 1991, Craig Venter's development of expressed sequence tags *(8)* as a means of pinpointing the protein coding regions within the genome proved so valuable that the majority of the protein coding genes notated in the National Institutes of Health Genbank repository, have been discovered using this methodology *(9)*. In 1998, Venter left NIH and founded a private company with the expressed purpose of fully mapping the entire human genome. When approached by NIH for possible collaboration in this endeavor, Venter, perhaps evincing some of the well-documented acerbic wit of James Watson, the previous head of genomics at NIH, is reported to have replied, "You can sequence the mouse." Thus ensued one of the great races in scientific endeavor of recent times, that of sequencing the entire human genome. Both Venter and Francis Collins of the NIH Human Genome Project succeeded in sequencing the entire human genome, with the race officially declared a draw in 2001 when both independently published complete draft maps of the human genome *(10, 11)*.

The publication of the human genome has had a profound, as yet only partially realized, impact on the state of medical knowledge and our approach to potential therapeutic strategies. While the number of protein coding genes is a moving target, most estimates now put it between 20,000 and 25,000 *(12)*. Despite the extremely rapid pace of advance, there are at present an estimated 6,000 characterized monogenic diseases *(13)*. Clearly there is more work to be done. Indeed, the ease of sequencing genetic material continues to increase at an exponential rate. If such a trend continues, in forty years physicians might order a complete individual genetic profile as easily as they now order a complete blood count. It is the recognition of these trends, and the potential improvement in clinical outcomes from reasoned application of this burgeoning wealth of genomic knowledge, that drives the rise of personalized medicine and pharmacogenomic approaches to therapy.

While we are in the midst of an embarrassment of riches of genomic data our fundamental understanding of genomic disease remains far from complete. This is seen in our inadequate understanding of genetic regulation, especially in higher organisms, an ignorance which has contributed to the lack of success of gene-based therapies for clearly defined rare diseases. It is now apparent that only some 1–2% of the genome codes for proteins; however, there is evidence that more of the genome is expressed than is transcribed *(14)*; there is also the mystery of evolutionarily preserved noncoding regions of the genome *(15)*. With advances in genomics we also begin to perceive an astonishing complexity not only in how a gene may interact with myriad others within its own genome, but also how these genes interact in complex ways with other organisms and the environment.

No discussion of the background of rare, monogenic diseases would be complete without mention of the Office of Orphan Products Development (OOPD). The OOPD has for nearly 25 years promoted the development to market of drugs for rare diseases. Through a basket of incentives granted to sponsors who meet the criteria for orphan designation, OOPD assists in the clinical development of promising rare disease therapies. The legislative definition for a "rare" disease in the United States is one with a prevalence of less than 200,000 persons *(16)* or, if over 200,000 persons, one for which there is no reasonable expectation of recovering drug development costs within seven years of market approval—a relatively generous definition when compared with that of other nations. This threshold may be seen then to capture all of the rare monogenic diseases. Perhaps equally important to our discussion is that, while there may be occasional rare disease market approvals which did not receive orphan designation, historically, the majority of rare disease products approved for market were so approved under the auspices of the Orphan Drug Act (ODA). This may be inferred from the simple finding that in the decade subsequent to the passage of the ODA, the number of drugs for rare diseases which were approved for marketing increased tenfold *(17)*, with the majority of this increase directly attributable to orphan-designated products. With the increasing visibility of the orphan drug program, it would seem even more unlikely that large numbers of sponsors of rare disease therapies would attempt, in recent times, such a difficult marketing challenge without taking advantage of the assistance provided by orphan designation. Such assistance is generally all the more crucial in the often ultra-rare diseases that constitute many of the monogenic rare diseases. In our overview and survey of the state of pharmacogenomic medicine as it relates to the rare monogenic diseases, we will rely extensively on publicly available data provided by the OOPD.

2 Why Study Pharmacogenomics in Relation to the Rare Monogenic Diseases?

Put simply, in attempting to make sense of the voluminous and confusing amount of recently available genomic data, it is worthwhile to begin with the clearly apparent cases of genetic disease, the rare monogenic disorders. One does not generally consider pharmacogenomics as it relates to the rare monogenic diseases. More likely, one would note efforts to, for instance, determine genetic variation in the metabolism of various drugs. Or one also might consider efforts such as the International HapMap Project *(18)* or the single nucleotide polymorphism database which now lists some 60,000 protein-coding SNPs *(19)*. More recently, one might look toward the Genes and the Environment Health Initiative established by the National Institutes of Health in February, 2006, to examine the interplay of SNPs, the environment, and the risk of chronic disease *(20)*. Efforts such as these are already leading to more numerous and exciting new discoveries than may be adequately addressed here.

In a very real sense, however, the rare monogenic diseases provide the low-hanging fruit for the application of pharmacogenomic therapeutic approaches. This is the case for a variety of reasons. First, the rare monogenic diseases are usually quite serious, often leading to death in childhood or early adulthood. As such, they also reveal the fundamental and crucial human metabolic pathways. No one would dispute the importance or clinical relevance of the recently reported finding that genetic variation in the vitamin K epoxide reductase complex accounts for some 55% of the variability in warfarin metabolism rates *(21)*. However, a single nucleotide polyporphism (SNP) which results in death in childhood, such as is seen in Fabry's disease, Pompe's disease, or a vast number of other rare diseases, is of even greater clinical relevance. Moreover, with diseases which so gravely compromise health, the cause and effect relationship between genetic lesion and pathology may be more clearly perceived. Often, though not always, the biological relationship between genetic lesion and pathology in a rare disease is well characterized, bringing one closer to the application of a reasoned therapeutic advance.

Indeed, the pivotal trial leading to approval of the first enzyme replacement therapy was performed in a total of ten patients *(22)*. In light of the seriousness of so many rare monogenic diseases, it also goes without saying that such patients are in dire need of and greatly deserving of therapeutic advances.

An additional reason for investigating pharmacogenomics in relation to the rare monogenic diseases is one that is independent of medicine. It is simply that time and again, the advance of science has taken fundamental and broad based steps forward due to the diligent investigation of exceptional findings and outlier data. Even some 400 years ago the eminent physician William Harvey commented upon this principle as it relates to medicine when he stated that there is no

> "... better way to advance the proper practice of medicine than to give our minds to the discovery of the usual laws of Nature by careful investigation of cases of rarer forms of disease *(23)*."

One recent illustrative example may be seen in the Nobel Prize winning work of doctors Brown and Goldstein. By diligent study of the rare monogenic disorder familial hypercholesterolemia, these researchers gained a fundamental understanding of cholesterol metabolism and its relation to heart disease *(24)*. This research into an obscure, monogenic disease also led directly to the development of the statin drugs, the most widely prescribed class of medications in the United States *(25)*.

One may also consider that single nucleotide polymorphisms present a wide spectrum of variation within any given allele. While organ systems such as the kidney or the liver exhibit great spare capacity, such that only 25–30% of normal function is compatible with health, there is even greater leeway in most crucial enzymatic systems. In general, 5% or greater function for a particular enzyme system is compatible with health. Function less than 3% usually leads to frank disease expression. A level of function in the 3–5% range may manifest itself as a mild or chronic disease. One well documented instance of this is the association of mild Fabry's disease with congestive heart failure. Approximately one out of twenty cases of congestive heart failure is believed to be the result of mild Fabry's disease *(26)*. A similarly well characterized, and in this instance treatable condition, is the association of alpha-1 antitrypsin deficiency with the subsequent development of early onset emphysema. In such light, the investigation of the more mild variants of the known rare monogenic diseases is an eminently logical place to begin a search for single nucleotide polymorphisms which contribute to chronic disease.

Finally, as shall be considered in more detail in a moment, a number of rare monogenic diseases are now seen to result from balanced genetic polymorphism. A well known example is the evolutionary compromise of selective advantage for the sickle cell trait in areas of highly endemic malaria. What follows, and is perhaps worthy of more avid scientific investigation, is that when one understands the genomics and proteomics of sickle cell anemia, one then has a logical path towards developing a treatment for malaria.

3 The Genomics of Rare Diseases: The Big Picture

Sickle cell anemia arises from a single nucleotide polymorphism (SNP) which leads to the production of hemoglobinS (HbS). The homozygous condition leads to sickle cell anemia with all of its attendant increases in morbidity and mortality.

The heterozygous condition, however, offers an approximate tenfold reduced risk of severe malaria as compared with the complete absence of HbS *(27)*. Therefore, as noted. a balanced polymorphism is established between the competing scenarios of no HbS leading to normal health but also normal susceptibility to malaria, all HbS leading to sickle cell disease, and one HbS gene and one normal gene leading to nearly normal health and greatly increased protection from malaria. Interestingly then, without treatment, in areas of highly prevalent malaria, the sickle cell allele is not unfit from an evolutionary standpoint; it is rather a tragic compromise. In areas of high malaria endemicity, one finds the HbS gene maintained at an approximately 10% level *(28)*. While the most common SNP is the exchange of glutamic acid for valine on the hemoglobin beta chain, there are at least 4 haplotypes, which arise independently on chromosome 11, in response to endemic malaria *(29)*.

The relationship between the sickle cell trait and malaria is by no means an isolated example. In a recent review of the influence of malaria on population genomics, Dominic Kwiatkowski comments on the incredible selective pressure exerted by malaria:

> "Malaria is the evolutionary driving force behind sickle-cell disease, thalassemia, glucose-6-phosphatase deficiency, and other erythrocyte defects that together comprise the most common Mendelian diseases of humankind *(30)*"

Considering only malaria then, one finds at least a half dozen known examples where there is selection for a balanced polymorphism that, if present in the homozygous state, leads to a rare monogenic disorder.

Nor is malaria somehow unique in exerting this pressure. Phenylketonuria, an inborn error of metabolism resulting from an inability to metabolize the amino acid phenylalanine, untreated, leads to severe mental retardation and early death. In the heterozygous carrier state, however, there is a nonpathologic increase in phenylalanine levels. It has been speculated that this heterozygous condition provides a measure of protection against the fungal toxin, ochratoxin A, found on moldy bread, which otherwise predisposes to spontaneous abortions *(31, 32)*. Similarly, cystic fibrosis, the most common genetic disease of Caucasians, with some one in twenty-five persons carrying the allele, leads to dysfunction of the chloride ion channel and, untreated, to death in childhood. Studies from laboratory mice indicate that the heterozygous state confers a significant degree of protection against cholera *(33)*, which exerts its pathologic effects by acting upon the chloride ion channel. Tay-Sachs disease in the heterozygous state has been reported to lead to increased resistance to tuberculosis *(34)*. If it were possible to grant greater dignity to those afflicted by a rare serious genetic disease, it might be pointed out that in the case of balanced polymorphism, viewed from the community level, the presence of such disease traits leads to greater survival within the population as a whole.

Certainly spontaneous mutations, founder effects, and genetic drift play a large role in the establishment and prevalence of many rare diseases. However, unless one presupposes that certain stretches of DNA are more mechanically prone to mutation, then in the absence of some form of evolutionary pressure, it is difficult to reconcile the widely disparate prevalences seen in rare monogenic diseases. Phenylketonuria has a prevalence more than tenfold that of tyrosinemia, while both are diseases of amino acid metabolism and closely related metabolically. With the dramatic documented effect which malaria has exerted on the human genome, what has been the influence from other equally prevalent and serious scourges such as tuberculosis, cholera, influenza, black plague, small pox, etc?

A corollary to the role of balanced polymorphism in rare diseases is also perhaps at present underemphasized. As noted earlier, if one understands the genetic adaptive response of the genome which led to genomic disease, does one not also have a rational starting point for developing a therapy for the highly prevalent disease? Such reverse engineering of nature's pharmacogenomic response to highly prevalent diseases is only just starting to be applied. The Duffy antigen, while not a rare disease causing polymorphism, has been found in the homozygous negative state to provide protection from *Plasmodium vivax* infection. Subsequent research determined the Duffy antigen (CD234) to be the erythrocyte transmembrane protein which mediates invasion of the merozoite form of *Plasmodium vivax (35)*. Those who are Duffy antigen negative are thus spared infection from this form of malaria. This genomic understanding has led to a major effort to develop a malaria vaccine directed against the Duffy antigen/*Plasmodium vivax* receptor. Hopefully, in future, the expanding genomic understanding of rare monogenic diseases may also lead to additional insights into the treatment of highly prevalent diseases.

A cautionary note may also be seen in the great complexity of the interaction of the human genome with the environment. A gene does not merely interact with the thousands of others in its own genome, it also interacts with its environment. Without a perfect understanding of the environment, one can never say with perfect certainty what the effect of any human genetic manipulation might be. There remain scientific as well as ethical grounds for the position that the human germ cell line remain inviolate. Of course some might say this is a Luddite perspective, and followed to its logical conclusion precludes any form of genetic engineering. The benefits of genetic manipulation of organisms are clear, dramatic, and widespread. However, in the altering of the genome of any replicating organism there is a risk benefit analysis and, with such a powerful technology, room for an abundance of caution. To stray afield of our topic for a moment, two recent examples illustrate this necessary risk-benefit analysis. In 2001, researchers in Australia attempted to create a contraceptive for the burgeoning mouse population by inserting the gene for IL-4 into the mousepox virus. This single manipulation, it was theorized, would lead to an attenuated smallpox virus that would cause sterility. To their surprise, researchers discovered that the modified mousepox proved fatal in 100% of the mice exposed to it. The fatality rate in mice immunized against mousepox proved to be 50% *(36, 37)*. The potential relevance of this unfortunate finding to human smallpox has not gone unnoticed. Researchers have also explored attenuated viruses as a potential oncology therapy. One variation on this approach involves first attenuating an adenovirus as a treatment for malignant glioma. However, in a second step, the tropism of the attenuated virus is expanded *(38)* by the addition of a motif which allows for cellular entry through the integrin receptor, seen commonly in malignant glioma, though also found to a lesser extent in other tissues. In commenting on this approach the National Institutes of Health Recombinant Advisory Committee noted that, not being merely a theoretical concern, it was to be expected that in production there would be recombination of the expanded tropism virus with wild-type virus. In returning to the topic at hand, it might be summed up that with any technology as powerful as that of genomics, an abundance of caution is in order lest we find ourselves in the position of the sorcerer's apprentice of Goethe's poem, unable to shut off the magic broom.

4 Genomic Advance and the Challenge of Disease Classification

The genetic heterogeneity apparent even in the rare monogenic diseases and the rate of scientific advance in characterizing these variations are nothing less than astonishing. If we consider again the work of Garrod in alkaptonuria and the metabolism of phenylalnine and tyrosine, we find that a related, more serious rare disease would not even be categorized for another half century. Maple syrup urine disease was first described only as recently as 1954, being named phenotypically for the sweet smelling urine of affected individuals *(39)*. The cause of this symptom, and the more serious mental retardation and rapidly progressive clinical course associated with it, was later discovered to be a blockage in the metabolism of branched chain amino acids such as tyrosine and phenylalanine *(40)*. The genetic lesion underlying this inborn error of metabolism was subsequently mapped to four different genes, all on different chromosomes *(41)*. Currently, there are five described disease subtypes. In one disease subtype alone, a recent paper classified nine separate genetic mutations.

Certainly a disease remains a clinical definition; however, the increase in genomic knowledge sometimes leads one to question whether certain relevant disease groupings may be made based on underlying genomics, independent of disease phenotype. One example of this might be seen in the discovery of compounds such as gentamicin, which promote the skipping of stop codons during ribosomal translation of messenger RNA (mRNA). It is estimated that some 5–10% of numerous monogenic diseases are caused by nonsense mutations leading to inappropriate stop codons on the mRNA transcript, the resultant truncated protein being nonfunctional. Preliminary studies in the enzyme deficiency disease Hurler's syndrome indicate an increase from a baseline 1% enzyme activity to 3% enzyme activity in those patients with a misplaced stop codon *(42)*. While such a change might not seem overwhelming, it is sufficient to convert a very serious case of the disease to one with a mild phenotypic expression. This approach is also being explored in diseases such as cystic fibrosis, Duchenne's muscular dystrophy, and Rett syndrome *(43, 44)*. If such a therapy were to prove safe and efficacious, would the more clinically relevant grouping be to speak of "aberrant stop codon disease," a genetic disease which may express itself phenotypically as Hurler's syndrome, cystic fibrosis, Huntington's disease, or any number of other rare monogenic diseases? An analogous example is seen in the development of molecular chaperone-based therapies for certain subsets of rare disease patients. Fabry's disease is a lysozomal storage disease with some 191 characterized genetic mutations of the enzyme alpha galactosidase *(45)*. In a subset of these, it is speculated that the enzyme remains functional; however, an altered three-dimensional configuration prevents the enzyme being shunted to the lysozome and it is instead destroyed *(46, 47)*.

In 2004, researchers presented a case report in the *New England Journal of Medicine* of a Fabry's disease patient who improved upon infusion of galactose, a competitive inhibitor to the enzyme galactosidase *(48)*. By infusing galactose, the researchers proposed to force the mutant enzyme into its proper three-dimensional configuration, thus "rescuing" the enzyme and allowing it unimpeded transit to the lysozome. If such an approach proves broadly applicable to lysozomal storage diseases, the relevant clinical distinction again might not be the phenotype of the disease, but rather whether it was one which was amenable to enzyme rescue through molecular chaperoning.

5 Background on Some Pharmacogenomic Successes in Rare Monogenic Disease therapies

Prior to 1990 there were no FDA-approved enzyme replacement therapies for rare monogenic diseases. This changed with the approval of a bovine-derived, polyethelene, glycol-coated adenonsine deaminase to treat severe combined immunodeficiency caused by a deficiency of adenisone deaminase (SCID-ADA). SCID-ADA has a prevalence of about 40 persons in the United States, while the pivotal trial for market approval was performed in about 10 patients *(49)*. The approval of pegademase was also groundbreaking in that it was the first use of a polyethylene glycol-treated therapy designed to decrease drug immunogenicity and prolong drug half-life *(50)*. This technique of pegylation has subsequently seen widespread adoption in more prevalent diseases, one of the more well known being the development of pegylated interferon in the treatment of hepatitis C, a disease with an estimated prevalence of some 2.7 million people in the United States *(51)* and 170 million worldwide *(52)*. While drugs such as pegademase provide new hope for diseases that are generally fatal in childhood, the underlying genetic lesion remains, and enzyme replacement therapies are not curative. Along with the need for continuous therapy difficulties with drug distribution, immunogenicity and tissue penetration allow for continued disease expression.

The advent of enzyme replacement therapies has also benefited from the concomitant development of recombinant drug production technologies. A full discussion of the impact, depth, and breadth of this development is far beyond the scope of this paper, though the production of recombinant insulin and its impact on the lives of millions serves to illustrate the point. To produce a recombinant protein, the underlying gene must first be isolated. This gene is then amplified, spliced, and ligated, or recombined, into a segment of DNA that, when inserted into a new organism, will allow for its constitutive expression in a propagating, now transgenic, organism. Organisms harnessed to produce human proteins include bacterium such as *E. coli*, yeast, Chinese hamster ovary cells, and, more rarely, higher vertebrates such as cows. These varied approaches may lead to posttranslational protein changes such as different glycosylation patterns. One might almost view recombinant drugs as gene therapy by proxy. Undoubtedly, this important advance is entirely dependent on the ability to manipulate the genome at the molecular level and on an underlying genomic understanding of the disease. While the enzyme replacement therapy pegademase, discussed earlier, is a bovine-derived product, nearly all newer enzyme replacement therapies are produced using recombinant techniques. Indeed, because of the improved safety profile and ease of production as compared with isolation from pooled serum, most enzymes, cell factors, and cell signaling proteins are now made in this manner.

Before surveying the products which have been approved to treat rare monogenic disorders, it is worthwhile to examine how one determines whether a therapy has been influenced by an underlying genomic disease understanding. Consider the rare autosomal recessive disease xeroderma pigmentosa (XP), caused by an inability to repair ultraviolet-induced DNA dimers. A physician 500 years ago might, from empiric experience, tell such a patient to wear hats and avoid the sun. If a modern physician were to prescribe a skin moisturizer, one would conclude the same. However, if the moisturizer were also a sunscreen prescribed on the basis of an understanding that the genomic error in XP leads to the lack of a necessary DNA repair enzyme, such an advance, while seemingly mundane, would necessarily have to be considered a pharmacogenomic one.

6 Survey of Orphan Products Approved to Treat Rare Monogenic Diseases

Since its inception in 1983 the Office of Orphan Products has designated over 300 products to treat rare diseases which have subsequently been approved to market *(53)*. Of these 300, fifty-four may conservatively be said to be primarily for the treatment of a rare monogenic disorder. Some products, such as treatments for Cushing's syndrome, are excluded from consideration. While Cushing's syndrome generally arises as a result of a pituitary adenoma, or adrenal carcinoma, it should be noted that in a minority of instances Cushing's syndrome will arise from a rare monogenic disease, such as multiple endocrine neoplasia. There is some necessary judgment and perhaps a possibility of bias in these distinctions, as a disease such as hypogonaditrophic hypogonadism, which arises very frequently from the genetic disease Kallman syndrome, is included; though empty sella syndrome, pituitary tumors, or head injury might also result in the identical presentation. Other diseases such as Paget's disease, central precocious puberty, primary pulmonary hypertension, Zollinger-Ellison syndrome, polycystic ovarian disease, Sjogren's syndrome, juvenile rheumatoid arthritis, or idiopathic growth hormone deficiency, all of which have seen approved orphan therapies, are currently speculated to possibly have a specific, important monogenic component; however, further research is needed.

Of the 54 products approved to treat rare monogenic diseases, the majority, 34, are biologically derived therapies. Of these 34 products the majority again, 23 products, are produced through recombinant techniques. These biologic products to treat rare monogenic diseases are listed below in Table 21.1.

One caveat to note is that for brevity's sake, the approved indication has been shortened to the relevant disease being treated, thus for instance the full indication

Table 21.1 Biologically derived products approved as orphan products to treat rare monogenic diseases

Generic Name	*Trade Name*	How Derived	Disease	Date Approved
Coagulation Factor IX	*BeneFix*	Recombinant	Hemophilia B.	11-Feb-97
Dornase alfa	*Pulmozyme*	Recombinant	To reduce mucous viscosity and enable the clearance of airway secretions in patients with cystic fibrosis.	30-Dec-93
Interferon gamma 1-b	*Actimmune*	Recombinant	Chronic granulomatous disease.	20-Dec-90
Antihemophilic factor	*Kogenate*	Recombinant	hemophilia A (congenital factor VIII deficiency).	25-Feb-93
Coagulation factor VIIa	*NovoSeven*	Recombinant	Hemophilia A or B patients with inhibitors to Factor VIII or Factor IX.	25-Mar-99
Imiglucerase	*Cerezyme*	Recombinant	Types I, II, and III Gaucher's disease.	23-May-94
Ceramide tri-hexosidase/ alpha-galac-tosidase A	*Fabrazyme*	Recombinant	Fabry's disease.	24-Apr-03
Interferon gamma-1b	*Actimmune*	Recombinant	Severe, malignant osteopetrosis.	10-Feb-00
Antihemophilic factor	*Refacto*	Recombinant	hemophilia A (congenital factor VIII deficiency).	06-Mar-00
human acid alpha-glu-cosidase	*Myozyme*	Recombinant	Glycogen storage disease type II.	28-Apr-06
Coagulation factor VIIa	*NovoSeven*	Recombinant	Hemophilia A or B.	12-Aug-05
Idursulfase	*Elaprase*	Recombinant	Mucopolysaccharidosis II (Hunter Syndrome).	24-Jul-06
N-acetylgalac-tosamine-4-sulfatase	*Naglazyme*	Recombinant	Mucopolysaccharidosis Type VI (Maroteaux-Lamy syndrome).	31-May-05
Coagulation factor VIIa	*NovoSeven*	Recombinant	Congenital factor VII deficiency.	11-Jul-05
Laronidase	*Aldurazyme*	Recombinant	Treatment of patients with mucopoly saccharidosis-I.	30-Apr-03
Somatropin	*Humatrope*	Recombinant	Short stature associated with Turner syndrome.	30-Dec-96

(continued)

Table 21.1 (continued)

Generic Name	*Trade Name*	How Derived	Disease	Date Approved
Somatropin	*Genotropin*	Recombinant	Short stature in patients with Prader-Willi syndrome.	20-Jun-00
Human luteinizing hormone	*Luveris*	Recombinant	chronic anovulation due to hypogonadotropic hypogonadism.	08-Oct-04
Coagulation factor VIIa	*NovoSeven*	Recombinant	Congenital factor VII deficiency.	11-Jul-05
Somatropin for injection	*Nutropin*	Recombinant	Short stature associated with Turner's syndrome.	30-Dec-96
Lepirudin	*Refluden*	Recombinant	heparin-associated thrombocytopenia type II.	06-Mar-98
Mecasermin	*Increlex*	Recombinant	growth hormone insensitivity syndrome.	30-Aug-05
Mecasermin rinfabate	*iPLEX*	Recombinant	growth hormone insensitivity syndrome (GHIS).	12-Dec-05
Hemin	*Panhematin*	Processed Red Blood cells	Acute intermittent porphyria, porphyria variegata and hereditary coproporphyria.	20-Jul-83
Coagulation factor IX	*AlphaNine*	Pooled Human Plasma	Hemophilia B.	31-Dec-90
Coagulation factor IX	*Mononine*	Pooled Human Plasma	Hemophilia B.	20-Aug-92
Alpha1-proteinase inhibitor	*Prolastin*	Pooled Human Plasma	Alpha-1-proteinase inhibitor congenital deficiency state.	02-Dec-87
Antithrombin III	*ATnativ*	Pooled Human Plasma	Hemophilia A (congenital factor VIII deficiency).	13-Dec-89
Antithrombin III	*Thrombate III*	Pooled Human Plasma	Congenital deficiency of AT-III.	30-Dec-91
Antihemophilic factor	*Alphanate*	Pooled Human Plasma	Von Willebrand's disease.	31-Jan-07
Antihemophilic factor/von Willebrand factor complex	*Humate-P*	Pooled Human Plasma	Von Willebrand's disease.	01-Apr-99
Alglucerase injection	*Ceredase*	Placenta Derived	Gaucher's disease type I.	05-Apr-91
Pegademase	*Adagen*	Bovine Derived	ADA deficiency in patients with severe combined immunodeficiency.	21-Mar-90
Sacrosidase	*Sucraid*	Baker's Yeast	Congenital sucrase-isomaltase deficiency.	09-Apr-98

for Refacto® would read "For the control and prevention of hemorrhagic episodes and for surgical prophylaxis in patients with hemophilia A (congenital factor VIII deficiency or classic hemophilia)." In some cases this leads to a product such as NovoSeven® being approved for two indications in the same disease state at different dates. Likewise we see multiple treatments for hemophilia B from different brands of identical generic therapies. Nonetheless, the list is an impressive demonstration of the positive effect developments in biologic therapies have had on rare diseases. If one counts as separate diseases those products which treat multiple rare monogenic diseases, then 26 different rare monogenic diseases have seen the approval of biologic therapies. Likewise, 23 separate generic biologic approaches to therapy are listed. One also can perceive the increasing influence of recombinant drug production technology on therapy. Since February 1993, when the first recombinant product was marketed, only three biologic therapies have been marketed that were not produced by recombinant means.

In general, the biologic products are very highly influenced, if not directed entirely, by an underlying genomic understanding of disease. However, one might consider approaches such as recombinant growth hormone for short stature secondary to Turner's syndrome or Prader-Willi syndrome, or recombinant dornase alpha, a DNA degradative enzyme employed as a mucolytic in cystic fibrosis, to be based more on an empirical approach rather than a pharmacogenomic one. Occasionally, as in the case of Panhematin®, derived from pooled red blood cells, the mechanism of action is not fully understood.

A large number of the biological products are enzyme replacement therapies of one form or another. Progress in this area is especially evident in those diseases in which some essential blood component is missing, such as hemophilia A, hemophilia B, von Willebrand's disease, and congenital antithrombin III deficiency. Another notable pharmacogenomic advance is seen in the approval of recombinant alpha-one antitrypsin to prevent early onset emphysema in patients with this enzyme deficiency. As noted earlier, enzyme replacement therapies for various inborn errors of metabolism, often the lysozomal storage diseases, have seen great and continuing advances from the development of pharmacogenomically-based therapies. At present a total of eight such enzyme replacement therapies have been marketed to treat SCID-ADA, Maroteaux-Lamy syndrome, Fabry's disease, Gaucher's disease, urea cycle disorders, Pompe's disease, and most recently, Hunter's syndrome, the last being approved to market in May 2006 *(54)*. Additional enzyme replacement therapies are in the developmental pipeline, with clinical trials currently ongoing in Niemann-Pick disease and Hurler's disease *(55)*.

Of the remaining 20 products approved as orphans to treat rare monogenic disorders, the large majority are small molecule therapeutics. These drugs are listed in Table 21.2.

In some cases the influence of pharmacogenomics on the development of these therapies is less apparent. Indeed, in cases such as Felbamate or Lamotrigine for the

Table 21.2 Non-biologically derived orphan products approved to treat rare, monogenic diseases

Generic Name	*Trade Name*	How Received	Disease	Date Approved
Anagrelide	*Agrylin*	Small Molecule	Essential thrombocythemia.	14-Mar-97
Benzoate/pheny-lacetate	*Ucephan*	Combination Product	carbamylphosphate synthetase, ornithine, transcarbamylase, or argininosuccinate synthetase deficiency.	23-Dec-87
Benzoate/pheny-lacetate	*Ammonul*	Combination Product	Urea cycle enzyme deficiencies.	17-Feb-05
Betaine	*Cystadane*	Small Molecule	Homocystinuria.	25-Oct-96
Cysteamine	*Cystagon*	Small Molecule (Amino Acid)	Nephropathic cystinosis.	15-Aug-94
Desmopressin acetate		Vassopressin analogue	Mild hemophilia A and von Willebrand's disease.	07-Mar-94
Felbamate	*Felbatol*	Small Molecule	Lennox-Gastaut syndrome.	29-Jul-93
Hydroxyurea	*Droxia*	Small Molecule	Sickle cell anemia (hemoglobin S).	25-Feb-98
Lamotrigine	*Lamictal*	Small Molecule	Lennox-Gastaut syndrome.	24-Aug-98
Levocarnitine	*Carnitor*	Small Molecule	Primary and secondary carnitine deficiency of genetic origin.	16-Dec-92
Levocarnitine	*Carnitor*	Small Molecule	Treatment of genetic carnitine deficiency.	10-Apr-86
Miglustat	*Zavesca*	Small Molecule	Gaucher's disease.	31-Jul-03
Nitisinone	*Orfadin*	Small Molecule	Tyrosinemia type 1.	18-Jan-02
Potassium citrate	*Urocit-K*	Small Molecule	Prevention of calcium renal stones in patients with hypocitraturia.	30-Aug-85
Sodium phenyl-butyrate	*Buphenyl*	Small Molecule	Urea cycle enzyme deficiencies.	30-Apr-96
Tiopronin	*Thiola*	Small molecule Chelating Agent	Prevention of cystine nephrolithiasis in patients with homozygous cystinuria.	11-Aug-88
Tobramycin for inhalation	*TOBI*	Antibiotic	Treatment of bronchopulmonary infections of Pseudomonas aeruginosa in cystic fibrosis patients.	22-Dec-97
Topiramate	*Topamax*	Small Molecule	Lennox-Gastaut syndrome.	28-Aug-01
Trientine HCl	*Syprine*	Small molecule Chelating Agent	Wilson's disease.	08-Nov-85
Zinc acetate	*Galzin*	Small Molecule	Wilson's disease.	28-Jan-97

treatment of Lennox-Gastaut syndrome, or hydroxurea for the treatment of sickle-cell anemia, the precise mechanism of action remains unclear. In other instances, such as the chelating agents trietine HCL and tiopronin for the treatment of Wilson's disease and cystinuria, respectively, it is difficult to conclude where empiric influences might end and genomic insights begin. Nor does this discussion by any means intend to discount the many tremendous advances that have occurred without an underlying genomic disease understanding. The approvals of dornase alpha discussed earlier, and inhaled tobramicin for the treatment of cystic fibrosis, have greatly extended and improved the quality of life in patients afflicted with this serious disease.

Nonetheless, in a number of the nonbiological products, one perceives the clear, guiding influence of pharmacogenomics in product development. One example of this is the development of nitisinone as a treatment for tyrosinemia, a disease which leads to hepatic failure and, untreated, generally death in childhood. Nitisinone languished as a failed herbicide in Europe before a researcher there realized its potential as a therapeutic. Hearkening again back to Garrod's investigations, we see that in contrast to the relatively nontoxic buildup of homogenistate in alkaptonuria, in tyrosinemia the specific metabolic blockage in tyrosine metabolism leads to accumulation of toxic metabolites. Nitisinone ameliorates this pathology by blocking an enzyme upstream of the metabolism of tyrosine, which does not lead to the accumulation of toxic secondary metabolites *(56)*. So successful was this drug in initial trials that it became known colloquially as the "Lazarus drug" for people with this disease. Tyrosinemia has an estimated prevalence of some 2,500 cases in the United States. The story of nitisinone also illustrates the new types of pharmaceutical companies being spawned in part in response to orphan drug legislation. By taking advantage of the incentives of the Orphan Drug Act, Rare Disease Therapeutics, which developed this drug, was able to bring this product to market for a very serious and ultra-rare disease.

A very similar approach is seen in the product miglustat, approved to treat Gaucher's disease. Gaucher's disease is a lysozomal storage disorder caused by a deficiency of the enzyme glucoceribrosidase, which breaks down glucosylceramide. Miglustat, in turn, is a competitive inhibitor of the enzyme glucosylceramide synthase. By decreasing the production of glucosylceramide it is intended that in those patients with somewhat milder disease, residual glucoceribrosidase activity may be sufficient to prevent pathologic glucosylceramide accumulation *(57)*. This approach of substrate reduction may show more broad applicability throughout a variety of lysozomal storage diseases *(58)*.

7 Pharmacogenomic Therapeutic Approaches in Development

Of course the preceding list discusses only those therapies which have been approved to market in recent years. Some of the most cutting edge and interesting approaches to therapy are still in the developmental stages. With some thousand designated orphan products currently in development, we can here only touch upon some of the more novel therapeutic approaches.

Unfortunately, the initial hopes of gene therapy for providing definitive cures in large numbers of rare genetic diseases remain elusive. Despite the diligent efforts of numerous researchers spanning some three decades, and the expenditure of large sums of money, there has to date been no FDA approval of a gene therapy. Difficulties with understanding complex mammalian DNA regulatory systems, with achieving adequate and persistent expression of the corrected gene, and with unintended side effects of commonly employed vectors, have all stymied therapeutic development. September of 1999 also saw the first death of a gene therapy patient in a clinical trial *(59)*. In this study, the use of an adenovirus vector injected intrahepatically to attempt to correct the rare metabolic disease ornithine transcarbamylase deficiency led to rapidly progressive and ultimately fatal multiorgan system failure. While it is speculated that there was some form of allergic response to the injected therapy, the cause of death remains incompletely understood. This development led to an FDA-imposed temporary moratorium on all gene therapy research. More recently, enthusiasm for the notable success of researchers in France in applying gene therapy to cure x-linked severe combined immunodeficiency in 11 children was tempered by the subsequent development of T-cell leukemia in three of these children. It is speculated that the adenoviral vector may have inserted within an oncogene *(60)*, or that the viral delivery system may have inadvertently allowed the inserted gene, IL2RG, to function as an oncogene in promoting T-cell leukemia. This development again led to a temporary moratorium on gene therapy research. Despite these setbacks, it is worth noting that the majority of children in this study did not develop leukemia and are considered cured of their serious immunodeficiency. Currently there are some 36 clinical trials utilizing gene therapy either ongoing in the United States or set to begin recruiting patients soon *(61)*. While the majority of these trials focus on cancer indications, a broad variety of rare monogenic diseases are being actively researched as well, including severe combined immunodeficiency caused by adenosine deaminase deficiency, urea cycle disorders, Leber's congenital amaurosis, alpha-1 antitrypsin deficiency, and x-linked severe combined immunodeficiency.

Vectors which have been commonly employed in gene therapy trials include adenoviruses, adenoassociated viruses, plasmids, and retroviruses. One promising recent avenue of gene therapy exploration concerns the use of zinc finger protein motifs as vectors for gene insertion. Zinc fingers are a class of molecules with specificity for certain DNA base patterns. By pairing a zinc finger to an endonuclease, researchers have been able to cause double-stranded DNA breaks within specific targeted genes. By further attaching a copy of a corrected DNA sequence to the zinc finger, this approach makes use of an organism's native homologous recombination techniques for repairing double-stranded DNA breaks *(62)*. This approach has the advantage of not randomly inserting a specific gene into the genome, but rather of actually correcting the diseased gene. There remain questions over whether sufficient correction rates can be achieved using this approach, and concerns over whether zinc fingers would have sufficient specificity not to introduce unintended excess double-stranded DNA breaks. In June of 2005, however, researchers reported using a zinc finger vector to achieve correction rates of 18% in cultured human cells with x-linked severe combined immunodeficiency *(63)*. Interestingly, as zinc fingers are somewhat analogous to artificially created transcription factors, they are also being explored as a means of regulating gene expression.

Antisense molecules are single-stranded nucleic acid segments which are complementary to the sense strand of a particular mRNA. Upon binding to the mRNA, cellular enzymes digest the double stranded RNA, and protein translation is reduced. Although being investigated in oncology primarily as a means of silencing aberrant cancerous protein overexpression, one clinical trial is currently examining antisense therapy in Duchenne's muscular dystrophy *(64)*. In 1998 the FDA approved the first antisense therapy, fomiversen (Vitravene) for the treatment of cytomegalovirus retinitis *(65)*. In January of 2006 the US Army Medical Research Institute reported that an antisense therapy directed against Ebola virus reduced mortality in monkeys from 80% to approximately 25% *(66)*. Difficulties with antisense therapies, including enzymatic digestion and nontherapeutic intracellular concentrations, are being addressed with various modifications to the oligonucleotide backbone of the antisense molecule *(67)*.

An even more recent means of modifying gene expression, and one that has generated great interest in the research community, is the use of short interfering RNA (siRNA) segments. Unexpectedly, the introduction of short gene-specific segments of double-stranded RNA appears to activate a native system for potentiating the gene silencing activity of these gene-specific siRNA molecules *(68)*. While still in their infancy, these siRNA approaches show great promise for developing research models with specifically silenced genes, and for treating conditions such as cancer, characterized by aberrant protein overexpression.

References

1. Mendel G (1866) Versuche über pflanzen-hybriden. Verh Naturforsch Ver Brünn 4:3–47 (in English (1901) J R Hortic Soc 26:1–32).
2. Avery OT, Mac Leod CM, McCarty M (1944) Studies on the chemical nature of the substance inducing transformation of pneumonococcal types: induction of transformation by a desoxyribonucleic acid fraction isolated from pneumococcus type III. J Exp Med 79:137–158 .
3. Watson JD, Crick FH (1953) Molecular structure of nucleic acids. Nature 171:737–738 .
4. Bearn AG, Miller ED (1979) Archibald Garrod and the development of the concept of inborn errors of metabolism. Bull Hist Med 53(3):315–28.
5. Garrod A (1902) The incidence of alkaptonuria: a study in chemical individuality. Lancet 2:1616–1620.
6. Berg J, Tymoczko J, Styrey L (2002) Biochemistry, Fifth Ed. http://www.ncbi.nlm.nih.gov/books/bv.fcgi?rid=stryer.section.3259 (accessed March 17, 2008).
7. Pollak MR, Chou Y-HW, Cerda J J, Steinmann B, La Du BN, Seidman JG, Seidman CE (1993) Homozygosity mapping of the gene for alkaptonuria to chromosome 3q2. Nature Genet 5:201–204.
8. Adams MD, Dubnick M, Kerlavage AR, Moreno R, Kelley JM, Utterback TR, Nagle JW, Fields C, Venter JC (1992) Sequence identification of 2,375 human brain genes. Nature 355(6361):632–4.
9. National Center for Biotechnology Information. http://www.ncbi.nlm.nih.gov/About/primer/est.html (accessed May 19, 2007).
10. Venter JC, Adams MD, Myers EW et al (2001) The sequence of the human genome [published erratum appears in Science 2001 Jun 5;292(5523):1838]. Science 291(5507):1304–51.
11. Collins FS, Green ED, Guttmacher AE et al (2003) A vision for the future of genomics. Nature 422(6934):835–47.
12. Stein LD (2004) Human genome: end of the beginning. Nature 431:915–916.

13. Human Genome Project Information. http://www.ornl.gov/sci/techresources/Human_Genome/medicine/assist.shtml (accessed March 17, 2008).
14. Nekrutenko A (2004) Reconciling the numbers: ESTs versus protein-coding genes. Mol Biol Evol 21(7):1278–1282.
15. Gaffney DJ, Keightley PD (2004) Unexpected conserved noncoding DNA blocks in mammals. Trends Genet 20(8):332–337.
16. Orphan Drug Act. (1982) Pub L. No. 97–414, 96 Stat. 2049.
17. Rados C (2003) Orphan products: hope for people with rare diseases. FDA consumer magazine. Nov–Dec 2003.
18. http://www.hapmap.org/ (accessed May 19, 2007).
19. Chiche JD, Cariou A, Mira JP (2002) Bench-to-bedside review: fulfilling the promises of the Human Genome Project. Crit Care 6(3):212–215.
20. http://www.gei.nih.gov/ (accessed May 14, 2007).
21. Scone EA, Khan TI, Wynne HA et al (2005) The impact of CYP2C9 and VKORC1 genetic polymorphism and patient characteristics upon warfarin dose requirements: proposal for a new dosing regime. Blood 106:2329–2333.
22. Abuchowski A. Severe combined immuonogenicity disease: enzyme therapy. OOPD, Rockville, MD. Grant no. FDR-000285–01. Available online at: http://www.fda.gov/orphan/grants/previous.htm. (accessed March 17, 2008).
23. Quoted in "Adopting orphan diseases: rare medical disorders repay researchers' attention tenfold, with medical insights and useful drugs." Red Herring. January 22, 2001.
24. Brown MS, Goldstein JL (1986) A receptor-mediated pathway for cholesterol homeostasis. Science 232(4746):34–47.
25. Brown MS, Goldstein JL (1996) Heart attacks: gone with the century? Science 272: 629.
26. Breunig F, Weidemann F, Beer M et al (2003) Fabry disease: diagnosis and treatment. Kidney Int Suppl 63(84):S181–5.
27. Hill AV, Allsopp CE, Kwiatkowski D, Anstey NM, Twumasi P, Rowe PA, Bennett S, Brewster D, McMichael AJ, Greenwood BM (1991) Common West African HLA antigens are associated with protection from severe malaria. Nature 352:595–600.
28. Flint J, Harding RM, Boyce AJ, Clegg JB (1998) The population genetics of the haemoglobinopathies. Baillieres Clin Haematol 11:1–51.
29. Nagel RL, Fleming AF (1992) Genetic epidemiology of the betas gene. Baillieres Clin Haematol 5:331.
30. Kwiatkowski DP (2005) How malaria has affected the human genome and what human genetics can teach us about malaria. Am J Hum Genet 77(2):171–192.
31. Woo SLC (1989) Molecular basis and population genetics of phenylketonuria. Biochemistry 28:1–7.
32. Woolf LI (1986) The heterozygote advantage in phenylketonuria. Am J Hum Genet 38(5):773–775.
33. Gabriel SE et al (1994) Cystic fibrosis heterozygote resistance to cholera toxin in the cystic fibrosis mouse model. Science 266(5182):107–9.
34. Spyropoulos B, Moens PB, Davidson J, Lowden JA (1981) Heterozygote advantage in Tay-Sachs carriers? Am J Human Genet 3:375–80.
35. Miller H, Mason SJ, Clyde DF, McGinniss MH (1976) The resistance factor to Plasmodium vivax in blacks. The Duffy-blood-group genotype, FyFy. N Engl J Med 295(6):302–4.
36. Nowak R (2001) Disaster in the making. New Sci 169:4–5.
37. Christensen CD, Beaton S, Hall DF, Ramshaw IA (2001) Expression of mouse interleukin-4 by a recombinant ectromelia virus suppresses cytolytic lymphocyte responses and overcomes genetic resistance to mousepox. J Virol 75(3):1205–1210.
38. Fueyo J, Alemany R, Gomez-Manzano C (2003) Preclinical characterization of the antiglioma activity of a tropism-enhanced adenovirus targeted to the retinoblastoma pathway. J Natl Cancer Inst 95(9):652–60.
39. Menkes JH, Hurst PL, Craig JM (1954) A new syndrome: progressive familial infantile cerebral dysfunction associated with an unusual urinary substance. Pediatrics 14:462–467.
40. Westall RG, Dancis J, Miller S (1957) Maple syrup urine disease. Am J Dis Child 94: 571–572.

41. National Center for Biotechnology Information. Online Mendellian Inheritance in Man (OMIM) #248600: Maple syrup urine disease. http://www.ncbi.nlm.nih.gov/entrez/dispomim.cgi?id=248600 (accessed March 17, 2008).
42. Stephenson J (2001) Antibiotics show promise as therapy for genetic disorders. JAMA 285:2067–8.
43. Bidoul L et al (2004) Premature stop codons involved in muscular dystrophies show a broad spectrum of read through efficiencies in response to gentamicin treatement. Gene Ther 11:619–27.
44. Wilschanski M, Yahav Y, Yaacov Y et al (2003) Gentamicin-induced correction of CFTR function in patients with cystic fibrosis and CFTR stop mutations. N Engl J Med 349:1433–41.
45. Garman SC, Garboczi DN (2002) Minireview: structural basis of Fabry disease. Mol Genet Metab 77:3–11.
46. Helenius A, Marquardt T, Braakman I (1992) The endoplasmic reticulum as a protein folding compartment. Trends Cell Biol 2:227–31.
47. Fan JQ (2003) A contradictory treatment for lysosomal storage disorders: inhibitors enhance mutant enzyme activity. Trends Pharmacol Sci 24:356–36.
48. Frustaci A, Chimenti C, Ricci R et al Improvement in cardiac function in the cardiac variant of Fabry's disease with galactose infusion therapy. N Engl J Med 2001;345:25–32.
49. ibid., ref. 23.
50. Chaffee S, Hersfield MS (1990) Imuune response to polyethylene glycol modified bovine adenosine deaminase (PEG-ADA). Pediatr Res 27(4 Pt 2):155A.
51. Alter MJ, Kruszon-Moran D, Nainan OV et al (1999) The prevalence of hepatitis C virus infection in the United States, 1988 through 1994. N Engl J Med 341(8):556–62.
52. World Health Organization. Fact Sheet N164. http://www.who.int/mediacentre/factsheets/fs164/en/ (accessed May17, 2007).
53. http://www.fda.gov/orphan/designat/list.htm (accessed May 15, 2007).
54. FDA News. FDA approves first treatment for pompe disease. P06–63. April 28, 2006.http://www.fda.gov/bbs/topics/NEWS/2006/NEW01365.html (accessed May17, 2007).
55. ClinicalTrials.gov. Search field: Experimental Treatment; search field: Enzyme replacement (accessed March 17, 2008).
56. Neergaard L (2002) FDA OKs drug to fight liver disease. Associated Press: http://www.communities.ninemsn.com/tyrosinemia/ntbc.msnw.
57. Mehta A (2006) Clinical experience with substrate reduction therapy. Eur J Intern Med 17(Suppl):S13–5.
58. Aerts JM, Hollak CE, Boot RG, Groener JE, Maas M (2006) Substrate reduction therapy of glycosphingolipid storage disorders. J Inherit Metab Dis 29(2–3):449–56.
59. Couzin J, Kaiser J (2005) Gene therapy: as Gelsinger case ends, gene therapy suffers another blow. Science 307(5712):1028.
60. Hacein-Bey-Abina S, von Kalle C, Schmidt M et al (2003) LMO2-associated clonal T proliferation in two patients after gene therapy for SCID-X. Science 302(5644):415–9.
61. ClinicalTrials.gov. Search field: Experimental Treatment; search field: Enzyme replacement (accessed March 17, 2008).
62. Kaiser J (2005) Putting the fingers on gene repair. Science 310(5756):1894–189.
63. Urnov FD, Miller JC, Lee Y-L et al (2005) Highly efficient endogenous human gene correction using designed zinc-finger nucleases. Nature 435:646–651 .
64. Safety and efficacy study of antisense oligonucleotides in Duchenne muscular dystrophy. ClinicalTrials.gov Identifier: NCT00159250 http://clinicaltrials.gov/ct/show/NCT00159250?order=2 (accessed May 19, 2007).
65. FDA Consumer Information (1998) Vitravene [package insert]. FDA, Rockville, MD.
66. U.S. Army Medical Research. Institute of Infectious Diseases (2006) Gene-specific ebola therapies protect nonhuman primates from lethal disease. Fort Detrick, MD. http://www.usamriid.army.mil/press%20releases/warfield_press_release.pdf (accessed March 17, 2008).
67. Gleave ME, Monia BP. (2005) Antisense therapy for cancer. Nat Rev Cancer 5:468–479.
68. Bantounas I, Phylactou LA, Uney JB (2004) RNA interference and the use of small RNA to study gene function in mammalian systems. J Mol Endocrinol 33:545–57.

Index

FSC
www.fsc.org
MIX
Papier | Fördert gute Waldnutzung
FSC® C083411

Kolibri 360 GmbH
Ferdinand-Jühlke-Straße 7
99095 Erfurt, Deutschland
produktsicherheit@kolibri360.de